DYSLIPIDEMIA - FROM PREVENTION TO TREATMENT

Edited by **Roya Kelishadi**

Dyslipidemia - From Prevention to Treatment

Edited by Roya Kelishadi

Published by InTech

Janeza Trdine 9, 51000 Rijeka, Croatia

Publishing Process Manager Marko Rebrovic

Technical Editor Teodora Smiljanic

Cover Designer InTech Design Team

Dyslipidemia - From Prevention to Treatment, Edited by Roya Kelishadi
p. cm.
ISBN 978-953-307-904-2

For EU product safety concerns:
IN TECH d.o.o., Prolaz Marije Krucifikse Kozulić 3, 51000 Rijeka, Croatia,
info@intechopen.com or visit our website at intechopen.com.

Meet the editor

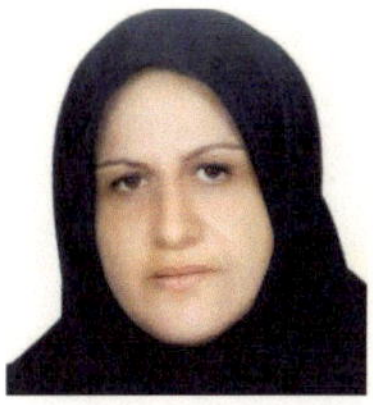

Roya Kelishadi, MD, is a University Professor at the Faculty of Medicine, and Child Health Promotion Research Center, Isfahan University of Medical Sciences, Isfahan, Iran. Her main field of study is primordial and primary prevention of non-communicable early life diseases. She has published more than 250 papers in peer reviewed biomedical journals, and 20 chapters in books. She has been awarded several times as distinguished researcher or physician. Many of her studies regarding the ethnic differences in metabolic parameters, and the association of lifestyle habits and environmental factors on the beginning and progress of atherosclerotic changes, have been acknowledged as the first of their kind.

Contents

Preface

The term dyslipidemia origins from dys- + lipid (fat) + -emia (in the blood), and essentially refers to serum lipid disorders. By definition, dyslipidemia is a disorder of lipoprotein metabolism in terms of either lipoprotein overproduction or deficiency. It may be expressed by increased serum total cholesterol, low-density lipoprotein cholesterol and/or triglycerides, a decrease in high-density lipoprotein cholesterol concentration, and/or various combinations of such disorders. Lipoproteins, which contain lipids and proteins (apolipoproteins), are mainly responsible for transporting plasma lipids from the intestines and liver to peripheral tissues.

Dyslipidemia has a complex pathophysiology consisting of various genetic, lifestyle, and environmental factors. It has many adverse health impacts, and has a pivotal role in the development of chronic non-communicable diseases.

Significant ethnic differences exist due to the prevalence and types of lipid disorders. While elevated serum total and LDL-cholesterol are the main concern in Western populations, in other countries hypertriglyceridemia and low HDL-cholesterol are more prevalent. The latter types of lipid disorders are considered as components of the metabolic syndrome, which is a clustering of dyslipidemia, hypertension, dysglycemia, and obesity. The rapid escalating trend of obesity at global level, which is associated with obesogenic milieus through high-calorie intake and sedentary lifestyle, as well as the environmental factors, will result in increasing prevalence of dyslipidemia, and will make it a global medical and public health threat.

This situation is not limited to adults, and the pediatric age group is being involved more and more. The results of longitudinal studies support the association of risk factors cluster in children and adolescents with future chronic diseases.

However, the processes by which lipids and lipoproteins participate in the development of non-communicable diseases at different life stages continue to be an area of controversy. Several experimental and clinical research studies are being conducted regarding issues related to the underlying mechanisms and therapeutic modalities.

The current book is providing a general overview of dyslipidemia from diverse aspects of pathophysiology, ethnic differences, prevention, health hazards, and treatment.

Prof. Roya Kelishadi
Faculty of Medicine & Child Health Promotion Research Center,
Isfahan University of Medical Sciences, Isfahan,
Iran

1

Obesity Related Lipid Profile and Altered Insulin Incretion in Adolescent with Policystic Ovary Syndrome

Annamaria Fulghesu and Roberta Magnini
Department of Obstetrics and Gynecology, University of Cagliari, Cagliari, Italy

1. Introduction

Polycystic ovary syndrome (PCOS) is the most common female endocrine disorder, present in 5 - 7% of women of reproductive age. The diagnosis of PCOS was made according to Rotterdam criteria in presence of at least two of the following: 1) oligomenorrhea and/or anovulation; 2) hyperandrogenism (clinical and/or biochemical); 3) polycystic ovaries with the exclusion of other etiologies (1). The disorder is characterized by irregular menstrual cycle, chronic anovulation and hyperandrogenism. Women with PCOS demonstrate marked clinical heterogeneity: the commonly associated features of hirsutism, acne, polycystic-appearing ovaries, obesity and acanthosis nigricans are neither uniform nor universal (2-3). In time the disorder may lead to onset of hyperinsulinemia, insulin resistance, gestational diabetes, early onset of type 2 diabetes mellitus (DM), dyslipidemia and cardiovascular disease (CVD) (4-5).
PCOS is characterized by a complex physiology implicating an interaction with environmental and genetic factors, resulting in a broad spectrum of reproductive and metabolic disorders. (6-7) Adult females with PCOS may be at increased risk for atherosclerotic cardiovascular disease (CVD) due to increased prevalence of obesity and central adiposity as well as to hypertension, hyperinsulinemia, type 2 DM, and dyslipidemia in these patients (8).The prevalence of obesity and consequently the presence of metabolic abnormalities reported in Italian and American published studies differs considerably, underlining the presence of important ethnic differences. (9, 10, 11, 12).
A percentage ranging from 30-75% of women with PCOS are obese, European women generally weighing less than their American counterparts (20,21). Hyperinsulemia and/or insulin resistance (IR) are frequently manifested in obese, and to a lesser extent (50%) in lean, PCOS patients (3, 13, 14). Hyperandrogenaemia, hyperinsulemia and obesity are considered as risk factors for the development of hypertension and dyslipidemia, diabetes mellitus and coronary disease in PCOS (15-16). The causes of metabolic disorders in PCOS remain to be clarified, but include obesity-related IR, an intrinsic abnormality of postreceptor insulin signaling (e.g. excess serine phosphorylation), and abnormal insulin secretion. On the other hand, increased resistance to insulin is a hallmark of the onset of normal pubertal development with natural to pre-pubertal values at the end of puberty in non-obese subjects. Consequently, in early adolescence a physiological resistance to insulin should be taken into account (12).

Dyslipidemia in PCOS is frequently manifested and is characterized by elevated plasma levels of low- density lipoproteins (LDL), very-low-density lipoproteins (VLDL) and triglycerides with concomitantly reduced concentration of high-density lipoproteins (HDL) in obese subjects (17, 18). A decrease in HDL, rise in triglyceride, VLDL, and LDL levels, as well as qualitative disorders of the LDL have all been described in young and adult PCOS (19). Moreover, recent data have shown a higher prevalence of metabolic syndrome in adolescent PCOS compared to controls (20) as well as an early impairment of endothelial structure and function even in non-dyslipidemic subjects with PCOS syndrome (21). Nevertheless, metabolic disorders in PCOS have not been extensively studied in the adolescent population. Several studies have shown how both lean and obese adolescents with PCOS appear to present an increased risk of both metabolic disorders and impaired glucose tolerance and diabetes (22), similar to their adult counterparts. A previous study carried out by our group demonstrated that the Italian young PCOS population is characterized by a high incidence of insulin alterations also in presence of normal weight and normal peripheral insulin resistance (12). Although the prevalence of dyslipidemia differs between PCOS subjects and young healthy girls, it however remains to be clarified whether dissimilarities in dyslipidemia occur in relation only to BMI or also to alterations to the insulinmetabolism and/or hyperandrogenemia.

Carmina recently demonstrated that MBS in women with PCOS is less common in Southern Italy compared to rates reported in the USA, the former reaching only 8.2% compared to a prevalence of 43-46% reported by US authors (23). The prevalence of MBS in the adult Italian PCOS population is higher than in control population matched for BMI, suggesting that body weight may be only in part responsible for this metabolic disorder (24).

Although few studies have investigated the latter condition in adolescents, it could prove to be of considerable importance in view of the health implications involved, requiring medical counseling to implement an adequate change in lifestyle. Likewise, obesity rate in adolescent PCOS subjects differs between Europe and the USA. In Sardinia, the incidence of obesity is lower than throughout the rest of Italy, with only 3-4% of high school female population presenting a BMI >25 (25). A combination of genetic factors, different lifestyle and diet are likely involved. In view therefore of the regional peculiarity, the patient population attending our Clinic was deemed to be of interest.

Therefore it is important to understand the relationship between lipid pattern and BMI, hyperinsulinemia and/or insulin resistance and circulating androgens in adolescent PCOS. In a study carried out in July 2005 to the Adolescent Center for gynecological diseases of the Department of Obstetrics and Gynecology, University of Cagliari, San Giovanni di Dio Hospital seventy-one adolescent (age 13-18) subjects affected by PCOS were recruited for this study. On the basis of the various aspects linking PCOS dyslipidemia and CVD risk, the present study was designed to investigate the influence of BMI and insulin metabolism derangement on lipid levels. All subjects were screened for other causes of hyperandrogenism, such as androgen secreting tumors and congenital adrenal hyperplasia (tested by evaluation of 17- dydroxyprogesterone). All subjects were euthyroid and devoid of hyperprolactinemia, diabetes mellitus and cardiovascular disease. No subjects had taken hormonal contraceptives or other type of medication or been on a diet that may have affected lipid profile, carbohydrate metabolism or insulin levels for at least 3 months preceding the study. No subjects were either smokers or drinkers. No subjects practiced sports on a regular basis (3 or more 20-min sessions of aerobic exercise per week).

These patients were linked with a control group consisting of healthy patients referred to the Adolescent centre for ultrasound screening of ovarian disease.
Control subjects and PCOS were studied 5 to 8 days following menstrual bleeding, which was progestin-induced in amenorrhoic patients. All patients were studied at least 15 days following Medrossi-Progesteron-Acetate administration (MAP 10 mg for 5 days). At the time of admittance to the study the presence of a dominant follicle, recent ovulation, or luteal phase was excluded by ultrasound examination and serum P evaluation. Height and weight were measured on the morning of testing. Waist and hip circumference were measured as previously referred. Blood pressure was measured in the second position and in the right arm (26) after 15 minutes resting.The hormonal study (after 12 hours overnight) included baseline plasma determination of LH, FSH, Estradiol (E2), Androstenedione (A), Testosterone (T), Dehydroepiandrosteronesulphate (DHEAS), 17hydroxyprogesterone (17-OHP) and Sex-hormone-binding globulin (SHBG). Lipid assay was performed to measure total cholesterol level, high-density lipoprotein cholesterol level (HDL), low-density lipoprotein cholesterol level (LDL) and triglyceride level. Homocysteine levels were also determined.
Adolescents meeting three or more of the following criteria were diagnosed with MBS: waist circumference of at least 90th percentile for age and gender; systolic or diastolic blood pressure at least 90th percentile for age, height and gender; fasting TG at least 110mg/dl (90th percentile for age); fasting HDL not exceeding 40mg/dl (10th percentile for age); and fasting glucose at least 110mg/dl.
Subsequently, patients underwent a 75-g oral glucose tolerance test (OGTT). Insulin, C-peptide, and glucose serum concentrations were analyzed prior to (time 0) and 30, 60, 90, 120 and 180 min after oral glucose load. A normal glycemic response to OGTT was defined according to the criteria of the National Diabetes Data Group (27). Insulin, C-peptide and glucose response to glucose load were expressed as area below the curve (AUC), calculated according to the trapezoidal rule. The homeostatic index of IR (HOMA) was calculated as follows: HOMA = [fasting insulin (μU/ml) x fasting glucose (mmol/L/22, 5)]. (28) The body mass index (BMI) was calculated according to the following formula: body weight in kilograms/ height in m2. Normal weight was considered as $18 \leq BMI \geq 25$. The degree of hirsutism was quantified using Ferriman and Gallwey (F-G) score (28).
No differences were observed with regard to the presence of overweight and obese subjects between PCOS and controls (30% vs. 23%); a similar finding was obtained also for waist measurement and WHR, confirming that obesity is not a common finding in young PCOS subjects in the population studied.Moreover, no subjects affected by metabolic Syndrome or diabetes either among PCOS or in the control group were detected. No differences were revealed in lipid levels between PCOS and controls. In addition, no differences were reported for any of the fasting metabolic parameters (i.e. Glucose fasting insulin, HOMA ratio), whilst a higher insulin response under OGTT was obtained for PCOS subjects. On the other hand, statistical correlations clearly demonstrated the influence produced by BMI and waist measurement on HDL, triglyceride and LDL levels. However, dividing the population into tertiles for BMI and waist measurement significant differences were revealed for both HDL and LDL levels in lean overweight and obese subjects and in relation to the presence of visceral fat.The above features have also been reported by several authors carrying out studies on young subjects.
Glueck published a study regarding PCOS and regular cycling adolescents in USA demonstrating a higher prevalence of obesity and dyslipidemia in PCOS.

However, when subjects were matched one-by-one for BMI and age, differences in lipids were no longer significant. In a recent paper on young obese subjects Shroff failed to demonstrate any difference in lipid as well as traditional CV factors in PCOS and control populations, but demonstrated a higher BMI in subjects presenting subclincal coronary atherosclerosis (CAC) (10). In young subjects from southern Italy, Orio demonstrated normal lipid levels in lean PCOS even in the presence of increased dimensions of heart ventricles.The above findings all seem to indicate that rather than being an insulin-correlated factor BMI may well be implicated in lipid alteration. On the other hand, the presence of increased waist measurements in PCOS population suggests that the presence of visceral fat may represent an additional risk factor, independent from BMI in PCOS. The influence of insulin on lipid profile was also determined.

Indeed, to date very few authors have investigated this aspect: Mather found a significant increase in traditional CV risk factors in PCOS women with fasting hyperinsulinemia in respect to their normoinsulinemic counterparts; this difference persisted when BMI was included as covariate. (29) Through reduction of hyperinsulinemia by means of metformin treatment Banazewska obtained a significant increase of HDL and reduction of triglycerides in a group of 43 adult PCOS. Our group recently published a paper on the peculiar insulin derangement observed in a population of normal weight young PCOS demonstrating a low incidence of insulin resistance but high incidence of hyperinsulinemia under OGTT (30). This peculiar metabolic alteration was confirmed in the present sample, thus allowing the separation of hyperinsulinemia from peripheral insulin resistance in data analysis.

Ibanez et al. also demonstrated higher serum insulin levels after OGTT with normal insulin sensitivity in a population of adolescent girls with PCOS. The causes underlying the increased response of β-cells in these subjects are, as yet, unknown. It is not clear whether high levels of insulin necessarily indicate the presence of a disorder although it may be hypothesized that adaptation to the chronic risk of hypoglycemia in hyperinsulinemic subjects could lead to IR after some time. Moreover, our group recently demonstrated that a normal HOMA score is not sufficient to exclude earlymetabolic abnormalities such as hyperinsulinemia in young lean PCOS subjects. Hyperinsulinemia per se could contribute toward onset of hyperandrogenism independently of peripheral IR.(12)

In this study was found a significant negative correlation between HDL and fasting insulin and HOMA, but this correlation was no longer significant when the influence of BMI was excluded, whereas insulin AUC was not related to any lipid parameters.

Furthermore, although the PCOS sample studied here was divided into tertiles on the basis of both insulin resistance and insulin AUC levels, the data obtained clearly indicate the failure to detect any relationship between insulin levels and lipid profile. Nevertheless, surprisingly a positive correlation was observed between A levels and HDL and a negative correlation between A and triglycerides. Reports present in literature did not afford any explanation for this result. A negative effect of A on HDL levels has previously been reported in males to whom A supplements had been administered (31). Moreover, exogenous T is reported to influence negatively HDL via hepatic lipase (HL) (31) an enzyme that increases the clearance of HDL. Less is known about the regulation of HDL by endogenally-derived androgens. A study performed in women with PCOS was not able to demonstrate any correlation between T and HDL. Considerable controversy exists as to the effect of androgens on lipoprotein lipase (LPL) activity.

In obese women LPL activity correlated positively with plasma free testosterone (32), whereas in women with PCOS a correlation with LPL activity was demonstrated.

Other authors have attributed to coexisting (29) insulin resistance the negative effect of androgen observed on lipid profile. In this case, the low incidence of insulin resistant subjects in a population may explain this unexpected result.
In conclusion, no lipid differences were revealed between our population of adolescent PCOS from southern Italy and controls.
Anthropometric characteristics (BMI, waist measurement and WHR) are the main parameters correlated to lipid derangement, confirming the importance of treating obesity at an early age to prevent onset of complex metabolic syndromes in the future. The latter may be of particular importance in PCOS populations in which insulin alterations (hyperinsulinemia and insulin resistance) are well known peculiarities potentially capable of influencing the long-term evolution of this endocrine disorder towards CVD and diabetes mellitus. A targeted support program should be set up for these young patients aimed at altering life style with the specific aim of reducing BMI and preventing onset of dyslipidemia.

	PCOS (n°71)	**CONTROLLI (n°94)**	**P**
Age (years) (M±ES) (range 13-19)	18,61 ± 0,4	18,10 ± 0,38	NS
BMI (kg\m²) (M±ES)	23,97 ± 0,72	22,56 ± 0,50	NS
Overweight (BMI 25 - 29) (%)	10%	11%	
Obesity (BMI > 29) (%)	20%	13%	
Waist (cm) (M±ES)	78,60 ± 1,79	75,56 ± 1,18	NS
WHR (M±ES)	0,77 ± 0	0,77 ± 0	NS
Hirsutism (score F&G) (M±ES)	11,24 ± 0,67	6,7 ± 0,45	0,005°
LH (IU/L)(M±ES)	5,21 ± 0,55	4,19 ± 0,36	NS
FSH (IU/L)(M±ES)	6,42 ± 0,63	5,96 ± 0,19	NS
E_2 (pmol/L)(M±ES)	129,30 ± 20,58	136,81 ± 13,25	NS
A (nmol/L)(M±ES)	0,08 ± 0	0,05 ± 0	0,005°
Tot T(nmol/L)(M±ES)	0,02 ± 0	0,01 ± 0	0,005°
17OHP (ng/mL)(M±ES)	1,49 ± 0,18	1,18 ± 0,07	NS
DHEAS (µmol/L)(M±ES)	2,05 ± 0,12	1,6 ± 0,09	NS
SHBG (nmol/L)(M±ES)	65,83 ± 4,54	71,18 ± 3,35	NS

°P < 0,05

Table 1. Shows the clinical and hormonal characteristics of PCOS population vs. Control group. No significant differences were revealed in age, body weight, waist and WHR between PCOS and control group. Likewise, no differences were observed in the incidence of overweight or obesity in the two groups. As expected, the prevalence of hirsutism and circulating androgen levels were higher amongst PCOS.

	PCOS (n° 71)	CONTROLLI (n°94)	P
Fasting Glucose (mmol/L)(M±ES)	81,13 ± 0,65	88,00 ± 3,27	NS
Fasting Insulin (pmol/L)(M±ES)	119,98 ± 6,14	96,68 ± 4,73	NS
HOMA (M±ES)	61,02 ± 3,09	57,81 ± 2,41	NS
I-AUC 180 min (UI/ml)(M±ES)	21069 ± 978,39	16578 ± 729,37	0,05°
Cholesterol (mg/dl)(M±ES)	166,48 ± 3,53	169,51 ± 2,62	NS
HDL-Cholesterol (mg/dl)(M±ES)	54,26 ± 1,44	51,25 ± 0,89	NS
LDL-Cholesterol (mg/dl)(M±ES)	96,78 ± 3,08	104,55 ± 2,34	NS
Cholesterol/ HDL (mg/dl)(M±ES)	3,16 ± 0,09	3,37 ± 0,07	NS
Triglycerides (mg/dl)(M±ES)	73,91 ± 3,75	78,35 ± 3,86	NS
Homocysteine (µmol/L) (M±ES)	8,16 ± 0,20	7,68 ± 0,25	NS
PCR (M±ES)	2,04 ± 0,36	0,89 ± 0,11	NS

° P < 0,05

Table 2. Reports the metabolic features of PCOS and control group. Fasting metabolic indexes detected for glucose, insulin and HOMA were similar between the two groups. On the contrary, insulin secretion after glucose load (I-AUC) was significantly higher in PCOS subjects. Total cholesterol, HDL, LDL, triglycerides and homocysteine levels did not differ between PCOS and control groups

	Cholesterol	LDL-Cholesterol	HDL-Cholesterol	Triglycerides
BMI (kg\m²)	R = 0,0727	R = 0,2579•	R = - 0,404▪	R = 0,1576
WAIST (cm)	R = 0,0869	R = 0,2960•	R = - 0,5934▪	R = 0,1704
WHR (cm)	R = 0,1645	R = 0,2872•	R = - 0,1853	R = 0,1362
A (nmol/L)	R = 0,0136	R = - 0,0523	R = 0,3705▪	R = -0,2948•
Tot T (nmol/L)	R = - 0,1016	R = - 0,0948	R = 0,0012	R = - 0,0157
FSH (mIU/L)	R = - 0,0134	R = - 0,0143	R = 0,0623	R = - 0,0687
E2(pmol/L)	R = - 0,1011	R = - 0,0895	R = 0,0698	R = - 0,1984
DHEAS (µmol/L)	R = - 0,0498	R = - 0,0022	R = - 0,0447	R = - 0,0441
HOMA	R = 0,0762	R = 0,1770	R = -0,3335	R = - 0,0214
I-AUC 180 min(UI/ml)	R = - 0,0098	R = - 0,0272	R = - 0,0701	R = - 0,0287
SHBG (nmol/L)	R = - 0,0689	R = - 0,1514	R = 0,1102	R = 0,1013
17OHP (nmol/L)	R = 0,0418	R = 0,0582	R = 0,0854	R = - 0,1720
Homocysteine (µmol/L)	R = - 0,0670	R = - 0,0786	R = 0,0463	R = - 0,1108▪
Fasting Glucose	R = 0,0049	R = 0,0260	R = -0,0829	R = 0,0643
Fasting Insulin	R = 0,0586	R = 0,1557	R = -0,3314	R = -0,0174

P < 0,05
P < 0,01
P < 0,001

Table 3. Illustrates linear regression relationship featured between lipid and physical, hormonal and metabolic parameters. Total cholesterol levels were significantly related to WHR but not to other antropometric parameters. On analyzing cholesterol fractions LDL levels were found to correlate positively with BMI, Waist, WHR and HOMA but not with I-AUC. HDL results correlated in a markedly negative manner with the same physical parameters as BMI, WHR and waist circumference. Moreover, HDL was negatively correlated with both fasting insulin and HOMA but not I-AUC. Finally, HDL was positively correlated with circulating A and negatively with circulating T levels.

Triglycerides appeared to correlate positively with BMI, Waist and WHR, and negatively with A levels. Homocysteine levels correlated positively with plasma triglyceride content. In view of the potential capacity of BMI to affect insulin sensitivity, conditional regression analysis was performed on HOMA and lipid assays to exclude any possible influence of BMI: HOMA resulted as being no longer correlated with any lipid parameter.To determine whether lipid alterations were primarily caused by increased BMI, lipid assay was repeated stratifying the population into 3 weight categories: normal weight, overweight and obese, and waist measurements were classified (normal and excessive).

BMI (kg\m²)

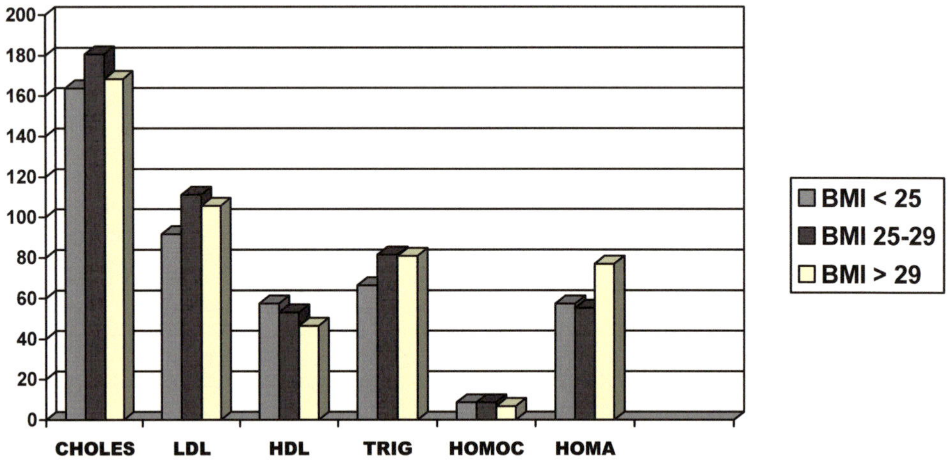

(mg/dl) (mg/dl) (mg/dl) (mg/dl) (µmol/L)

P < 0,05 LDL BMI < 25 VS BMI 25-29
P < 0,05 LDL BMI < 25 VS BMI > 29
P < 0,05 HDL BMI < 25 VS BMI > 29

WAIST (cm)

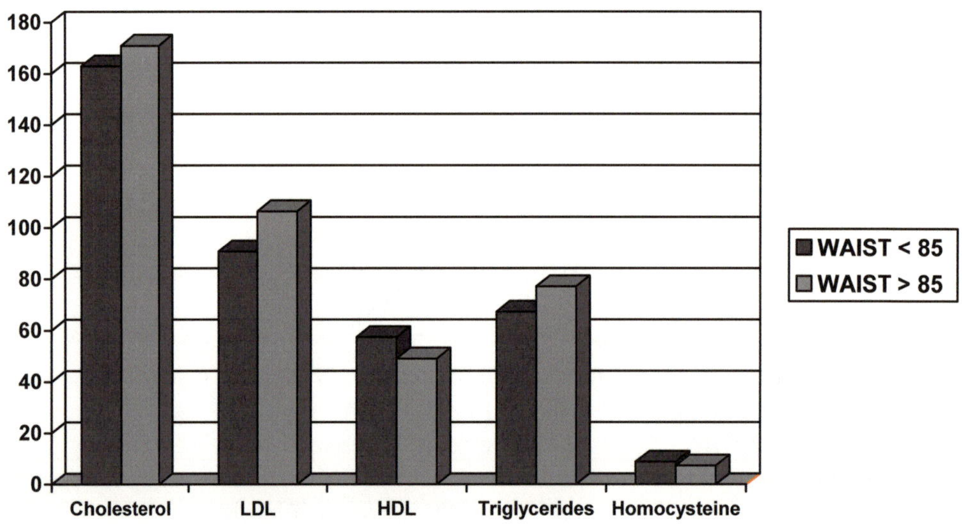

(mg/dl) (mg/dl) (mg/dl) (mg/dl) (µmol/L)

P < 0,05 LDL WAIST < 85 VS LDL WAIST > 85
P < 0,05 HDL WAIST <85 VS HDL WAIST > 85

Fig. 1. Shows the lipid levels in relation to the BMI and the waist of PCOS group.Normal weight and normal waist subjects featured lower LDL and Higher HDL compared to increased waist overweight or obese counterparts. On the other hand, in order to evaluate the influence of metabolic alteration subjects were also stratified on the basis of both HOMA and Insulin AUC values (fig.2).

HOMA

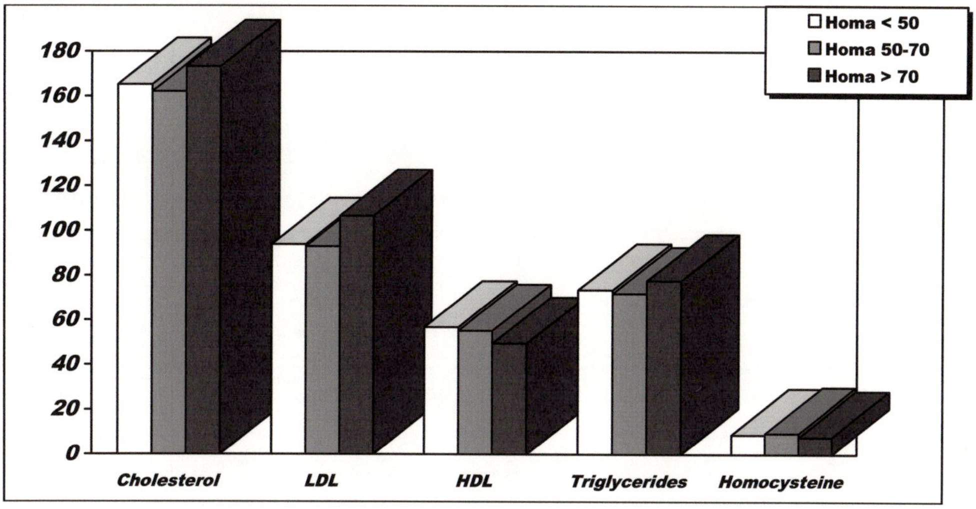

(mg/dl) (mg/dl) (mg/dl) (mg/dl) (μmol/L)

I-AUC (UI/ml)

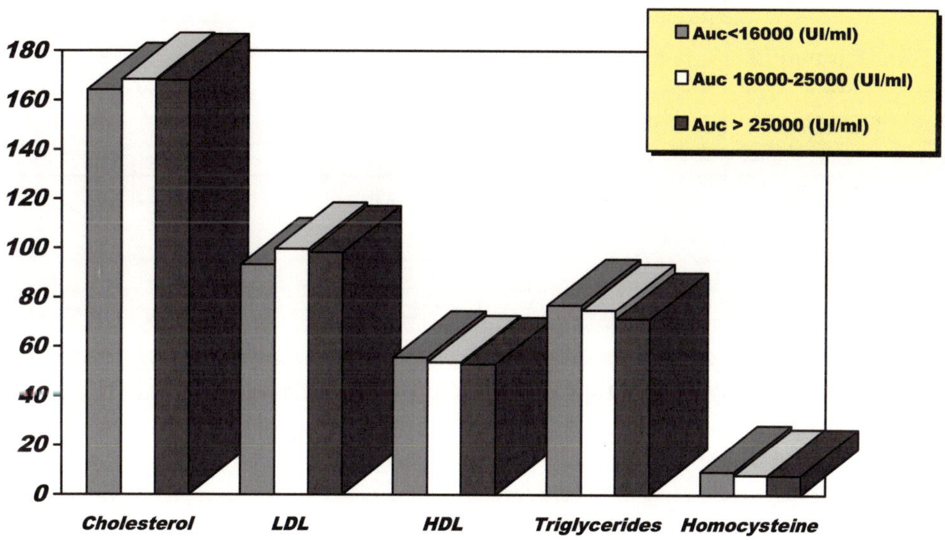

(mg/dl) (mg/dl) (mg/dl) (mg/dl) (μmol/L)

Fig. 2. Shows lipid levels in subjects divided into tertiles for both HOMA and Insulin AUC levels. Similar lipid values were demonstrated in all subjects.

	Cholesterol	LDL-Cholesterol	HDL-Cholesterol	Triglycerides
BMI (kg\m^2)	R = 0,0800	R = - 0,0017	R = - 0,4762▪	R = 0,6962
WAIST (cm)	R = 0,1410	R = 0,0753	R = - 0,4253▪	R = 0,6765
WHR (cm)	R = 0,0326	R = - 0,1535	R = - 0,1878	R = 0,4262
A (nmol/L)	R = - 0,1921	R = - 0,0280	R = - 0,1845	R = 0,0007
Tot T (nmol/L)	R = - 0,3425	R = - 0,4544▪	R = - 0,1377	R = 0,3692
FSH (IU/L)	R = 0,3094	R = 0,3909▪	R = 0,3711▪	R = - 0,1603
E2(pmol/L)	R = 0,0150	R = 0,0124	R = - 0,0264	R = - 0,0876
DHEAS (µmol/L)	R = 0,1230	R = 0,1925	R = - 0,1793	R = 0,2206
SHBG (nmol/L)	R = - 0,2226	R = - 0,2834	R = 0,0655	R = - 0,0942
17OHP (nmol/L)	R = - 0,0925	R = - 0,0586	R = 0,1667	R = - 0,3703▪
HOMA	R = 0,4724	R = 0,5140	R = 0,2293	R = - 0,0123
I-AUC 180 min(UI/ml)	R = - 0,0021	R = 0,0331	R = - 0,3391	R = 0,2882
Homocysteine (µmol/L)	R = 0,2148	R = 0,1214	R = - 0,2604	R = 0,5656▪
Fasting Glucose	R = 0,0440	R = 0,1325	R = - 0,1952	R = - 0,0396
Fasting Insulin	R = 0,1226	R = 0,1315	R = 0,0435	R = 0,0972

P < 0,05
P < 0,01
P < 0,001

Table 4. Linear relationships between lipid assays and phisical endocrine and metabolic parameters in CONTROLS.

	Cholesterol	LDL-Cholesterol	HDL-Cholesterol	Triglycerides
BMI (kg\m^2)	R = 0,1058	R = 0,2252	R = - 0,3930	R = 0,2933
WAIST (cm)	R = 0,1298	R = 0,2624	R = -0,3756	R = 0,2856
WHR (cm)	R = 0,2174	R = 0,3039	R = - 0,1924	R = 0,2063
E2(pmol/L)	R = - 0,0912	R = - 0,0912	R = 0,0541	R = - 0,1495
A (nmol/L)	R = - 0,0401	R = - 0,0953	R = 0,2933	R = -0,2400
Tot T (nmol/L)	R = - 0,1848	R = - 0,2191	R = 0,0181	R = 0,0085
SHBG (nmol/L)	R = - 0,1260	R = -0,1973	R = 0,1038	R = 0,0368
Fasting Glucose	R = 0,0107	R = 0.0800	R = - 0,1425	R = -0,0092
Fasting Insulin	R = 0,0773	R = 0,1239	R = - 0,1960	R = 0,0109
HOMA	R = 0,1349	R = 0,2269	R = - 0,2800▪	R = 0,0021
I-AUC 180 min(UI/ml)	R = 0,0324	R = 0,0550	R = - 0,0930	R = 0,0123
Homocysteine (μmol/L)	R = 0,0764	R = 0,0209	R = - 0,0656	R = 0,2863▪

P < 0,05
P < 0,01
P < 0,001

Table 5. Linear relationships between lipid assays and phisical endocrine and metabolic parameters in all patients.

2. References

[1] The Rotterdam ESHRE/ASRM sponsored PCOS consensus workshop group. Revised 2003 consesus on diagnostic criteria and long-term health risks related to polycystic ovary syndrome (PCOS). Human Reproduction 19: 41,47

[2] Hacihanefioglou B. Polycystic ovary syndrome nomenclature: chaos? Fertility and Sterility 2000 73, 1261-1262.2.

[3] Ancien P, Quereda F, Matallin P, Villarroya E, Lopez-Fernandez JA, Ancien M, Mauri M, Alfayate R. Insulin, androgens and obesity in women with and without Policystic ovary syndrome: a heterogeneous group of disorders. Fertility and Sterility 1999 72, 32-40

[4] Franks S. Policystic ovary syndrome. The New England Journal of Medicine 1995 333: 853-861

[5] Ehrmann DA, Barnes RB, Rosenfield RI, Cavaghan MK, Imperial J. Prevalence of impaired glucose tollerance and diabetes in women with Policystic ovary syndrome. Diabetes Care 1999 22: 141-14626.

[6] Diamanti-Kandarakis E, Piperi C. Genetics of polycystic ovary syndrome: searching for the way out of the labyrinth. Human. Reproduction. Update 2005 11, 631-643

[7] Diamanti-Kandarakis E, Piperi C, Spina J, Argyrakopoulou G, Papanastasiou L, Bergiele A, Panidis D. Polycystic ovary syndrome: the influence of environmental and genetics factors. Hormones (Athens) 2006 5, 17-3428.

[8] Conway GS, Agrawal R, Betteridge DJ, Jacobs HS. Risk factors for coronary artery disease in lean and obese women with the polycystic ovary syndrome. Clinical Endocrinology (Oxf) 1992 37: 119-125

[9] Teimuraz Apridonidze, Paulina A. Essah, Maria J. Iuorno and John E. Nestler. Prevalence and Characteristics of the Metabolic Syndrome in Women with Polycystic Ovary Syndrome. Journal of Clinical Endocrinology and metabolism 2005 Apr;90(4):1929-35

[10] Shroff R, Kerchner A, Maifeld M, Van Beek EJ, Jagasia D, Dokras A. Young obese women with polycystic ovary syndrome have evidence of early coronary atherosclerosis. Journal of Clinical Endocrinology and metabolism 2007 Dec;92(12):4609-14

[11] Carmina E, Orio F, Palomba S, Cascella T, Longo RA, Colao AM, Lombardi G, and Lobo RA. Evidence of altered adipocyte function in policystyc ovary sindrome. European Journal of Endocrinology 2005 Mar;152(3):389-94

[12] Fulghesu AM, Angioni S, Portoghese E. Milano F, Batetta B, Paoletti AM, Melis GB. Failure of the homeostatic model assessment calculation score for detecting metabolic deterioration in young patients with polycystic ovary syndrome. Fertility and Sterility. 2006 Aug;86(2):398-404

[13] Chang RJ, Nakamura RM, Judd HL, & Kaplan SA. Insulin resistence in nonobese patients with Policystic ovarian disease. Journal of Clinical Endocrinology and Metabolism 1983 57, 356-359 7.

[14] Morin-Papunen LC, Vauhkonen I, Koivunen RM, Ruokonen A, & Tapanainen JS. Insulin sensitivity, insulin secretion, and metabolic and hormonal parameters in healthy women and women with Policystic ovary syndrome.Human Reproduction 2000 15, 1266-1274

[15] Dunaif A, Graf M, Mandeli J, Laumas V, & Dobrjansky A. Characterization of group of hyperandrogenic women with acanthosis nigricans impaired glucose tolerance, and/or hyperinsulinemia. Journal of Clinical Endocrinology and Metabolism 1987 65, 499-507

[16] Diamanti-Kandarakis E, Kouli CR, Bergiele AT, Filandra FA, Tsianateli TC, Spina GG, Zapanti Ed, & Bartzis MI. A survey of the Policystic ovary syndrome in the greck island of Lesbos: hormonal and metabolic profile. Journal of Clinical Endocrinology and Metabolism 1999 84, 4006-4011

[17] Wild RA, Painter PC, Counlson PB, Carruth KB, Ranney GB. Lipoprotein lipid concentrations and cardiovascular risk in women with Policystic ovary syndrome. Journal of Clinical Endocrinology and Metabolism 1985; 61,946-51 11.
[18] Holte J, Bergh T, Berne C, Lithell H. Serum lipoprotein lipid profile in women with the Policystic ovary syndrome:relation to anthropometric, endocrine and metabolic variables. Clinical Endocrinology 1994; 41: 463-71
[19] Diamanti-Kandarakis E, Papavassiliou AG, Kandarakis SA, Chrousos GP. Patophysiology and types of dylipidemia in PCOS, Trends in Endocrinology and Metabolism 2007 Sep;18(7):280-5
[20] Coviello AD, Richard S, Legro, Dunaif A. Adolescent girls with polycystic ovary syndrome have an increased risk of the metabolic syndrome associated with increasing androgen levels independent of obesity and insulin resistance. Journal of Clinical Endocrinology and metabolism 2006 Feb;91(2):492-7.
[21] Orio F Jr, Palomba S, Cascella T, Tauchmanovà L, Nardo LG, Di Biase S, Labella D, Russo T, Savastano S, Tolino A, Zullo F, Colao A, Lombardi. Is plasminogen activator inhibitor-1 a cardiovascular risk factor in young women with polycystic ovary syndrome? Reprod Biomed Online Journal. 2004 Nov;9(5):505-10
[22] Lewy UD, Danadian K, Witchel SF, Arslanian S. Early metabolic abnormalities in adolescent girl with polycystic ovarian syndrome. Journal of Pediatric 2001 138: 38-44
[23] Carmina E, Legro RS, Stamets K, Lowell J, Lobo RA. Difference in body weight between American and Italian women ith polycystic ovary syndrome: influence of the diet. Hum Reprod 2003 18: 2289-93
[24] Carmina E, Lobo RA. Policystic ovary syndrome (PCOS): arguably the most common endocrinopathy is associated with significant morbidity in women. Journal of Clinical Endocrinology and metabolism 1999 84:1897-1899
[25] Piccione E, Dei M Donna Domani, CIC Edizioni Internazionali
[26] Palmert MR, Gordon CM, Kartashov AI, Legro RS, Emans SJ; Dunaif A. Screening for abnormal glucose tolerance in adolescents with polycistic ovary syndrome. Journal of Clinical Endocrinology and metabolism 2002 87:1017-1023
[27] Matthews DR, Hosker JP, Rudenski AS, Naylor BA, Treacher DF, Turner RC. Homeostasis model assessment: insulin resistence and βcell function from fasting plasma glucose and insulin concentrations in man. Diabetologia 1985 28; 412-419
[28] Ferriman D, Gallwey JD. Clinical Assesmentof body hair growth in women. Journal of Clinical Endocrinology and metabolism 1960 21:1440 - 1447
[29] Mather KJ, Verma S, Corenblum B, Anderson TJ. Normal endothelial function despite insulin resistance in healthy women with the polycystic ovary syndrome. Journal of Clinical Endocrinology and metabolism 2000 May;85(5)
[30] Pasquali R. Obesity and androgens: facts and perspectives; Fertil Steril 2006 May;85(5):1319-40
[31] Brown GA, Vukovich MD, Martini ER, Kohut ML, Franke WD, Jackson DA, King DS. Endocrine responses to chronic androstenedione intake in 30- to 56-year-old men. Journal of Clinical Endocrinology and metabolism 2000 Nov;85(11):4074-80

[32] Tan KC, Shiu SW, Kung AW.Alterations in hepatic lipase and lipoprotein subfractions with transdermal testosterone replacement therapy. Clinical Endocrinology (Oxf) 1999 51, 765-769

2

Ethnic Difference in Lipid Profiles

Lei Zhang[1,2,3,4], Qing Qiao[1,4] and Yanhu Dong[2,3]
[1]*Hjelt Institute, University of Helsinki, Helsinki,*
[2]*Qingdao Endocrine & Diabetes Hospital, Qingdao,*
[3]*Weifang Medical University, Weifang,*
[4]*National Institute for Health and Welfare, Helsinki,*
[1,4]*Finland*
[2,3]*China*

1. Introduction

Dyslipidaemia is a major cardiovascular disease (CVD) risk factor that plays an important role in the progress of atherosclerosis, the underlying pathology of CVD. To keep lipids and lipoproteins levels within ideal range has been recommended by different national, regional, or global (2001; Graham et al. 2007; World Health Organization 2007) guidelines on the prevention and management of CVD. The prevalence and pattern of lipid disorder, however, differ between ethnicities and populations.

As a component of the metabolic syndrome, dyslipidaemia often coexists with diabetes, the coronary heart disease (CHD) risk equivalent. An atherogenic lipid profiles consists of high triglycerides (TG) and small dense low-density lipoprotein cholesterol (LDL-C) and low high-density lipoprotein cholesterol (HDL-C). The importance of dyslipidaemia on risk of CVD in patients with diabetes has been extensively studied in numerous studies. Reduced HDL-C is well documented as an independent predictor of CVD events (Wilson et al. 1988; Cooney et al. 2009). In contrast, the role of TG as an independent risk factor for CVD is more controversial (Patel et al. 2004; Psaty et al. 2004; Barzi et al. 2005; Sarwar et al. 2007; Wang et al. 2007). Recently, the interest to use novel parameters such as total cholesterol (TC) to HDL ratio (TC/HDL-C), non-HDL-cholesterol (non-HDL-C), apolipoprotein B (apoB) and apolipoprotein A (apoA) to assess CVD risk has increased (Barzi et al. 2005; Pischon et al. 2005; Charlton-Menys et al. 2009). As a CVD risk predictor, the non-HDL-C has been considered to be superior to LDL-C (Cui et al. 2001; Schulze et al. 2004; Liu et al. 2005; Ridker et al. 2005). However, there are racial and geographic disparities in lipid profiles not only in general populations but also in individuals with different glucose categories. The Third Report of the National Cholesterol Education Program Expert Panel on Detection, Evaluation, and Treatment of High Blood Cholesterol in Adults (NCEP-ATP III) has recommended that certain factors be recognized when clinicians evaluate the lipid profile of different population groups (Adult Treatment Panel III 2002). Although management of lipids using NCEP-ATP III guidelines is applicable to all populations, unique aspects of risk factor profile call for special attention to certain features in different racial/ethnic groups.

2. Ethnic differences in lipid profiles in general populations

The prevalence of dyslipidaemia varies depending on the population studied, geographic location, socioeconomic development and the definition used (Wood et al. 1972; Mann et al. 1988; Onat et al. 1992; Berrios et al. 1997; Ezenwaka et al. 2000; Foucan et al. 2000; Hanh et al. 2001; Zaman et al. 2001; Azizi et al. 2003; Florez et al. 2005; Li et al. 2005; Hertz et al. 2006; Pang et al. 2006; Pongchaiyakul et al. 2006; Tekes-Manova et al. 2006; Zhao et al. 2007; Erem et al. 2008; Steinhagen-Thiessen et al. 2008). Caucasians generally have higher mean TC concentrations than do populations of Asian or African origin (Fuentes et al. 2003; Tolonen et al. 2005). In general populations, the highest prevalence of hypercholesterolaemia (TC ≥ 6.5mmol/l) has been seen in Malta (up to 50% in women) and the lowest in China (2.7% in men) in the World Health Orgnization (WHO) Inter-Health Programme (Berrios et al. 1997). However, inhabitants of the developing world now have had access to more fats in their diets and more sedentary lives; therefore the disease is becoming an increasing problem there.

Ethnic differences in the risk of CVD and type 2 diabetes have consistently been identified, with the most studies comparing the risk between African-Americans and Whites. African-Americans usually display a more favorable lipid profile compared with Whites, despite having the highest overall mortality rates from CVD. In general, African-American men have similar or lower LDL-C and TG but higher HDL-C levels compared with White men. There is evidence that the difference in HDL-C between African-American and White men may be due to a relatively lower hepatic lipase activity in African-Americans (Vega GL 1998). The difference in TG may be related to increased activity of lipoprotein lipase in African-Americans (Sumner AE 2005). However, compared with Whites, Hispanics and Asians, African-Americans have less favorable levels of lipoprotein(a) (Lp[a]), which is structurally similar to LDL-C, with an additional disulfide linked glycoprotein termed ApoA. A number of studies have suggested that Lp(a) may be an important risk factor for CVD (Danesh J 2000; The Emerging Risk Factors C 2009).

Compared to non-Hispanic Whites, Hispanics, specifically Mexican-Americans, have demonstrated lower HDL-C and higher TG levels (Sundquist J 1999). Data from the Dallas Heart Study and a smaller cross-sectional analysis of healthy individuals confirm that levels of Lp(a) are likely similar or even lower in Hispanics compared with Whites (Tsimikas S 2009). Although Lp(a) levels have been associated with endothelial dysfunction in Hispanics, the relationship with coronary artery disease in this population is less clear.

Asian Indians exhibit a higher prevalence of diabetes mellitus than Chinese and Malays (Tan et al. 1999). They also have higher serum TG concentrations and lower HDL-C concentrations than Chinese (Gupta M 2006). In the HeartSCORE and IndiaSCORE studies (Mulukutla et al. 2008) where lipids were measured with the same assay procedures for Asian Indians as for Whites and Blacks, Asian Indians had lowest TC and HDL-C and highest TG among all the ethnic groups studied. In another multi-ethnic study of the 1992 Singapore National Health Survey (Tan et al. 1999), Asian Indians appeared to have lower HDL-C but higher TG levels compared with the Chinese group. Data in other racial/ethnic groups are somewhat limited. Mean total cholesterol and LDL-C levels are lower in American Indians compared with the US average, and levels of Lp(a) are reported to be lower than in Whites (Wang W 2002). East Asians tend to have lower LDL-C, HDL-C and TG as compared with non-Asians (Karthikeyan et al. 2009). East Asians have been reported to have low Lp(a) levels, whereas south Asians have higher mean Lp(a) levels (Geethanjali FS 2003; Berglund L 2004).

Globalization of the western lifestyle contribute to worldwide increases of adiposity and type 2 diabetes not only in adults but also in children and adolescents (Kelishadi et al. 2006; Schwandt et al. 2010). In the BIG Study comparing the prevalence of the metabolic syndrome components in children and adolescents of European, Asian and South-American ethnicities, Iranian and Brazilian youths had considerably higher prevalence of dyslipidaemia than German youths. The most remarkable ethnic difference detected in this study is the high prevalence of low HDL-C levels in Iranian children and adolescents (38%) compared with German youths (7%) (Schwandt et al. 2010). Future longitudinal studies should seek the clinical importance of these ethnic differences.

3. Ethnic differences in lipid profiles in the state of hyperglycaemia

3.1 Lipid disorder and CVD risk in individuals with hyperglycaemia

Lipids and lipoproteins abnormalities are major metabolic disorders, commonly including elevated levels of TC, LDL-C, Lp(a) and TG and reduced levels of HDL-C. In patients with type 2 diabetes, a CHD equivalent (Juutilainen et al. 2005), it is most commonly characterized by elevated TG and reduced HDL-C (Goldberg, I. J. 2001; Krauss 2004; Kendall 2005). There is increasing evidence that the diabetic dyslipidaemia pattern is common not only in patients with overt diabetes (Barrett-Connor et al. 1982) but also in individuals with different glucose categories, i.e., impaired glucose tolerance (IGT) or impaired fasting glucose (IFG) (Meigs et al. 2002; Novoa et al. 2005; Chen et al. 2006; Pankow et al. 2007). These abnormalities can be present alone or in combination with other metabolic disorders. It is well known that the risk of morbidity and mortality from CVD is increased by two- to four-fold in diabetic patients compared with the general population (Kannel 1985; Morrish et al. 1991; Almdal et al. 2004). A number of studies have determined the association of dyslipidaemia with cardiovascular risk in people with hyperglycaemia, and most of them were conducted in patients with diabetes. There is a large body of evidence linking dyslipidaemia and cardiovascular risk in patients with diabetes against quite few negative reports (Vlajinac et al. 1992; Roselli della Rovere et al. 2003) on this issue. Cross-sectional studies have found positive associations of atherosclerotic vascular disease with TC (Ronnemaa et al. 1989; Jurado et al. 2009), LDL-C (Reckless et al. 1978; Agarwal et al. 2009; Jurado et al. 2009), non-HDL-C (Jurado et al. 2009), TG (Santen et al. 1972; Ronnemaa et al. 1989; Gomes et al. 2009), apoB (Ronnemaa et al. 1989) and Lp(a) (Mohan et al. 1998; Murakami et al. 1998; Smaoui et al. 2004), but inverse associations with HDL-C (Reckless et al. 1978; Ronnemaa et al. 1989; Smaoui et al. 2004; Grant and Meigs 2007; Gomes et al. 2009; Jurado et al. 2009) and apoA-I (Seviour et al. 1988; Ronnemaa et al. 1989).

Prospective data have provided with further evidence. The UKPDS study (Turner et al. 1998) has demonstrated that high LDL-C and low HDL-C are potentially modifiable risk factors for coronary artery disease (CAD) in patients with type 2 diabetes. TG, however, was not independently associated with CAD risk in this study, possibly because of its close inverse relationship with HDL-C. Results from the MRFIT (Stamler et al. 1993), in which 356,499 nondiabetic and 5163 diabetic men without CHD at baseline were followed for 12 years, indicated that serum cholesterol is an independent predictor of CHD mortality in men with diabetes. Rosengren et al. (Rosengren et al. 1989) showed similar results in a prospective study of 6897 middle aged diabetic men. Patients with TC > 7.3 mmol/l had a significantly higher incidence of CHD during the 7-year follow up than those with TC ≤ 5.5 mmol/l (28.3% vs. 5.4%, $p<0.05$). Long term follow-up of the London cohort of the WHO

Multinational Study of Vascular Disease in Diabetics, consisting of 254 type 2 diabetic patients, has showed that TC was associated with incidence of MI (Morrish et al. 1991) and overall cardiovascular mortality (Morrish et al. 1990). The role of TC in predicting CHD was also confirmed in women patients with diabetes (Schulze et al. 2004).

3.2 Ethnic difference in lipid profiles across glucose categories

Although the ethnic variation in lipid patterns has been wided studied in general populations, the ethnic differences in lipid profiles given the same glucose levels have not been well investigated. This issue has been recently studied in the DECODE (Diabetes Epidemiology: Collaborative analysis Of Diagnostic criteria in Europe) and DECODA (Diabetes Epidemiology: Collaborative analysis Of Diagnostic criteria in Asia) study, which consisted of 64 cohorts of mainly population-based from 24 countries and regions around the world, with about 84 000 Europeans and 84 207 Asians of Chinese, Japanese, Indians, Mongolians and Filipinos.

In the collaborative analysis of seven ethnic groups of European and Asian populations (studies included see Appendix 1), considerable ethnic differences in lipid profiles were observed within each glucose category. Asian Indians exhibited an adverse lipid pattern consisting of low HDL-C and high TG across all glucose categories as compared with other ethnic groups. Reduced HDL-C is prevalent even in Asian Indians with desirable LDL-C levels regardless of the diabetic status. In addition, in most of the ethnic groups, individuals detected with undiagnosed diabetes had a worse lipid profile than did diagnosed cases. Age-, cohort- and BMI adjusted mean TC, LDL-C and TG increased while the mean HDL-C decreased with more pronounced glucose intolerance in most of the ethnic groups in individuals without a prior history of diabetes (Fig. 1 a-h). Subjects with undiagnosed diabetes, however, had a worse lipid profile than those with known disease. Within individuals with normoglycaemia, mean lipid and lipoprotein concentrations differed among the ethnic groups. The Europeans had highest TC (Fig. 1 a-b) and LDL-C (Fig. 1 c-d), while Qingdao Chinese had highest HDL-C levels among all ethnic groups (Fig. 1 e-f). In contrast, Asian Indians had the lowest TC (Fig. 1 a-b), LDL-C (Fig. 1 c-d) and HDL-C (Fig. 1 e-f) but the highest TG (Fig. 1 g-h) among the ethnic groups ($p < 0.05$ for all comparisons). These ethnic differences were consistently found in all glucose categories.

The multivariate-adjusted odds ratio (95% CI) of having low HDL-C was significantly higher for Asian Indians, Mauritian Indians, Hong Kong Chinese and Southern Europeans but lower for Qingdao Chinese compared with Central & North (C&N) Europeans, across all glucose categories from normal to diabetes (Table 1). Asian Indians and Mauritian Indians tended to have higher but Southern Europeans lower odds ratios for having high-TG compared with the reference group. Unlike that for HDL-C or TG, the odds ratio for having high LDL-C was consistently lower in all Asian ethnic groups compared with the reference, across most of the glucose categories.

In the HeartSCORE and IndiaSCORE studies (Mulukutla et al. 2008) where lipids were measured with the same assay procedures for Asian Indians as for whites and blacks, Asian Indians had lowest TC and HDL-C and highest TG among all the ethnic groups studied. In another multi-ethnic study of the 1992 Singapore National Health Survey (Tan et al. 1999), Asian Indians appeared to have lower HDL-C but higher TG levels compared with Chinese. The findings of these previous studies are consistent with ours although glucose status was not controlled in the previous studies.

Similar to others (Harris and Eastman 2000; Hadaegh et al. 2008), we observed a worse lipid profile in individuals with undiagnosed diabetes than that of previously diagnosed patients in most of the ethnic groups, indicating individuals with undiagnosed diabetes are at increased CVD risk and need to be identified and treated early. On the other hand, glycaemic control is shown to be an important determinant of diabetic dyslipidaemia (Ismail et al. 2001). The better lipid profile in diagnosed diabetes as compared with undiagnosed diabetes might imply a benefit of lifestyle intervention or drug treatment targeting favorable metabolic profiles and hemoglobin A1c (HbA1c), a surrogate measure for average blood glucose. However, to what extent the levels of HbA1c have contributed to the differences is unknown due to the lack of information in the current study. In addition, the data on lipid-lowering treatment is not available for most of the earlier studies conducted in the 1990s because the statins were not widely prescribed at that time. These deserve further investigation in future studies.

In contrast to the lower HDL-C and higher TG profiles, Asian Indians had considerably lower TC and LDL-C concentrations than others. As shown in Table 2, 71% non-diabetic and 57.6% diabetic Asian Indians had low LDL-C (< 3.0 mmol/l), while the corresponding figures were 19.2% and 24.6% ($p < 0.01$) for C&N Europeans and 46.6% and 38.8% ($p < 0.01$) for Qingdao Chinese. However, even within the low LDL-C category, there was still a higher proportion of Asian Indians having low HDL-C compared with others (Table 2). The results were confirmed in the same analysis conducted separately for men and women.

There is a large body of evidence showing that diabetes is associated with a high prevalence of dyslipidaemia (Kannel 1985; Cowie et al. 1994; 1997; Jacobs et al. 2005; Bruckert et al. 2007; Abdel-Aal et al. 2008; Ahmed et al. 2008; Okafor et al. 2008; Surana et al. 2008; Agarwal et al. 2009; Jurado et al. 2009; Papazafiropoulou et al. 2009; Roberto Robles et al. 2009; Temelkova-Kurktschiev et al. 2009; Zhang et al. 2009; Seyum et al. 2010). In the Framingham Heart Study (Kannel 1985), the prevalence of low HDL-C (21% vs. 12% in men and 25% vs. 10% in women, respectively) and high TG levels (19% vs. 9% in men and 17% vs. 8% in women, respectively) in people with diabetes was almost twice as high as the prevalence in non-diabetic individuals. By contrast, TC and LDL-C levels did not differ from those of non-diabetic counterparts. A similar pattern of lipid profiles was observed in the UK Prospective Diabetes Study (UKPDS) (1997). In this study, the plasma TG levels were substantially increased whereas HDL-C levels were markedly reduced in both men and women with diabetes compared with the non-diabetic controls. Higher prevalence has been reported in other studies. Data from a primary care-based 7692 patients with type 2 diabetes in the United States showed nearly half of the patients had low HDL-C (Grant and Meigs 2007). The figure was even worse in an urban Indian cohort of 5088 type 2 diabetes patients, with more than half having low HDL-C (52.3%) or high TG (57.9%) (Surana et al. 2008). In addition to the traditional lipid measurement, increased levels of apoB were also seen in patients with diabetes compared with non-diabetic individuals (Bangou-Bredent et al. 1999).

It has been shown that the prevalence of lipid and/or glucose abnormality differs between ethnic groups. It is clear that certain ethnic groups have differences in lipid profiles in general. Elevated TG and reduced HDL-C, as the components of the metabolic syndrome and atherogenic dyslipidaemia, was seen more common in Asian Indians than in the Whites (Anand et al. 2000; Razak et al. 2005; Chandalia et al. 2008; Mulukutla et al. 2008), Chinese (Tan et al. 1999; Anand et al. 2000; Razak et al. 2005; The DECODA Study Group 2007; Karthikeyan et al. 2009), Japanese (The DECODA Study Group 2007; Karthikeyan et al. 2009) or Africans (Mulukutla et al. 2008). In a nationally representative sample of seven ethnic groups in the UK (Zaninotto et al. 2007), the prevalence of low HDL-C was highest in south Asian groups such as Bangladeshi, Indian and Pakistani, followed by Chinese, Irish and those from the general population living in private households; In contrast, the lowest prevalence was seen in Black Caribbean. Similar finding was reported in another study where the comparison was made between non-South-Asians and South Asians (France et al. 2003). In addition, African Americans have been reported to have less adverse lipid profiles than Whites or Hispanics despite the presence of diabetes (Werk et al. 1993; Cowie et al. 1994; Sharma and Pavlik 2001). The causes of ethnic difference in levels of CVD risk factor are complex and may include genetic, environmental and cultural factors (Zaninotto et al. 2007). However, little is known about such ethnic differences in lipid profiles at comparable glucose tolerance status.

4. Causes of ethnic differences

There are several factors that contribute to the development of dyslipidaemia (2001), including genetic factors (Cohen et al. 1994) and acquired factors (Chait and Brunzell 1990; Devroey et al. 2004; Ruixing et al. 2008) such as overweight and obesity (Denke et al. 1993; Denke et al. 1994; Brown et al. 2000), physical inactivity (Berg et al. 1997; Hardman 1999), cigarette smoking (Criqui et al. 1980; Cade and Margetts 1989; Umeda et al. 1998; Fisher et al. 2000; Wu et al. 2001; Maeda et al. 2003; Mammas et al. 2003; Venkatesan et al. 2006; Grant and Meigs 2007; Arslan et al. 2008; Batic-Mujanovic et al. 2008), high fat intake (Hennig et al. 2001; Millen et al. 2002; Tanasescu et al. 2004), very high carbohydrate diets (> 60 percent of total energy) (McNamara and Howell 1992) and certain drugs (Lehtonen 1985; Fogari et al. 1988; Roberts 1989; Middeke et al. 1990; Stone 1994) (such as beta-blockers, anabolic steroids, progestational agents, et al.). Excess alcohol intake is also documented as a risk factor (Umeda et al. 1998; Wu et al. 2001; Mammas et al. 2003) despite that moderate alcohol consumption may have a beneficial effect on improving HDL-C concentrations (De Oliveira et al. 2000; Shai et al. 2004). In addition, glycaemic control is an important determinant of dyslipidaemia in patients with diabetes (Ismail et al. 2001; Grant and Meigs 2007; Ahmed et al. 2008; Gatti et al. 2009). Among these acquired factors, overweight, obesity and physical inactivity appear to be most important (Denke et al. 1993; Denke et al. 1994; Berg et al. 1997; Hardman 1999; Brown et al. 2000). They are also the most important lifestyle variables that decrease insulin action and increase the risk of diabetes.

The causes of ethnic difference in cardiovascular risk profile are complex. Possible contributors include genetic, environmental, psychosocial, cultural and unmeasured factors and many are not well clarified (Zaninotto et al. 2007). It is clear that the observed ethnic differences in lipid profiles cannot be explained by genetics alone and may be more indicative of lifestyle-related factors such as dietary pattern and physical activity (Ruixing et al. 2008; McNaughton et al. 2009; Sisson et al. 2009). To what extent is ethnic-specific lifestyle pattern associated with different lipid profiles deserves further investigation.

4.1 Genetic factors

An adverse lipid profile in Asian Indians has been reported to be associated with the greater susceptibility to insulin resistance (Tan et al. 1999; Anand et al. 2000; Bhalodkar et al. 2005; Palaniappan et al. 2007), and a higher percentage of body fat for the same BMI as compared with Whites (McKeigue et al. 1991), which may contribute to the high prevalence of CVD

(Kuller 2004) and diabetes (Ramachandran et al. 2008; Snehalatha and Ramachandran 2009) in this ethnic group. In addition, it may also reflect the genetic variation, for example, at the apoE locus (Tan et al. 2003) and an excess of other risk factors such as homocysteine, Lp(a) or dietary fat (France et al. 2003).

4.2 Environmental factors

As suggested by previous research, dietary factors may play a role in both lipid and insulin profiles, although these patterns may be mediated by body fat content (Ku CY 1998). Total fat (and saturated fat) intake has been shown to adversely affect total cholesterol concentrations in children, adolescents, and young adults (Post GB 1997). The difference in HDL-C concentrations between Qingdao and Hong Kong Chinese subgroups observed in the DECODA study cannot be simply explained by the difference in assay methods. It may largely attribute to the differences in dietary structure and preference, geographic and environmental factors. Shellfish and beer, for example, are commonly consumed all the year round in Qingdao. Nevertheless, whether other factors exist and contribute to the high HDL-C in Qingdao needs to be further investigated.

Mexican Americans have been previously reported to have greater adiposity, higher TG levels and lower HDL-C levels than Anglos. The relationship between behavioral variables (caloric balance, cigarette and alcohol consumption, exercise, post-menopausal estrogen or oral contraceptive use) and lipid pattern has been investigated in the San Antonio Heart Study (1979–1982) (n=2,102) to explain the ethnic difference in lipids and lipoproteins. Adjustment for caloric balance (as reflected by body mass index) narrowed the ethnic difference in TG and HDL-C levels for both sexes, while adjustment for smoking widened the ethnic difference. For females, the ethnic difference was also decreased by adjustment for alcohol and estrogen use. However, adjustment for these behavioral variables did not completely eliminate the ethnic difference in lipids and lipoproteins in either sex. Increased central adiposity, more characteristic of Mexican Americans than Anglos, was positively associated with triglycerides and negatively associated with HDL-C levels, especially in females. Fat patterning made a more important contribution to the prediction of TG and HDL-C levels than did the other behavioral variables (except for caloric balance) and, in general, eliminated ethnic differences in lipids and lipoproteins (Steven H 1986). Epidemiologists should consider the use of a centrality index to distinguish different types of adiposity since it is easy and inexpensive to measure.

5. Implications for management and prevention of dyslipidaemia

Epidemiological investigations of human populations have revealed a robust relationship between lipids and CVD risk. Furthermore, the benefit of lipid-modifying strategy on cardiovascular events has been demonstrated from a large number of randomized clinical trials (Thavendiranathan et al. 2006; Mills et al. 2008), especially from those using 3-hydroxy-3-methyl-glutaryl-CoA (HMG-CoA) reductase inhibitors (i.e., statins) (Goldberg, R. B. et al. 1998; Collins et al. 2003; Colhoun et al. 2004; Pyorala et al. 2004; Sever et al. 2005; Knopp et al. 2006; Shepherd et al. 2006). Intensive control of dyslipidaemia has been greatly emphasized in the prevention and management of CVD. Current guidelines from the National Cholesterol Education Program Adult Treatment Panel III (ATP III) (Adult Treatment Panel III 2002), the European Society of Cardiology (Graham et al. 2007) and the American Diabetes Association (American Diabetes Association 2009) consistently

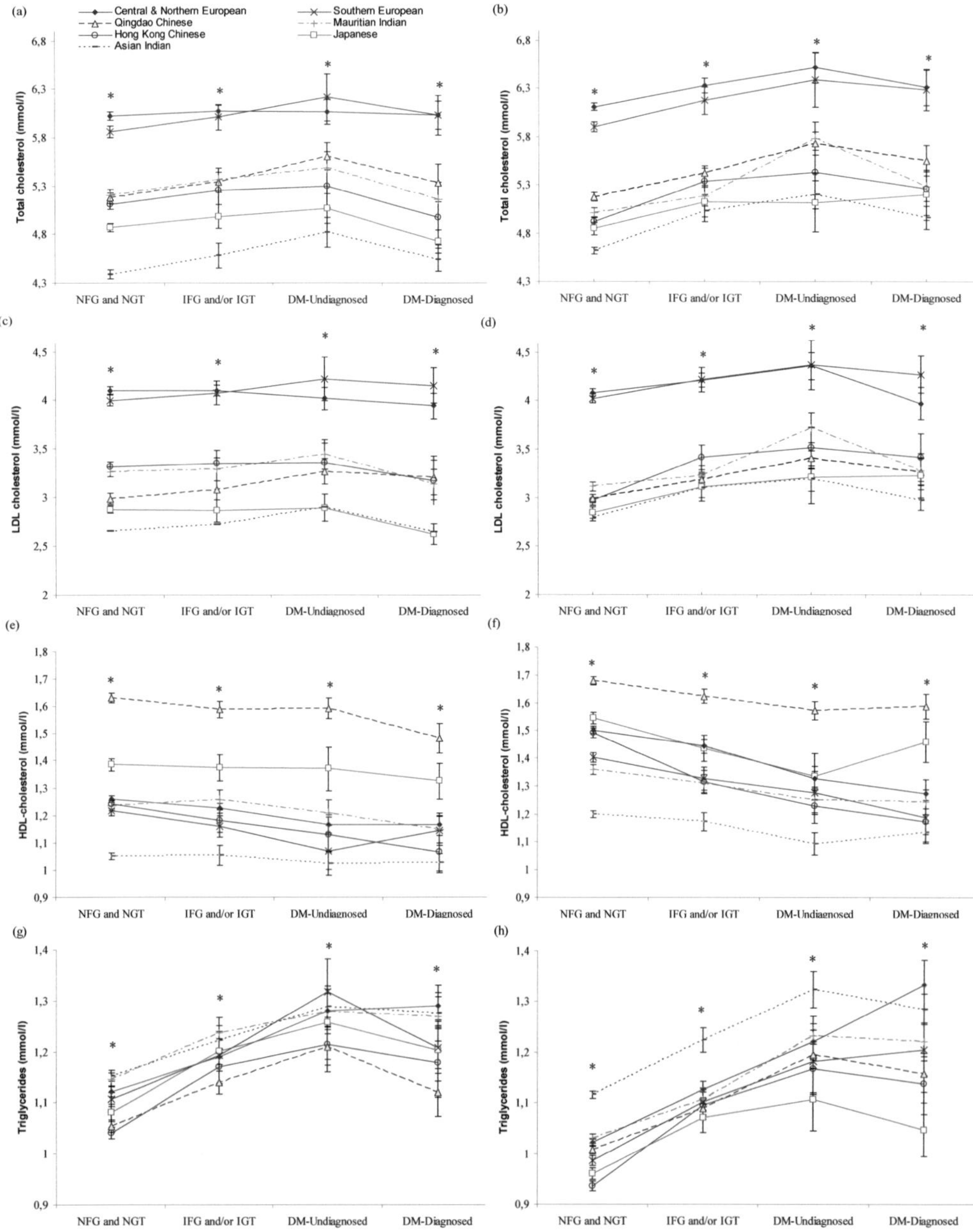

Fig. 1. Age-, study cohort- and body mass index-adjusted mean lipid (geometric means for triglycerides) and lipoprotein concentrations and 95% CIs (vertical bars) in men (figure 1-a, c, e and g) and women (figure 1-b, d, f and h) by ethnicities and glucose categories.* p for trend < 0.05 within each glucose category.

	HDL-C < 1.03 in men and < 1.29 in women (mmol/l)				TG ≥ 1.7 mmol/l				LDL-C ≥ 3 mmol/l			
	NFG and NGT	IFG and/or IGT	Undiagnosed diabetes	Diagnosed diabetes	NFG and NGT	IFG and/or IGT	Undiagnosed diabetes	Diagnosed Diabetes	NFG and NGT	IFG and/or IGT	Undiagnosed diabetes	Diagnosed diabetes
Men												
Central & Northern European [a]	1	1	1	1	1	1	1	1	1	1	1	1
Hong Kong Chinese	1.63 (1.41-1.87)	2.75 (2.09-3.62)	1.82 (1.20-2.76)	2.57 (1.48-4.46)	0.75 (0.64-0.87)	1.16 (0.88-1.53)	1.05 (0.70-1.58)	0.63 (0.36-1.12)	0.51 (0.44-0.58)	0.61 (0.46-0.82)	0.51 (0.33-0.78)	0.86 (0.49-1.52)
Qingdao Chinese	0.12 (0.09-0.16)	0.07 (0.04-0.13)	0.11 (0.07-0.20)	0.16 (0.08-0.32)	0.68 (0.58-0.79)	0.81 (0.66-1.00)	0.81 (0.61-1.09)	0.40 (0.26-0.63)	0.23 (0.20-0.26)	0.30 (0.24-0.37)	0.44 (0.32-0.60)	0.57 (0.37-0.86)
Asian Indian	4.74 (4.19-5.37)	5.05 (3.88-6.56)	3.07 (2.15-4.40)	2.37 (1.67-3.35)	1.40 (1.23-1.58)	1.53 (1.19-1.97)	1.24 (0.88-1.75)	1.42 (1.01-2.00)	0.12 (0.10-0.13)	0.17 (0.13-0.22)	0.23 (0.16-0.33)	0.29 (0.20-0.41)
Mauritian Indian	1.82 (1.58-2.09)	2.04 (1.58-2.63)	1.27 (0.89-1.81)	1.16 (0.78-1.74)	1.47 (1.28-1.69)	1.55 (1.23-1.98)	1.18 (0.85-1.65)	1.06 (0.72-1.57)	0.39 (0.34-0.45)	0.38 (0.30-0.49)	0.49 (0.34-0.70)	0.75 (0.50-1.12)
Japanese	0.87 (0.73-1.03)	1.29 (0.98-1.70)	0.73 (0.44-1.20)	0.57 (0.36-0.90)	0.99 (0.84-1.15)	1.31 (1.02-1.68)	1.36 (0.88-2.09)	1.02 (0.68-1.53)	0.26 (0.23-0.30)	0.35 (0.27-0.44)	0.36 (0.23-0.57)	0.77 (0.51-1.16)
Southern European	1.21 (1.06-1.37)	1.49 (1.15-1.93)	1.79 (1.19-2.70)	1.13 (0.78-1.63)	0.78 (0.69-0.88)	0.83 (0.65-1.07)	1.16 (0.77-1.75)	0.58 (0.40-0.84)	0.87 (0.75-1.00)	0.99 (0.73-1.36)	1.80 (1.01-3.23)	1.52 (0.99-2.31)
Women												
Central & Northern European [a]	1	1	1	1	1	1	1	1	1	1	1	1
Hong Kong Chinese	2.23 (1.93-2.57)	3.79 (2.88-4.98)	3.02 (1.88-4.85)	3.03 (1.68-5.48)	0.86 (0.69-1.08)	1.16 (0.85-1.58)	0.98 (0.61-1.57)	0.69 (0.39-1.21)	0.41 (0.35-0.47)	0.64 (0.48-0.86)	0.61 (0.36-1.04)	1.21 (0.66-2.22)
Qingdao Chinese	0.66 (0.57-0.76)	0.52 (0.41-0.65)	0.27 (0.19-0.38)	0.20 (0.13-0.31)	1.29 (1.11-1.50)	1.06 (0.87-1.30)	0.99 (0.73-1.36)	0.57 (0.39-0.84)	0.40 (0.36-0.45)	0.45 (0.37-0.55)	0.48 (0.33-0.69)	0.67 (0.45-0.99)
Asian Indian	10.91 (9.68-12.30)	7.80 (5.99-9.94)	8.64 (5.62-13.29)	4.34 (2.93-6.44)	2.76 (2.39-3.18)	2.21 (1.71-2.87)	3.13 (2.15-4.55)	1.29 (0.90-1.85)	0.22 (0.20-0.25)	0.36 (0.28-0.47)	0.36 (0.24-0.54)	0.41 (0.28-0.60)
Mauritian Indian	4.41 (3.88-5.02)	3.80 (3.05-4.74)	2.65 (1.82-3.88)	2.26 (1.53-3.35)	1.38 (1.16-1.65)	1.15 (0.91-1.47)	1.54 (1.07-2.23)	0.81 (0.56-1.19)	0.48 (0.42-0.55)	0.50 (0.40-0.63)	0.78 (0.51-1.21)	0.85 (0.57-1.27)
Japanese	2.40 (2.12-2.73)	3.07 (2.44-3.87)	2.65 (1.62-4.34)	1.07 (0.67-1.72)	0.92 (0.77-1.09)	1.19 (0.93-1.53)	0.72 (0.43-1.21)	0.41 (0.25-0.68)	0.58 (0.51-0.66)	0.67 (0.52-0.87)	0.56 (0.31-0.99)	2.24 (1.27-3.93)
Southern European	1.50 (1.34-1.68)	1.62 (1.26-2.08)	0.93 (0.56-1.52)	1.70 (1.13-2.56)	0.70 (0.60-0.81)	0.80 (0.61-1.05)	0.60 (0.36-1.01)	0.53 (0.35-0.79)	0.98 (0.87-1.11)	1.39 (1.01-1.93)	1.38 (0.70-2.72)	2.67 (1.62-4.42)

Model adjusted for age, study cohort, body mass index, systolic blood pressure and smoking status. NFG, normal fasting glucose; NGT, normal glucose tolerance. [a] Reference group

Table 1. Odds ratio (95% confidence interval) of having dyslipidaemia in relation to ethnicity by glucose categories.

	LDL-C < 3 mmol/l				LDL-C ≥ 3 mmol/l			
	Normal HDL-C and normal TG, %	Low HDL-C [a] alone, %	High TG [b] alone, %	both, %	Normal HDL-C and normal TG, %	Low HDL-C [a] alone, %	High TG [b] alone, %	both, %
Non-diabetic population								
Hong Kong Chinese	29.3	9.9	1.6	4.2	32.1	12.9	3.7	6.2
Qingdao Chinese	31.0	5.4	8.3	1.9	40.5	2.4	9.8	0.7
Asian Indian	23.2	33.6	3.2	11.0	9.2	10.7	2.8	6.4
Mauritian Indian	23.9	15.8	5.0	4.7	23.2	14.7	5.7	7.0
Japanese	25.2	6.4	3.4	3.5	38.2	13.0	5.0	5.3
Central & Northern European	13.3	2.3	2.0	1.6	48.6	9.7	12.6	10.0
Southern European	14.2	4.3	1.1	2.1	45.5	15.1	7.8	10.0
Diabetic population								
Hong Kong Chinese	12.4	9.6	1.4	11.0	22.6	18.1	7.6	17.2
Qingdao Chinese	21.1	3.5	11.1	3.1	37.9	2.7	19.1	1.5
Asian Indian	12.8	17.4	6.0	21.4	8.1	12.4	7.2	14.7
Mauritian Indian	12.4	8.6	6.4	10.2	21.2	15.5	10.2	15.5
Japanese	14.3	6.0	7.1	5.1	34.3	11.6	12.2	9.4
Central & Northern European	10.5	2.8	4.9	6.4	30.4	9.3	16.4	19.4
Southern European	7.5	3.3	6.0	10.2	24.4	11.2	12.8	14.8

a < 1.03 mmol/l in men and < 1.29 mmol/l in women
b ≥ 1.70 mmol/l

Table 2. Proportions (%) of individuals according to lipid levels stratified by diabetic status in each ethnic group.

recommend that LDL-C should be the primary target of therapy not only in patients with CHD or diabetes but also in individuals with increased cardiovascular risk. In addition, non-HDL-C is set by ATP III as a secondary target of therapy and HDL-C and TG as potential target. The Current guideline, mainly based on the data of Whites, consistently recommend that LDL-C < 2.6 mmol/l should be the primary target of therapy in patients with diabetes. As shown in our study and others' (Mulukutla et al. 2008; Karthikeyan et al. 2009), the Asian Indian population had significantly lower TC and LDL-C than did Whites. The threshold of LDL-C for treatment target for Whites may be too high for Asian Indians. Further studies are warranted to verify this hypothesis and determine the threshold applicable to this ethnic group.

In contrast to LDL-C, HDL-C has been either dropped from (Graham et al. 2007) or set as a secondary (American Diabetes Association 2010) or tertiary (Expert Panel on Detection 2001) target in the major guidelines despite the strong evidence of reduced HDL-C as an independent risk factor for CVD (Boden 2000). This may change if more therapy choices developed to increase HDL-C levels and improve HDL function are shown to prevent CVD (Singh et al. 2007; Duffy and Rader 2009; Sorrentino et al. 2010) or reduce the residual cardiovascular risk (Fruchart J 2008). Most recently, the ARBITER 6-HALTS (Arterial Biology for the Investigation of the Treatment Effects of Reducing Cholesterol 6-HDL and LDL Treatment Strategies in Atherosclerosis) trial has shown a significant improvement in serum HDL-C levels and regression of carotid intima-media thickness when ERN was conbined with statin therapy in patients with CHD or CHD equivalent (Taylor et al. 2009; Villines et al. 2010). Considering the high proportion of Asian Indians with adverse HDL-C levels, appropriate approaches to increasing HDL-C and/or improving HDL function may become an important treatment target in Asian Indians in order to reduce their excess CVD risks.

6. Appendix 1

Countries and studies	Blood sample	Total cholesterol	High-density lipoprotein cholesterol	Triglycerides
China				
Hong Kong Cardiovascular DiseaseRisk Factor Prevalence Study	Plasma	Cholesterol oxidase (CHOD) method; Hitachi 717 analyser (Hitachi Instruments, California, USA).	Measured after precipitation of very-low density lipoprotein (VLDL) and low-density lipoprotein (LDL) by polyethylene glycol PEG 6000.	Lipase/glycerol kinase method;
Hong Kong Workforce Survey on CVD Risk Factors	Venous Plasma	Enzymatic method, with reagents (Baker Instruments Corporation, Allentown, PA 18103, USA) with Cobas Mira analyzer (Hoffman-La Roche and Co., Basle Switzerland).	Enzymatic method after precipitation with dextran sulphate-$MgCl_2$ on Cobas Mira analyzer (Hoffman-La Roche and Co., Basle Switzerland)	Enzymatic method, with reagents (Baker Instruments Corporation, Allentown, PA 18103, USA) with Cobas Mira analyzer (Hoffman-La Roche and Co., Basle Switzerland)
Qingdao Diabetes Survey 2002	Venous Plasma	Enzymatic method (AMS Analyzer Medical System, SABA-18, Rome, Italy)	Enzymatic method after precipitation (AMS Analyzer Medical System, SABA-18, Rome, Italy)	Enzymatic method (AMS Analyzer Medical System, SABA-18, Rome, Italy)
Qingdao Diabetes Study 2006	Serum	Enzymatic method (Olympus reagent) With OLYMPUS-AU640 Automatic Analyzers (Olympus Optical. Tokyo, Japan)	Direct method (Olympus reagent) with OLYMPUS-AU640 Automatic Analyzers (Olympus Optical. Tokyo, Japan)	Enzymatic method (Olympus reagent) with OLYMPUS-AU640 Automatic Analyzers (Olympus Optical. Tokyo, Japan)

Finland				
East-West men	Serum	Enzymatic techniques (Monotest, Boehringer Mannheim GmbH, FRG) Olli C3000 photometer (Kone Oy, Finland)	Enzymetic method after precipitation of VLDL and LDL by means of dextran-magnesium-chloride, with Olli C3000 photometer (Kone Oy, Finland)	Enzymatic techniques (Monotest, Boehringer Mannheim GmbH, FRG) Olli C3000 photometer (Kone Oy, Finland)
National FINRISK Study 87, 92	Serum	Enzymatic techniques (Cholesterol oxidase-peroxidase-amidopyrine, CHOD-PAP, Boehringer-Mannheim, Mannheim, Germany)	Enzymatic method after dextran sulfate magnesium chloride precipitation of apolipoprotein B (apoB)-containing lipoproteins	Enzymatic techniques (CHOD-PAP, Boehringer-Mannheim, Mannheim, Germany)
National FINRISK Study 2002	Serum	Enzymatic method (CHOD-PAP; Thermo Elektron Oy, Finland);	Enzymatic method (CHOD-PAP; Thermo Elektron Oy, Finland) after precipitation by the PTA-precipitation method	Enzymatic techniques (Glycerol phosphate oxidase-peroxidase-amidopyrine, GPO-PAP; Thermo Elektron Oy)
Oulu Study	Serum	Enzymatic method (CHOD-PAP, Boehringer Mannheim, Mannheim, Germany).	Enzymatic CHOD-PAP method after precipitation of LDL and VLDL with a reagent containing phosphotungstic acid and $MgCl_2$ (Boehringer Mannheim)	Enzymatic method (CHOD-PAP, Boehringer Mannheim, Mannheim, Germany)
Savitaipale Study	Plasma	Enzymatic colorimetric method (CHOD-PAP) Cobas Integra 400/700 analyzer	Enzymatic colorimetric method (CHOD-PAP) Cobas Integra 400/700 analyzer	Enzymatic colorimetric method (CHOD-PAP) Cobas Integra 400/700 analyzer
Vantaa Study	Serum	Enzymatic techniques (Boehringer-Mannheim)	Enzymatic method after precipitation with polyethylenglycol	Enzymatic techniques (Boehringer-Mannheim)
India				
Chennai 94	Serum	Enzymatic method; Hitachi 704 autoanalyser, using Boehringer Mannheim (Mannheim, Germany) reagents	Phosphotungstate-magnesium precipitation method. Hitachi 704 autoanalyser, using Boehringer Mannheim (Mannheim, Germany) reagents	Enzymatic method. Hitachi 704 autoanalyser, using Boehringer Mannheim (Mannheim, Germany) reagents

Chennai 97	Venous Plasma	CHOD-PAP method (Boehringer Mannheim, Germany); Corning Express Plus Auto Analyser (Corning, medfied, MA, USA)	Phosphotungstic acid method after precipitation of LDL and chylomicrons (Boehringer Mannheim, Germany); Corning Express Plus Auto Analyser (Corning, medfied, MA, USA)	GPO-PAP method (Boehringer Mannheim, Germany); Corning Express Plus Auto Analyser (Corning, medfied, MA, USA)
CURES	Serum	CHOD-PAP method with Hitachi-912 Autoanalyser (Hitachi, Mannheim, Germany) using kits supplied by Roche Diagnostics (Mannheim, Germany).	Direct method (polyethylene glycol–pretreated enzymes) with Hitachi-912 Autoanalyser (Hitachi, Mannheim, Germany) using kits supplied by Roche Diagnostics (Mannheim, Germany).	GPO-PAP method; Hitachi-912 Autoanalyser (Hitachi, Mannheim, Germany) using kits supplied by Roche Diagnostics (Mannheim, Germany).
Chennai 2006	Serum	Standard enzymatic procedures (Roche Diagnostics, Mannheim, Germany)	Direct assay method (Roche Diagnostics, Mannheim, Germany)	Standard enzymatic procedures (Roche Diagnostics, Mannheim, Germany)
Italy				
Cremona Study	Plasma	Enzymatic techniques (Boehringer-Mannheim, Mannheim, Germany) with CIBA Corning 550 Express Auto-analyser	Precipitation with PEG using a Colortest kit (Roche, Basel, Switzerland).	Enzymatic techniques (Boehringer-Mannheim, Mannheim, Germany) with CIBA Corning 550 Express Auto-analyser
Japan				
Funagata Study	Plasma	Cholesterol oxidase method (L-type Wako CHO-H [Wako Pure Chemical Industries, Osaka, Japan]) with TBA 80FR (Toshiba medical system corporation, Tokyo)	Direct method (Cholesterol N HDL [Daiichi Pure Chemicals, Tokyo, Japan]) with TBA 80FR (Toshiba medical system corporation, Tokyo)	GPO HDAOS method (Pureauto S TG-N [Daiichi Pure Chemicals, Tokyo, Japan]) with TBA 80FR (Toshiba medical system corporation, Tokyo)
Hisayama Study	Serum	Enzymatic techniques (TBA-80S; Toshiba Inc., Tokyo, Japan)	Enzymatic method after precipitation of of VLDL and LDL with dextran sulfate and magnesium (TBA-80S; Toshiba Inc., Tokyo, Japan)	Enzymatic techniques (TBA-80S; Toshiba Inc., Tokyo, Japan)
Mauritius				

Mauritius 1987	Venous plasma	Manual enzymatic colorimetric method (Coulter Minikem Spectrophotometer), (Boeringer Cat no 701912)	Manual enzymatic colorimetric method (Coulter Minikem Spectrophotometer), (Boeringer Cat no 701912) Precipitation method (Biomerieux)	Manual enzymatic colorimetric method(Coulter Minikem Spectrophotometer) (Boeringer Cat nr 400971)
Mauritius 1992	Venous plasma	Automated enzymatic method with Chemistry Profile Analyser Model LS (Coulter- France)	Automated enzymatic method, Chemistry Profile Analyser Model LS (Coulter- France) Precipitation method (Biomerieux)	Automated enzymatic method with Chemistry Profile Analyser Model LS (Coulter-France)
Mauritius 1998	Venous plasma	Automated enzymatic methods; Cobas Mira analyzer (Roche Diagnostics, France)	Automated enzymatic methods; Cobas Mira analyzer (Roche Diagnostics, France) Direct method (Biomerieux)	Automated enzymatic methods; Cobas Mira analyzer (Roche Diagnostics, France)
Poland				
POLMONICA	Serum	Direct Liebermann-Burchard method (Boehringer-Mannheim)	Determined in the supernatant after precipitation with heparin manganese (Boehringer-Mannheim)	Enzymatic method (Boehringer-Mannheim)
Republic of Cyprus				
Nicosia Diabetes Study	Whole Blood	Cobas Micra Plus Roche	Cobas Micra Plus Roche	Cobas Micra Plus Roche
Spain				
The Guía Study	Plasma	Standard enzymatic methods (Boehringer-Mannheim Hitachi 717 autoanalyser, Tokyo, Japan)	Phosphotungstate precipitation (Boehringer-Mannheim Hitachi 717 autoanalyser, Tokyo, Japan)	Standard enzymatic methods (Boehringer-Mannheim Hitachi 717 autoanalyser, Tokyo, Japan)
The Viva Study	Plasma	Enzymatic techniques (Boehringer-Mannheim)	Enzymatic techniques (Boehringer-Mannheim)	Enzymatic techniques (Boehringer-Mannheim)
Sweden				
MONICA	Serum	Enzymatic techniques (Boehringer-Mannheim GmbH, Germany)	Phosphotungstate-Mg^{2+} precipitation method	Enzymatic method (CHOD-PAP, Boehringer-Mannheim GmbH, Germany)
The Uppsala Longitudinal Study of Adult	Serum	Enzymatic techniques using IL Test Cholesterol Trinders's	Separated by precipitation with magnesium chloride/	Enzymatic techniques using IL Test Cholesterol

Men (ULSAM)		Method and IL Test Enzymatic-colorimetric Method for use in a Monarch apparatus (Instrumentation Laboratories, Lexington, USA). (http://www.pubcare.uu.se/ULSAM/invest/70yrs/meth70.htm#09)	phosphotumgstate.	Trinders's Method and IL Test Enzymatic-colorimetric Method for use in a Monarch apparatus (Instrumentation Laboratories, Lexington, USA).
The Netherlands				
The Hoorn Study	Serum	Enzymatic techniques (Boehringer-Mannheim, Mannheim, Germany);	Enzymatic techniques after precipitation of the low and very low-density lipoproteins (Boehringer-Mannheim, Mannheim, Germany)	Enzymatic techniques (Boehringer-Mannheim, Mannheim, Germany);
Zutphen	Serum	Enzymatic techniques (CHOD-PAP mono-test kit,Boehringer-Mannheim)	Enzymatic method after precipitation of apoB-containing particles by means of dextran magnesium sulphate.	Enzymatic techniques (CHOD-PAP mono-test kit,Boehringer-Mannheim)
U.K.				
Isle of ELY Diabetes Project	Plasma	Enzymatic techniques, RA 1000 (Bayer Diagnostics, Basingstoke, Hants, UK)	Enzymatic methods	Standard automated enzymatic method with the RA1000 (Bayer Diagnostics, Suffolk, U.K.),
Newcastle Heart Project	Plasma	Cholesterol oxidase/peroxidase method with Cobas Bio centrifugal analyzer (Roche Products Ltd, Welwyn Garden City, UK)	Measuring the supernatant cholesterol concentration after precipitation of apoB-containing lipoproteins with heparin and manganese. Cobas Bio centrifugal analyzer (Roche Products Ltd, Welwyn Garden City, UK)	Lipase/glycerol kinase method. Cobas Bio centrifugal analyzer (Roche Products Ltd, Welwyn Garden City, UK)
The Goodinge Study	Plasma	Cholesterol esterase method (Boehringer Mannheim, Lewes, Sussex, U.K.)	Enzymatic spectrophotometric method (Roche Diagnostics, Hatfield, Herts, U.K.) after precipitation of LDL by the addition of phosphotungstic acid in the presence of magnesium ions.	Enzymatic spectrophotometric method (Roche Diagnostics, Hatfield, Herts, U.K.).

Measures of lipid components in each study.

7. References

Abdel-Aal, N. M., A. T. Ahmad, E. S. Froelicher, A. M. Batieha, M. M. Hamza, et al. (2008). "Prevalence of dyslipidemia in patients with type 2 diabetes in Jordan." Saudi Med J 29(10): 1423-1428.

Adult Treatment panel III (2002). "Third Report of the National Cholesterol Education Program (NCEP) Expert Panel on Detection, Evaluation, and Treatment of High Blood Cholesterol in Adults (Adult Treatment Panel III) final report." Circulation 106(25): 3143-3421.

Agarwal, A. K., S. Singla, R. Singla, A. Lal, H. Wardhan, et al. (2009). "Prevalence of coronary risk factors in type 2 diabetics without manifestations of overt coronary heart disease." J Assoc Physicians India 57: 135-142.

Ahmed, N., J. Khan and T. S. Siddiqui (2008). "Frequency of dyslipidaemia in type 2 diabetes mellitus in patients of Hazara division." J Ayub Med Coll Abbottabad 20(2): 51-54.

Almdal, T., H. Scharling, J. S. Jensen and H. Vestergaard (2004). "The independent effect of type 2 diabetes mellitus on ischemic heart disease, stroke, and death: a population-based study of 13,000 men and women with 20 years of follow-up." Arch Intern Med 164(13): 1422-1426.

American Diabetes Association (2009). "Standards of medical care in diabetes--2009." Diabetes Care 32 Suppl 1: S13-61.

American Diabetes Association (2010). "Standards of medical care in diabetes--2010." Diabetes Care 33 Suppl 1: S11-61.

Anand, S. S., S. Yusuf, V. Vuksan, S. Devanesen, K. K. Teo, et al. (2000). "Differences in risk factors, atherosclerosis, and cardiovascular disease between ethnic groups in Canada: the Study of Health Assessment and Risk in Ethnic groups (SHARE)." Lancet 356(9226): 279-284.

Arslan, E., T. Yakar and I. Yavasoglu (2008). "The effect of smoking on mean platelet volume and lipid profile in young male subjects." Anadolu Kardiyol Derg 8(6): 422-425.

Azizi, F., M. Rahmani, A. Ghanbarian, H. Emami, P. Salehi, et al. (2003). "Serum lipid levels in an Iranian adults population: Tehran Lipid and Glucose Study." Eur J Epidemiol 18(4): 311-319.

Bangou-Bredent, J., V. Szmidt-Adjide, P. Kangambega-Nouvier, L. Foucan, A. Campier, et al. (1999). "Cardiovascular risk factors associated with diabetes in an Indian community of Guadeloupe. A case control study." Diabetes Metab 25(5): 393-398.

Barrett-Connor, E., S. M. Grundy and M. J. Holdbrook (1982). "Plasma lipids and diabetes mellitus in an adult community." Am J Epidemiol 115(5): 657-663.

Barzi, F., A. Patel, M. Woodward, C. M. Lawes, T. Ohkubo, et al. (2005). "A comparison of lipid variables as predictors of cardiovascular disease in the Asia Pacific region." Ann Epidemiol 15(5): 405-413.

Batic-Mujanovic, O., A. Beganlic, N. Salihefendic, N. Pranjic and Z. Kusljugic (2008). "Influence of smoking on serum lipid and lipoprotein levels among family medicine patients." Med Arh 62(5-6): 264-267.

Berg, A., M. Halle, I. Franz and J. Keul (1997). "Physical activity and lipoprotein metabolism: epidemiological evidence and clinical trials." Eur J Med Res 2(6): 259-264.

Berglund L, R. R. (2004). "Lipoprotein(a): an elusive cardiovascular risk factor." Arterioscler. Thromb. Vasc. Biol 24(12): 2219-2226.

Berrios, X., T. Koponen, T. Huiguang, N. Khaltaev, P. Puska, et al. (1997). "Distribution and prevalence of major risk factors of noncommunicable diseases in selected countries: the WHO Inter-Health Programme." Bull World Health Organ 75(2): 99-108.

Bhalodkar, N. C., S. Blum, T. Rana, R. Kitchappa, A. N. Bhalodkar, et al. (2005). "Comparison of high-density and low-density lipoprotein cholesterol subclasses and sizes in Asian Indian women with Caucasian women from the Framingham Offspring Study." Clin Cardiol 28(5): 247-251.

Boden, W. E. (2000). "High-density lipoprotein cholesterol as an independent risk factor in cardiovascular disease: assessing the data from Framingham to the Veterans Affairs High--Density Lipoprotein Intervention Trial." Am J Cardiol 86(12A): 19L-22L.

Brown, C. D., M. Higgins, K. A. Donato, F. C. Rohde, R. Garrison, et al. (2000). "Body mass index and the prevalence of hypertension and dyslipidemia." Obes Res 8(9): 605-619.

Bruckert, E., M. Baccara-Dinet and E. Eschwege (2007). "Low HDL-cholesterol is common in European Type 2 diabetic patients receiving treatment for dyslipidaemia: data from a pan-European survey." Diabet Med 24(4): 388-391.

Cade, J. and B. Margetts (1989). "Cigarette smoking and serum lipid and lipoprotein concentrations." Bmj 298(6683): 1312.

Chait, A. and J. D. Brunzell (1990). "Acquired hyperlipidemia (secondary dyslipoproteinemias)." Endocrinol Metab Clin North Am 19(2): 259-278.

Chandalia, M., V. Mohan, B. Adams-Huet, R. Deepa and N. Abate (2008). "Ethnic difference in sex gap in high-density lipoprotein cholesterol between Asian Indians and Whites." J Investig Med 56(3): 574-580.

Charlton-Menys, V., D. J. Betteridge, H. Colhoun, J. Fuller, M. France, et al. (2009). "Apolipoproteins, cardiovascular risk and statin response in type 2 diabetes: the Collaborative Atorvastatin Diabetes Study (CARDS)." Diabetologia 52(2): 218-225.

Chen, L. K., M. H. Lin, Z. J. Chen, S. J. Hwang, S. T. Tsai, et al. (2006). "Metabolic characteristics and insulin resistance of impaired fasting glucose among the middle-aged and elderly Taiwanese." Diabetes Res Clin Pract 71(2): 170-176.

Cohen, J. C., Z. Wang, S. M. Grundy, M. R. Stoesz and R. Guerra (1994). "Variation at the hepatic lipase and apolipoprotein AI/CIII/AIV loci is a major cause of genetically determined variation in plasma HDL cholesterol levels." J Clin Invest 94(6): 2377-2384.

Colhoun, H. M., D. J. Betteridge, P. N. Durrington, G. A. Hitman, H. A. Neil, et al. (2004). "Primary prevention of cardiovascular disease with atorvastatin in type 2 diabetes in the Collaborative Atorvastatin Diabetes Study (CARDS): multicentre randomised placebo-controlled trial." Lancet 364(9435): 685-696.

Collins, R., J. Armitage, S. Parish, P. Sleigh and R. Peto (2003). "MRC/BHF Heart Protection Study of cholesterol-lowering with simvastatin in 5963 people with diabetes: a randomised placebo-controlled trial." Lancet 361(9374): 2005-2016.

Cooney, M. T., A. Dudina, D. De Bacquer, L. Wilhelmsen, S. Sans, et al. (2009). "HDL cholesterol protects against cardiovascular disease in both genders, at all ages and at all levels of risk." Atherosclerosis 206(2): 611-616.

Cowie, C. C., B. V. Howard and M. I. Harris (1994). "Serum lipoproteins in African Americans and whites with non-insulin-dependent diabetes in the US population." Circulation 90(3): 1185-1193.

Criqui, M. H., R. B. Wallace, G. Heiss, M. Mishkel, G. Schonfeld, et al. (1980). "Cigarette smoking and plasma high-density lipoprotein cholesterol. The Lipid Research Clinics Program Prevalence Study." Circulation 62(4 Pt 2): IV70-76.

Cui, Y., R. S. Blumenthal, J. A. Flaws, M. K. Whiteman, P. Langenberg, et al. (2001). "Non-high-density lipoprotein cholesterol level as a predictor of cardiovascular disease mortality." Arch Intern Med 161(11): 1413-1419.

Danesh J, C. R., Peto R. (2000). "Lipoprotein(a) and coronary heart disease: meta-analysis of prospective studies." Circulation 102(10): 1082-1085.

De Oliveira, E. S. E. R., D. Foster, M. McGee Harper, C. E. Seidman, J. D. Smith, et al. (2000). "Alcohol consumption raises HDL cholesterol levels by increasing the transport rate of apolipoproteins A-I and A-II." Circulation 102(19): 2347-2352.

Denke, M. A., C. T. Sempos and S. M. Grundy (1993). "Excess body weight. An underrecognized contributor to high blood cholesterol levels in white American men." Arch Intern Med 153(9): 1093-1103.

Denke, M. A., C. T. Sempos and S. M. Grundy (1994). "Excess body weight. An under-recognized contributor to dyslipidemia in white American women." Arch Intern Med 154(4): 401-410.

Devroey, D., N. De Swaef, P. Coigniez, J. Vandevoorde, J. Kartounian, et al. (2004). "Correlations between lipid levels and age, gender, glycemia, obesity, diabetes, and smoking." Endocr Res 30(1): 83-93.

Duffy, D. and D. J. Rader (2009). "Update on strategies to increase HDL quantity and function." Nat Rev Cardiol 6(7): 455-463.

Erem, C., A. Hacihasanoglu, O. Deger, M. Kocak and M. Topbas (2008). "Prevalence of dyslipidemia and associated risk factors among Turkish adults: Trabzon lipid study." Endocrine 34(1-3): 36-51.

Expert Panel on Detection, E., and Treatment of High Blood Cholesterol in Adults (2001). "Executive Summary of The Third Report of The National Cholesterol Education Program (NCEP) Expert Panel on Detection, Evaluation, And Treatment of High Blood Cholesterol In Adults (Adult Treatment Panel III)." Jama 285(19): 2486-2497.

Ezenwaka, C. E., N. Premanand and F. A. Orrett (2000). "Studies on plasma lipids in industrial workers in central Trinidad and Tobago." J Natl Med Assoc 92(8): 375-381.

Fisher, S. D., W. Zareba, A. J. Moss, V. J. Marder, C. E. Sparks, et al. (2000). "Effect of smoking on lipid and thrombogenic factors two months after acute myocardial infarction." Am J Cardiol 86(8): 813-818.

Florez, H., E. Silva, V. Fernandez, E. Ryder, T. Sulbaran, et al. (2005). "Prevalence and risk factors associated with the metabolic syndrome and dyslipidemia in White, Black, Amerindian and Mixed Hispanics in Zulia State, Venezuela." Diabetes Res Clin Pract 69(1): 63-77.

Fogari, R., A. Zoppi, C. Pasotti, L. Poletti, F. Tettamanti, et al. (1988). "Effects of different beta-blockers on lipid metabolism in chronic therapy of hypertension." Int J Clin Pharmacol Ther Toxicol 26(12): 597-604.

Foucan, L., P. Kangambega, D. Koumavi Ekouevi, J. Rozet and J. Bangou-Bredent (2000). "Lipid profile in an adult population in Guadeloupe." Diabetes Metab 26(6): 473-480.

France, M. W., S. Kwok, P. McElduff and C. J. Seneviratne (2003). "Ethnic trends in lipid tests in general practice." QJM 96(12): 919-923.

Fruchart J, S. F., Hermans M, Assmann, G, Brown W, Ceska R, Chapman M, Dodson P, Fioretto P, Ginsberg H (2008). "The residual risk reduction initiative: a call to action to reduce residual vascular risk in dyslipidaemic patients." Diabetes&Vascular Disease Research 5(4): 319-335.

Fuentes, R., T. Uusitalo, P. Puska, J. Tuomilehto and A. Nissinen (2003). "Blood cholesterol level and prevalence of hypercholesterolaemia in developing countries: a review of population-based studies carried out from 1979 to 2002." Eur J Cardiovasc Prev Rehabil 10(6): 411-419.

Gatti, A., M. Maranghi, S. Bacci, C. Carallo, A. Gnasso, et al. (2009). "Poor glycemic control is an independent risk factor for low HDL cholesterol in patients with type 2 diabetes." Diabetes Care 32(8): 1550-1552.

Geethanjali FS, L. K., Lingenhel A. (2003). "Analysis of the apo(a) size polymorphism in Asian Indian populations: association with Lp(a) concentration and coronary heart disease." Atherosclerosis 169(1): 121-130.

Goldberg, I. J. (2001). "Clinical review 124: Diabetic dyslipidemia: causes and consequences." J Clin Endocrinol Metab 86(3): 965-971.

Goldberg, R. B., M. J. Mellies, F. M. Sacks, L. A. Moye, B. V. Howard, et al. (1998). "Cardiovascular events and their reduction with pravastatin in diabetic and glucose-intolerant myocardial infarction survivors with average cholesterol levels: subgroup analyses in the cholesterol and recurrent events (CARE) trial. The Care Investigators." Circulation 98(23): 2513-2519.

Gomes, M. B., D. Giannella-Neto, M. Faria, M. Tambascia, R. M. Fonseca, et al. (2009). "Estimating cardiovascular risk in patients with type 2 diabetes: a national multicenter study in Brazil." Diabetol Metab Syndr 1(1): 22.

Graham, I., D. Atar, K. Borch-Johnsen, G. Boysen, G. Burell, et al. (2007). "European guidelines on cardiovascular disease prevention in clinical practice: executive summary. Fourth Joint Task Force of the European Society of Cardiology and other societies on cardiovascular disease prevention in clinical practice (constituted by representatives of nine societies and by invited experts)." Eur J Cardiovasc Prev Rehabil 14 Suppl 2: E1-40.

Grant, R. W. and J. B. Meigs (2007). "Prevalence and treatment of low HDL cholesterol among primary care patients with type 2 diabetes: an unmet challenge for cardiovascular risk reduction." Diabetes Care 30(3): 479-484.

Gupta M, S. N., Verma S. (2006). "South Asians and cardiovascular risk: what clinicians should know." Circulation 113(25): E924-E929.

Hadaegh, F., M. R. Bozorgmanesh, A. Ghasemi, H. Harati, N. Saadat, et al. (2008). "High prevalence of undiagnosed diabetes and abnormal glucose tolerance in the Iranian urban population: Tehran Lipid and Glucose Study." BMC Public Health 8: 176.

Hanh, T. T. M., T. Komatsu, N. T. Hung, V. N. Chuyen, Y. Yoshimura, et al. (2001). "Nutritional status of middle-aged Vietnamese in Ho Chi Minh City." J Am Coll Nutr 20(6): 616-622.

Hardman, A. E. (1999). "Physical activity, obesity and blood lipids." Int J Obes Relat Metab Disord 23 Suppl 3: S64-71.

Harris, M. I. and R. C. Eastman (2000). "Early detection of undiagnosed diabetes mellitus: a US perspective." Diabetes Metab Res Rev 16(4): 230-236.

Hennig, B., M. Toborek and C. J. McClain (2001). "High-energy diets, fatty acids and endothelial cell function: implications for atherosclerosis." J Am Coll Nutr 20(2 Suppl): 97-105.

Hertz, R. P., A. N. Unger and C. M. Ferrario (2006). "Diabetes, hypertension, and dyslipidemia in Mexican Americans and non-Hispanic whites." Am J Prev Med 30(2): 103-110.

Ismail, I. S., W. Nazaimoon, W. Mohamad, R. Letchuman, M. Singaraveloo, et al. (2001). "Ethnicity and glycaemic control are major determinants of diabetic dyslipidaemia in Malaysia." Diabet Med 18(6): 501-508.

Jacobs, M. J., T. Kleisli, J. R. Pio, S. Malik, G. J. L'Italien, et al. (2005). "Prevalence and control of dyslipidemia among persons with diabetes in the United States." Diabetes Res Clin Pract 70(3): 263-269.

Jurado, J., J. Ybarra, P. Solanas, J. Caula, I. Gich, et al. (2009). "Prevalence of cardiovascular disease and risk factors in a type 2 diabetic population of the North Catalonia diabetes study." J Am Acad Nurse Pract 21(3): 140-148.

Juutilainen, A., S. Lehto, T. Ronnemaa, K. Pyorala and M. Laakso (2005). "Type 2 diabetes as a "coronary heart disease equivalent": an 18-year prospective population-based study in Finnish subjects." Diabetes Care 28(12): 2901-2907.

Kannel, W. B. (1985). "Lipids, diabetes, and coronary heart disease: insights from the Framingham Study." Am Heart J 110(5): 1100-1107.

Karthikeyan, G., K. K. Teo, S. Islam, M. J. McQueen, P. Pais, et al. (2009). "Lipid profile, plasma apolipoproteins, and risk of a first myocardial infarction among Asians: an analysis from the INTERHEART Study." J Am Coll Cardiol 53(3): 244-253.

Kelishadi, R., G. Ardalan, R. Gheiratmand and A. Ramezani (2006). "Is family history of premature cardiovascular diseases appropriate for detection of dyslipidemic children in population-based preventive medicine programs? CASPIAN study." Pediatr Cardiol 27(6): 729-736.

Kendall, D. M. (2005). "The dyslipidemia of diabetes mellitus: giving triglycerides and high-density lipoprotein cholesterol a higher priority?" Endocrinol Metab Clin North Am 34(1): 27-48.

Knopp, R. H., M. d'Emden, J. G. Smilde and S. J. Pocock (2006). "Efficacy and safety of atorvastatin in the prevention of cardiovascular end points in subjects with type 2 diabetes: the Atorvastatin Study for Prevention of Coronary Heart Disease Endpoints in non-insulin-dependent diabetes mellitus (ASPEN)." Diabetes Care 29(7): 1478-1485.

Krauss, R. M. (2004). "Lipids and lipoproteins in patients with type 2 diabetes." Diabetes Care 27(6): 1496-1504.

Ku CY, G. B., Nagy TR, Goran MI. (1998). "Relationships between dietary fat, body fat, and serum lipid profile in prepubertal children." Obes Res(6): 400-407.

Kuller, L. H. (2004). "Ethnic differences in atherosclerosis, cardiovascular disease and lipid metabolism." Curr Opin Lipidol 15(2): 109-113.

Lehtonen, A. (1985). "Effect of beta blockers on blood lipid profile." Am Heart J 109(5 Pt 2): 1192-1196.

Li, Z., R. Yang, G. Xu and T. Xia (2005). "Serum lipid concentrations and prevalence of dyslipidemia in a large professional population in Beijing." Clin Chem 51(1): 144-150.

Liu, J., C. Sempos, R. P. Donahue, J. Dorn, M. Trevisan, et al. (2005). "Joint distribution of non-HDL and LDL cholesterol and coronary heart disease risk prediction among individuals with and without diabetes." Diabetes Care 28(8): 1916-1921.

Maeda, K., Y. Noguchi and T. Fukui (2003). "The effects of cessation from cigarette smoking on the lipid and lipoprotein profiles: a meta-analysis." Prev Med 37(4): 283-290.

Mammas, I. N., G. K. Bertsias, M. Linardakis, N. E. Tzanakis, D. N. Labadarios, et al. (2003). "Cigarette smoking, alcohol consumption, and serum lipid profile among medical students in Greece." Eur J Public Health 13(3): 278-282.

Mann, J. I., B. Lewis, J. Shepherd, A. F. Winder, S. Fenster, et al. (1988). "Blood lipid concentrations and other cardiovascular risk factors: distribution, prevalence, and detection in Britain." Br Med J (Clin Res Ed) 296(6638): 1702-1706.

McKeigue, P. M., B. Shah and M. G. Marmot (1991). "Relation of central obesity and insulin resistance with high diabetes prevalence and cardiovascular risk in South Asians." Lancet 337(8738): 382-386.

McNamara, D. J. and W. H. Howell (1992). "Epidemiologic data linking diet to hyperlipidemia and arteriosclerosis." Semin Liver Dis 12(4): 347-355.

McNaughton, S. A., G. D. Mishra and E. J. Brunner (2009). "Food patterns associated with blood lipids are predictive of coronary heart disease: the Whitehall II study." Br J Nutr 102(4): 619-624.

Meigs, J. B., D. M. Nathan, R. B. D'Agostino, Sr. and P. W. Wilson (2002). "Fasting and postchallenge glycemia and cardiovascular disease risk: the Framingham Offspring Study." Diabetes Care 25(10): 1845-1850.

Middeke, M., W. O. Richter, P. Schwandt, B. Beck and H. Holzgreve (1990). "Normalization of lipid metabolism after withdrawal from antihypertensive long-term therapy with beta blockers and diuretics." Arteriosclerosis 10(1): 145-147.

Millen, B. E., P. A. Quatromoni, B. H. Nam, C. E. O'Horo, J. F. Polak, et al. (2002). "Dietary patterns and the odds of carotid atherosclerosis in women: the Framingham Nutrition Studies." Prev Med 35(6): 540-547.

Mills, E. J., B. Rachlis, P. Wu, P. J. Devereaux, P. Arora, et al. (2008). "Primary prevention of cardiovascular mortality and events with statin treatments: a network meta-analysis involving more than 65,000 patients." J Am Coll Cardiol 52(22): 1769-1781.

Mohan, V., R. Deepa, S. P. Haranath, G. Premalatha, M. Rema, et al. (1998). "Lipoprotein(a) is an independent risk factor for coronary artery disease in NIDDM patients in South India." Diabetes Care 21(11): 1819-1823.

Morrish, N. J., L. K. Stevens, J. H. Fuller, R. J. Jarrett and H. Keen (1991). "Risk factors for macrovascular disease in diabetes mellitus: the London follow-up to the WHO Multinational Study of Vascular Disease in Diabetics." Diabetologia 34(8): 590-594.

Morrish, N. J., L. K. Stevens, J. H. Fuller, H. Keen and R. J. Jarrett (1991). "Incidence of macrovascular disease in diabetes mellitus: the London cohort of the WHO Multinational Study of Vascular Disease in Diabetics." Diabetologia 34(8): 584-589.

Morrish, N. J., L. K. Stevens, J. Head, J. H. Fuller, R. J. Jarrett, et al. (1990). "A prospective study of mortality among middle-aged diabetic patients (the London Cohort of the WHO Multinational Study of Vascular Disease in Diabetics) II: Associated risk factors." Diabetologia 33(9): 542-548.

Mulukutla, S. R., L. Venkitachalam, O. C. Marroquin, K. C. Kip, A. Aiyer, et al. (2008). "Population variation in atherogenic dyslipidemia: A report from the HeartSCORE and IndiaSCORE Studies." Journal of Clinical Lipidology 2(6): 410-417.

Murakami, K., S. Ishibashi, Y. Yoshida, N. Yamada and Y. Akanuma (1998). "Lipoprotein(a) as a coronary risk factor in Japanese patients with Type II (non-insulin-dependent) diabetes mellitus. Relation with apolipoprotein(a) phenotypes." Diabetologia 41(11): 1397-1398.

Novoa, F. J., M. Boronat, P. Saavedra, J. M. Diaz-Cremades, V. F. Varillas, et al. (2005). "Differences in cardiovascular risk factors, insulin resistance, and insulin secretion in individuals with normal glucose tolerance and in subjects with impaired glucose regulation: the Telde Study." Diabetes Care 28(10): 2388-2393.

Okafor, C. I., O. A. Fasanmade and D. A. Oke (2008). "Pattern of dyslipidaemia among Nigerians with type 2 diabetes mellitus." Niger J Clin Pract 11(1): 25-31.

Onat, A., G. Surdum-Avci, M. Senocak, E. Ornek and Y. Gozukara (1992). "Plasma lipids and their interrelationship in Turkish adults." J Epidemiol Community Health 46(5): 470-476.

Palaniappan, L. P., A. C. Kwan, F. Abbasi, C. Lamendola, T. L. McLaughlin, et al. (2007). "Lipoprotein abnormalities are associated with insulin resistance in South Asian Indian women." Metabolism 56(7): 899-904.

Pang, R. W., S. Tam, E. D. Janus, S. T. Siu, O. C. Ma, et al. (2006). "Plasma lipid, lipoprotein and apolipoprotein levels in a random population sample of 2875 Hong Kong Chinese adults and their implications (NCEP ATP-III, 2001 guidelines) on cardiovascular risk assessment." Atherosclerosis 184(2): 438-445.

Pankow, J. S., D. K. Kwan, B. B. Duncan, M. I. Schmidt, D. J. Couper, et al. (2007). "Cardiometabolic risk in impaired fasting glucose and impaired glucose tolerance: the Atherosclerosis Risk in Communities Study." Diabetes Care 30(2): 325-331.

Papazafiropoulou, A., A. Sotiropoulos, E. Skliros, M. Kardara, A. Kokolaki, et al. (2009). "Familial history of diabetes and clinical characteristics in Greek subjects with type 2 diabetes." BMC Endocr Disord 9: 12.

Patel, A., F. Barzi, K. Jamrozik, T. H. Lam, H. Ueshima, et al. (2004). "Serum triglycerides as a risk factor for cardiovascular diseases in the Asia-Pacific region." Circulation 110(17): 2678-2686.

Pischon, T., C. J. Girman, F. M. Sacks, N. Rifai, M. J. Stampfer, et al. (2005). "Non-high-density lipoprotein cholesterol and apolipoprotein B in the prediction of coronary heart disease in men." Circulation 112(22): 3375-3383.

Pongchaiyakul, C., P. Hongsprabhas and V. Pisprasert (2006). "Rural-urban difference in lipid levels and prevalence of dyslipidemia: a population-based study in Khon Kaen province, Thailand." J Med Assoc Thai 89(11): 1835-1844.

Post GB, K. H., Twisk J, van Mechelen W. (1997). "The association between dietary patterns and cardiovascular disease risk indicators in healthy youngsters: results covering fifteen years of longitudinal development." Eur J Clin Nutr 51: 387-393.

Psaty, B. M., M. Anderson, R. A. Kronmal, R. P. Tracy, T. Orchard, et al. (2004). "The association between lipid levels and the risks of incident myocardial infarction, stroke, and total mortality: The Cardiovascular Health Study." J Am Geriatr Soc 52(10): 1639-1647.

Pyorala, K., C. M. Ballantyne, B. Gumbiner, M. W. Lee, A. Shah, et al. (2004). "Reduction of cardiovascular events by simvastatin in nondiabetic coronary heart disease patients with and without the metabolic syndrome: subgroup analyses of the Scandinavian Simvastatin Survival Study (4S)." Diabetes Care 27(7): 1735-1740.

Ramachandran, A., S. Mary, A. Yamuna, N. Murugesan and C. Snehalatha (2008). "High prevalence of diabetes and cardiovascular risk factors associated with urbanization in India." Diabetes Care 31(5): 893-898.

Razak, F., S. Anand, V. Vuksan, B. Davis, R. Jacobs, et al. (2005). "Ethnic differences in the relationships between obesity and glucose-metabolic abnormalities: a cross-sectional population-based study." Int J Obes (Lond) 29(6): 656-667.

Reckless, J. P., D. J. Betteridge, P. Wu, B. Payne and D. J. Galton (1978). "High-density and low-density lipoproteins and prevalence of vascular disease in diabetes mellitus." Br Med J 1(6117): 883-886.

Ridker, P. M., N. Rifai, N. R. Cook, G. Bradwin and J. E. Buring (2005). "Non-HDL cholesterol, apolipoproteins A-I and B100, standard lipid measures, lipid ratios, and CRP as risk factors for cardiovascular disease in women." Jama 294(3): 326-333.

Roberto Robles, N., S. Barroso, G. Marcos and J. F. Sanchez Munoz-Torrero (2009). "[Lipid control in diabetic patients in Extremadura (Spain)]." Endocrinol Nutr 56(3): 112-117.

Roberts, W. C. (1989). "Recent studies on the effects of beta blockers on blood lipid levels." Am Heart J 117(3): 709-714.

Ronnemaa, T., M. Laakso, V. Kallio, K. Pyorala, J. Marniemi, et al. (1989). "Serum lipids, lipoproteins, and apolipoproteins and the excessive occurrence of coronary heart disease in non-insulin-dependent diabetic patients." Am J Epidemiol 130(4): 632-645.

Roselli della Rovere, G., A. Lapolla, G. Sartore, C. Rossetti, S. Zambon, et al. (2003). "Plasma lipoproteins, apoproteins and cardiovascular disease in type 2 diabetic patients. A nine-year follow-up study." Nutr Metab Cardiovasc Dis 13(1): 46-51.

Rosengren, A., L. Welin, A. Tsipogianni and L. Wilhelmsen (1989). "Impact of cardiovascular risk factors on coronary heart disease and mortality among middle aged diabetic men: a general population study." Bmj 299(6708): 1127-1131.

Ruixing, Y., W. Jinzhen, H. Yaoheng, T. Jing, W. Hai, et al. (2008). "Associations of diet and lifestyle with hyperlipidemia for middle-aged and elderly persons among the Guangxi Bai Ku Yao and Han populations." J Am Diet Assoc 108(6): 970-976.

Santen, R. J., P. W. Willis, 3rd and S. S. Fajans (1972). "Atherosclerosis in diabetes mellitus. Correlations with serum lipid levels, adiposity, and serum insulin level." Arch Intern Med 130(6): 833-843.

Sarwar, N., J. Danesh, G. Eiriksdottir, G. Sigurdsson, N. Wareham, et al. (2007). "Triglycerides and the risk of coronary heart disease: 10,158 incident cases among 262,525 participants in 29 Western prospective studies." Circulation 115(4): 450-458.

Schulze, M. B., I. Shai, J. E. Manson, T. Li, N. Rifai, et al. (2004). "Joint role of non-HDL cholesterol and glycated haemoglobin in predicting future coronary heart disease events among women with type 2 diabetes." Diabetologia 47(12): 2129-2136.

Schwandt, P., R. Kelishadi and G. M. Haas (2010). "Ethnic disparities of the metabolic syndrome in population-based samples of german and Iranian adolescents." Metab Syndr Relat Disord 8(2): 189-192.

Schwandt, P., R. Kelishadi, R. Q. Ribeiro, G. M. Haas and P. Poursafa (2010). "A three-country study on the components of the metabolic syndrome in youths: the BIG Study." Int J Pediatr Obes 5(4): 334-341.

Sever, P. S., N. R. Poulter, B. Dahlof, H. Wedel, R. Collins, et al. (2005). "Reduction in cardiovascular events with atorvastatin in 2,532 patients with type 2 diabetes: Anglo-Scandinavian Cardiac Outcomes Trial--lipid-lowering arm (ASCOT-LLA)." Diabetes Care 28(5): 1151-1157.

Seviour, P. W., T. K. Teal, W. Richmond and R. S. Elkeles (1988). "Serum lipids, lipoproteins and macrovascular disease in non-insulin-dependent diabetics: a possible new approach to prevention." Diabet Med 5(2): 166-171.

Seyum, B., G. Mebrahtu, A. Usman, J. Mufunda, B. Tewolde, et al. (2010). "Profile of patients with diabetes in Eritrea: results of first phase registry analyses." Acta Diabetol 47(1): 23-27.

Shai, I., E. B. Rimm, M. B. Schulze, N. Rifai, M. J. Stampfer, et al. (2004). "Moderate alcohol intake and markers of inflammation and endothelial dysfunction among diabetic men." Diabetologia 47(10): 1760-1767.

Sharma, M. D. and V. N. Pavlik (2001). "Dyslipidaemia in African Americans, Hispanics and whites with type 2 diabetes mellitus and hypertension." Diabetes Obes Metab 3(1): 41-45.

Shepherd, J., P. Barter, R. Carmena, P. Deedwania, J. C. Fruchart, et al. (2006). "Effect of lowering LDL cholesterol substantially below currently recommended levels in patients with coronary heart disease and diabetes: the Treating to New Targets (TNT) study." Diabetes Care 29(6): 1220-1226.

Singh, I. M., M. H. Shishehbor and B. J. Ansell (2007). "High-density lipoprotein as a therapeutic target: a systematic review." Jama 298(7): 786-798.

Sisson, S. B., S. M. Camhi, T. S. Church, C. K. Martin, C. Tudor-Locke, et al. (2009). "Leisure time sedentary behavior, occupational/domestic physical activity, and metabolic syndrome in U.S. men and women." Metab Syndr Relat Disord 7(6): 529-536.

Smaoui, M., S. Hammami, R. Chaaba, N. Attia, K. B. Hamda, et al. (2004). "Lipids and lipoprotein(a) concentrations in Tunisian type 2 diabetic patients; Relationship to glycemic control and coronary heart disease." J Diabetes Complications 18(5): 258-263.

Snehalatha, C. and A. Ramachandran (2009). "Cardiovascular risk factors in the normoglycaemic Asian-Indian population--influence of urbanisation." Diabetologia 52(4): 596-599.

Sorrentino, S. A., C. Besler, L. Rohrer, M. Meyer, K. Heinrich, et al. (2010). "Endothelial-vasoprotective effects of high-density lipoprotein are impaired in patients with type 2 diabetes mellitus but are improved after extended-release niacin therapy." Circulation 121(1): 110-122.

Stamler, J., O. Vaccaro, J. D. Neaton and D. Wentworth (1993). "Diabetes, other risk factors, and 12-yr cardiovascular mortality for men screened in the Multiple Risk Factor Intervention Trial." Diabetes Care 16(2): 434-444.

Steinhagen-Thiessen, E., P. Bramlage, C. Losch, H. Hauner, H. Schunkert, et al. (2008). "Dyslipidemia in primary care--prevalence, recognition, treatment and control: data from the German Metabolic and Cardiovascular Risk Project (GEMCAS)." Cardiovasc Diabetol 7: 31.

Steven H, M. M., Helen H, Marc R, J.AVA K. (1986). "The role of behavioral variables and fat patterning in explaining ethnic differences in serum lipids and lipoproteins." Am. J. Epidemiol 123(5): 830-839.

Stone, N. J. (1994). "Secondary causes of hyperlipidemia." Med Clin North Am 78(1): 117-141.

Sumner AE, V. G., Genovese DJ, Finley KB, Bergman RN, Boston RC. (2005). "Normal triglyceride levels despite insulin resistance in African Americans: role of lipoprotein lipase." Metabolism 54(7): 902-909.

Sundquist J, W. M. (1999). "Cardiovascular risk factors in mexican american adults: a transcultural analysis of NHANES III, 1988-1994." Am. J. Public Health 89(5): 723-730.

Surana, S. P., D. B. Shah, K. Gala, S. Susheja, S. S. Hoskote, et al. (2008). "Prevalence of metabolic syndrome in an urban Indian diabetic population using the NCEP ATP III guidelines." J Assoc Physicians India 56: 865-868.

Tan, C. E., S. C. Emmanuel, B. Y. Tan and E. Jacob (1999). "Prevalence of diabetes and ethnic differences in cardiovascular risk factors. The 1992 Singapore National Health Survey." Diabetes Care 22(2): 241-247.

Tan, C. E., E. S. Tai, C. S. Tan, K. S. Chia, J. Lee, et al. (2003). "APOE polymorphism and lipid profile in three ethnic groups in the Singapore population." Atherosclerosis 170(2): 253-260.

Tanasescu, M., E. Cho, J. E. Manson and F. B. Hu (2004). "Dietary fat and cholesterol and the risk of cardiovascular disease among women with type 2 diabetes." Am J Clin Nutr 79(6): 999-1005.

Taylor, A. J., T. C. Villines, E. J. Stanek, P. J. Devine, L. Griffen, et al. (2009). "Extended-release niacin or ezetimibe and carotid intima-media thickness." N Engl J Med 361(22): 2113-2122.

Tekes-Manova, D., E. Israeli, T. Shochat, M. Swartzon, S. Gordon, et al. (2006). "The prevalence of reversible cardiovascular risk factors in Israelis aged 25-55 years." Isr Med Assoc J 8(8): 527-531.

Temelkova-Kurktschiev, T. S., D. P. Kurktschiev, L. G. Vladimirova-Kitova, I. Vaklinova and B. R. Todorova (2009). "Prevalence and type of dyslipidaemia in a population at risk for cardiovascular death in Bulgaria." Folia Med (Plovdiv) 51(2): 26-32.

Thavendiranathan, P., A. Bagai, M. A. Brookhart and N. K. Choudhry (2006). "Primary prevention of cardiovascular diseases with statin therapy: a meta-analysis of randomized controlled trials." Arch Intern Med 166(21): 2307-2313.

The DECODA Study Group (2007). "Prevalence of the metabolic syndrome in populations of Asian origin. Comparison of the IDF definition with the NCEP definition." Diabetes Res Clin Pract 76(1): 57-67.

The Emerging Risk Factors C (2009). "Lipoprotein(a) concentration and the risk of coronary heart disease, stroke, and nonvascular mortality." Jama 302(4): 412-423.

Tolonen, H., U. Keil, M. Ferrario and A. Evans (2005). "Prevalence, awareness and treatment of hypercholesterolaemia in 32 populations: results from the WHO MONICA Project." Int J Epidemiol 34(1): 181-192.

Tsimikas S, C. P., Brilakis ES. (2009). "Relationship of oxidized phospholipids on apolipoprotein B-100 particles to race/ethnicity, apolipoprotein(a) isoform size, and cardiovascular risk factors: results from the Dallas Heart Study." Circulation 119(13): 1711-1719.

Turner, R. C., H. Millns, H. A. Neil, I. M. Stratton, S. E. Manley, et al. (1998). "Risk factors for coronary artery disease in non-insulin dependent diabetes mellitus: United Kingdom Prospective Diabetes Study (UKPDS: 23)." Bmj 316(7134): 823-828.

U.K. Prospective Diabetes Study Investigators (1997). "U.K. Prospective Diabetes Study 27. Plasma lipids and lipoproteins at diagnosis of NIDDM by age and sex." Diabetes Care 20(11): 1683-1687.

Umeda, T., S. Kono, Y. Sakurai, K. Shinchi, K. Imanishi, et al. (1998). "Relationship of cigarette smoking, alcohol use, recreational exercise and obesity with serum lipid atherogenicity: a study of self-defense officials in Japan." J Epidemiol 8(4): 227-234.

Vega GL, C. L., Tang A, Marcovina S, Grundy SM, Cohen JC. (1998). "Hepatic lipase activity is lower in African-American men than in white American men: effects of 5' flanking polymorphism in the hepatic lipase gene (LIPC)." J Lipid Res 39(1): 228-232.

Venkatesan, A., A. Hemalatha, Z. Bobby, N. Selvaraj and V. Sathiyapriya (2006). "Effect of smoking on lipid profile and lipid peroxidation in normal subjects." Indian J Physiol Pharmacol 50(3): 273-278.

Villines, T. C., E. J. Stanek, P. J. Devine, M. Turco, M. Miller, et al. (2010). "The ARBITER 6-HALTS Trial (Arterial Biology for the Investigation of the Treatment Effects of Reducing Cholesterol 6-HDL and LDL Treatment Strategies in Atherosclerosis) Final Results and the Impact of Medication Adherence, Dose, and Treatment Duration." J Am Coll Cardiol: doi:10.1016/j.jacc.2010.1003.1017.

Vlajinac, H., M. Ilic and J. Marinkovic (1992). "Cardiovascular risk factors and prevalence of coronary heart disease in type 2 (non-insulin-dependent) diabetes." Eur J Epidemiol 8(6): 783-788.

Wang, J., S. Ruotsalainen, L. Moilanen, P. Lepisto, M. Laakso, et al. (2007). "The metabolic syndrome predicts cardiovascular mortality: a 13-year follow-up study in elderly non-diabetic Finns." Eur Heart J 28(7): 857-864.

Wang W, H. D., Lee ET. (2002). "Lipoprotein(a) in American Indians is low and not independently associated with cardiovascular disease: the Strong Heart Study." Ann. Epidemiol. 12(2): 107-114.

Werk, E. E., Jr., J. J. Gonzalez and J. E. Ranney (1993). "Lipid level differences and hypertension effect in blacks and whites with type II diabetes." Ethn Dis 3(3): 242-249.

Wilson, P. W., R. D. Abbott and W. P. Castelli (1988). "High density lipoprotein cholesterol and mortality. The Framingham Heart Study." Arteriosclerosis 8(6): 737-741.

Wood, P. D., M. P. Stern, A. Silvers, G. M. Reaven and J. von der Groeben (1972). "Prevalence of plasma lipoprotein abnormalities in a free-living population of the Central Valley, California." Circulation 45(1): 114-126.

World Health Organization (2007). "Prevention of cardiovascular disease: guideline for assessment and management of cardiovascular risk." WHO Press.

Wu, D. M., L. Pai, P. K. Sun, L. L. Hsu and C. A. Sun (2001). "Joint effects of alcohol consumption and cigarette smoking on atherogenic lipid and lipoprotein profiles: results from a study of Chinese male population in Taiwan." Eur J Epidemiol 17(7): 629-635.

Zaman, M. M., N. Yoshiike, M. A. Rouf, M. H. Syeed, M. R. Khan, et al. (2001). "Cardiovascular risk factors: distribution and prevalence in a rural population of Bangladesh." J Cardiovasc Risk 8(2): 103-108.

Zaninotto, P., J. Mindell and V. Hirani (2007). "Prevalence of cardiovascular risk factors among ethnic groups: results from the Health Surveys for England." Atherosclerosis 195(1): e48-57.

Zhang, X., Z. Sun, D. Zhang, L. Zheng, J. Li, et al. (2009). "Prevalence and association with diabetes and obesity of lipid phenotypes among the hypertensive Chinese rural adults." Heart Lung 38(1): 17-24.

Zhao, W. H., J. Zhang, Y. Zhai, Y. You, Q. Q. Man, et al. (2007). "Blood lipid profile and prevalence of dyslipidemia in Chinese adults." Biomed Environ Sci 20(4): 329-335.

3

Nutrigenetics and Dyslipidemia

Maryam Shalileh
Islamic Azad University of Hamedan Branch
Iran

1. Introduction

Dyslipidemia is an abnormal amount of lipids (abnormality in any of the lipoprotein fractions), especially elevated Low Density Lipoprotein (LDLs) and decreased High Density Lipoprotein (HDLs) in the blood (Shalileh et al., 2009). In developed countries, most dyslipidemias are hyperlipidemias; that is, an elevation of lipids in the blood, are often due to diet and lifestyle (Wikipedia., 2011; Shalileh et al., 2009). According to the Katharina studie's, elevated cholesterol levels and dyslipoproteinemia are metabolic abnormalities that are becoming increasingly significant in industrialized countries, but also worldwide (Shalileh et al., 2009).

There is a proportional increase in the risk of Coronary Heart Disease (CHD) with rising serum cholesterol levels (Shalileh et al., 2009). Dyslipidaemia is an important risk factor for Cardiovascular Disease (CVD) (Masson & McNeili., 2005).

CVD is a common killer in both the Western and the developing world and is the leading cause of death globally (Lovegrove & Gitau., 2008).

More people die annually from CVDs than from any other cause. An estimated 17. 1 million people died from CVDs in 2004, representing 29%of all global deaths. Of these deaths, an estimated 7. 2 million were due to CHD and 5. 7 million were due to stroke. By 2030, almost 23. 6 million people will die from CVDs, mainly from heart disease and stroke (WHO. 2011).

Atherosclerosis is the most common cause of CHD and related mortality (Debra., 2008; Shalileh et al., 2009) .Endothelial dysfunction initiates atherosclerosis (Shalileh et al., 2009) . The first observable event in the process of atherosclerosis is the accumulation of plaque (cholesterol from low-density lipoproteins, calcium, and fibrin) in the endothelium in large and medium arteries (Debra., 2008).

One of the factors that causes endothelial dysfunction is dyslipidemia (Shalileh et al., 2009).

2. Treatment

CVD represents the paradigm of multi factorial disorders encompassing multiple genetic and non modifiable risk factors, for example older age and modifiable risk factors such as elevated total and LDL-cholesteroland and triglycerides concentrations, reduced HDL-cholesterol concentrations (Ordovas & Corella., 2004; Ordovas., 2009; Perez-Martinez et al, 2011; Lovegrove & Gitau, 2008). The interactions of those modulate plasma lipid concentrations and potentially CVD risk (Ordovas., 2009; Lovegrove & Gitau., 2008).

The link between serum cholesterol and the development of atherosclerosis was established a few decades ago and is now widely accepted. The National Cholesterol Education Program (NCEP) Adult Treatment Panel (ATP) publishes updated guidelines for treating lipid disorders. The latest version is the ATP III (Ordovas & Corella., 2004; Debra., 2008).
The current recommendations aim to reduce the classical modifiable risk factors, and much emphasis has been placed on controlling high-plasma cholesterol levels (Ordovas & Corella., 004).
Physicians are encouraged to refer patients to Registered Dietitians (RDs) to help patients meet goals for therapy (NCEP) based on LDL cholesterol levels. So the ATP III recommended the therapeutic lifestyle change (TLC) dietary pattern as the cornerstone for primary and secondary prevention of CHD. These guidelines consider dietary modification of treatment with emphasis on reducing the high saturated fat atherogenic diet and increased content of polyunsaturated fatty acid (PUFA) as well as controlling other behavioral factors. These therapies are used primarily to lower elevated blood levels of LDL-C, raise HDL -C and lower triglycerides (TGs) (Rubin & Berglund., 2002; Debra., 2008; Ordovas & Orella., 2004).

3. Response to the diet therapy

Although dietary recommendations have been implemented to improve health and diminish the risk of CVD, type 2 diabetes and obesity, these recommendations have been established based on populations and not the individual. On the other hand the approach has been surprisingly unsuccessful in reducing CVD risk and the drastically different inter individual responses to a diet (Ordovas & Corella., 2004).
So this clearly highlights the limitations of population-based nutritional recommendations and suggests that our understanding of the mechanisms responsible for inter-individual differences are far from being understood (Much et al., 2005).
Recent clinical evidence suggests dramatic inter-individual differences and existence of consistent hypo- and hyperresponders in response of plasma lipids to dietary manipulations, ranging from reduced LDL-C levels and TGs in some, to decreased HDL-C levels to elevated TGs. So in some, a low-fat diet has caused a shift to a lipid pattern that is more atherogenic than the original one. This supports the hypothesis that responsiveness is related to genetic variation and existence of nutrient–gene interactions or persons genotype (defined by the term 'nutrigenetics') (DeBusk, 2008; Perez-Martinez et al., 2011; Masson et al., 2003; Rideout., 2011; Ordovas et al., 2007).
A classic example of this is the large variation in the concentration of serum low-density lipoprotein-cholesterol (LDL-C) in response to fish oil supplementation. The cardio protective effects of the fatty acids in fish oil, Eicosapentaenoic Acid (EPA) and Docosahexaenoic Acid (DHA) are well recognized. However, a potentially deleterious increase in LDL-C (5–10%) has been consistently reported after moderate to high doses of fish oil (>2 g day−1 EPA + DHA) (Lovegrove & Gitau., 2008).
Despite this small, but significant increase in LDL-C, closer examination of the responses revealed a noticeable inter-individual variation. There was a mean increase in LDL-C of 4. 1%, yet the spread of individual responses was substantial, with 33 of the 74 subjects demonstrating a lower serum LDL-C and the remaining 41 demonstrating a higher LDL-C (range −40 to +113%) following fish oil intervention. This heterogeneous response to a change in dietary fat, may be attributed to a number of factors; including age, gender,

baseline LDL-C levels, disease status and drug use. However, recent evidence strongly suggests that variations in a number of key genes may also be important (Lovegrove & Gitau., 2008). For example, individuals with specific of genetic variants in a gene may experience different type of lipoprotein changes when placed on a particular diet, whereas individuals with other variants in the gene may be resistant to the effects of the same diet. Although data is sparse in regard to whether such interactions exist, some limited work suggests that interactions may play an important role in determining lipoprotein profiles and may thus be informative for CVD risk prediction. For example, knowledge of a patient's genetic information may allow medical providers and nutritional counselors to predict what lipoprotein changes are likely to occur if the patient starts a particular dietary intervention and, thus, better advise the patient regarding lifestyle changes (Musunuru., 2010; Ordovas & Corella., 2004).

Lipoproteins are macromolecular complexes of lipids and proteins that originate mainly in the liver and intestine and are involved in transporting and redistributing lipids in the body. Lipid homeostasis is achieved by the coordinated action of numerous nuclear factors, enzymes, apolipoproteins, binding proteins, and receptors. Lipid metabolism is also linked with energy metabolism and is subject to many hormonal controls essential for adjusting to environmental and internal conditions. Genetic variability exists in humans for most of these components, and some of these mutations result in abnormal lipid metabolism and plasma lipoprotein profiles that may contribute to the pathogenesis of atherosclerosis. Many of these genes have been explored in terms of gene-diet interactions (Ordovas & Corella., 2004).

So the shift towards personalized nutritional advice is a very attractive proposition, where, in principle, an individual can be given dietary advice specifically tailored to their genotype. However, the evidence-base for the impact of interactions between nutrients and fixed genetic variants on biomarkers of CVD risk is still very limited (Lovegrove & Gitau., 2008; Ordovas., 2006; Masson et al., 2003; Masson & Mc Neil., 2005; Fisler & Warden., 2005).

With the advent of nutritional genomics, it's becoming clear that an individual's genetic makeup (genotype) is an important factor in this response and that dietary interventions must be matched to genotypes to effect the intended lipid-lowering responses (DeBusk., 2008).

A number of such genes have already been identified and include those involved with postprandial lipoprotein and triglyceride responses, homocysteine metabolism, hypertension, blood-clotting, and inflammation (Ordovas & Corella., 2004; DeBusk., 2008).

Genetic polymorphism in human populations is part of the evolutionary process that results from the interaction between the environment and the human genome. Recent changes in diet have upset this equilibrium, potentially influencing the risk of most common morbidities such as cardiovascular diseases, diabetes, and cancer. Reduction of these conditions is a major public health concern, and such a reduction could be achieved by improving our ability to detect disease predisposition early in life and by providing more personalized behavioral recommendations for successful primary prevention. In terms of cardiovascular diseases, polymorphisms at multiple genes have been associated with differential effects in terms of lipid metabolism. The integration of genetic and environmental complexity into current and future research will drive the field toward the implementation of clinical tools aimed at providing dietary advice optimized for the individual's genome (Ordovas., 2009; Engler., 2009).

The recognition that nutrients have the ability to interact and modulate molecular mechanisms underlying an organism's physiological functions has prompted a revolution in the field of nutrition (Much et al., 2005).
For the field of nutrition, this would encompass the ongoing efforts to understand the relationships between the genome and diet, currently termed nutrigenomics and nutrigenetics (Much et al., 2005; Ommen., 2004)

4. Nutritional genomics

Nutrigenetics and nutrigenomics are promising multidisciplinary fields that focus on studying the interactions between nutritional factors, genetic factors and health outcomes. Their goal is to achieve more efficient individual dietary intervention strategies aimed at preventing disease, improving quality of life and achieving healthy aging (Ordovas., 2004).
In contrast to most single gene disorders, chronic disorders (e. g., cardiovascular disease, cancer, diabetes) are far more complex. First, they involve multiple genes, each of which comes in more than one variation, that likely contribute in small ways to the overall condition rather than have the dramatic impact that is more typical with single gene disorders. Second, the genes are more likely to be influenced by environmental factors, which make the resulting phenotype murkier than with single-gene disorders. An individual might have gene variants that predispose to a particular chronic disorder but, depending on that individual's nutritional and other lifestyle choices, the disorder may or may not develop (DeBusk., 2008).
Nutritional genomics or nutrigenomics is the newly developing field of science that focuses on the complex interaction among genes and environmental factors, specifically bioactive components in food and how a person's diet interacts with his or her genotype to influence the balance between health and disease (DeBusk., 2009; Much et al., 2005; Fisler & Warden., 2005).
Nutritional genomics is the umbrella term (Ryan-Harshman., 2008). There are two major subcategories of nutritional genomics: nutrigenetics and nutrigenomics (Much et al., 2005).
The creation of nutrigenomics and nutrigenetics, two fields with distinct approaches to elucidate the interaction between diet and genes but with a common ultimate goal to optimize health through the personalization of diet, provide powerful approaches to unravel the complex relationship between nutritional molecules, genetic polymorphisms, and the biological system as a whole (Much et al., 2005).
Thus, nutrition in the 21st century is poised to be an exciting and highly relevant field of research, as each new day is accompanied by advances in our understanding of how the interactions between lifestyle and genotype contribute to health and disease, taking us one step closer to achieving the highly desirable goal of personalized nutrition (Much et al., 2005).

4.1 Nutrigenetics

Nutrigenetics term was used first time by Dr R. O Brennan in 1975 (Farhud et al., 2010). Nutrigenetics is concerned with the effect of gene variations or gene variant or individual's genetic make-up on the organism's functional ability, specifically its ability to digest, absorb, and use food (DeBusk., 2009; Ordovas & Corella., 2004; Lovegrove & Gitau., 2008). Nutrigenetics embodies the science of identifying and characterizing gene variants associated with differential responses to nutrients or dietary pattern, functional food or supplement on a specific health outcome, and relating this variation to disease states (Much et al., 2005; Michael., 2008). The particular gene variants a person has to determine the nutritional requirements for that person and the gene-based differences in response to dietary components and developing nutraceuticals that are most compatible with health based on individual genetic makeup (DeBusk., 2009; Subbiah., 2007). Nutrigenetics will assist clinicians in identifying the optimal diet for a given individual, i. e., personalized nutrition (Much et al., 2005; Svacina., 2007; Zak & Slaby., 2007; Gillies., 2003).

Furthermore, the concept is that if an individual is genotyped at various genes for disease-associated risk alleles, a genotype-based diet or nutritional supplement regimen may be useful to overcome the genetic variation and reduce risk or prevent the disease altogether (Wood., 2008; Xacur-GarcAa et al., 2008; Kussmann & Fay., 2008).

4.2 Nutrigenomics

Nutrigenomics, is concerned with how bioactive components within food affect genes. The field of nutritional genomics is still evolving, and it is common to see "nutrigenomics" used as a shorthand version of "nutritional genomics ". However, keeping the concepts separate can be helpful when sorting out the underlying mechanisms involved (DeBusk., 2009). Nutrigenomics will unravel the optimal diet from within a series of nutritional alternatives, whereas nutrigenetics will help clinicians in identifying the optimal diet for a given individual, i. e., personalized nutrition (Much et al., 2005).

Although these two concepts are intimately associated, they take a fundamentally different approach to understanding the relationship between genes and diet. Despite the immediate goals differing, the long-term goal of improving health and preventing disease with nutrition requires the amalgamation of both disciplines (Much et al., 2005)

Nutrigenetics is the more familiar of the two subtypes of nutritional genomics (DeBusk., 2009) At one end of the spectrum of nutritional genomics are the highly penetrant monogenic disorders that give rise to inborn errors of metabolism such as phenylketonuria (DeBusk., 2009). More recently less penetrant, more subtle variations have been identified that also affect the gene-encoded protein's function. However, such variations do not in themselves cause disease. Instead, they alter a person's susceptibility for developing a disease. Depending on the specific gene variant, the person's likelihood of developing a disorder may be increased or reduced. These genes are the primary focus of nutritional genomics, because they are common within the global population, they affect dietary recommendations about the types and amounts of food that best fit a person, and practical interventions are possible. These interventions can potentially improve the health potential of individual people and, by extrapolation, the populations in which they live (DeBusk., 2009).

Current nutrition recommendations, directed towards populations, are based on estimated average nutrient requirements for a target population and intend to meet the needs of most individuals within that population. They also aim at preventing common diseases such as obesity, diabetes and cardiovascular disease. So diet has been reported as a major contributor to alarming prevalence of obesity (Shalileh et al, 2010). For infants with specific genetic polymorphisms, e. g. some inborn errors of metabolism such as phenylketonuria, adherence to current recommendations will cause disease symptoms and they need personalized nutrition recommendations (Hernell & West., 2008; Farhud & Shalileh., 2008).

Some other monogenic polymorphisms, e. g. adult hypolactasia, are common but with varying prevalence between ethnic groups and within populations. Ages at onset as well as the degree of the resulting lactose intolerance also vary, making population-based as well as personalized recommendations difficult. The tolerable intake is best set by each individual based on symptoms. For polygenetic diseases such as celiac disease, and allergic disease, current knowledge is insufficient to suggest personalized recommendations aiming at primary prevention for all high-risk infants, although it may be justified to provide such recommendations on an individual level should the parents ask for them.

New technologies such as nutrigenetics and nutrigenomics are promising tools with which current nutrition recommendations can possibly be refined and the potential of individualized nutrition be explored. It seems likely that in the future it will be possible to offer more subgroups within a population personalized recommendations (hernell & West., 2008).

The possibility of offering personalized nutritional advice to the individual is an attractive option for dietitians and nutrition scientists and is becoming practicable with the emergence of nutritional genomics. This developing field promises to revolutionize dietetic practice, with dietary advice prescribed according to an individual's genetic makeup to prevent, mitigate or cure chronic disease (Lovegrove & Gitau., 2008). It has been also termed "personalized nutrition" or "individualized nutrition" (Ordovas & Corella., 2004; Perez-Martinez et al., 2011). The practical applications of this research include a new set of tools that nutrition professionals can use to identify disease susceptibilities and a growing body of knowledge that will form the basis for developing strategies for disease prevention and intervention that are specifically targeted to the underlying genetic mechanisms (DeBusk., 2008).

Nutrigenetics and personalized nutrition are components of the concept that in the future genotyping will be used as a means of defining dietary recommendations to suit the individual. Over the last two decades there has been an explosion of research in this area, with often conflicting findings reported in the literature (Rimbach & Minihane., 2009).

According to WHO reports, diet factors influence occurrence of more than 2/3 of diseases. Most of these factors belong to the categories of nutrigenetics and nutrigenomics. In the future both, nutrigenetics and nutrigenomics, will induce many changes in preventive medicine and also in clinical medicine (Svacina., 2007).

Nutrients interact with the human genome to modulate molecular pathways that may become disrupted, resulting in an increased risk of developing various chronic diseases. Understanding how genetic variations influence nutrient digestion, absorption, transport, biotransformation, uptake and elimination will provide a more accurate measure of exposure to the bioactive food ingredients ingested. Furthermore, genetic polymorphisms in the targets of nutrient action such as receptors, enzymes or transporters could alter molecular pathways that influence the physiological response to dietary interventions. Knowledge of the genetic basis for the variability in response to these dietary factors should result in a more accurate measure of exposure of target tissues of interest to these compounds and their metabolites. Examples of how 'slow' and 'fast' metabolizers respond differently to the same dietary exposures will be discussed. Identifying relevant diet-gene interactions will benefit individuals seeking personalized dietary advice as well as improve public health recommendations by providing sound scientific evidence linking diet and health (EL-Sohemy, 2007; Amouyel., 2000).

A really personalized diet will be a diet considering the nutritional status, the nutritional needs based on age, body composition, work and physical activities, but also considering the genotype. That is, define the "nutritional phenotype (Perez-Martinez et al., 2011; Miggiano & De Sanctis., 2006). It is clear that integrating knowledge of gene variants into dietary recommendations for populations and individuals will increasingly play a role in nutrition counseling and policy making (DeBusk., 2008).

Nutrigenetics will provide the basis for personalized dietary recommendations based on the individual's genetic makeup. This approach has been used for decades for certain single gene diseases; such as phenylketonuria, however, the challenge is to implement a similar concept for common multi factorial disorders and to develop tools to detect genetic predisposition and to prevent common disorders decades before their manifestation. The preliminary results involving gene-diet interactions for cardiovascular diseases and cancer are promising, but mostly inconclusive. Success in this area will require the integration of different disciplines and investigators working on large population studies designed to adequately investigate gene-environment interactions (Ordovas & Corella., 2004; Ordovas & Mooser., 2004).

4.3 Nutritional genomics and lipid metabolism

From a health perspective, the major concerns regarding genes and lipid metabolism center on susceptibility to vascular disease. Genes involved with cholesterol homeostasis offer examples of how genetic variations affect lipid metabolism and, thereby, disease risk (DeBusk., 2009).

The blood lipid response to diet is influenced by polymorphisms within genes for the apolipoproteins as well as within those for enzymes, such as hepatic lipase, that are involved in lipid metabolism (fisler & Warden., 2005).

The major focus of nutritional genomics research is on identifying (1) gene-disease associations, (2) the dietary components that influence these associations, (3) the mechanisms by which dietary components exert their effects, and (4) the genotypes that benefit most from particular dietary choices (DeBusk., 2008).

The following section takes a brief look at some of the key diet-related genes and their known variants and how these variants affect the person's response to diet. Keep in mind that chronic diseases involve complex interactions among genes and bioactive food components, and unraveling the details will require population and intervention studies large enough to have the statistical power needed to draw meaningful conclusions. Although what is known today is but the tip of the iceberg compared to what will come in the years ahead (DeBusk., 2008).

Over the last two decades there has been an explosion of research in this area, with often conflicting findings reported in the literature (Rimbach & Minihan., 2009).

5. Candidate gene approach

The candidate gene approach involves the selection and study of biologically relevant genes. Genetic polymorphisms in these genes, known as Single-Nucleotide Polymorphism (SNPs), can alter susceptibility to a disease. Candidate or "susceptibility" genes should meet one or more of the following conditions: genes that are chronically activated during a disease state and have been previously demonstrated to be sensitive to dietary intervention; genes with

functionally important variations; genes that have an important hierarchical role in biological cascades; polymorphisms that are highly prevalent in the population (usually >10% for public health relevance); and/or genes with associated biomarkers, rendering clinical trials useful (Lovegrove & Gitau., 2008).
Many studies have investigated this possibility and have largely focused on genes whose products affect lipoprotein metabolism, eg, apolipoproteins, enzymes, and receptors. Although there have been several reviews of such studies, many of them may have led to articles being omitted and introduced bias toward positive findings (Ordovas., 2006).

5.1 Apolipoprotein A-I (Apo AI)

The Apo AI gene, codes for apolipoprotein A-I, is a major structural and functional component of HDL constituting about 70% to 80% of HDL protein mass, and is the main activator of the enzyme lecithin cholesterol acyl transferase (LCAT) (Ordovas & Corella., 2004; Lovegrove & Gitau., 2008; Much et al., 2005; DeBusk., 2008).
Plasma HDL-cholesterol plays a protective role for CVD (Lovegrove & Gitau., 2008; Much et al., 2005). Its gene product Apo A-I plays a central role in lipid metabolism and CVD risk. Pedigree studies have reported associations between genetic variation at the Apo A1 locus and plasma lipid and lipoprotein levels (Ordovas & Corella., 2004). One of the variants that has been identified to be diet-related is -75G>A, in which the typical guanine has been replaced with an adenine at position 75 within the regulatory region of the Apo *A-I* gene (DeBusk., 2008).
It was reported that this polymorphism was associated with Apo A-I and HDL-C concentrations, and individuals carrying the A-allele presented with the highest levels, compared with subjects homozygotes for the G allele (G/G) but many studies have had contradictory results (Lovegrove & Gitau., 2008; Ordovas & Corella., 2004).
In the context of the Framingham Heart Study, individuals with a polymorphism in the Apo A1 gene promoter region (–75 G/A) were found to respond differently to dietary PUFA (Much et al., 2005; Lovegrove & Gitau., 2008).
The inconsistencies in reported studies outcomes are not necessarily a result of inherent differences, but are a result of a nutrient–gene interaction, i. e. a classic example of where individualized dietary advice could be important in relation to exerting a positive influence on HDL-C levels and CVD risk (Lovegrove & Gitau., 2008; Much et al., 2005). In brief, that individuals with the A allele showed an increase in HDL levels following an increased consumption of PUFA. In contrast, those with the more common G allele showed an inverse relationship between HDL levels and PUFA consumption. This study revealed that differences in sex also mediate the response. Indeed, men did not show a relationship between HDL and PUFA consumption, irrespective of their Apo A1 polymorphism (Lovegrove & Gitau., 2008; Much et al., 2005).
A common practice in treating dyslipidemia is to reduce the saturated fat content of the diet and increase the polyunsaturated fat content. Typically, HDL levels fall in women with the more common G allele as the polyunsaturated content of the diet increases, an effect counter to the desired one. These women would benefit from a fat modified diet that keeps amounts of both saturated and polyunsaturated fat low and increases amounts of monounsaturated fat. Women with the A allele, increasing polyunsaturated dietary fat leads to increased HDL levels, and the effect is "dose-dependent; so in women with the more common G allele,

increasing dietary Polyunsaturated Fat (PUFA) levels from less than 4% of total energy to 4% to 8% to greater than 8% resulted in a corresponding decline in HDL levels as PUFA levels increase. However, in women with the A allele, increasing PUFA concentrations (>8% of energy derived from PUFA) increased HDL levels and the increase is more dramatic in the presence of two copies of the A alleles than it is with just one. For these women, a diet low in saturated fat, moderate in polyunsaturated fat (8% or greater of total calories), and supplying the rest in monounsaturated fat has the greatest benefit in raising HDL levels. Clearly, whether a person has the -75G>A *Apo AI* variant, and how many copies are present, will affect any therapeutic intervention developed to correct dyslipidemia (DeBusk., 2009; Much et al., 2005; Debra., 2008).

Juo et al (Hank Juo., 1999) used a meta analysis approach to show the lack of consistency between the less common A-allele and higher HDL-cholesterol concentrations. In view of the significant gene-diet interaction observed for those intervention studies, they examined whether these results could be extrapolated to a free living population, consisting of about 1600 Framingham Offspring Study participants (Ordovas et al., 2002). The results from the straightforward association between genotype and phenotype were disappointing and suggested that the G/A polymorphism was not associated with HDL-cholesterol, Apo A-I concentrations, nor with any other anthropometrical or plasma lipid variable examined. To examine the potential modifying effect of dietary fat on these associations, they fitted multivariate linear regression models, including interaction terms for fat intake [total, Saturated Fatty Acid (SFA), Monounsaturated Fat (MUFA), and PUFA fat]. No significant interactions were observed between the G/A polymorphism, total, SFA, and MUFA fat intakes. However, in women, HDL-cholesterol concentrations were associated with a significant interaction between PUFA intake and Apo A1 genotype ($p = 0.005$). Using PUFA as a dichotomous variable, their data show that G/G women consuming <6% PUFA/day had higher HDL-cholesterol (1. 48 ± 0. 40 m mol/L) than A-carriers (1. 43 ± 0. 40 m mol/L). Conversely, when consuming ≥6% PUFA/day, G/G had lower HDL-cholesterol concentrations (1. 44 ± 0. 39 m mol/L) than A-carriers (1. 49 ± 0. 39 m mol/L). In men, the situation was more complex because the effects were observed using three-way interactions, including smoking and alcohol consumption, in the analyzes (Ordovas & Corella., 2004).

The most evident application of these results may be to help us make more efficacious dietary recommendations based on genetic profile. It is clear that subjects with the A-allele at this Apo A1-75 (G/A) polymorphism will benefit from diets containing a high percentage (it is important to underscore that we are talking about percent in the diet and not about total amounts) of PUFA (i. e., vegetable oils, fish, nuts, and so on). According to their data, this should result in higher HDL-cholesterol concentrations, which in turn should lower CVD risk. These findings suggest that the expression of the Apo A1 gene may be regulated by PUFA (Ordovas & Corella., 2004).

On the other hand, of 13 reports, 5 found that the presence of the Apo A-I-75 (*G/A*) A allele instead of the common G allele resulted in greater LDL-cholesterol responses to changes in dietary. In addition, significant interactions between the *G/A* genotype and diet were found for changes in total and LDL cholesterol when subjects changed from a low-fat diet to a diet high in MUFAs. No significant interactions between diet and other polymorphisms in the Apo A-I gene were shown (Ordovas & Corella., 2004).

5.2 Apolipoprotein A-IV (APOA4)

Apo A-IV is a 46-Kd plasma glycoprotein that is synthesized by intestinal enterocytes during lipid absorption and is incorporated into nascent chylomicrons. Apo A-IV enters circulation on lymph chylomicrons, but then dissociates from their surface and circulates primarily as a lipid-free protein. Several genetically determined isoforms of Apo A-IV have been detected; amino acid positions 360 and 347 of the mature protein are the most common. The polymorphism at position 360 is due to a CAG → CAT substitution at codon 360 in the Apo A4 gene and encodes a Q360H (Gln → His) substitution in the carboxyl terminus, and produces an isoform, originally known as Apo A-IV-2, one charge unit more basic than the common isoform, Apo A-IV-. In some population studies the Apo A-IV-2 allele is associated with higher levels of HDL-cholesterol and or Apo A-I and/or lower triglyceride (TG) levels, as well as lower LDL-cholesterol, lower Lp (a), and higher fasting glucose and insulin levels, but no associations have been observed in other studies (Ordovas & Corella., 2004).

The other common mutation (Thr347→Ser) is due to an ACT→TCT substitution at codon 347 in the human Apo A-IV gene, it is found within subjects with the apoA-IV-1 isoform. Several population studies note that carriers of the 347S allele have lower plasma, total, LDL-cholesterol, Apo B levels, and Lp (a) levels, than 347T/T homozygotes. The results of many reports showing that male carriers of the less common allele at the Gln360His polymorphism were less responsive to changes in dietary fat and cholesterol or cholesterol alone (Ordovas & Corella., 2004).

Several studies have focused on the interaction between the Apo *A4* locus and dietary factors, both in the fasting and postprandial states. Similar to the findings for other genes, the data are conflicting when it comes to the effect of Apo A-IV polymorphisms on the LDL response to dietary cholesterol. However, according to Weinberg (Weinberg., 2002), the results from different studies can be partially reconciled if one assumes that the dietary fatty acid effects dominate over the allele effects. Therefore, if dietary cholesterol intake is the principal variable, and total fat intake is moderate and constant, Q/H subjects display an attenuated response of LDL-cholesterol. However, when dietary cholesterol intake is changed in the setting of a higher baseline dietary fat intake or with a change in fat saturation, the fatty acid effects on LDL levels predominate and overrule the allele effect. The impact of the Q360H polymorphism on cholesterol absorption may be greater on a high PUFAs intake. However, dietary PUFA counteract the effect of dietary cholesterol on the expression of hepatic LDL receptors. Thus, the final effect of Apo AIV alleles on the LDL response to dietary cholesterol may be determined by the relative amounts of cholesterol, saturated fatty acids (SAFAs), and PUFAs in the diet (winberg et al., 2000; Weggemans., 2000; Lopez-Miranda., 1998; Ordovas & Corella., 2004; Hockey., 2001).

There is more consistency and probably less complexity regarding the impact of Apo A-IV polymorphisms on HDL-cholesterol: When total fat intake is raised or lowered, Q/H subjects have an exaggerated, and Threonine /Serine (T/S) subjects an attenuated, response in plasma HDL levels. It has been suggested, and Weinberg demonstrated, that a high-PUFA intake may amplify this effect (Ordovas & Corella., 2004; Winberg et al., 2000).

Given the relationships between plasma TG and plasma HDL-cholesterol levels, it is possible that the response of plasma HDL-cholesterol levels to changes in dietary fat is mediated by Apo A-IV allele effects on postprandial triglyceride-rich lipoprotein metabolism. These studies clearly illustrate the extreme complexity associated with the

interpretation of results from studies involving gene-diet interactions (Ordovas & Corella., 2004).
The presence of serine instead of threonine at position 347 in the Apo A-IV gene was associated with increased total and LDL-cholesterol responsiveness when subjects switched from a high-SFA diet to a National Cholesterol Education Program Step I diet. When the same subjects changed from the National Cholesterol Education Program Step I diet to a high-MUFA diet, subjects with the *Thr /Thr* genotype had a 1% decrease in total cholesterol concentrations, whereas subjects with the *Ser* allele had a 5% increase in total cholesterol concentrations. When the Thr347Ser and the Apo A-I–75 (*G/A*) genotypes were combined, carriers of the *A* and *Ser* alleles showed greater LDL-cholesterol responses to changes in dietary fat. However, Carmena-Ramon et al (Carmena-Ramon et al., 1998) investigated both the Gln360His and Thr347Ser polymorphisms and found no gene-diet or haplotype-diet interactions (Masson et al., 2003). The evidence that exists for an interaction between diet and the Apo A-IV glutamine-histidine mutation at position 360 (Gln360His) suggests that *Gln / Gln* subjects show significantly greater total and LDL-cholesterol responses and that *Gln /His* subjects show greater HDL-cholesterol responses to changes in dietary fat, cholesterol, or both. Although Wallace et al found no significant differences in LDL-cholesterol responses between genotypes, dense LDL cholesterol decreased more in subjects carrying the *His* allele when polyunsaturated fatty acids (PUFAs) replaced SFAs in the diet (Wallace et al, 2000). In the same study, there was a significant difference in HDL-cholesterol responses between genotype groups such that concentrations decreased in *Gln /Gln* subjects and increased in *Gln /His* subjects (Masson et al., 2003).

5.3 Apolipoprotein B (Apo B)

Apolipoprotein B is the main protein component of low-density-lipoprotein (LDL) and contains several domains. The human Apo B is 43 kb in length with 81 bp signal sequence. Numerous polymorphisms have been identified on this gene (Heilbronn et al., 2000).
The evidence for an interaction between the *Xba*I polymorphism and diet is inconsistent. In 2 studies, *X-X-* subjects showed greater LDL-cholesterol responses, whereas Tikkanen et al, found that subjects carrying the *X+* allele had greater total, LDL-, and HDL-cholesterol responses. However in, analysis of these data, the *Xba*I polymorphism only explained a significant proportion of variance of the change in HDL cholesterol (Tikkanen et al., 1995). In one research they found no significant effect on LDL-cholesterol responsiveness, although *X-X*-subjects showed the greatest HDL_2- and VLDL-cholesterol responses. Finally, in another study researchers studied the effect of the *Xba*I polymorphism in subjects with the common Apo *E3/3* genotype and found that *X-X-* subjects showed the greatest triacylglycerol response. Rantala et al conducted a meta-analysis of all published dietary trials. In their analysis of 8 studies, *X-X+* subjects had greater LDL responses than did *X+X+* subjects and no significant differences in the responses of total or HDL cholesterol or triacylglycerol were found between genotypes (Masson et al., 2003; Rantala., 2000). Two of 7 intervention studies found that the *Eco*RI *R-* allele was associated with significantly greater total and LDL-cholesterol responses to changes in dietary fat and cholesterol. Only one study found an interaction between the *Msp*I polymorphism and response to diet. Ten intervention studies found no significant effects of the Apo B signal peptide insertion/deletion (*I/D*) polymorphism on dietary responsiveness; however, 2 studies reported a significantly greater responsiveness in subjects homozygous for the *I* allele. In a

study, 43 men and women were observed to compare the effects of insoluble and soluble fiber on plasma lipids. Their statistical model identified gene-diet interactions. However, they did not look specifically at differences between genotype groups. It was found that *D/D* subjects had similar decreases in HDL cholesterol after consumption of the insoluble- and soluble-fiber diets. However, *I/I* subjects had larger HDL-cholesterol decreases with the soluble-fiber diet, whereas *I/D* subjects had larger HDL-cholesterol decreases with the insoluble-fiber diet. The gene-diet interaction was significant (P = 0. 021) (Masson et al., 2003; Rantala., 2000).

In response, low-fat, low-cholesterol diet, *I/I* subjects showed the greatest decrease in HDL_2. In addition, *I/I* and *I/D* subjects showed increased VLDL-cholesterol and decreased LDL-cholesterol concentrations, whereas *D/D* subjects showed decreased VLDL-cholesterol and increased LDL-cholesterol concentrations. The *I/D* polymorphism showed no significant effect on the responsiveness of total, LDL, or HDL cholesterol or triacylglycerol in a meta-analysis of 7 studies (Masson et al., 2003).

5.4 Apolipoprotein E (APO E)

Apo E gene variants have implications for nutrition therapy related to preventing and treating CVD and the responses to dietary fat, soluble fiber, and alcohol. The impact of Apo E genotype on individual variability in its LDL cholesterol response to diet interventions and CVD risk has been extensively investigated over the past 30 years. Apo E contains 299 amino acids, considering Apo E's key role in lipoprotein metabolism, being involved in chylomicron metabolism, very low-density lipoprotein synthesis and secretion, and in the cellular removal of lipoprotein remnants from the circulation. Apo E serves as a ligand for multiple lipoprotein receptors. This gene locus is polymorphic, with 84 gene variants being characterized to date. The prevalence of this SNP varies in different populations (Lovegrove & Gitau., 2008; Rubin & Berglund., 2002; Ordovas & Corella., 2004; DeBusk., 2009).

Apo E is present in a subfraction of lipoprotein (a). The receptor-binding properties reside in the N-terminal part of Apo E, whereas the lipid-binding domain resides in the C-terminal portion. It was recognized that Apo E was present as three different Apo E isoforms (E2, E3, and E4), coded by three different alleles (e2, e3, and e4), resulting in six homo and heterozygous genotypes (e2/e2, e2/e3, e2/e4, e3/e3, e3/e4, e4/e4). Apo E2 differs from the wild type, Apo E3, by a substitution of arginine for cysteine at amino acid 158, and Apo E4 differs from Apo E3 by a substitution of cysteine for arginine at amino acid 112. In addition, several other genetic variants have been described at the Apo E locus (Rubin & Berglund., 2002; Lovegrove & Gitau., 2008; Masson et al., 2003; Farhud et al., 2010).

Persons with E4 variant respond to a high-fat diet negatively with an increased risk for coronary heart disease (CHD). In these individuals, low-fat diet should be useful (Farhud et al., 2010; Sheweta et al., 2011).

Population studies show that plasma cholesterol, LDL cholesterol, and Apo B levels are highest in subjects carrying the Apo E4, intermediate in those with the Apo E3, and lowest in those with the Apo E2 isoform. An initial observation was that the association of the Apo E4 isoform with elevated serum cholesterol levels was greater in populations consuming diets rich in saturated fat and cholesterol than in other populations (Ordovas & Corella., 2004).

Corella and Ordovas reviewed the numerous studies that have investigated the diet-gene interaction for Apo E variants. People with at least one E4 allele have the highest basal levels of various lipids and show the greatest lipid-lowering response to a low-fat diet. Taking into account which Apo E alleles a person has is helpful in developing diet and lifestyle interventions for improving serum lipid levels (DeBusk., 2009).

In 46 studies that examined the Apo E locus and alterations in dietary fat content, significantly different responses in total and LDL cholesterol by Apo E genotype were reported in 8 and 11 studies, respectively, with the Apo E4 individuals generally being the most responsive (Lovegrove & Gitau., 2008; Masson et al., 2003).

Note that despite the numerous studies examining the relation between Apo E genetic variability and LDL-cholesterol response to diet intervention, there is considerable inconsistency regarding the magnitude and significance of the reported associations, and this locus continues to be the subject of intense research (Ordovas & Corella., 2004).

In a study, there are 29 intervention studies that examine Apo E-diet interactions. A total of 3224 subjects participated in these studies, ranging from 16 to 420 subjects per study. Of the 29 studies, 12 demonstrated no significant Apo E-diet interactions, 15 reported significant interactions (E4 was usually associated with increased dietary response), and 2 were undefined. Using the same available literature, but different selection criteria, Masson, reviewed 62 dietary intervention periods, including 3223 subject-by-diet interventions (Masson et al., 2003). Again, the range of the studies varied between 8 and 210 subjects per dietary intervention. According to this review, 42 of the diet interventions did not demonstrate significant Apo E-diet interactions, and only 19 provided evidence for significant interactions, clearly demonstrating the diversity of the results presented in the original papers as well as those obtained from review papers (Ordovas & Corella., 2004; Masson et al., 2003).

The heterogeneous response to changes in dietary fat may be attributed to a number of factors including age, gender, baseline LDL-C levels, disease status and drug use (Lovegrove & Gitau., 2008).

One difference between the negative studies and those reporting significant Apo E gene–diet interactions relates to the baseline lipid levels of the subjects. Studies reporting significant associations often included subjects who were moderately hypercholesterolemic and/or had significant differences in base total cholesterol and LDL-cholesterol among the Apo E genotype groups. This suggests that the significant gene-diet interaction is apparent only in subjects susceptible to hypercholesterolemia. Concerning differences in dietary interventions, there were significant interactions in studies in which total dietary fat and cholesterol were modified. Several mechanisms are proposed to explain these Apo E-related differences in individual response to dietary therapy. Some studies show that intestinal cholesterol absorption is related to Apo E phenotype, with Apo E4 carriers absorbing more cholesterol than non-Apo E4 carriers. Other mechanisms such as different distribution of Apo E on the lipoprotein fractions, LDL Apo B production, bile acid, and cholesterol synthesis, and postprandial lipoprotein clearance may also be involved (Ordovas & Corella., 2004).

On the other hand although the obvious dietary factors implicated in gene-diet interactions affecting plasma lipid levels are dietary fats and cholesterol, other dietary components have revealed significant interactions. This is the case for alcohol intake.

Although the raising effect of alcohol consumption on high-density lipoprotein (HDL)-cholesterol levels is well established, the effect on LDL-cholesterol is still unclear. It is possible that the reported variability will be due to interactions between genetic factors and alcohol consumption. Using cross-sectional analysis, researcher examined whether variation at the Apo E locus modulates the association between alcohol consumption and LDL-cholesterol levels in a healthy population based sample of 1014 male and 1133 female participants in the Framingham Offspring Study (Corella et al., 2001). In male nondrinkers, LDL-cholesterol levels were not different across Apo *E* groups; however, in male drinkers, there were differences in LDL-cholesterol, with Apo E2 subjects displaying the lowest levels. When LDL cholesterol levels were compared among the Apo E subgroups by drinking status, LDL-cholesterol levels in Apo E2 male drinkers were lower than in Apo E2 non drinkers. Conversely, in Apo E4 males, LDL-cholesterol was higher in drinkers than in nondrinkers. This Apo E-alcohol interaction remained significant after controlling for age, BMI, smoking, fat, and energy intake. In women, the expected effect of Apo E alleles on LDL-cholesterol levels was present in both drinkers and nondrinkers. Multiple linear regression models showed a negative association between alcohol and LDL-cholesterol levels in Apo E2 men, with alcohol intake a continuous variable. Conversely, in Apo E4 men, this association was positive. There were no statistically significant associations in either Apo E3 men or in women. These data suggest that in men, variability at the Apo E locus partially modulates the effects of consuming alcoholic beverages on LDL-cholesterol levels (Ordovas & Corella., 2004).

The effect of alcohol was also investigated in the Copenhagen City Heart Study (Frikke-Schmidt., 2000). In that study, there was an interaction between alcohol and Apo E among women, in which higher triglyceride levels were associated with both the E2 and E4 alleles among women who regularly consumed alcohol. For men, increased triglyceride levels among E2 and E4 carriers were seen across the entire alcohol distribution spectrum, perhaps because of some degree of alcohol consumption among all men. Overall, the results suggested that metabolic stresses, such as the postprandial situation or alcohol consumption, might contribute to uncover underlying differences between Apo E genotypes in cholesterol, triglyceride or lipoprotein metabolism (Frikke-Schmidt., 2000).

The effect of the Apo E gene on lipoproteins may differ with age. In elderly individuals as well as in children, there is less difference in LDL cholesterol levels in individuals carrying the E4 allele versus non-E4 carriers. Interestingly, in both of these age groups, the presence of the Apo E2 allele was associated with lower LDL cholesterol levels. An age-dependent variation between Apo E and plasma lipids was also seen by Jarvik et al (Jarvik et al, 1997). By longitudinally following male Caucasian twins, the authors demonstrated that whereas E4 carriers initially had higher triglyceride and cholesterol levels compared with E3 homozygotes, this difference disappeared over an 18-year period (Rubin & Berglund., 2002).

A sex-specific association between Apo E2 and HDL cholesterol levels has been described in Turkish individuals. In Turkish women, but not men, the frequency of the Apo E2 allele increased almost six fold from the lowest to the highest HDL cholesterol tertiary (Rubin & Berglund., 2002). The available information show, significant diet–Apo E gene interactions occurred in male-only studies. In studies including men and women, significant effects were noted only in men, suggesting a significant gene-sex interaction (Ordovas & Corella., 2004).

As pointed out above, in studies in which an Apo E gene nutrient interaction was found, it was generally more common among men than women, suggesting a modulation by sex. Interestingly, in the study by Mahley et al, on HDL levels in Turkish individuals, the authors suggested that the association of Apo E2 with higher HDL cholesterol levels found in women but not in men may be caused by a sex difference in hepatic lipase. Among women, a lower hepatic lipase activity might allow the detection of the modulating effect of Apo E genotypes, whereas this effect might be overwhelmed by a higher enzyme activity in men (Mahley et al., 2000). This is an analogous situation to the suggestion above that differences in susceptibility might be uncovered by a metabolic challenge (Rubin & Berglund., 2002).

Other causes for the observed differences between studies may be the presence of confounders, the type of dietary intervention used, the population studied and, importantly, the number of subjects in the respective studies. A small number of subjects limits the possibility of detecting differences, or could alternatively lead to spurious associations. Although the number of studies addressing the gene nutrient interaction for Apo E is growing, in most studies so far this has been a secondary endpoint, usually analyzed post hoc. Perhaps the most likely possibility is that a number of dietary interventions will elicit variable responses across Apo E genotypes, but that the ability to detect such differences will depend on the strength and type of intervention as well as on specific recipient factors (type of population, presence of hyperlipidemia, etc.). In the end, however, our ability to confirm or refute the presence of Apo E gene nutrient interactions as well as to understand their metabolic basis fully will require larger and more detailed studies (Rubin & Berglund., 2002).

Inconsistency in nutrient–gene interactions in relation to Apo E polymorphisms may be a result, in part, of retrospective genotyping of small study cohorts, for which the genotype–diet–LDL-C interactions were not the primary outcome. This factor has resulted in the under-representation of the less-frequent genotypes and, although trends may have been evident, many of the studies were clearly under-powered to detect significant genotype–treatment effects. The prospective genotyping of larger study cohorts has been used as an alternative approach to increase statistical power (Lovegrove & Gitau., 2008).

However, recent evidence strongly suggests that variations in a number of key genes may also be important, including common variants of the Apo E gene. The most convincing evidence to date for genotypic effects on dietary response comes from the extensively studied Apo E gene variant (Lovegrove & Gitau., 2008).

A metaanalysis has been published recently that summarizes the overall findings from studies using a variety of end-point measures. A mean 40–50% increase in CHD risk was observed in E4 carriers (overall OR 1. 42) relative to the wild-type E3/E3 genotype, with no apparent differences for either the E2 and E3 subgroups (OR 0. 98). Although a causal mechanism to link E4 with increased CHD risk has not been fully elucidated, the association has been ascribed to a higher concentration of LDL-C. This higher LDL-C is believed to arise from the Apo E4 isoform having a relatively higher affinity for its membrane (LDL/chylomicron remnant) receptor and feedback inhibition of receptor activity in E4 carriers Other mechanisms relating to reduced antioxidant status may also be operative (Lovegrove & Gitau., 2008).

There is the large variation that is observed in the concentration of serum LDL-cholesterol (LDL-C) in response to fish oil supplementation. The cardioprotective effects of the fatty acids in fish oil include eicosapantanoiec acid (EPA) and docosahesanoiec acid (DHA) are well recognized. However, a potentially deleterious increase in LDL-C (5–10%) has been consistently reported after moderate to high doses of fish oil (>2 g EPA+ DHA/d). These data showed the DHA rather than the EPA in fish oils that is responsible for the LDL-C raising effects in E4 individuals (Lovegrove & Gitau., 2008).

In contrast, those with one or more E4 alleles have the highest serum total cholesterol, LDL-, and Apo B levels, the lowest HDL-C levels, and have elevated fasting and postprandial triglyceride levels. They respond best to a low-fat diet but are the least responsive to soluble fiber for lowering serum lipids or to exercise for increasing HDL levels. Fish oil supplementation in these people increases total cholesterol and reduces HDL. Whether a person has the *U* allele or the E4 allele appears to make a difference in the diet and lifestyle recommendations that would be appropriate for improving vascular health (DeBusk., 2009).
Two prospectively genotyped studies designed to test the hypothesis that Apo E polymorphism has a significant effect on the LDL-C response to EPA and DHA have recently been completed (Lovegrove & Gitau., 2008).
Overall, the triglyceride response to the fat load was lower during fish oil supplementation, and interestingly the decrease in the incremental area under the curve for triglyceride levels was significantly higher for E2 carriers compared with E3 homozygotes and E4 carriers (Rubin & Berglund., 2002).
Although a number of previous studies have observed effects of Apo E genotype in response to dietary total fat and saturated fatty acid (SFA) manipulation, only one study to date has examined the Apo E genotype–dietary fat-LDL-C association using prospective recruitment by genotype. A study reported a significant effect of Apo E genotype on the plasma lipid response to a low fat diet, with a 5%, 13% and 16% reduction in LDL-C in E3/E3, E3/E4 and E4/E4 males, respectively. Other studies have examined the association between Apo E genotype and fish oil (EPA/DHA) on LDL-C responses. In a retrospectively genotyped study it was observed that a mean increase of 7. 1% in LDL-C for the group as a whole was solely attributable to a 16% rise in LDL-C in the Apo E4 participants, and it was speculated that Apo E genotype may, in part, predict the blood lipid response to fish oil intervention. Variable effects of EPA and DHA on LDL-C have been reported previously (Kobayashi et al., 2001; Lovegrove & Gitau., 2008).
The ApoE gene locus accounts for approximately 7% of the population variance in total and LDL cholesterol levels; in general, E4 carriers have higher and E2 carriers have lower LDL cholesterol levels. It has also been suggested that Apo E variations impact triglyceride levels, as higher triglyceride levels have been reported for both E4 and E2 carriers compared with E3 homozygotes (Rubin & Berglund, 2002).
In a recent study of more than 9000 individuals from the Copenhagen City Heart Study, Frikke-Schmidt and colleagues demonstrated that the association between the Apo E locus and cholesterol or plasma Apo B levels was invariant, i. e. present in most contexts (e. g. present in both men and women), whereas associations between Apo E and other lipoproteins such as triglycerides, Apo A-I, HDL cholesterol and lipoprotein (a) were found to be context dependent (Frikke-Schmidt., 2000). As the associations of Apo E with Apo B remained significant when adjusting for cholesterol but not the other way around, this suggested that Apo B is the factor primarily associated with Apo E genotype. It should be pointed out, however, that in their study triglyceride levels represented nonfasting conditions, and LDL cholesterol was not included in the analysis (Rubin & Berglund., 2002).
Furthermore, the Apo E2 allele was more common in individuals with high LpA-I levels, i. e. HDL with Apo AI but not Apo A-II. This HDL subfraction generally corresponds to the larger HDL2 subpopulation, which interestingly, in a study by Isasi et al, was associated with Apo E2 in children (Isasi et al., 2000). In view of their results, Mahley et al, suggest that HDL containing Apo E2 might be a poorer substrate for hepatic lipase compared with HDL

with Apo E3 or E4, leading to an accumulation of HDL in plasma. In addition, there might be a difference in the clearing mechanisms between HDL containing Apo E2 compared with Apo E3 or E4 (Mahley et al., 2000).

This mixed pattern was recently addressed by Weggemans et al, who performed a meta-analysis of 26 controlled clinical diet trials conducted. The effect of Apo E genotypes on response to dietary change in 395 healthy subjects, well balanced for sex, was evaluated. The authors pooled data in the response of LDL and HDL cholesterol from four types of trials; replacement of cis-unsaturated fat for saturated fat (n = 7 studies), replacement of cis-unsaturated fat for trans unsaturated fat (n = 2), changes in dietary cholesterol (n = 8) and changes in coffee diterpenes (n = 9). Overall, there were small, non-significant differences between Apo E genotypes in the response of LDL cholesterol, and results were unchanged after adjusting for age, sex and body mass index. For HDL cholesterol, a sex difference was noted, as the response to trans fat and cholesterol differed across Apo E genotypes in men but not in women (Weggemans et al., 2001).

Appropriately, the authors caution against the over interpretation of this result because of chance associations (Rubin & Berglund., 2002).

Friedlander et al, compared plasma levels across Apo E genotypes in response to two diets, a high saturated fat/high cholesterol and a low saturated fat/low cholesterol diet, in 214 free-living individuals in two kibbutz settlements in Israel. Although the baseline total and LDL cholesterol levels were higher among E4 carriers and lower among E2 carriers compared with E3 homozygotes, the plasma lipid response to the diet intervention did not differ across Apo E genotypes (Friedlander et al., 2000).

Loktionov et al, investigated 132 free-living healthy individuals participating in the European Prospective Investigation of Cancer study, a cohort study with approximately 25 000 subjects. The reported subgroup was part of a quality control study on the dietary methods used. In the 132 subjects, serum cholesterol levels correlated with the intake of total and saturated fat. For LDL cholesterol, a significant correlation with relative saturated fat intake was seen only for Apo E 4/3, and not for Apo E3/3 or 3/2 (Loktionov et al., 2000).

In another recent study, researchers analyzed lipid levels in relation to Apo E genotypes in 420 randomly selected free-living Costa Rican individuals consuming a low fat intake (53% of energy). In accordance with most previous studies, E2 carriers had lower, and E4 carriers higher LDL cholesterol and Apo B levels compared with E3 homozygotes. The population was dichotomized in two groups depending on the intake of saturated fat. High saturated fat intake (mean intake 13. 5% of energy) was associated with increased VLDL cholesterol, decreased HDL cholesterol and smaller LDL sizes in Apo E2 carriers, whereas the opposite was found for Apo E4 carriers. Effects on LDL size had previously been noted by Dreon et al, in which a more pronounced decrease in large, buoyant LDL particles during reduced fat intake was seen for Apo E4 carriers (Dreon et al, 1995). The findings of Campos et al suggested, as pointed out by the authors, that in E2 carriers, a high saturated fat intake may result in increased VLDL production and delayed clearance. Such a metabolic challenge might thus unmask a relative susceptibility in E2 carriers (Campos et al, 2001).

Finally, the study on plasma lipid response to dietary fat and carbohydrate in men and women with coronary heart disease provided further support for the association of triglyceride metabolism with Apo E2. Overall, E2 carriers had lower LDL cholesterol as well as a tendency to higher triglyceride levels than E3 and E4 carriers. In addition, there was a positive association between dietary sucrose (6±7% of the total energy intake) and plasma triglyceride levels among E2 carriers (Rubin & Berglund., 2002).

Postprandial studies as Apo E have important functions in chylomicron remnant metabolism, there has been substantial interest in the role of Apo E genotypes in the postprandial setting. Furthermore, a postprandial challenge could serve as a tool to uncover more precisely the differences between different Apo E alleles (Rubin & Berglund., 2002).
In a study of normolipidemic adults by Rubin & Berglund, the Apo E2 allele was associated with an increased postprandial triglyceride response. A similar response has also been demonstrated in other studies. Regarding the Apo E4 allele, more controversial results have been obtained (Rubin & Berglund., 2002).
However, although such studies are compatible with a faster clearance of VLDL and chylomicron remnants in E4 compared with E3 carriers, the meta-analysis showed higher triglyceride and lower HDL cholesterol levels among E4/3 individuals compared with E3 homozygotes. This would perhaps suggest an impaired postprandial clearance among E4 carriers (Rubin & Berglund., 2002). In support of this, another study found an impaired clearance of chylomicron and VLDL remnants in normolipidemic male E4 carriers compared with E3/3. Furthermore, several recent studies have also reported an increased postprandial triglyceride excursion in E4 carriers. In children, they did not observe any difference in triglyceride or retinyl palmitate response between E3/3 and E4 carriers, although a non-significant trend towards higher baseline triglyceride levels as well as higher triglyceride and retinyl palmitate levels 3 h postprandially among E4 carriers was seen (Couch et al., 2000). Another research found no significant effects of the Apo E4 allele on the postprandial triglyceride response after adjusting for baseline triglyceride levels, although a delayed retinyl palmitate clearance in E2 carriers was observed (Rubin & Berglund., 2002). In a recent study by Kobayashi et al, individuals with the E3/3 and E3/4 genotypes were matched for intra-abdominal visceral fat accumulation. Postprandial triglyceride levels did not differ between the two genotypes when adjusting for baseline levels, whereas retinyl palmitate levels among lipoproteins with Sf 5400 were higher among male E3/4 subjects, indicating a slower remnant clearance. As pointed out by the authors, there were fewer women in the study, which might contribute to the non-significant finding in this sex group (Kobayashi et al., 2001).
In a study, the researchers investigated postprandial fat load tolerance in 55 healthy volunteers with an atherogenic lipid profile, defined as triglyceride levels of 1. 5±4 m M, cholesterol 5±8 m M and HDL cholesterol less than 1. 1 m M, as part of a double-blind placebo-controlled crossover study with the consumption of either 6 g of fish oil or 6 g of olive oil supplements for 6 weeks. At the end of each period, a postprandial study was carried out. The difference in LDL cholesterol levels among Apo E genotypes is associated with differences in LDL receptor activity, with Apo E2 carriers having higher and Apo E4 carriers lower activity compared with Apo E3 homozygotes. Conditions with increased stress of this system, such as the increased intake of cholesterol and saturated fat, could therefore result in a variable response in LDL cholesterol levels across Apo E genotypes. In addition, E2 carriers may have decreased lipolytic function with an inhibition of the conversion of VLDL to LDL, as well as a compromised clearance system for triglyceride-rich lipoproteins. Therefore, even a modestly increased VLDL production in response to increased precursor availability might result in differences in plasma triglyceride levels across Apo E genotypes (Rubin & Berglund., 2002).
Although the results from postprandial studies are generally in agreement with the established metabolic differences between Apo E2 and E3, it is currently more difficult to

explain the reduced postprandial clearance in E4 carriers. However, it is possible that a differential distribution of the varying Apo E isoforms over different lipoprotein fractions, as well as variations in Apo E levels, could play a role. In addition, a lower LDL receptor activity in E4 carriers may contribute to a decreased postprandial clearance (Rubin & Berglund., 2002).

How could we reconcile these varying results? Even if most studies have established associations between Apo E and baseline lipoprotein levels, the absolute differences between the Apo E genotypes are relatively modest. It might thus be expected that inter-genotype differences in response to nutrient variations may generally be even smaller in magnitude, and thus more difficult to detect, although they might be enhanced by metabolic challenges affecting the synthetic or clearance systems in lipoprotein metabolism described above. Examples of such metabolic stresses in which Apo E gene nutrient interactions may be more readily detectable may be hyperlipidemia, an increased intake of saturated fat or cholesterol, the postprandial state, or alcohol intake. In agreement with this, studies indicating Apo E gene nutrient interactions have been more common in hyperlipidemic settings, whereas it has been more difficult to detect differences across Apo E genotypes in normolipidemic individuals or populations. However, Apo E gene± nutrient interaction has not been seen in all hyperlipidemic states. In familial heperlipidemia heterozygotes, no difference in plasma lipid response to a step 1 diet was seen across Apo E genotypes, indicating that the modulating effects of Apo E may be overwhelmed by other genetic defects, such as LDL receptor deficiency (Rubin & Berglund., 2002).

In conclusion, Apo E has important functions in lipoprotein metabolism and the Apo E polymorphism is associated with plasma lipoprotein levels. Although a large number of studies have addressed whether there is an interaction between Apo E genotypes and diet in affecting plasma lipid levels, this issue is presently unresolved. Most studies to date have involved a small number of subjects, analyzed the Apo E polymorphism post hoc, or included populations in which the effects might be modest, making discrepancies difficult to detect. Studies conducted with conditions representing a metabolic challenge have generally been more successful in finding differential effects across Apo E genotypes, and such studies may be helpful in the future to clarify Apo E gene nutrient relationships. The mixed results obtained indicate that, at present, it is premature to suggest the use of genotyping of Apo E in the design of therapeutic diet interventions (Rubin & Berglund., 2002).

All studies have demonstrated a strong association between plasma cholesterol and Apo E phenotypes in the following order: E4/E4 > E4/E3 > E3/E3 > E3/E2. It has been thought possible that the Apo E gene might be involved in the modulation of dietary plasma cholesterol responses, perhaps explaining the differences in cholesterol concentrations. Some dietary intervention studies have suggested that Apo E4 individuals react to dietary change with exaggerated cholesterol responses. In one study, Apo E4/E4 individuals responded by increased cholesterol reductions during low fat intake, and by increased cholesterol elevations during a switchback to high fat diet. Plausible mechanisms have been postulated which could explain such differences. However, other studies have reported no differences in plasma lipid responses among Apo E phenotypes. The studies cannot be directly compared because of different designs and study populations with differing Apo E allele frequencies (Tikkanen., 1995).

Although Tikkanen et al, found that subjects with the E4/4 phenotype showed the greatest total and LDL-cholesterol responses to dietary change (Tikkanen et al., 1995) Xu et al

analyzed the same data and concluded that the Apo E polymorphism did not explain a significant proportion of the variation of the response (Xu et al., 1990). In a meta-analysis of 9 studies involving 612 subjects and found that the presence of the E4 allele was associated with a significantly greater LDL response to dietary intervention (Masson et al, 2003).
Four studies found significantly different HDL-cholesterol responses between genotype groups: one study found that carriers of the E4 allele had the smallest HDL-cholesterol response, whereas the other 3 studies found that carriers of the E4 allele had the largest response (Masson et al., 2003).
However, recent evidence strongly suggests that variations in a number of key genes may also be important, including common variants of the Apo E gene. The most convincing evidence to date for genotypic effects on dietary response comes from the extensively studied Apo E gene variant (Lovegrove & Gitau., 2008).

5.5 Cholesteryl ester transfer protein (CETP)

Another gene that affects HDL levels is CETP, encoding for the cholesteryl ester transfer protein that exchanges cholesteryl esters and triglycerids from HDL to other lipoproteins. This protein is also called the "lipid transfer protein:' People with two copies of a common allele at position 279 of this gene tend to have low HDL levels and elevated levels of LDL and VLDL. A variation (279G>A) that decreases plasma levels of CETP is associated with increased HDL levels, decreased LDL and VLDL levels, and a lower risk of cardiovascular disease than the more common (GG) form (DeBusk, 2009; Musunuru., 2010).
A recent meta-analysis which confirms that the I405V and TaqIB variants are indeed associated with lower CETP activity and higher high-density lipoprotein-cholesterol levels (Boekholdt., 2004).
The currently available evidence suggests that several genetic variants in the CETP gene are associated with altered CETP plasma levels and activity, high-density lipoprotein-cholesterol plasma levels, low-density lipoprotein and high-density lipoprotein particle size, and perhaps the risk of coronary heart disease (Boekholdt., 2004).

5.6 Hepatic lipase (LIPC)

Hepatic lipase (HL) is a lipolytic enzyme involved in the hydrolysis of triacylglycerols present in circulating chylomicrons providing nonesterified fatty acids and 2-monoacylglycerol for tissue utilization and phospholipids from plasma lipoproteins that participates in metabolizing intermediate-density lipoprotein and large LDL into smaller, denser LDL particles, and in converting HDL2 to HDL3 during reverse cholesterol transport (Ordovas & Corella., 2004; Fisler, Warden, 2005; Ordovas., 2006; Much et al., 2005). It may suggest a role to play as a ligand for cell-surface proteoglycans in the uptake of lipoproteins by cell-surface receptors (Fisler & Warden., 2005; Ordovas & Corella., 2004).
Given the wide spectrum of effects that HL exerts on lipoprotein metabolism, and the significance of the promoter variant (s), it is reasonable to hypothesize that genetic variation at this locus may also be involved in variability in the response to dietary therapy (Ordovas & Corella., 2004). HL deficiency is characterized by mildly elevated concentrations of triglyceride-rich LDL and HDL particles, as well as impaired metabolism of postprandial triglyceride-rich lipoproteins, which may result in premature atherosclerosis. Conversely, increased HL activity is associated with increased small, dense LDL particles and decreased HDL2 concentrations, which may also result in increased CAD risk. Four common single

nucleotide polymorphisms (SNPs) on the 5_-flanking region of the HL gene (*LIPC*) [−763 (A/G), −710 (T/C), −514 (C/T), and -250 (G/A)] are in total linkage disequilibrium and define a unique haplotype that is associated with variation in HL activity and HDL-cholesterol levels (Fisler & Warden., 2005; Ordovas & Corella., 2004).
The less common A-allele of the SNP at position−250 is associated with lower HL activity and buoyant LDL particles. Normal and CAD subjects heterozygous for the A-allele have lower HL activity and significantly more buoyant LDL particles. Homozygosity for this allele (AA) is associated with an even lower HL activity. The A-allele is associated with higher HDL2-cholesterol (Ordovas & Corella., 2004).
An early intervention study with a low-saturated-fat, low-cholesterol diet found that, although significant improvements in fasting lipids occurred, there was no difference in response between genotypes at the hepatic lipase gene (LIPC) polymorphism measured. However, the study of 83 subjects may not have had adequate power to detect a modest effect of genotype (Fisler & Warden., 2005; Masson & McNeill., 2005; Ordovas., 2006).
Dietary information collected from Framingham Heart Study participants shows that subjects carrying the CC genotype react to higher contents of fat in their diets by increasing the concentrations of HDL-cholesterol, which could be interpreted as a "defense mechanism" to maintain the homeostasis of lipoprotein metabolism. Conversely, carriers of the TT genotype cannot compensate, and experience decreases on the HDL-cholesterol levels. These data could identify a segment of the population especially susceptible to diet-induced atherosclerosis. Considering the higher frequency of the T allele among certain ethnic groups (i. e., African-Americans), these data could shed some light on the impaired ability of certain ethnic groups to adapt to new nutritional environments, as clearly seen for Native Americans and Asian Indians. In this regard, they replicated the significant gene-diet interaction demonstrated in the Caucasian population of Framingham in another multiethnic cohort that consisted of Chinese, Malays, and Indians representing the population of Singapore. In addition to the significant gene-diet interactions reported in these papers, these data provides clues about the reasons why genotype-phenotype association studies fail to show consistent results. In theory, this polymorphism at the hepatic lipase gene will show dramatically different outcomes in association studies depending on the dietary environment of the population studies. The impact of these interactions will be magnified in populations with a high prevalence of the T-allele, as it is with Asians and African-Americans (Ordovas & Corella., 2004).
Three larger observational studies on the effect of a common polymorphism in the LIPC promoter gene -514C→T on the response of HDL cholesterol to dietary fat intake have been published. In examining the effects of the -514C→T LIPC polymorphism x dietary fat interaction on HDL in 2130 men and women participating in the Framingham Study, Ordovas et al found that the rarer *TT* genotype was associated with significantly higher HDL-cholesterol concentrations only in subjects consuming <30% of energy from fat. This same interaction was found for saturated and monounsaturated fats but not for polyunsaturated fat. A second association study, in an Asian population of 2170 subjects, found that Asian Indian subjects with a total fat intake of <30% of energy and with *TT* genotype at the -514C→T polymorphism had the highest HDL-cholesterol concentrations. This interaction, however, did not apply to the Chinese or Malay subjects in that study, and the significant interactions found for saturated or monounsaturated fats found by Ordovas et al were not found in the study by Tai et al. However, these 2 studies are consistent with

other studies showing that the *TT* genotype at -514C→T is associated with higher HDL concentrations, although, in 1 of those studies, this effect was attenuated by visceral obesity (Fisler & Warden., 2005).

The third association study of the interaction between dietary fat and the -514C→T polymorphism, by Zhang et al that, from a study population of 18159 men, Zhang et al selected 780 men with confirmed type 2 diabetes. After adjustment for age, smoking, alcohol intake, exercise, and BMI, higher HDL-cholesterol concentrations were found in men with the *CT* or *TT* genotype, which is consistent with previous studies. However, they found significantly higher HDL-cholesterol concentrations in men with the *CT/TT* genotype who consumed large amounts of dietary fat (≥32% of energy), saturated fat, and monounsaturated fat, a result that is apparently opposite to the findings of the other 2 association studies. Thus, the interaction effect of dietary fat with the -514C→T polymorphism was not replicated (Zhang et al., 2005).

Two researcher discussed causes of nonreplication of genetic association studies in obesity and diabetes research that should apply to studies of dyslipidemias as well. An important cause of nonreplication is a lack of statistical power. For any polygenic model, such as models with complex phenotypes (eg, obesity, dyslipidemia, or type 2 diabetes), the effect size for any marker will be small to moderate. Thus, larger sample sizes are needed to ensure adequate power to observe an effect. In the study of Zhang et al, the problem of small sample size (despite the fact that >18000 men were screened to identify ≈800 men with type 2 diabetes) is compounded by the fact that the *TT* genotype is rare, especially in a white population. Thus, only 30 subjects in that study had homozygous *TT* genotype at -514C→T LIPC, and subjects with either the *CT* or *TT* genotype were pooled for analysis. Examination of the data of Ordovas et al and Tai et al found that the slope of predicted values for HDL cholesterol versus total fat intake as a percentage of energy is steeply negative in persons with the *TT* genotype, whereas it is positive for persons with the *CT* genotype (Ordovas, et al, 2002; Tai et al, 2003). Assuming that the data of Zhang et al followed the same pattern, combining the smaller number (n = 30) of persons with the *TT* genotype with the larger number (n = 247) of persons with the *CT* genotype would mask the effects of percentage of dietary fat and the *TT* genotype on HDL-cholesterol concentrations. An additional complexity is that BMI and obesity phenotypes may also interact with dietary fat and LIPC genotype to modulate HDL-cholesterol concentrations (Tai et al., 2003; Zhang., 2005). Thus, the nonreplication in the study by Zhang et al of the findings of Ordovas et al and Tai et al is likely due to the small number of persons with the *TT* genotype who were available in the study of Zhang et al (Fisler & Warden., 2005).

5.7 Lipoprotein lipase (LPL)

LPL, encoding lipoprotein lipase, which hydrolyzes triglycerides in chylomicrons and VLDL particles, converting the latter to LDL particles, as well facilitating cellular lipoprotein uptake (Musunuru, 2010).

Several polymorphisms have been described that disrupt normal LPL function and contribute to the premature development of CHD, primarily through the increased levels of circulating TGs (Much et al., 2005).

Indeed, several of the common LPL polymorphisms described by Merkel et al have recently been established to influence circulating lipid levels in pregnant women, whom are often characterized with high levels of circulating TGs and increased total cholesterol (Merkel et al., 2011). Although TG levels were unaffected, certain LPL SNPs modulated HDL levels and may alter the susceptibility of pregnant women to developing CHD. However, further studies are required to definitively define a relationship between lipid levels, CHD, and pregnant women. Therefore, the importance of LPL in the whole-body regulation of lipid metabolism has been avidly demonstrated and merits further exploration.

One common LPL polymorphism, known as T495G *Hind* III, has been extensively examined and demonstrates the complexity of disease prediction associated with a single SNP. Indeed, preliminary indications suggest that this polymorphism may play a role in the onset of several important diseases, such as CHD, diabetes and obesity. This SNP has been associated with the higher plasma TG and lower HDL levels characteristic with the early onset of diabetes. Preliminary results have also suggested a positive association between the *Hind* III polymorphism and a predisposition to developing obesity. Finally, this polymorphism has been associated with variations in lipid levels and heart disease, and that these alterations were attenuated by such environmental factors as physical exercise and low calorie diets, reiterating the important interactions arising between lifestyle, nutrition, and disease. Although these associations are not conclusive, they do suggest that LPL variants play a critically important role in the regulation of whole-body lipid metabolism that may predispose an individual to the onset of several metabolic diseases.

A relationship was established between a low calorie diet and the circulating lipid profile in obese individuals with the *Hind* III polymorphism. Homozygotes (H2H2) were found to have significantly higher levels of plasma VLDL-TG and Apo B than heterozygotes. Caloric restriction reduced lipid levels in both H2H2 and H1 individuals to a point where no difference was observed between the groups. Although H2H2 individuals responded more strongly (larger decreases in plasma lipids) to the low calorie diet, these preliminary results identify an important relationship between LPL polymorphisms, function, and diet (Much et al., 2005).

As such, it is difficult to draw any firm conclusions from any one gene-diet study in the absence of replication by another study that examined the same question using similar methodologies. For example, one study demonstrated that a Mediterranean-style, MUFA-rich diet compared to a high-carbohydrate diet increased LDL size in individuals with certain Apo E gene variants but decreased LDL size in those with other Apo E variants; this is potentially a clinically important observation, but no confirmatory study has yet emerged, calling this observation into doubt. As pointed out by others, the field would greatly benefit from increased collaboration and coordination of studies among international nutrition researchers (Musunuru., 2010).

6. Magnitude of the response

Because of the heterogeneity in the type and duration of the interventions described the magnitude of the lipid response to dietary interventions varied widely: in one study the change in LDL cholesterol in the Apo B *Eco*RI *R-R-* genotype group was as large as 59% of the baseline concentration. In the studies that showed a significant difference in response between genotype groups, the results also varied widely: in some studies, the difference in response between 2 genotype groups was ≈20% of the baseline lipid concentration (Rantala et al., 2000; Clitfon., 1997). However, the magnitude of these differences cannot be estimated with any accuracy, largely because most studies had only a small number of subjects in the rare genotype group (Masson et al, 2003). The proportion of variance in the lipid response attributable to a single polymorphism is not likely to be > 10% (Xu et sal., 1990). Therefore, individual genes contribute only a small part to the variation in the lipid response; however, when several genes are considered, the proportion of variance explained could be larger (Masson et al, 2003).

7. Evidence for a gene-diet interaction

Evidence suggests that variation in the genes for apolipoproteins A-I, A-IV, B, and E may contribute to the heterogeneity in the lipid response to dietary intervention. Many studies were unable to show significantly different responses between these genotype groups, and the genotypes showing the greatest response are not necessarily consistent between studies. There was insufficient evidence to assess whether lipid responsiveness is affected by variation in the genes for Apo C-III, lipoprotein lipase, hepatic lipase, the cholesteryl ester transfer protein. Although each of these gene products is essential in lipid metabolism, only a handful of studies have investigated variation in these genes, and most of these studies were unable to show significant gene-diet interactions (Masson et al, 2003).

8. Publication bias

Publication bias is a problem with any review because "studies with results that are significant, interesting, from large well-funded studies, or of higher quality are more likely to be submitted, published, or published more rapidly than work without such characteristics" (Sutton, 2000). Therefore, it is possible that other relevant dietary intervention studies with genotype information exist but were not included in this review because they have not been published. It is possible that the literature strategy for this review missed studies because the genotype analyses were not mentioned in their title, abstract, or subject headings (Masson et al, 2003).

In the search for explanations for the heterogeneity in lipid responses, reviewers may tend to highlight studies showing significant effects of genetic variation while ignoring a large proportion of studies that found no such results. Studies showing nonsignificant or conflicting results cannot be ignored, especially because they outnumber the studies showing significant effects, notwithstanding the unpublished studies that could have nonsignificant and uninteresting results. Therefore, one has to ask the question "If genetic variability plays a role in the heterogeneity of lipid and lipoprotein responses to dietary change, why have so many studies been unable to demonstrate this with statistical significance?" (Masson et al, 2003).

9. Possible reasons for conflicting results

There are many possible reasons why studies have been unable to show statistically significant gene-diet interactions. First, it is highly probable that lipid responses to dietary change are under polygenic control, with each gene contributing a relatively small effect. However, most studies have attempted to find only single-gene effects (Masson et al, 2003). Most of the studies summarized in this review lacked sufficient statistical power to detect any but a very strong effect because the sample sizes were too small, particularly for genotypes with low frequencies of the rare allele. However, many of the studies were retrospective and were not designed to examine gene-diet interactions, but data were reexamined after the availability of new information from genotype analyses. Therefore, it is perhaps not surprising that significant effects were not found in many studies because the numbers of individuals in each genotype group were so small. In many studies there were too few subjects homozygous for the rare allele to allow an analysis that would take into account differences in the response between heterozygote's and homozygote's. For Apo E, where there are 6 possible genotypes, differences in the grouping of these could also lead to differences in results between studies. This illustrates that meta-analyses are important because they can detect effects with greater power and greater precision because of their inflated sample size (Rantala et al., 2000; Lopez-Miranda et al., 1994). In addition, in studies with small sample sizes, genotype misclassification of one individual may significantly affect the interpretation and validity of the results. Conflicting results may also occur because of the different dietary protocols that were followed. The studies reviewed varied widely in the composition and length of the baseline and experimental diets. The dietary factors responsible for the changes seen in each genotype group are not clear because many studies modified several dietary factors, and so the dietary content in future studies should be tightly controlled and compliance must be strictly measured not only for cholesterol and the amount and type of fatty acids but also for other influential dietary components such as fiber and plant sterols. In addition, these studies investigated fasting lipid and lipoprotein concentrations; however, the effect of genetic variation may be more evident in the postprandial state than in the less-common fasting state). Differences in the age, sex, body mass index, menopausal status, dietary backgrounds, and baseline lipid values of the participants could also have contributed to the discrepancies between the results. For instance, subjects with the E4 allele tend to have higher baseline total and LDL-cholesterol concentrations, and so greater responses in these subjects could reflect the regression to the mean phenomenon. It is also possible that weight change could account for differences in lipid and lipoprotein changes. In addition, a significant effect may not reflect a causal relation but the allele may be in linkage disequilibrium with another one that does. For example, the base change that results in the *Xba* I site in the gene for Apo B does not alter the amino acid, and so it may be in linkage disequilibrium with another functional mutation (Masson et al., 2003).

The studies varied widely in terms of the number and type of study participants, the composition and duration of the dietary interventions, the nutrients studied and dietary assessment methods used in the observational studies, and the polymorphisms analyzed - some of which had not been studied before with regard to the lipid response to diet (Masson et al., 2005).

10. Conclusion

Evidence suggests that genetic variation may contribute to the heterogeneity in lipid responsiveness. At present, the evidence is limited but suggestive and justifies the need for future studies with much larger sample sizes based on power calculations, with carefully controlled dietary interventions, and that investigate the effects of polymorphisms in multiple genes rather than in single genes. Investigating gene-diet interactions will increase our knowledge of the mechanisms involved in lipid metabolism and improve our understanding of the role of diet in reducing cardiovascular disease risk (Masson et al., 2003).

Future studies will have to be large in order to assess the effects of multiple polymorphisms, and will have to control for many factors other than diet. At present, it is premature to recommend the use of genotyping in the design of therapeutic diets. However, such studies may be useful in identifying the mechanisms by which dietary components influence lipid levels (Masson & McNeill., 2005).

However, current knowledge is still very limited and so is the potential benefit of its application to clinical practice. Thinking needs to evolve from simple scenarios (e. g., one single dietary component, a single nucleotide polymorphism and risk factor) to more realistic situations involving multiple interactions. One of the first situations where personalized nutrition is likely to be beneficial is in patients with dyslipidemia who require special intervention with dietary treatment. This process could be more efficient if the recommendations were carried out based on genetic and molecular knowledge. Moreover, adherence to dietary advice may increase when it is supported with information based on nutritional genomics, and a patient believes the advice is personalized. However, a number of important changes in the provision of health care are needed to achieve the potential benefits associated with this concept, including a teamwork approach with greater integration among physicians, food and nutrition professionals, and genetic counselors (Ordovas., 2006).

The ultimate goal of nutritional genomics is to provide sufficient knowledge to allow diagnosis and nutritional treatment recommendations based on an individual's genotype. Defining the interaction effects of nutrients and genes on complex phenotypes will be the challenge of this field of nutrition research for some time to come (Fisler & Warden, 2005; Gregori et al, 2011; Ordovas & Corella., 2004).

11. Ethic

Although an increased understanding of how these and other genes influence response to nutrients should facilitate the progression of personalized nutrition, the ethical issues surrounding its routine use need careful consideration (Lovegrove & Gitau., 2008).

The study of nutrigenetics is in its infancy. Many studies published in this area have only considered one SNP in a single gene, with little consideration being given to multiple nutrient-gene-environmental interactions. Although this is scientifically valid, and invaluable for the elucidation of causative mechanisms in disease, multiple gene-nutrient-environment-gender interactions will be required for developing specific personalized nutritional advice. The collation of data in haplotype databases and biobanks is expensive and difficult to establish, but is a necessity if nutrigenetic research is to progress (Lovegrove & Gitau., 2008).

Standardized protocols in nutrigenetics are not yet established, the comparison of studies is challenging and conclusions are often difficult to draw. As discussed previously, studies are often retrospective in design and thus of insufficient power to detect nutrient-gene associations. Prospective genotyping increases the power to resolve these associations and should be used whenever possible. With any research, publication bias results in positive associations being reported more often than negative associations. This has applied to nutrigentic studies and created a false impression of the level of significance of many nutrient-gene interactions (Lovegrove & Gitau., 2008).

There are numerous ethical issues and unavoidable assumptions that need to be considered before personalized nutritional can become routine practice. First, it is important to consider whether the genetic tests and personalized food products would be affordable, cost-effective and socially acceptable. It is also of concern that only the well educated and affluent would benefit. The open accessibility of genetic information to third parties has major implications for the availability of health insurance and increased premiums (Lovegrove, Gitau, 2008).

Moreover, it is still unknown whether people will want to undertake genetic tests or even understand the concept of such technology. A survey was conducted by Cogent Research in 2003 on 1000 Americans in which 62% of respondents reported they had never heard of 'nutrigenomics'. However, if specific products did arise from nutrigenomic research, those interviewed did express interest in an in-depth well-being assessment and also a strong interest in vitamins, fortified foods and natural foods. More research is required to determine whether individuals would want to undergo such tests, and for understanding the value to the individual of an increased awareness of personalized nutrition regimens. There is already a large gap between the existing dietary guidelines and what people actually eat. Knowledge of being at higher than average risk of CVD may motivate people to actually make positive changes to their diets. However, genetic testing could undermine current healthy eating messages, by implying that only those with the 'risky gene' need to eat a healthy diet. These are important unanswered questions that must be addressed if personalized nutritional advice is ever to become part of mainstream disease prevention and treatment. It may be that the interactions between genotype-phenotype and the environment are just too complex to be properly understood from human dietary intervention studies (Lovegrove, Gitau, 2008).

There is resistance to the use and perceived effectiveness of personalized nutrition that is based on genomics, and whether this can offer a solution to diseases caused by a diet that is inappropriate for health (Canon & Leitzmann, 2005). It has been suggested that it may be more beneficial to use current risk factors as a basis for population screening and the management of CVD (McCluskey et al., 2007). There has also been dialogue on the social, economic and environmental causes of CVD, shifting the emphasis away from dietary intake to food manufacturing as being more effective in disease management (Canon & Leitzmann, 2005; Lovegrove & Gitau., 2008).

Progression of knowledge in the fields of nutrient-gene interactions promises a future revolution in preventative health care. However, although there is increasing evidence for interactions between diets/nutrients, genes and environmental factors, there are inconsistencies in the evidence that will limit the application of nutrigenetics in diet-related disease in the immediate future. In addition to the need for adequately powered intervention studies, greater attention should be given to ethical issues, such as the public's acceptance of genetic testing and the economics of this relatively new science (Lovegrove & Gitau., 2008).

Ethical issues fall into a number of categories: (1) why nutrigenomics? Will it have important public health benefits? (2) questions about research, e. g. concerning the acquisition of information about individual genetic variation; (3) questions about who has access to this information, and its possible misuse; (4) the applications of this information in terms of public health policy, and the negotiation of the potential tension between the interests of the individual in relation to, for example, prevention of conditions such as obesity and allergy; (5) the appropriate ethical approach to the issues, e. g. the moral difference, if any, between therapy and enhancement in relation to individualised diets; whether the 'technological fix' is always appropriate, especially in the wider context of the purported lack of public confidence in science, which has special resonance in the sphere of nutrition (Chadwick., 2004).

12. References

Amouyel, P. (2000). Genomics and cardiovascular diseases. *Bull Acad Natl Med.* 184 (7):1431-8.

Boekholdt, SM. & Kuivenhoven, JA. & Hovingh, GK. & Jukema, JW. & Kastelein, JJ. & van, Tol A. (2004). CETP gene variation: relation to lipid parameters and cardiovascular risk. *Curr Opin Lipidol.* 15 (4):393-8.

Campos, H. & D'Agostino, M. & Ordovas, JM. (2001). Gene±diet interactions and plasma lipoproteins: role of apolipoprotein E and habitual saturated fat intake. *Genet Epidemiol;* 20:117±128.

Canon, G. & Leitzmann, C. (2005). The new nutrition science Progect. *Public Health Nutr.* : 8 (6A):673-694.

Carmena-Ramon, R. & Ascaso, J F. & Real, J T. & Ordovas, J M. (1998). Genetic Variation at the ApoA-IV Gene Locus and Response to Diet in Familial Hypercholesterolemia. *Arteriosclerosis, Thrombosis, and Vascular Biology.* 18:1266- 1274.

Chadwick, R. (2004). Nutrigenomics, individualism and public health. *Proc Nutr Soc.* 63 (1):161-6.

Clifton, P. & Kind, K. & Jones, C. & , Noakes, M. (1997). Response to dietary fat and cholesterol and genetic polymorphisms. *Clin Exp Pharmacol Physiol;*24:A21–5.

Corella, D. & Tucker, K. & Lahoz, C. & Coltell, O. & Cupples, L A. & Wilson, P WF. & Schaefer, E J. & Ordovas, J M. (2001). Alcohol drinking determines the effect of the *APOE* locus on LDL-cholesterol concentrations in men: the Framingham Offspring Study. *American Journal of Clinical Nutrition.* 73 (4): 736-745.

Couch, SC. & Isasi, CR. & Karmally. W, et al. (2000). Predictors of postprandial triacylglycerol response in children: the Columbia University Biomarkers Study. *Am J Clin Nutr.* 72:1119±1127.

Debra A. K. (2008). Medical Nutrition Therapy For Cardiovascular Disease. In Mahan KL, Escoott- Stump S (eds). *Krause's Food Nutrition and Diet Therapy.* Suanders. 12th ed. Philadelphia. 833-864. DeBusk, R. . (2008). Nutritional genomic. In Mahan KL, Escoott-Stump S (eds). *Krause's Food Nutrition and Diet Therapy.* 12th ed. Suanders. Philadelphia. Pp: 364- 382.

DeBusk, R M. (2009). Nutritional Genomics: The Foundation for Personalized Nutrition, What Is Nutritional Genomicsl. *In Advanced nutrition and human metabolism.* Sareen S. G, Jack L. Smith, James L. G. FIFTH EDITION. *WADSWORTH-CENGAGE Learning*". USA. pp 29-32.

Dreon, DM. & Fernstrom, HA. & Miller, B. & , Krauss, RM. (1995). Apolipoprotein E isoform phenotype and LDL subclass response to a reduced-fat diet. *Arterioscler Thromb Vasc Biol;* 15:105±111.

El-Sohemy, A. (2007). Nutrigenetics. *Forum Nutr.* 60:25-30.

Engler, M B. (2009). Nutrigenomics in Cardiovascular Disease: Implications for the Future. *Progress in Cardiovascular Nursing.* 24 (4): 190–195.

Farhud, D. & Shalileh, M. (2008). Phenylketonuria and its Dietary Therapy in Children. Iran J Pediatr. 18 (Suppl 1):88-98.

Farhud, DD. & Zarif Yeganeh, M. & Zarif Yeganeh, M. *(2010).* Nutrigenomics and Nutrigenetics. *Iranian J Public Health.* 39 (4) :1-14.

Fenech, M. (2008). Genome health nutrigenomics and nutrigenetics-dignosis and nutritional treatment of genome damage on an individual basis. *FdChem Tox*. 46 (4):1365-70.

Fisler, J S. & Warden, C H. (2005). Dietary fat and genotype: toward individualized prescriptions for lifestyle changes. *American Journal of Clinical Nutrition*. 81 (6): 1255-1256.

Friedlander, Y. & Leitersdorf, E. & Vecsler, R. et al. (2000). The contribution of candidate genes to the response of plasma lipids and lipoproteins to dietary challenge. *Atherosclerosis*. 152:239±248.

Frikke-Schmidt R. (2000). Context-dependent and invariant associations between APOE genotype and levels of lipoproteins and risk of ischemic heart disease: a review. *Scand J Clin Lab Invest*. 60 (Suppl. 233):3±26.

Gillies, P J. (2003). Nutrigenomics : the Rubicon of molecular nutrition. *J am Diet Ass*. 103 (12 suppl 2):50-55.

Gregori, D. & Foltran, F. & Verduci, E. & Ballali, S. & Franchin, L. & Ghidina, M. &. Halpern, G M. & Giovannini, M. (2011). A Genetic Perspective on Nutritional Profiles: Do We Still Need Them?. *J Nutrigenet Nutrigenomic*. 4 (1):25-35.

Hank Juo, S-H. & Wyszynski, D F. & Beaty, T H. & Huang, H-Y. & Bailey-W, J E. (1999). Mild association between the A/G polymorphism in the promoter of the apolipoprotein A-I gene and apolipoprotein A-I levels: A meta- analysis. *American Journal of Medical Genetics*. 82 (3):235-241.

Heilbronn a, L. K., & Noakes b, M. & Morris a, A. M. & Kind b, K. L. & Clifton, P. M. (2000). 360His polymorphism of the apolipoproteinA-IV gene and plasma lipid response to energy restricted diets in overweight subjects. *Atherosclerosis*. 150: 187–192.

Hernell, O. & West. C. (2008). Do we need personalized recommendations for infants at risk of developing disease? *Nestle Nutr Workshop ser Pediatr Program*. 62:239-49; discussion 249-52.

Hockey, K. J. & Anderson, R. A. & Cook, V. R. & Hantgan, R. R. & Weinberg R. B. (2001)Effect of the apolipoprotein A-IV Q360H polymorphism on postprandial plasma triglyceride clearance. *J. Lipid Res.* . 42: 211–217.

Isasi, CR. & Couch, SC. & Deckelbaum, RJ. et al. (2000). The apolipoprotein e2 allele is associated with an anti- atherogenic lipoprotein profile in children: the Columbia University Biomarkers Study. *Pediatrics*; 106:568±575.

Jarvik, GP., & Goode, EL. & Austin, MA, et al. (1997). Evidence that the apolipoprotein Egenotype effects on lipid levels can change with age in males: a longitudinal analysis. *Am J Hum Genet*; 61:171±181.

Kobayashi, J. & Saito, Y. & Taira, K. & Hikita, M. & , Takahashi, K. & Bujo, H. & Morisaki, N. & Saito, Y. (2001). Effect of apolipoprotein E3.4 phenotype on postprandial triglycerides and retinyl palmitate metabolism in plasma from hyperlipidemic subjects in Japan. *Atherosclerosis*. 154; 539–546.

Kusmann, M. & Fsy, L B. (2008). nutrigenomics and personalized nutrition:science and concept. *Personalized Medicine*. 5 (5):447-455.

Loktionov, A. & Scollen, S. & McKeown, N. & Bingham S. (2000). Gene±nutrient interactions: dietary behavior associated with high coronary heart disease risk particularly affects serum LDL cholesterol in apolipoprotein E (4-carrying free-living individuals. *Br J Nutr*. 84:885±890.

Lopez-Miranda, J. & Ordovas, JM. & Mata, P, et al. (1994). Effect of apolipoprotein E phenotype on diet-induced lowering of plasma low density lipoprotein cholesterol. *J Lipid Res*. 35:1965–75.

Lovegrove, J. A. & Gitau, R. (2008). Personalized nutrition for the prevention of cardiovascular disease: a future perspective. *Journal of Human Nutrition and Dietetics*. 21 (4) : 306–316.

Mahley, RW. & PeÂ, pin J. & Erhan, Paraoglu K, et al. (2000). Low levels of high density lipoproteins in Turks, a population with elevated hepatic lipase: high density lipoprotein characterization and gender-specific effects of apolipoprotein E genotype. *J Lipid Res*. 41:1290±1301.

Masson, L F. & McNeill, G. & Avenell, A. (2003). Genetic variation and the lipid response to dietary intervention: a systematic review. *American Journal of Clinical Nutrition*. 77 (5): 1098-1111.

Masson, L F. & McNeill, G. (2005). The effect of genetic variation on the lipid response to dietary change: recent findings. *Current Opinion in Lipidology*. 16 (1):61-67.

McCluskey, S. & Baker, D. & Perey, D. & Lewis, P. & Middleton, E. (2007). Reduction in cardiovascular risk in association with population screening : a 10- year longitudinal study. *J Public Heaht (oxf)*. 29:379-387.

Merkel, M. & Eckel, R H. & Goldberg, I J. (2011). Lipoprotein lipase: genetics, lipid uptake and regulation
URL:www. jlr. org. on July 26.

Miggiano, GA. & De Sanctis, R. (2006). Nutritional genomics: toward a personalized diet. *Clin Ter*. 157 (4):355-61.

Musunuru, K. (2010). Atherogenic Dyslipidemia: Cardiovascular Risk and Dietary Intervention. *Lipids*. 45:907–914.

Mutch, D M. & Wahli, W. & Gary, W. (2005). Nutrigenomics and nutrigenetics: the emerging faces of nutrition. *The FASEB Journal*. 19:1602-1616.

Ordovas, J. M. (2002). Gene-diet interaction and plasma lipid responses to dietary intervention. *Biochemical Society Transactions*. 30: (68–73).

a.Ommen, B V. (2004). Nutrigenomics: Exploiting Systems Biology in the Nutrition and Health Arenas. *Nutrition*. 20:4–8.

b.Ordovas, JM. (2004). The quest for cardiovascular health in the genomic era : nutrigenetics and plasma lipoproteins. *Proc Nutr Soc*. 63 (1):145-152.

Ordovas JM, Corella D. (2004). Nutritional genomics. *Annu Rev Genomics Hum Genet*. 5:71-118.

Ordovas JM, Mooser V. (2004). Nutrigenomics and nutrigenetics. *Curr Opin Lipidol*. 15 (2):101-8.

Ordovas, J. M. (2006). Nutrigenetics, plasma lipids and cardiovascular risk. *Journal Of The American Dietetic Association*. 106 (7):1074-81.

Ordovas. J M. & Kaput, J. & Corella, D. (2007). Nutrition in the genomics era: Cardiovascular disease risk and the Mediterranean diet. *Molecular Nutrition & Food Research*. 51 (10) :1293–1299.

Ordovas, J M. (2009). Genetic influences on blood lipids and cardiovascular disease risk: tools for primary prevention. *American Journal of Clinical Nutrition*. 89 (5):1509S-1507S.

Perez-Martinez, P. & Garcia-Rios, A. & Delgado-Lista, J. & Perez-Jimenez, F. & Lopez-Miranda, J. (2011). Nutrigenetics of the postprandial lipoprotein metabolism: evidences from human intervention studies. *Curr Vasc Pharmacol.* 9 (3):287-91.

Rantala, M. & Rantala, TT. & Savolainen, MJ. & Friedlander, Y. & Kesaniemi, YA. (2000). Apolipoprotein B gene polymorphisms and serum lipids: meta-analysis of the role of genetic variation in responsiveness to diet. *Am J Clin Nutr.* 71:713–24.

Rideout, T C. (2011). Getting personal: considering variable interindividual responsiveness to dietary lipid-lowering therapies. *Current Opinion in Lipidology.* 22 (1): 37–42 .

Rimbach, G. & Minihane, A M. (2009). nutrigenetics and personalized nutrition:how far have we progressed and are we likely to get there? *Proceedings of the Nutrition Society.* 68 (2): 162-172.

Rubin, J. & Berglund, L. (2002). Apolipoprotein E and diets: a case of gene-nutrient interaction? *Current Opinion in Lipidology.* 13:25±32.

Ryan-Harshman, M. & Vogel, E. & Jones-Taggart, H. & Green-Johnson, J. & Castle, D. & Austin, Z. & Anderson, K. (2008). Nutritional genomics and dietetic professional practice. Kristin Anderson Can J Diet Pract Res. 69 (4):177-82.

Shalileh, M. & , Shidfar, F. & Eghtesadi, SH. & Haghani, H. & Heidari, I. (2009). The Effects of Calcium Supplement on Serum Lipoprotein in Obese Adults Receiving Energy Restricted Diet. *Iranian J Publ Health. 38 (4):10-20.*

Shalileh, M. & , Shidfar, F. & Haghani, H. & Eghtesadi, SH. & Heidari, I. (2010). The influence of calcium supplement on body composition, weight loss and insulin resistance in obese adults receiving low calorie diet. JRMS; 15 (4):1-11.

Sheweta, B. & Deepak, M. & BS Khatkar. (2011). Nutrigenomics :The emerging face of nutrition. *International Journal of Current Research and Review.* 3 (6) :108-113.

Subbiah, M T R. (2007). Nutrigenetics and nutraceuticals: the next wave riding on personalized medicine. *Transl res.* 149 (2):55-61.

Sutton, A J. & Duval, S J. & Tweedie, R L. & Abrams, K R. & Jones, D R. *(2000).* Empirical assessment of effect of publication bias on meta-analyse. *BMJ.* 320 : 1574

Svacina, S. (2007)Nutrigenetics and nutrigenomics. *Cas Lek Cesk.* 146 (11):837-9.

Tai, E S. & Corella, D. & Deurenberg-Yap, M. & Cutter, J. & Chew Kai, S. & Tan, C E. & Ordovas, J M. (2003). Dietary Fat Interacts with the -514C>T Polymorphism in the Hepatic Lipase Gene Promoter on Plasma Lipid Profiles in a Multiethnic Asian Population: The 1998 Singapore National Health Survey. *J Nutr.* 133:3399-3408.

Tikkanen, M. & Huttunen, JK. & Pajukanta, PE. & Pietinen, P. (1995). Apolipoprotein E polymorphism and dietary plasma cholesterol response. *Can J Cardiol.* 11:93G-96G.

URL: en. wikipedia. org/wiki/Dyslipidemia.

URL : http://www. who. int/mediacentre/factsheets/fs317/en/index. html

Wallace, A J. & E Humphries, S. & Fisher, R M. & Mann, J I. & Chisholm, A. & Sutherland, W H F. (2000). Genetic factors associated with response of LDL subfractions to change in the nature of dietary fat. *Atherosclerosis.* ; 149 (2) : 387-394.

Weggemans, RM. & Zock, PL. & Ordovas JM, et al. (2001). Apoprotein E genotype and the response of serum cholesterol to dietary fat, cholesterol and cafestol. *Atherosclerosis.* 154:547±555.

Weinberg, R B. & Geissinger, B W. & Kasala, K. & Hockey, K J. & James G, T. & Easter, L. & Crouse, R. (2000). Effect of apolipoprotein A-IV genotype and dietary fat on cholesterol absorption in humans. *J Lipid Res.* 41: 2035–2041.

Weinberg RB. (2002). Apolipoprotein A-IV polymorphisms and diet-gene interactions. *Curr Opin Lipidol.* 13 (2):125-34.

Wood, Philip A. (2008). Potential of nutrigenetics in the treatment of metabolic disorders. Expert Review of Endocrinology and Metabolism. 3 (6): 705-713.

Xacur-García F, Castillo-Quan JI, Hernández-Escalante VM, Laviada-Molina H. (2008). Nutritional genomics: an approach to the genome-environment interaction. *Rev Med Chil.* Nov. 136 (11):1460-7.

Xu, CF. & Boerwinkle, E. & Tikkanen, MJ. & Huttunen, JK. & Humphries, SE. & Talmud, PJ. (1990). Genetic variation at the apolipoprotein gene loci contribute to response of plasma lipids to dietary change. *Genet Epidemiol;* 7:261–75.

Zak, A. & Slaby, A. (2007). Gene - diet interactions in atherogenic dyslipidemias (part1). *Cas Lek Cesk.* 146 (12):896-901.

Zhang, C. & Lopez-Ridaura, R. & Rimm, E B. & Rifai, Nr. & Hunter, D J. & Hu, F B. (2005). Interactions between the -514C→T polymorphism of the hepatic lipase gene and lifestyle factors in relation to HDL concentrations among US diabetic men. *American Journal of Clinical Nutrition.* 81 (6):1429-1435.

4

Impact of Climate Change and Air Pollution on Dyslipidemia and the Components of Metabolic Syndrome

Roya Kelishadi[1] and Parinaz Poursafa[2]
[1]*Faculty of Medicine & Child Health Promotion Research Center, Isfahan University of Medical Sciences, Isfahan,*
[2]*Environment Research Center, Isfahan University of Medical Sciences, Isfahan, Iran*

1. Introduction

Environmental factors, notably climate change and air pollution influence health before conception, and continue during pregnancy, childhood, and adolescence. Experts have suggested that such health hazards may represent the greatest public health challenge humanity has faced. The accumulation of greenhouse gases such as carbon dioxide, primarily from burning fossil fuels results in warming, which has an impact on air pollution, particularly on levels of ozone and particulates. Heat-related health effects include increased rates of pregnancy complications, pre-eclampsia, eclampsia, low birth weight, renal effects, vector-borne diseases as malaria and dengue; increased diarrheal and respiratory disease, food insecurity, decreased quality of foods (notably grains), malnutrition, water scarcity, exposures to toxic chemicals, worsened poverty, natural disasters, and population displacement. Air pollution has many adverse health effects, which would have long-term impact on the components of the metabolic syndrome. In addition to short-term effects as premature labor, intrauterine growth retardation, neonatal and infant mortality rate, malignancies (notably leukemia and Hodgkin lymphoma), respiratory diseases, allergic disorders and anemia, exposure to criteria air pollutants from early life might be associated with dyslipidemia, increase in stress oxidative, inflammation and endothelial dysfunction which in turn might have long-term effects on chronic non-communicable diseases.

2. Environmental factors: Climate change and air pollution

2.1 Air pollutants

Air pollution is a mixture of solid particles and gases in the air. The six common and hazardous air pollutants consist of particulate matter, ground-level ozone, carbon monoxide, sulfur oxides, nitrogen oxides, and lead; of which, particle pollution and ground-level ozone are the most widespread health hazards (Samet & Krewski, 2007; Chen & Kan, 2008).

Particulate matter or PM consists of a diverse mixture of very small particles and liquid droplets suspended in air. The PM size is directly related to their potential for affecting health. Particles with diameter < 10 micrometers are the particles that usually pass through the throat and nose to enter the lungs. Then, they can affect different body organs especially the heart and lungs, and may cause serious health effects. According to the size, the particle pollution is grouped into: "inhalable coarse particles" which have a diameter of 2.5 to 10 micrometers, and are found near roadways and industries, and "fine particles" < 2.5 micrometers in diameter such as those found in smoke and haze; they can form when gases emitted from power plants, industries and automobiles react in the air. Ozone (O3) is a gas composed of three oxygen atoms. In the presence of sunlight, it is created at ground-level by a chemical reaction between oxides of nitrogen and volatile organic compounds. Ozone might have harmful effects when formed in the earth's lower atmosphere, i.e. at ground-level. Hot weather and sunlight cause ground-level ozone to form in harmful concentrations in the air. Carbon monoxide (CO) is an odorless and colorless gas formed by incomplete carbon combustion. It is mainly emitted from the motor vehicle exhaust followed by non-road engines as construction equipment, industrial processes and wood burning. The increasing number of cars has an important role in the increase in CO emission worldwide. Sulfur Dioxide (SO2) is a gas formed when fuel containing sulfur, such as coal and oil, is burned, and when gasoline is extracted from oil or metals are extracted from ore. Nitrogen oxides (Nox) are a group of highly reactive gases containing various levels of nitrogen and oxygen. Lead is usually emitted from motor vehicles and industrial sources (Chen & Kan, 2008; Brook et al., 2004). Other stationary sources are waste incinerators, utilities, and lead-acid battery manufacturers. In addition to exposure to lead in air, other major exposure pathways include ingestion of lead in drinking water and lead-contaminated food as well as incidental ingestion of lead-contaminated soil and dust. Lead-based paint remains a major exposure pathway in older homes. Some toys might contain considerable amounts of lead that would be harmful for children's health (Samet & Krewski, 2007; Han & Naeher, 2006).

2.2 Climate change

Climate change and global warming have various health hazards (Poursafa & Kelishadi 2011).

Climate change has an impact on levels of ozone and particulate matters, which are both associated with various health hazards. The accumulation of greenhouse gases such as carbon dioxide, primarily from burning fossil fuels results in warming. Heat increases ground level ozone production, which in turn augments morbidity and mortality (Bell et al., 2007). Moreover, warming increases water vapor and ground-level ozone formation, and will result in harmful ozone levels (Jacob & Winner, 2009). Warming modify the risk of forest fires, and may generate massive amounts of carcinogens, as formaldehyde and benzene, potent lung irritants, as acrolein and other aldehydes, carbon monoxide, and particulates (Wegesser et al., 2009).

3. Association of environmental factors and dyslipidemia

Environmental factors are associated with many chronic diseases. Air pollution and climate change are associated with risk factors of non-communicable diseases in children and adolescents (Kelishadi et al., 2009; Sheffield & Landrigan, 2011; Kelishadi & Poursafa, 2010; Mansourian et al., 2010; Poursafa et al., 2011; Kargarfard et al., 2011).

The effects of environmental factors on intrauterine growth retardation and preterm labor are well documented. In turn, low birth weight (Sinclair et al., 2007) and prematurity (Evensen et al., 2008) would increase the risk of chronic non-communicable diseases and their risk factors. Exposure to air pollutants is reported to be associated with stress oxidative and markers of insulin resistance (Kelishadi et al., 2010) as well as with diabetes mellitus (Brook et al., 2008). These systemic responses to environmental factors can potentially increase the risk for dyslipidemia, development of the metabolic syndrome, hypertension, and other chronic diseases.Moreover, it is documented that some environmental factors as increased humidity are associated with preeclampsia and eclampsia, and their related consequences (Subramaniam, 2007).

Several reports exist on the association of environmental factors with dyslipidemia and the components of metabolic syndrome. By applying generalized additive models, Secondary analyses of a Taiwanese survey in 2002 demonstrated that increased particulate matter with aerodynamic diameters <10 microm was associated with elevated systolic blood pressure, triglycerides, apolipoprotein B, hemoglobin A1c, and reduced high-density lipoprotein (HDL) cholesterol. Elevated ozone was associated with increased diastolic blood pressure, apolipoprotein B, and hemoglobin A1c (Chuang et al., 2010). Genetic-environment interactions may have a role in this regard (Eisenberg et al., 2010).

The associations of both obesity and air pollution with several age-related diseases remain poorly understood with regard to causality and underlying mechanisms. Exposure to both, excess body fat and particulate matter, is accompanied by systemic low-grade inflammation as well as alterations in insulin/insulin-like growth factor signaling and cell cycle control. Understanding the causality of exposure disease associations and differences in susceptibilities to environment and lifestyle is an important aspect for effective prevention (Probst-Hensch, 2010).

A case-control study evaluated the effects of urban pollution on the lipid balance of members of a municipal police force in comparison with controls. Mean and frequency distributions of HDL-cholesterol and triglycerides had significant difference between the exposed traffic police group and controls. This study suggested that some chemical agents, as carbon dioxide, of the urban pollution could cause dyslipidemia among exposed people (Tomao et al., 2002).

A study among asthmatic patients showed that with a 1-microg/m3 increase in coarse PM, triglycerides increased 4.8% ($p = 0.02$), and very low-density lipoprotein increased 1.15% ($p = 0.01$). This study suggested that small temporal increases in ambient coarse PM are sufficient to affect lipid profile in adults with asthma (Yeatts et al., 2007).

Hypercholesterolemia may potentiate diesel exhaust-related endothelial gene regulation. These regulated transcripts may implicate pathways involved in the acceleration of atherosclerosis by air pollution (Maresh et al., 2011). The systemic pro-inflammatory and pro-thrombotic response to the inhalation of fine and ultrafine particulate matters may be associated with platelet activation (Poursafa & Kelishadi, 2010 platelets).

A study conducted in Greece, explored the relations between ambient environmental factors and arterial stiffness, peripheral and central hemodynamics in a cohort of 1222 participants.It found that the exposure to lower environmental temperatures is related to impaired hemodynamics not only to the periphery but also to the aorta. In men, PM10 levels were associated with intensified amplitude of the reflection wave resulting in significant alterations in central-pulse pressure (Adamopoulos et al., 2010).

A study examined the associations of PM2.5 with heart rate variability, a marker of autonomic function, and whether metabolic syndrome modified these associations. It found significant correlations; which were stronger among individuals with metabolic syndrome than among those without it. This study proposed that autonomic dysfunction may be a mechanism through which PM exposure affects cardiovascular risk, especially among persons with metabolic syndrome (Park et al., 2010).

Exposure to high and low air temperatures are associated with cardiovascular mortality, the underlying mechanisms are still under investigation. In a cohort in the US, 478 men with a mean age of 74.2 years were followed up from 1995 to 2008. Associations of three temperature variables, i.e. ambient, apparent, and dew point temperature with serum lipid profile were studied with linear mixed models by including possible confounders such as air pollution and a random intercept for each individual. HDL decreased -1.76%, and -5.58% for each 5°C increase in mean ambient temperature. For the same increase in mean ambient temperature, LDL increased by 1.74% and 1.87%. Similar results were also found for apparent and dew point temperatures. No changes were found in total cholesterol or triglycerides in relation to temperature increase. This study suggested that changes in HDL and LDL levels, which are associated with an increase in ambient temperature, may be among the underlying mechanisms of temperature-related cardiovascular mortality (Halonen et al., 2011).

A study in Taiwan found that increased 1-year average ozone, PM and nitrogen dioxide were associated with elevated blood pressure, total cholesterol, fasting glucose, and HbA1c. PM2.5 was more significantly associated with end-point variables than other gaseous pollutants (Chuang et al., 2011). A study on the association of blood markers of cardiovascular risk and air pollution in a national sample of the U.S. population found that PM_{10}, but not gaseous air pollutants, is associated with blood markers of cardiovascular risk (Schwartz, 2001). In a study in Italy, the carboxyhaemoglobin concentration had an inverse correlation with HDL-C (Biava et al., 1992). In addition to the outdoor environment, the health hazards of indoor pollution should be considered (Kaplan, 2010).

In recent years, global climate change has affected many biological and environmental factors. Of its most important effects are the increasing levels of atmospheric carbon dioxide, ultraviolet radiation, and ocean temperatures. In turn, they have resulted in decreased marine phytoplankton growth and reduced synthesis of omega-3 polyunsaturated fatty acids. It is suggested that the detrimental effects of climate change on the oceans may reduce the availability of dietary omega-3, which may have detrimental effects on serum lipid profile (Kang, 2011).

4. Conclusion

Climate change may alter concentrations of air pollutants or alterations in mechanisms of pollutant transport and thus influence individual and public health. The potential impacts of climate change and air pollution on lipid disorders is considered as an important area of investigation. This is of special concern for low- and middle-income countries, where the burden of air pollution and climate-related health disorders, and the burden of non-communicable diseases are emerging. Effects of environmental factors on dyslipidemia should be considered in primordial and primary prevention of chronic diseases from early life.

5. References

Adamopoulos D, Vyssoulis G, Karpanou E, Kyvelou SM, Argacha JF, Cokkinos D, Stefanadis C, van de Borne P.Environmental determinants of blood pressure, arterial stiffness, and central hemodynamics. J Hypertens 2010;28(5):903-9.

Bell ML, Goldberg R, Hogrefe C, *et al.* Climate change, ambient ozone, and health in 50 US cities. Climatic Change 2007; 82:61-76.

Biava PM, Audisio R, Centonze A, Barbieri A, Bisanti L, Duca G. [An epidemiological study of the health conditions of Milan traffic police with respect to pollution from vehicular traffic]. Lav 1992;83(3):249-58.

Brook RD, Franklin B, Cascio W. Expert Panel on Population and Prevention Science of the American Heart Association. Air pollution and cardiovascular disease: a statement for healthcare professionals from the Expert Panel on Population and Prevention Science of the American Heart Association. Circulation 2004; 109: 2655-71.

Chen B, Kan H. Air pollution and population health: a global challenge.Environ Health Prev Med 2008;13:94-101.

Chuang KJ, Yan YH, Cheng TJ. Effect of air pollution on blood pressure, blood lipids, and blood sugar: a population-based approach. J Occup Environ Med 2010;52(3):258-62.

Eisenberg DT, Kuzawa CW, Hayes MG. Worldwide allele frequencies of the human apolipoprotein E gene: climate, local adaptations, and evolutionary history. Am J Phys Anthropol 2010;143(1):100-11.

Evensen KA, Steinshamn S, Tjønna AE, Stølen T, Høydal MA, Wisløff U, et al. Effects of preterm birth and fetal growth retardation on cardiovascular risk factors in young adulthood. Early Hum Dev 2008: 85:239-45.

Halonen JI, Zanobetti A, Sparrow D, Vokonas PS, Schwartz J. Outdoor temperature is associated with serum HDL and LDL. Environ Res 2011 ;111(2):281-7.

Han X, Naeher LP. A review of traffic-related air pollution exposure assessment studies in the developing world. Environ Int 2006; 32:106-20.

Jacob D, Winner D. Effect of climate change on air quality. Atmospheric Environ 2009; 43:51-63.

Kang JX.Omega-3: a link between global climate change and human health. Biotechnol Adv. 2011;29(4):388-90.

Kaplan C. Indoor air pollution from unprocessed solid fuels in developing countries. Reviews on Environmental Health 2010 ; 25(3) : 221-42.

Kargarfard M, Poursafa P, Rezanejad S, Mousavinasab F. Effects of exercise in polluted air on the aerobic power, serum lactate level and cell blood count of active individuals. Int J Prev Med 2011; 2(3): 145-50.

Kelishadi R, Mirghaffari N, Poursafa P, Gidding SS. Lifestyle and environmental factors associated with inflammation, oxidative stress and insulin resistance in children. Atherosclerosis 2009; 203: 311-9.

Kelishadi R, Poursafa P. Air pollution and non-respiratory health hazards for children. Arch Med Sci.2010; 6: 483-95.

Mansourian M, Javanmard SH, Poursafa P, Kelishadi R. Air pollution and hospitalization for respiratory diseases among children in Isfahan, Iran. Ghana Med J. 2010; 44(4):138-43.

Maresh JG, Campen MJ, Reed MD, Darrow AL, Shohet RV. Hypercholesterolemia potentiates aortic endothelial response to inhaled diesel exhaust. Inhal Toxicol2011;23(1):1-10.

Park SK, Auchincloss AH, O'Neill MS, Prineas R, Correa JC, Keeler J, Barr RG, Kaufman JD, Diez Roux AV. Particulate air pollution, metabolic syndrome, and heart rate variability: the multi-ethnic study of atherosclerosis (MESA). Environ Health Perspect. 2010 Oct;118(10):1406-11.

Poursafa P, Kelishadi R. Air pollution, platelet activation and atherosclerosis. Inflamm Allergy Drug Targets 2010;9 (5):387-92.

Poursafa P, Kelishadi R, Lahijanzadeh A, Modaresi M, Javanmard SH, Assari R, et al. The relationship of air pollution and surrogate markers of endothelial dysfunction in a population-based sample of children. BMC Public Health 2011;11:115.

Poursafa P, Kelishadi R, Moattar F, Rafiei L, Amin MM, Lahijanzadeh A, et al. Genetic variation in the association of air pollutants with a biomarker of vascular injury in children and adolescents in Isfahan, Iran. J Res Med Sci 2011;16(6)

Probst-Hensch NM. Chronic age-related diseases share risk factors: do they share pathophysiological mechanisms and why does that matter? Swiss Med Wkly 2010 1;140: w13072.

Samet J, Krewski D. Health effects associated with exposure to ambient air pollution. J Toxicol Environ Health A 2007; 70:227-42.

Schwartz J. Air pollution and blood markers of cardiovascular risk. Environ Health Perspect. 2001;109 Suppl 3:405-9

Sinclair KD, Lea RG, Rees WD, Young LE.The developmental origins of health and disease: current theories and epigenetic mechanisms. Soc Reprod Fertil 2007;Suppl. 64:425-43.

Sheffield PE, Landrigan PJ. Global climate change and children's health: threats and strategies for prevention. Environ Health Perspect 2011;119(3):291-8.

Subramaniam V. Seasonal variation in the incidence of preeclampsia and eclampsia in tropical climatic conditions. BMC Womens Health. 2007;7:18

Tomao E, Tiziana PB, Rosati V, Marcellini L, Tomei F. The effects of air pollution on the lipid balance of traffic police personnel. Ann Saudi Med 2002;22(5-6):287-90.

Yeatts K, Svendsen E, Creason J, Alexis N, Herbst M, Scott J, Kupper L, Williams R, Neas L, Cascio W, Devlin RB, Peden DB. Coarse particulate matter (PM2.5-10) affects heart rate variability, blood lipids, and circulating eosinophils in adults with asthma. Environ Health Perspect. 2007;115(5):709-14.

Wegesser TC, Pinkerton KE, Last JA. California Wildfires of 2008: coarse and fine particulate matter toxicity. Environ Health Perspect 2009; 117:893-7

5

Dyslipidemia and Type 2 Diabetes Mellitus: Implications and Role of Antiplatelet Agents in Primary Prevention of Cardiovascular Disease

Hasniza Zaman Huri
Department of Pharmacy, Faculty of Medicine, University of Malaya, Kuala Lumpur, Malaysia

1. Introduction

Dyslipidemia is the major risk factors for macrovascular complications leading to cardiovascular disease (CVD) in type 2 diabetes mellitus (T2DM). In addition to this, endothelial dysfunction, platelet hyperactivity, impaired fibrinolytic balance and abnormal blood flow may accelerate atherosclerosis and increased risk of thrombotic vascular events (Colwell & Nesto, 2003). Macrovascular disease is the most common cause of morbidity and mortality in T2DM (Koskinen, 1998). Macrovascular disease is defined as illnesses affecting the larger arteries supplying the heart, brain, and the legs, thereby causing ischemic heart disease, cerebrovascular disease, and peripheral vascular disease (Thompson, 1999). In patients with diabetes, alteration in distribution of lipid increased risk of atherosclerosis. Specifically, insulin resistance and insulin deficiency was identified as phenotype of dyslipidemia in diabetes mellitus (Taskinen, 2003; Krauss & Siri, 2004; Chahil & Ginsberg, 2006). This was characterized with high plasma triglyceride level, low HDL cholesterol level and increased level of small dense LDL-cholesterol (Mooradian, 2008). In these patient also, the increment of free fatty-acid release is due to insulin resistance. With the presence of adequate glycogen stores in the liver, this will promote triglyceride production, which stimulates the secretion of apolipoprotein B (Apo B) and VLDL cholesterol (Mooradian, 2008). Hepatic production of VLDL cholesterol is enhanced due to disability of insulin to inhibit the release of free fatty-acid. Low HDL cholesterol levels were also associated with hyperinsulinemia. There are several associations between dyslipidemia and the increased risk of cardiovascular disease in patients with type 2 diabetes mellitus. Low HDL cholesterol and increased triglyceride levels may contribute to the increased risk of cardiovascular disease. In conjunction with increased small dense LDL cholesterol and low HDL cholesterol levels, further evidence suggests that acceleration of atherosclerosis in diabetes mellitus and insulin-resistant conditions is regulated by hypertriglyceridemia. Nevertheless, the association between LDL cholesterol and CHD risk is stronger compared to the association between hypertriglyceridemia and CHD risk. Type 2 diabetes is also associated with insulin resistance and hyperinsulinemia or syndrome X comprises hypertension, dyslipidemia, decreased fibrinolysis and increased procoagulation factors (Serrano Rios, 1998). Besides dyslipidemia, platelet abnormalities contributed significantly to increased risk of CVD in these patients. In patients with type 2 diabetes, the platelet abnormalities are due to increased platelet aggregability and adhesiveness (Colwell & Nesto, 2003) and enhanced platelet aggregation activity may precede development of CVD (Halushka et al. 1981, Mandal et al. 1993). It has been well known that management of dyslipidemia in diabetes mellitus includes lifestyle changes such as increased physical activity and dietary modifications. Besides, various antihyperlipidemic agents have been utilized for this purpose. In contrast, antiplatelet agents are recommended mainly for primary and secondary prevention for cardiovascular disease in T2DM. Dyslipidemia is categorized as one of the cardiovascular risk factors besides others (family history CHD, hypertension, smoking, albuminuria) (American Diabetes Association, 2011). Patients with T2DM and having dyslipidemia are eligible for primary prevention of CVD with antiplatelet agents. This chapter will discuss on different types of antiplatelet agents used as primary prevention of cardiovascular disease in patients with T2DM. It will also emphasize appropriate selection of antiplatelet agents pertaining to clinical conditions of patients with T2DM and dyslipidemia.

2. Pathophysiology of dyslipidemia and platelet abnormalities in type 2 diabetes mellitus

Atherogenic dyslipidemia is characterized by three lipoprotein abnormalities: elevated VLDL, small LDL and decreased HDL cholesterol levels, named as atherogenic lipoprotein phenotype (Grundy, 1998). In patients with type 2 diabetes, the prothrombotic state is characterized by increased fibrinogen levels (Imperatore et al 1998), increased plasminogen activator inhibitor (PAI)-1 (Byberg et al., 1998) and abnormalities in platelet function (Trovati et al., 1988). The reason for three aforementioned phenotypes in athrogenic dyslipidemia is the increased free fatty-acid release from insulin-resistant fat cells (Taskinen, 2003; Krauss & Siri, 2004; Chahil & Ginsberg, 2006). The increased flux of free fatty acids into the liver in the presence of adequate glycogen stores promotes triglyceride production, which in turn stimulates the secretion of apolipoprotein B (ApoB) and VLDL cholesterol (Mooradian, 2008). The impaired ability of insulin to inhibit free fatty-acid release leads to enhanced hepatic VLDL cholesterol production (Frayn, 2001) which correlates with the degree of hepatic fat accumulation (Adiels et al., 2007). The increased number of plasma VLDL cholesterol and triglyceride levels decrease the level of HDL cholesterol and increase the concentration of small dense LDL cholesterol (Mooradian, 2008).

Platelet activation commenced with binding of thrombogenic substances (collagen, thrombin, components of atheromatous plaque) to receptors located on the platelet surface (Colwell & Nesto, 2003). Receptor binding triggers a series of events that include hydrolysis of membrane phospholipids, mobilization of intracellular calcium, and phosphorylation of important intracellular proteins (Colwell & Nesto, 2003). There are several platelet abnormalities seen in diabetes patients. Abnormalities of thromboxane A2 (TXA_2) production were among the earliest abnormalities in platelets of diabetes patients. TXA_2 is a potent activator and its synthesis is suppressed by aspirin (Natarajan et al., 2008). Platelets from patients with type 2 diabetes mellitus found to have increased expression of adhesion molecules CD31, CD36, CD49b, CD62P and CD63 (Eibl et al., 2004). Glycemic control improvement led to a significant decline in their expression (Eibl et al., 2004). In type 2 diabetes patients, platelets increased surface expressionof GP Ib and GP IIb/IIIa (Vinik et al., 2001). GP Ib mediates binding to von Willebrand factor (vWf) which is important in platelet-dependent thrombogenesis (Natarajan et al., 2008). Increased expression of GP IIb/IIIa on platelet surfaces leads to enhanced fibrinogen binding, platelet cross-linking and thrombogenesis (Colwell & Nesto, 2003). In patients with type 2 diabetes, decreased platelet insulin receptor number and affinity responsible for platelet hyperactivity (Vinik et al., 2001). Platelets have been shown to be targets of insulin action as they act as functional insulin receptor for insulin binding and autophosphorylation (Vinik et al., 2001). Insulin reduces platelet responses to the agonists' adenosine diphosphate (ADP), collagen, thrombin, arachidonate and platelet-activating factor. (Natarajan et al., 2008). In patients with type 2 diabetes also, platelets show disordered calcium homeostasis (Li et al., 2001). This may cause hyperactivity including platelet shape change, secretion, aggregation and thromboxane formation (Beckman et al., 2002). Furthermore, the deficiency of magnesium in diabetes has been associated with platelet hyperaggregability and adhesiveness (Gawaz et al., 1994). In type 2 diabetes patients, the reduced vascular synthesis of the anti-aggregants prostacyclin and nitric oxide by endothelium, shift the balance towards aggregation and vasoconstriction (Vinik et al., 2001; Ferroni et al., 2004). In type 2 diabetes patients with acute hyperglycaemia, shear stress-induced platelet activation and P-selection expression (Natarajan et al., 2008). Hyperglycaemia also causes non-enzymatic glycation of platelet membrane proteins resulting in changes in protein structure and conformation, as well as alterations of membrane lipid dynamics (Brownlee et al., 1988; Winocour et al., 1992). This could result in enhanced expression of certain crucial platelet receptors, for instance, P-selectin and GP IIb/IIIa, thus altering platelet activity (Ferroni et al., 2004). Glycated LDL causes an increase in intracellular calcium concentration and platelet nitric oxide (NO) production, as well as inhibition of the platelet membrane Na+/K+-adenosine triphosphatase (Na+/K+-ATPase) activity (Ferroni et al., 2004).

3. Implications of dyslipidemia and platelet abnormality in type 2 diabetes mellitus

In patients with type 2 diabetes mellitus, low HDL cholesterol and high triglyceride levels might contribute to the increased risk of cardiovascular disease (Mooradian, 2008). Based on the Expert panel on Detection, Evaluation and Treatment of High Blood Cholesterol in Adults (2011), hypertriglyceridemia, increased small dense LDL cholesterol and low HDL cholesterol found to be important in accelerating atherosclerosis in diabetes mellitus and insulin-resistant conditions. Abnormal platelet function is another important risk factors for cardiovascular disease in patients with diabetes (Colwell & Nesto, 2003). Atherosclerosis and thrombosis contribute significantly to the increased cardiovascular risk of diabetic patients (Colwell, 1997). The majority of ischemic coronary and cerebrovascular events are precipitated by vessel occlusion caused by atherosclerotic plaque disruption, platelet aggregation, platelet adhesion and thrombosis (Colwell & Nesto, 2003). Several systems that involved vasculature such as platelet, endothelial function, coagulation and fibrinolysis are impaired in patients with diabetes (Jokl & Colwell, 1997). Furthermore, increased platelet aggregability and adhesiveness are due to reduce membrane fluidity, increased intracellular Ca2+ and decreased intracellular Mg2+, increased arachidonic acid metabolism, increased

TXA_2 synthesis, decreased prostacyclin production, decreased NO production, decreased antioxidant levels and increased expression of activation-dependent adhesion molecules (Halushka et al., 1981; Mayfield et al., 1985; Watala et al., 1998; Martina et al., 1998; Trovati et al., 1997; Sarji et al., 1979; Tschoepe, et al., 1997; Leet et al., 1981). For patients with T2DM, the presence of dyslipidemia and platelet hyperactivity justifies the use of antiplatelet agents as primary prevention strategy of CVD.

4. Role of antiplatelet agents in primary prevention of CVD

Increased physical activity, dietary modifications and pharmacologic interventions are the key methods in management of dyslipidemia in type 2 diabetes mellitus (Mooradian, 2008). The Antithrombotic Trialists' Collaboration meta-analysis found that antiplatelet therapy reduces the relative risk of any serious vascular event by 25% in patients at high risk for a cardiovascular (CV) event (Antithrombotic Trialist' Collaboration, 2002). Antiplatelet agents are used for primary and secondary prevention of CVD in type 2 diabetes mellitus patients. Antiplatelet therapy is needed in the management of diabetes mellitus because there is an increase of platelet aggregability and adhesiveness due to platelet and endothelial dysfunction, impaired coagulation cascade, and fibrinolysis process among diabetic individuals compared to nondiabetic individuals (Colwell & Nesto, 2003). Consequently, the balance in normal hemostasis is shifted to favor thrombosis and accelerated atherosclerosis and results in increasing CVD (Colwell & Nesto, 2003). For primary prevention of cardiovascular diseases, type 2 diabetes mellitus patients with high risk acquiring cardiovascular events such as those with family history of cardiovascular disease, hypertension, obesity (BMI > 30 kg/m^2), smoking, dyslipidemia and albuminuria (Colwell, 2004). Several types of antiplatelet agents is being utilized for prevention of CVD which including aspirin, ticlopidine, clopidogrel and glycoprotein (Gp) IIb-IIIa antagonist such as abciximab, eptifibatide and tirofiban (Patrono et al., 2004; American Diabetes Association, 2006; Colwell & Nesto, 2003). Aspirin is one of the most common antiplatelet that been suggested in prevention of CVD in diabetes. Clopidogrel and ticlopidine are theinopyridine antiplatelet agents that generally suggested if patients are contraindicated to aspirin (American Diabetes Association, 2006). In contrast, Gp IIb-IIIa antagonist is usually given to diabetes patients who undergo precutaneous coronary intervention in order to intensify the antiplatelet therapy and to reduce the risk of procedure related thrombotic complication and reoccurrence of CV event (Patrono et al., 2004).

5. Types of antiplatelet

5.1 Aspirin

Aspirin selectively and irreversibly acetylates the COX-1 enzyme, thereby blocking the formation of thromboxane A2 in platelets and leads to inability of platelet to resynthesize COX-1 (Patrono et al., 2005). Aspirin has been used as a primary strategy to prevent CVD in type 2 diabetes due to its effectiveness in atherosclerosis prevention is well established. Various meta-analyses studies and large scale randomized controlled trials in T2DM support that low-dose aspirin therapy should be prescribed as prevention strategy in T2DM, if the contraindication is not exist (Colwell, 2004). Low dose of aspirin inhibits thromboxane production by platelets but has little or no effects on other sites of platelet activity (Colwell & Nesto, 2003). Several randomized controlled trials had been designed to assess the efficacy of aspirin in primary prevention of CVD which included Primary Prevention Project (PPP), US physicians' Health Study (USPHS), Early Treatment of Diabetes Retinopathy Study (ETDRS), Hypertension Optimal Treatment Trial (HOT), British Male Doctors' Trial (BMD) and the Thrombosis Prevention Trial (TPT) (Colwell & Nesto, 2003; Hayden et al., 2002). In Primary Prevention Project (PPP), a low dose aspirin (100 mg/day) was evaluated for the prevention of cardiovascular events in individuals with one or more of the following conditions such as hypertension, hypercholesterolemia, diabetes, obese, family history of premature myocardial infarction or being elderly. After a mean of 3.6 years follow-up, aspirin was found to significantly lower the frequency of cardiovascular death (from 1.4 % to 0.8 %); relative risk (RR) 0.56 [confidence interval (CI) 0.31-.99] and total cardiovascular events (from 8.2 to 6.3% ; RR 0.77 [0.62-0.95]). This trial involved large sample size (n = 4495) with the largest proportion of patients with diabetes mellitus (17%) (Collaborative Group of the Primary Prevention Project, 2001). Overall, PPP provides evidence to prove the efficacy of aspirin in diabetes; though participants were not blinded and were not given placebo pills. Additionally, a meta-analysis done by Hayden et al., (2002) also rated the quality of PPP as "fair" if compared to the rest of studies. In addition to PPP, a 5 years primary prevention trial in 22 701 healthy men; included 533 men with diabetes was conducted in US Physicians' Health Study (USPHS) in which a low-dose aspirin regimen (325 mg every other day) was given to treated group compared with placebo. A total of 44% significant risk reduction in CVD treated group was noted and the subgroup analyses in the diabetes reveals a reduction in myocardial infarction from 10.1 % (placebo) to 4.0 % (aspirin), yield a relative risk reduction of 0.39 for the diabetes men on aspirin therapy (Steering Committee of the Physicians' Health Study Research Group, 1989). Researcher and participants were blinded in this trial. In contrast with PPP, women were included in the study populations (2583 out of 4495 sample sizes). Hence, this study was more reliable compared to previous ones even though only 2% of the study population was diagnosed with diabetes. The Hypertension Optimal Treatment Trial (HOT) also examined the effects of low dose of aspirin (75 mg/day) versus placebo in 18 790 hypertension patients and 8% of them had diabetes. Results showed that aspirin significantly reduce cardiovascular event by 15% and myocardial infarction by 36% (Hansson et al., 1998). The HOT trial was another primary prevention study that included women, which was 46.6 % from total study population. Colwell (2004) commended that this study provided further evidence for the efficacy and safety of aspirin therapy in diabetes with systolic blood pressure less than 160 mmHg. Hayden et al., (2002) was in agreement with Colwell (2004) and concluded that HOT was a "good" quality of trial in their meta-analysis. Despite that, these findings were mirrored by Early Treatment of Diabetes Retinopathy Study (ETDRS) where they reported that although aspirin did not prevent progression of retinopathy but it did produce a significant reduction in risk for myocardial infarction (28%) over 5 years (P=0.038). This study may viewed as mixed primary and secondary prevention trials since those enrolled had a history of myocardial infarction and less than 50% had elevated blood pressure and history of CVD (ETDRS Investigators 1992). Conversely, the British Male Doctors' Trial (BMD) had conflicting results regarding aspirin effects in reducing the risk for myocardial infarction and adverse effects such as gastrointestinal bleeding and hemorrhagic stroke to diabetes patients. A total of 39 % of participants were discontinued therapy during the study due to adverse effect of aspirin (Hayden et al., 2002). Similar to PPP trial, participants in this study were not blinded thus results may be varies. Following this, a meta-analysis of these five randomized clinical trials (except ETDRS) was performed by Hayden et al., (2002) and systematic reviews on nine articles about the effect of aspirin on gastrointestinal bleeding and hemorrhagic stroke were conducted. They concluded that the net benefit of aspirin increase with CV risk. Nonetheless, this meta-analysis was found to have selection bias due to exclusion of 2 large trials that examined the effects of aspirin in patients with diabetes or stable angina. Sanmuganathan et al., (2001) also reached similar estimates of the beneficial effects of aspirin in primary prevention of CVD. The Japanese Primary Prevention of Atherosclerosis With Aspirin for Diabetes (JPAD) trial was the first prospectively designed trial to evaluate the use of aspirin (81 mg or 100 mg) in the primary prevention of cardiovascular events in patients with type 2 diabetes (n = 2539) aged 30–85 years in Japan (Ogawa et al., 2008). Among patients aged > 65 years (n =1363), aspirin was associated with a 32% reduction in the risk of the primary end point (6.3 vs. 9.2%; P = 0.047). Furthermore, in aspirin-treated patients, the incidence of fatal coronary and cerebrovascular events was significantly lower by 90% (0.08 vs. 0.8%; P = 0.0037). Paradoxically, there were no differences in nonfatal coronary and cerebrovascular events. Aspirin was well tolerated, with no significant increase in the composite of hemorrhagic stroke and severe gastrointestinal bleeding (Angiolillo, 2009). The outcome of this study was in opposite with the current recommendations on aspirin usage in primary prevention of CVD in diabetes patients (Angiolillo, 2009). However, the ASCEND and ACCEPT-D study are two ongoing trials will provide further insights to the appropriateness of aspirin usage in primary prevention of CVD in patients with diabetes. Another recent trial (POPADAD), failed to show any benefit with aspirin or antioxidants in primary prevention of cardiovascular events (Belch, 2008). The outcome of the study could be due to small number of patients with low event rates. A study on the utilization of antiplatelet therapy in type 2 diabetes patients revealed that many of the eligible patients did not receive the drugs as primary prevention strategy for CVD (Huri et al., 2008). Therefore, the recommendations on aspirin usage in primary prevention of CVD in type 2 diabetes patients must be fully justified after taking consideration against the benefit versus risk of its use. In another words, the recommendations should be base on individual patients' assessment and clinical judgment. Proper use of aspirin in primary prevention of CVD in type 2 diabetes patients may result in long-term benefits.

5.2 Clopidogrel

Clopidogrel is another type of antiplatelet agents used in primary prevention of CVD in type 2 diabetes when patients are intolerant to aspirin. It inhibits ADP-induced platelet aggregation by blocking the purinergic receptors and therefore prevents the activation of the GpIIb-IIIa receptor and subsequent binding to fibrinogen (Colwell & Nesto, 2003). Clopidogrel is preferable compared to ticlopidine because of its safety profile (Savi & Herbert, 2005; Bertrand et al., 2000). Nevertheless, the information regarding the usage of clopidogrel in primary prevention of CVD is limited than for secondary prevention of CVD in diabetes patients. Even though clopidogrel may be slightly more effective than aspirin, the size of any additional benefits is statistically uncertain and it has not been granted a claim of superiority against aspirin (Patrono et al., 2004). However, the publication of the Clopidogrel in Unstable Angina to Prevent Recurrent Events (CURE) recently had led to FDA approval of a new indication for clopidogrel in patients with acute coronary syndromes without ST-segment elevation (Patrono et al., 2004).The CURE trial examined CV outcomes with clopidogrel plus aspirin versus aspirin alone in patients with acute ischemic heart disease (IHD) (CURE Steering Committee, 2001). These findings demonstrated that clopidogrel has beneficial effects in patients with acute coronary syndromes without ST-segment elevation thus can be generalized as the study sample size (n =12,562) was large and patients were recruited from 482 centers in 28 countries. This trial also showed that 3.7% of patients in this combination therapy group had major bleeding and it was significant more compared with those solely on aspirin but there was no increase in life-threatening bleeds (CURE Steering Committee, 2001). Hence, a loading dose of 300mg clopidogrel should be used in this setting followed by 75 mg daily (Patrono et al., 2004). Bhatt et al., (2002) concluded that clopidogrel is an effective drug for secondary prevention in diabetes. Therefore, previous studies clearly justified the use of dual anti platelet therapy with aspirin and clopidogrel for secondary prevention of CVD in diabetes patients. Its role in primary prevention of CVD in diabetes patients is vague since no study has directly measure the outcome for this purpose.

5.3 Ticlopidine

Ticlopidine also inhibit ADP-induced platelet aggregation with no direct effects on the metabolism of arachidonic acid (Patrono, 1998). It has slower antiplatelet effect compared with clopidogrel (Patrono et al., 2004). Ticlopidine in Microangiopathy of Diabetes (TIMAD) study was conducted by involving 435 patients with nonproliferative diabetes retinopathy to evaluate for its effects on macrovascular disease in diabetes patients. Patients were randomized to receive ticlopidine, 250 mg twice daily and were followed up to 3 years. Ticlopidine was found significantly reduced annual microaneurysm progression by 67% and overall progression of retinopathy was significantly less severe with ticlopidine (TIMAD Study Group, 1990). However, this study was not designed to evaluate effect of ticlopidine on cardiovascular events. There are limited studies done on effect of ticlopidine in prevention of CVD in diabetes. In contrast to clopidogrel, ticlopidine does not have an approved indication for patients with a recent myocardial infarction (Patrono et al., 2004). Even though ticlopidine has lower cost compared to clopidogrel, (Drug Formulary University Malaya Medical Centre, 2005; Patrono et al., 2004), its role in primary prevention of CVD in type 2 diabetes patients have not been established.

5.4 Dipyridamole

Dipyridamole inhibits platelet cyclic-3′,5′-adenosine monophosphate and cyclic-3′, 5′-guanosine monophosphate phosphodiesterase (Natarajan et al. 2008). Overview of 25 trials among approximately 10000 high risks of CVD patients with the use of dipyridamole and aspirin, it was found that the addition of dipyridamole to aspirin has not been shown clearly to produce additional reductions in serious vascular events (Patrono et al., 2004). However, one of 25 trials suggested that there may be a worthwhile further reduction in stroke (Patrono *et al.* 2004). Patrono et al., (2004) also suggested that the combination of low dose aspirin and extended release dipyridamole (200 mg twice daily) is considered an acceptable option for initial therapy of patients with non-cardioembolic cerebral ischemic events and not in patients with ischemic heart attack. The benefits of dipyridamole in patients with diabetes have not been reported (Natarajan et al., 2008). Specifically, there are limited studies or trials conducted to examine the role of dipyridamole for primary and secondary prevention of CVD amongst T2DM patients.

5.5 GP IIb/IIIa inhibitors

The platelet glycoprotein (GP) IIb/IIIa complex receptor antagonists block activity at the fibrinogen binding site on platelet (Colwell & Nesto, 2003). These agents are useful in type 2 diabetes patients with acute coronary syndrome and in those undergoing percutaneous coronary interventions (Colwell & Nesto, 2003). These agents are administered intravenously with a rapid onset of action and short half-life (Natarajan et al., 2008). Numerous studies have been performed comparing various GP IIb/IIIa inhibitors. Currently, three different GP IIb/IIIa inhibitors (abciximab, eptifibatide, and tirofiban) are approved for clinical use. This group of drugs was mainly study for secondary prevention of CVD in diabetes patients. Evidence from three trials revealed that among 1,262 diabetes patients, use of these agents was associated with reduction in mortality from 4.5% to 2.5% (p=0.031) (Bhatt et al., 2000). In another meta-analysis of six large trials, with 6,458 patients with diabetes and acute coronary syndromes, GP IIb/IIIa inhibitor therapy was associated with a significant mortality reduction at 30 days, from 6.2% to 4.6% CI(0.59-0.92, p=0.007) (Roffi et al., 2001). Nonetheless, the role of GP IIb/IIIa inhibitors in primary prevention of CVD in type 2 diabetes mellitus has not been justified; therefore it is not recommended for this purpose.

6. Appropriate selection of antiplatelet agents for primary prevention of CVD in type 2 diabetes patients

Among all choices, there are considerations to be taken into account before types of antiplatelet agents chosen. According to American Diabetes Association (2011), aspirin (75-162mg/day) should be considered for primary prevention of cardiovascular disease in type 2 diabetes patients for men (>50 years) and women (>60 years) with at least one additional major risk factor (family history of cardiovascular disease, hypertension, smoking, dyslipidemia or albuminuria). The other types of antiplatelet agents either alone or combination with aspirin therapy has no established role in primary prevention of cardiovascular disease in type 2 diabetes patients. In contrast, aspirin should not be recommended for CVD prevention for diabetes patients with low CVD risk (10-year CVD risk <5%, such as in men <50 and women <60 years of age with no additional CVD risk factors, since the potential adverse effects from bleeding likely outweigh the potential benefits (ADA, 2011). A same recommendation goes to type 2 diabetes patients with multiple other risk factors (e.g. 10-year risk 5-10%), in which clinical judgment is required (American Diabetes Association, 2011).

7. Monitoring of aspirin efficacy and adverse effects

Aspirin once daily (75-100 mg) is recommended in primary prevention of CVD in type 2 diabetes patients when antiplatelet prophylaxis has a favorable benefit/risk profile (Patrono et al., 2004). For effectiveness of primary prevention strategy, patients should be followed on a regular basis and examined for signs and symptoms of any cardiovascular diseases. In consideration of dose-dependent GI toxicity and its potential impact on compliance, physicians are encouraged to use the lowest dose of aspirin that was shown to be effective in each clinical setting (Patrono et al., 2001). Aspirin should not be given to patients with gastrointestinal ulcerations; best tolerated after food. In conclusion, bleeding and gastrointestinal complications are the most common adverse effects of aspirin. Thus, the patients on aspirin should be monitored for stomach pain, heartburn, nausea and bleeding tendency.

8. Conclusion

Dyslipidemia is one of the risk factors for acquiring cardiovascular disease in patients with type 2 diabetes. In absent for contraindication, type 2 diabetes patients with dyslipidemia are eligible for primary prevention of cardiovascular disease although the routine use has not been documented. Aspirin plays a key role in primary prevention strategy of cardiovascular disease in type 2 diabetes patients. With limited studies and evidence for other antiplatelet agents, their role in primary prevention has not been established.

9. Summary

Dyslipidemia is one of the major risk factors for macrovascular disease leading to CVD in type 2 diabetes.

In type 2 diabetes patients with dyslipidemia, alteration in lipid distribution and platelet abnormalities increased risk of acquiring CVD.

Patients with type 2 diabetes with one of the following; dyslipidemia, family history of coronary heart disease, hypertension, smoking and albuminuria are at increased risk of CVD, thus eligible for primary prevention strategy of CVD.

With limited evidence, proper justification and clinical judgments of benefit versus risk, aspirin plays a key role as antiplatelet agent in primary prevention of CVD in patients with type 2 diabetes with dyslipidemia.

Patients with type 2 diabetes and dyslipidemia receiving aspirin for primary prevention strategy should be monitored for effectiveness of treatment (sign and symptoms of CVD) and adverse effects (stomach pain, heartburn, nausea and bleeding tendency).

10. References

Adiels, M., Westerbacka, J., Soro-Paavonen, A., Häkkinen, A.M., Vehkavaara, S., Caslake, M.J., Packard, C., Olofsson, S.O., Yki-Järvinen, H., Taskinen, M.R. & Borén, J. (2007). Acute suppression of VLDL1 secretion rate by insulin is associated with hepatic fat content and insulin resistance. *Diabetologia* Vol.50, No.11, (November 2007), pp. 2356-2365, ISSN 1432-0428

American Diabetes Association (2006). Standards of Medical Care in diabetes. *Diabetes Care* Vol.29, No.1, (January 2006), pp. 4-42, ISSN 1935-5548

American Diabetes Association (2011). Standard of Medical Care in Diabetes 2011. *Diabetes Care* Vol.34, No.1, (January 2011), pp. S11-S61, ISSN 1935-5548

Angiolillo, D.J. (2009). Antiplatelet therapy in diabetes: efficacy and limitations of current treatment strategies and future directions. *Diabetes Care* Vol.32, No.4, (April 2009), pp. 531-540, ISSN 1935-5548

Antithrombotic Trialists' Collaboration (2002): Collaboration meta-analysis of randomized trials of antiplatelet therapy for prevention of death, myocardial infarction, and stroke in high risk patients. *BMJ Vol.*324, No.7329, (January 2002), pp. 71–86, ISSN 1468-5833

Beckman, J.A., Creager, M.A. & Libby, P. (2002). Diabetes and atherosclerosis: epidemiology, pathophysiology, and management. *JAMA* Vol.287, No.19, (May 2002), pp. 2570-81, ISSN 1538-3598

Belch, J., MacCuish, A., Campbell, I., et al. (2008). The prevention of progression of arterial disease and diabetes (POPADAD) trial: factorial randomised placebo controlled trial of aspirin and antioxidants in patients with diabetes and asymptomatic peripheral arterial disease. *BMJ Vol.*337, (October 2008), pp. a1840, ISSN 1468-5833

Bertrand, M.E., Rupprecht, H.J., Urban, P. et al. (2000). Double-blind study of the safety of clopidogrel with and without a loading dose in combination with aspirin compared with ticlopidine in combination with aspirin after coronary stenting. The clopidogrel aspirin stent international cooperative study (CLASSICS). *Circulation* Vol.102, No.6, (August 2000), pp. 624–629, ISSN 1524-4539

Bhatt, D.L., Marso, S.P., Lincoff, A.M., Wolski, K.E., Ellis, S.G. & Topol, E.J. (2000). Abciximab reduces mortality in diabetics following percutaneous coronary intervention. *J Am Coll Cardiol* Vol.35, No.4, (March 2000), pp. 922-928, ISSN 1558-3597

Bhatt, D.L., Marso, S.P., Hirsch, A.T., et al. (2002). Amplified benefit of clopidogrel versus aspirin in patients with diabetes mellitus. *Am J Cardiol Vol.*90, No.6, (September 2002), pp. 625- 628, ISSN 0735-1097

Brownlee, M., Cerami, A. & Vlassara, H. (1988). Advanced products of nonenzymatic glycosylation and the pathogenesis of diabetic vascular disease. *Diabetes Metab Rev* Vol.4, No.5, (August 1988), pp. 437-51, ISSN 1520- 7560

Byberg, L., Siegbahn, A., Berglund, L., Mc-Keigue, P., Reneland, R. & Lithell, H. (1998). Plasminogen activator inhibitor-1 activity is independently related to both insulin sensitivity and serum triglycerides in 70-year-old men. *Arterioscler Thromb Vasc Biol* Vol.18, No.2, (February 1998), pp. 258 -264, ISSN 1079-5642

Chahil, T.J. & Ginsberg, H.N. (2006). Diabetic dyslipidemia. *Endocrinol Metab Clin North Am* Vol.35, No.3, pp. 491–510, ISSN 1558-4410

Collaborative Group of the Primary Prevention Project (2001). Low-dose aspirin and vitamin E in people at cardiovascular risk: a randomized trial in general practice. *Lancet Vol.*357, No.9250, (January 2001), 89–95, ISSN 1474-4465

Colwell, J.A. (1997). Multifactorial aspects of the treatment of the type II diabetic patient. *Metabolism* Vol.46, No.12, (December 1997), pp.1–4, ISSN 1532-8600

Colwell, J.A. & Nesto, R.W. (2003). The platelet in diabetes: focus on prevention of ischemic events. *Diabetes Care,* Vol.26, No.7, pp. 2181–2188, ISSN 1935-5548

Colwell, J.A. (2004). Aspirin therapy in diabetes. *Diabetes Care* Vol.27, No.1, (January 2004), pp. S72-S73, ISSN 1935-5548

CURE Steering Committee (2001). Effects of clopidogrel in addition to aspirin in patients with acute coronary syndromes without ST-segment elevation. *N Engl J Med* Vol.345, No.7, (August 2001), pp. 494–502, ISSN 1533-4406

Drug Formulary University Malaya Medical Centre (2005). Senarai Ubat-Ubatan. Malaysia: University Malaya Medical Centre; 2005.

ETDRS Investigators (1992). Aspirin effects on mortality and morbidity in patients with diabetes mellitus. *JAMA* Vol.268, No.10, (September 1992), pp. 1292–1300, ISSN 1538-3598

Eibl, N., Krugluger, W., Streit, G., Schrattbauer, K., Hopmeier, P. & Schernthaner, G. (2004). Improved metabolic control decreases platelet activation markers in patients with type-2 diabetes. *Eur J Clin Invest* Vol.34, No.3, (March 2004), pp. 205-209, ISSN 1365-2362

Ferroni, P., Basili, S., Falco, A. & Davi, G. (2004). Platelet activation in type 2 diabetes mellitus. *J Thromb Haemost* Vol.2, No.8, (August 2004), pp. 1282-1291, ISSN 1538-7836

Frayn, K.N. (2001) Adipose tissue and the insulin resistance syndrome. *Proc Nutr Soc* Vol.60, No.3, (August 2001), pp. 375–380, ISSN 1475- 2719

Gawaz, M., Ott, I., Reininger, A.J. & Neumann, F.J. (1994). Effects of magnesium on platelet aggregation and adhesion. Magnesium modulates surface expression of glycoproteins on platelets in vitro and ex vivo. *Thromb Haemost* Vol.72, No.6, (December 1994), pp. 912-918, ISSN 0340-6245

Grundy, S.M. (1998). Hypertriglyceridemia, atherogenic dyslipidemia, and the metabolic syndrome. *Am J Cardiol* Vol.81, No. 4A, (February 1998), pp. 18B–25B, ISSN 0002-9149

Halushka, P.V., Rogers, R.C., Loadholt, C.B. & Colwell, J.A. (1981). Increased platelet thromboxane synthesis in diabetes mellitus. *J Lab Clin Med* Vol.97, No.1, (January 1981), pp. 87–96, ISSN 1532-6543

Hansson, L., Zanchetti, A., Carruthers, S.G., Dahlof, B., Elmfeldt, D., Julius, S., Menard, J., Rahn, K.H., Wedel, H., Westerling, S., for the HOT Study Group (1998). Effects of intensive blood-pressure lowering and low-dose aspirin in patients with hypertension: principal results of the Hypertension Optimal Treatment (HOT) randomised trial. *Lancet* Vol.351, No.9118, (June 1998), pp. 1755–1762, ISSN 1474-547X

Hayden, M., Pignone, M., Phillips, C. & Mulrow, C. (2002). Aspirin for the primary prevention of cardiovascular events: a summary of the evidence for the U.S. Preventive Services Task Force. *Ann Intern Med* Vol.136, No.2, (January 2002), pp. 161-172, ISSN 1539-3704

Huri, H.Z., Yi, L.Q., Pendek, R. & Sulaiman, C.Z. 2008. Use of antiplatelet agents for primary and secondary prevention of cardiovascular disease amongst type 2 diabetic patients. *Journal of Pharmacy Practice*, Vol.21, No.4, (August 2008), pp. 287-301, ISSN 1531-1937

Imperatore, G., Riccardi, G., Iovine, C., Rivellese, A.A. & Vaccaro, O. (1998). Plasma fibrinogen: a new factor of the metabolic syndrome: a population-based study. *Diabetes Care* Vol.21, No.4, (April 1998), pp. 649–654, ISSN 1935-5548

Koskinen, S.V., Reunanen, A.R., Martelin, T.P. & Valkonen, T. (1998). Mortality in a large population-based cohort of patients with drug-treated diabetes mellitus. *Am J Publ Health* Vol.88, No.5, (May 1998), pp. 765-770, ISSN 1541-0048

Krauss, R.M. & Siri, P.W. (2004). Dyslipidemia in type 2 diabetes. *Med Clin North Am* Vol.88, No.4, pp. 897–909, ISSN 1557-9859

Jokl, R. & Colwell, J.A. (1997). Arterial thrombosis and atherosclerosis in diabetes. *Diabetes Metab Rev Vol.*5, pp. 1–15, ISSN 1520- 7560

Leet, H., Paton, R.C., Passa, P. & Caen, J.P. (1981). Fibrinogen binding and ADP-induced aggregation in platelets from diabetic subjects. *Thromb Res* Vol.24, No.1-2, (October 1981), pp. 143–150, ISSN 0049-3848

Li, Y., Woo, V. & Bose, R. (2001). Platelet hyperactivity and abnormal Ca(2+) homeostasis in diabetes mellitus. *Am J Physiol Heart Circ Physiol* Vol.280, No.4, (April 2001), pp. H1480-H1489, ISSN 1522-1539

Mandal, S., Sarode, R., Dash, S. & Dash, R.J. (1993) Hyperaggregation of platelets detected by whole blood platelet aggregometry in newly diagnosed noninsulindependent diabetes mellitus. *American Journal of Clinical Pathology*, Vol.100, No.2, (August 1993), pp. 103-107, ISSN 0002-9173

Martina, V., Bruno, G.A., Trucco, F., Zumpano, E., Tagliabue, M. & Di Bisceglie, C. (1998). Platelet cNOS activity is reduced in patients with IDDM and NIDDM. *Thromb Haemost* Vol.79, No. 3, (March 1998), pp. 520–522, ISSN 0340-6245

Mayfield, R.K., Halushka, P.V., Wohltmann, H.J., Lopes-Virella, M. & Chambers, J.K. (1985). Platelet function during continuous insulin infusion treatment in insulin-dependent diabetic patients. *Diabetes* Vol.34, No.11, (November 1985), pp. 1127–1133, ISSN 1939-327X

Mooradian, A.D (2008). Dsylipidemia in type 2 diabetes mellitus. Nature Clinical Practice *Endocrinology & Metabolism,* Vol.5, No.3, (March 2009), pp. 150-159, ISSN 1759-5029

Natarajan, A., Zaman, A.G. & Marshall, S.M. (2008). Platelet hyperactivity in type 2 diabetes: role of antiplatelet agents. *Diab Vasc Dis Res* Vol.5, No.2, (June 2008), pp. 138-144, ISSN 1752-8984

Ogawa H, Nakayama M, Morimoto T, et al. (2008). Low-dose aspirin for primary prevention of atherosclerotic events in patients with type 2 diabetes: a randomized controlled trial. *JAMA* Vol. 300, No.18, (November 2008), pp. 2134-2141, ISSN 1538-3598

Patrono, C., Coller, B., Dalen, J.E., Fuster, V., Gent, M., Harker, L.A., Hirsh, J. & Roth, G. (1998). Platetet-active drugs: the relationship among dose, effectiveness and side-effects. *Chest* Vol.114, No.5, (November 1998), pp. 470s-488s, ISSN 1931- 3543

Patrono, C., Coller, B. & Dalen, J.E. et al. (2001). Platelet-Active Drugs: The relationships among dose, effectiveness, and side effects. *Chest* Vol.119, No.1, (January 2001), pp. 39S–63S, ISSN 1931- 3543

Patrono, C., Bachmann, F., Baigent, C., Bode, C., Caterina, R.D., Charbonnier, B., Fitzgerald, D., Hirsh, J., Husted, S., Kvasnicka, J., Montalescot, G., Garcia Rodriguez, L.A., Verhueght, F., Vermylen, J., Wallentin, L. et al. (2004). Expert Consensus Document on the Use of Antiplatelet Agents. *European Heart Journal* Vol.25, No.2, (January 2004), pp. 166-181, ISSN 1522-9645

Patrono, C., Garcia Rodriguez, L.A., Landolfi, R. & Baigent, C. (2005). Low-dose aspirin for the prevention of atherothrombosis. *N Engl J Med* Vol.353, No.22, (December 2005), 2373–2383, ISSN 1533-4406

Roffi, M., Chew, D.P., Mukherjee, D., Bhatt, D.L., White, J.A., Heeschen, C., Hamm, C.W., Moliterno, D.J., Califf, R.M., White, H.D., Kleiman, N.S., Theroux, P. & Topol, E.J. (2001). Platelet glycoprotein IIb/IIIa inhibitors reduce mortality in diabetic patients with non-ST-segment-elevation acute coronary syndromes. *Circulation* Vol.104, No. 23, (December 2001), pp. 2767–2771, ISSN 0009-7322

Sanmuganathan, P.S., Ghahramani, P., Jackson, P.R., Wallis, E.J. & Ramsay, L.E. (2001). Aspirin for primary prevention of coronary heart disease: safety and absolute benefit related to coronary risk derived from meta-analysis of randomised trials. *Heart* Vol.85, No.3, (March 2001), pp. 265-271, ISSN 1468-201X

Sarji, K.E., Kleinfelder, J., Brewington, P., Gonzalez, J., Hempling, H. & Colwell, J.A. (1979). Decreased platelet vitamin C in diabetes mellitus: possible role in hyperaggregation. *Thromb Res* Vol.15, No.5-6, pp. 639–650, ISSN 0049-3848

Savi, P. & Herbert, J.M. (2005). Clopidogrel and ticlopidine: P2Y12 adenosine diphosphate-receptor antagonists for the prevention of atherothrombosis. *Semin Thromb Hemost* Vol.31, No.2, (April 2005), pp. 174 –183, ISSN 0094-6176

Serrano Rios, M. (1998). Relationship between obesity and the increased risk of major complications in non-insulin-dependent diabetes mellitus. *Eur J Clin Invest* Vol.28, No.2, (September 1998), pp. 14–18, ISSN 1365-2362

Steering Committee of the Physicians' Health Study Research Group (1989). Final report on the aspirin component of the ongoing Physicians' Health Study. *N Engl J Med* Vol.321, No.3, (July 1989), pp. 129–135, ISSN 1533-4406

Taskinen, M.R. (2003) Diabetic dyslipidaemia: from basic research to clinical practice. *Diabetologia* Vol. 46, No.6, pp. 733–749, ISSN 1432-0428

Thompson, D.M. (1999). Cardiovascular disease and diabetes. *BC Endocrine Research Foundation Newsletter* 1: 3, ISSN 1755-3245

TIMAD Study Group (1990). Ticlopidine treatment reduces the progression of nonproliferative diabetic retinopathy. *Arch Ophthalmol* Vol.108, pp. 1577–1583, ISSN 1538-3601

Trovati, M., Anfossi, G., Cavalot, F., Massucco, P., Mularoni, E. & Emanuelli, G. (1988). Insulin directly reduces platelet sensitivity to aggregating agents: studies in vitro and in vivo. *Diabetes* Vol.37, No.6, (June 1988), pp. 780–786, ISSN 1939-327X

Trovati, M., Anfossi, G., Massucco, P., Mattiello, L., Costamagna, C., Piretto, V., Mularoni, E., Cavalot, F., Bosia, A. & Ghigo, D. (1997). Insulin stimulates nitric oxide synthesis in human platelets and, through nitric oxide, increases platelet concentrations of both guanosine-3_, 5_-cyclic monophosphate and adenosine 3_, 5_ cyclic monophosphate. *Diabetes* Vol.46, No.5, (May 1997), pp. 742–749, ISSN 1939-327X

Tschoepe, D., Rauch, U. & Schwippert, B. (1997). Platelet-leukocyte-cross-talk in diabetes mellitus. *Horm Metab Res* Vol.29, No.12, (December 1997), pp. 631–635, ISSN 1439-4286

Vinik, A.I., Erbas, T., Park. T.S., Nolan, R. & Pittenger, G.L. (2001). Platelet dysfunction in type 2 diabetes. Diabetes Care Vol.24, No.8, (August 2001), pp. 1476-85, ISSN 1935-5548

Watala C, Boncer M, Golanski J, Koziolkiewcz W, Trojanowski Z, Walkowiak B: Platelet membrane lipid fluidity and intraplatelet calcium mobilization in type 2 diabetes. *Eur J Haematol* Vol.61, No.5, (November 1998), pp. 319–326, ISSN 1600-0609

Winocour, P.D., Watala, C. & Kinlough-Rathbone, R.L. (1992). Reduced membrane fluidity and increased glycation of membrane proteins of platelets from diabetic subjects are not associated with increased platelet adherence to glycated collagen. *J Lab Clin Med* Vol.120, No.6, (December 1992), pp. 921-928, ISSN 1532-6543

6

Dyslipidemia: Genetics and Role in the Metabolic Syndrome

Nora L. Nock and Aiswarya L.P. Chandran Pillai
Case Western Reserve University
USA

1. Introduction

Dyslipidemia is characterized by an aggregation of lipoprotein abnormalities including low high density lipoprotein cholesterol (HDL-C), high serum triglycerides (TG) and increased small low density lipoprotein cholesterol (LDL-C). Lipoproteins, which contain lipids and proteins (apolipoproteins, APO) are responsible, primarily, for transporting water insoluble lipids (cholesterol, TG) in plasma from the intestines and liver, where they are absorbed and synthesized, respectively, to peripheral tissues (muscle, adipose) for utilization, processing and/or storage (Kwan et al., 2007). There are several subtypes of lipoproteins with specific functions including, from smallest to largest: 1) chylomicrons, which transport dietary TG from the intestines to the peripheral tissue and liver; 2) very LDL (VLDL) particles, which transport TG from the liver to peripheral tissues; 3) intermediate density lipoproteins (IDL), which are produced from VLDL particle metabolism and may be taken up by the liver or further hydrolyzed to LDL; and, 4) HDL, which is key in 'reverse cholesterol transport' or shuttling cholesterol from peripheral cells to the liver (Kwan et al., 2007).

The Metabolic Syndrome (MetSyn) is a clustering of traits including dyslipidemia as well as hypertension (raised systolic and/or diastolic blood pressure), dysglycemia (high fasting glucose) and obesity (high body mass index (BMI) and/or waist circumference). Dyslipidemia is formally defined within the context of MetSyn. Various diagnostic definitions have been proposed for MetSyn by several organizations including the World Health Organization (WHO) (Alberti and Zimmet, 1998), European Group Insulin Resistance (EGIR) (Balkau and Charles, 1999), National Cholesterol Education Program Adult Treatment Panel III (NCEP ATP III, (2001), International Diabetes Federation (IDF, (Alberti et al., 2005), American Heart Association/National Heart, Lung, and Blood Institute (AHA/NHLBI) (Grundy et al., 2006) and, with the most recent joint interim statement proposed by the AHA/NHLBI, IDF and other organizations (Alberti et al., 2009). Although the recommendations differ widely on the obesity component, the dyslipidemia component has been fairly consistently defined as having TG $\geq$ 150 mg/l, HDL-C <40 mg/dL (1.03 mmol/l, in males) or <50 mg/dL (1.29 mmol/l in females) or drug treatment for elevated TG or low HDL-C (NCEP ATP III: (2001), IDF: (Alberti et al., 2005), Joint Statement: (Alberti et al., 2009)). However, the WHO (Alberti and Zimmet, 1998) proposed slightly lower limits for HDL-C (male: < 0.9 mmol/l (35 mg/dl); female: < 1.0 mmol/l (39 mg/dl)) and the EGIR (Balkau and Charles, 1999) recommended dyslipidemia be defined by HDL-C < 1.0 mmol/l (39 mg/dl) or TG > 2.0 mmol/l (177 mg/dl). There is currently no recommended value for

LDL-C levels in the context of MetSyn yet LDL-C remains the primary target of therapy for the management of high blood cholesterol per the most recent guidelines from the NCEP ATPIII, which recommended drug therapy for LDL-C values ranging from ≥100 mg/dl to ≥190 mg/dl depending on the presence/absence of other coronary heart disease (CHD) risk factors (Grundy et al., 2004). When LDL becomes lipid depleted, small dense LDL (sdLDL) particles are formed, which have a lower affinity for the LDL receptor (LDLR), more susceptibility to oxidation and a higher affinity for macrophages; and, thus, sdLDL particles contribute to the atherosclerotic process (Austin et al., 1990; Littlewood and Bennett, 2003) and likely MetSyn (Kruit et al., 2010).

Dyslipidemia and MetSyn are common in developed nations and the prevalence of both are rising worldwide, which may be attributed, in part, to the rising rates of overweight and obesity (Alberti et al., 2009; Halpern et al., 2010). According to the National Health and Nutrition Examination Survey (NHANES) III (1988-1994) in the United States (U.S.), which used the NCEP ATP III criteria, the age-adjusted prevalence of dyslipidemia defined by high TG or low HDL-C, was approximately 30.0% and 37.1%, respectively; and, the prevalence of MetSyn was approximately 23.7% (Ford et al., 2002). The prevalence of dyslipidemia and MetSyn generally increase with increasing age (Ford et al., 2002). However, in a more recent study that used the Health Survey for England (HSE) (2003-2006) survey data and NHANES (1999-2006) data with exclusion of persons over 80 years old, the prevalence of low HDL-C (defined in both males and females as <40 mg/dL) was 10.0% in England and 19.2% in the U.S. (Martinson et al., 2010). Thus, the prevalence can vary markedly depending on how these traits are defined (Cook et al., 2008). Interestingly, trends in the U.S. and England indicate during the past two decades an increase in the proportion of individuals diagnosed with high cholesterol (≥240 mg/dL) but who achieved therapeutic control (Roth et al., 2010). For example, in the U.S. in 2006, 54.0% of men (95% CI: 47.6–60.4) and 49.7% of women (95% CI: 44.3–55.0) with high total serum cholesterol were on cholesterol-lowering medication, as opposed to 10.8% of men (95% CI: 8.0–13.6) and 8.6% (95% CI: 6.7–10.6) of women in 1993 (Roth et al., 2010). In England, in 2006, 35.5% of men (95% CI: 32.8–38.3) and 25.7% of women (95% CI: 23.4–28.1) were on cholesterol-lowering medication as opposed to 0.6% of men (95% CI: 0.3–1.3) and 0.4% of women (95% CI: 0.1–0.7%) in 1993 (Roth et al., 2010). Thus, prevalence rates will also vary by whether or not relevant drug treatments have been considered and, perhaps, the list of relevant drugs should include cholesterol lowering therapies (e.g., statins) as well as other drugs (e.g., tamoxifen, glucocorticoids) known to alter TG and cholesterol levels (Garg and Simha, 2007).

Both dyslipidemia and MetSyn increase the risk of Type II diabetes mellitus (T2DM) (Adiels et al., 2006; Kruit et al., 2010) and cardiovascular disease (CVD) morbidity (Alberti et al., 2009; Linsel-Nitschke and Tall, 2005) and CVD mortality (Lewington et al., 2007). Patients with MetSyn have a five-fold increase in the risk of developing T2DM and are at twice the risk of developing CVD over the next 5 to 10 years compared to individuals without the syndrome (Alberti et al., 2009). In the presence of both MetSyn and T2DM, the prevalence of CVD is markedly increased with an odds ratio (OR) of 3.04 [95% confidence interval (CI) of OR: 1.98-4.11] in comparison to those with none of these conditions (Athyros et al., 2004). The importance of MetSyn is exemplified by its ICD-9 code (277.7), which was initially established as a diagnosis of "Dysmetabolic Syndrome X" (Einhorn et al., 2003; Kahn et al., 2005). In summary, both dyslipidemia and MetSyn are substantial public health problems, which require a better understanding of their respective etiologies to develop more effective lifestyle and therapeutic interventions.

Heritability estimates suggest there is a strong genetic component to dyslipidemia and MetSyn. Heritability estimates for dyslipidemia range from 0.20 to 0.60 (Edwards et al., 1997; Goode et al., 2007; Herbeth et al., 2010; Kronenberg et al., 2002; Wang and Paigen, 2005) and from 0.24 to 0.63 for MetSyn (Lin et al., 2005; Sung et al., 2009).
Multiple genetic variants in the form of single nucleotide polymorphisms (SNPs) (i.e., single DNA base changes) have been associated with manifestation of dyslipidemia and MetSyn. In this chapter, we review and summarize associations between common SNPs (i.e., those with a minor allele frequency (MAF) ≥0.05) in the most biologically plausible candidate genes and HDL-C, LDL-C and TG levels as well as MetSyn as a single, unifying trait. Previous estimates suggest all common variants together explain less than 10 percent of HDL-C levels in the general population (Kronenberg et al., 2002); however, more elegant statistical modeling methods that combine SNPs in a more biologically meaningful way may be needed to better understand the collective role of genetic variants in manifestation of dyslipidemia, MetSyn and other complex metabolic traits. As a result, at the end of this chapter, we review studies that have undertaken more complex modeling strategies to understand the aggregate effects of SNPs in manifestation of dyslipidemia and MetSyn and provide our insights for future directions in this field.

2. Genetic variants in lipid metabolism and HDL-C levels

As mentioned above, HDL-C is important for "reverse cholesterol transport" or the shuttling of cholesterol from peripheral cells to the liver. Many of the genetic variants associated with HDL-C levels have been summarized nicely in a recent comprehensive review by Boes et al. (Boes et al., 2009). In Table 1, we include common SNPs tabulated in Boes et al. (2009) review of large studies (ethnic group sample sizes ≥500) as well as common SNPs in large studies that have been identified since their review.

Gene	Polym.	rs Number	MAF	Ethn.	Sample Size	Results (Effect Size, p-value)	Reference
ABCA1	C (-297)T	rs2246298	0.25 (T)	A	1625 (GP)	p=0.0455	(Shioji et al. 2004b)
ABCA1	G (-273)C	rs1800976	0.40 (C)	A	1626 (GP) 735 (HBP)	+1.9/+2.7 mg/dl (1/2copies); p=0.03 +1.9 /+5.0 mg/dl (1/2 copies); p=0.03	(Shioji et al. 2004b)
ABCA1	G (-273)C	rs1800976	0.38 (T)	Tu	2332 (GP)	+0.7/+1.9 mg/dl (1/2 copies); p<0.02	(Hodoglugil et al. 2005)
ABCA1	G378C	rs1800978	0.13 (C)	W	5040 (GP)	-1.2/- 2.7 mg/dl (1/2 copies); p=0.03	(Porchay et al. 2006)
ABCA1		rs3890182	0.13 (A)	W	5287 (GP)	-1/-3 mg/dl (1/2 copies) ; p=0.003	(Kathiresan et al. 2008)
ABCA1		rs2275542		A	<1880 (GP)	p=0.006	(Shioji et al. 2004b)

ABCA1		rs2515602	0.27	B	1943 (P)	M; p=0.034; F; p<0.001	(Klos et al. 2006a)
ABCA1	G596A	rs2853578	0.28 (A)	W	2468 CVD 834 (Co)	0.2 / +2.8 mg/dl (1/2 copies); p=0.02	(Whiting et al. 2005)
ABCA1	2310G>A	rs2066718	0.03 (A)	W	9123 (P)	F: higher levels in carriers; p=0.02	(Frikke-Schmidt et al. 2004)
ABCA1	G2706A	rs2066718	0.05 (A)	Tu	2458 (GP)	M: +2.0 mg/dl for heterozygotes; p<0.01	(Hodoglugil et al. 2005)
ABCA1	2472G>A G2868A	rs2066718	0.06 (A)	Tu	2105 (GP)	F: +3.1 mg/dl for carriers; p=0.0005	(Hodoglugil et al. 2005)
ABCA1	1883M	rs4149313	0.12 (G)	W	9123 (P)	F: + heterozygotes; p=0.05	(Frikke-Schmidt et al. 2004)
ABCA1	32b.+30, ABC32			W	1543 (P)	-2.2 mg/dl for carriers ; p=0.0040	(Costanza et al. 2005)
ABCA1	R1587K	rs2230808	0.24 (A)	W	9123 (P)	M: - 1.5 mg/dl for heterozygotes; p=0.008	(Frikke-Schmidt et al. 2004)
ABCA1	4759G > A	rs2230808	0.26 (K)	W	779 (CVD)	-1.5 mg/dl for carriers; p=0.03	(Clee et al. 2001)
ABCA1	50b.3038, ABC50	rs41474449	.	W	1543 (P)	+1.6 mg/dl for carriers; p=0.043	(Costanza et al. 2005)
ABCA1		rs3890182	0.12 (A)	EA	25,167	p= 4.53E-07	(Dumitrescu et al. 2011)
APOA1	T84C (HaeIII)	rs5070	0.23 (C)	A	1637 (GP)	+1.9 / +5.4 mg/dl (1/2copies); p=0.0005	(Shioji et al. 2004a)
APOA1	MspI RFLP	rs5069	0.31 (C)	B	3831 (P)	M/F; p=n.s/0.022	(Brown et al. 2006)
APOA1		rs28927680	0.93 (G)	EA	25,167	p= 8.61E-09	(Dumitrescu et al. 2011)
APOA1		rs964184	0.86 (C)	EA	25,167	p= 6.08E-10	(Dumitrescu et al. 2011)
APOA5	- 1131T > C	rs662799	0.06 (C)	UK	1696 (P)	-1.5 mg/dl / -5.4 mg/dl (1/2 copies) ; p=0.04	(Talmud et al. 2002a)
APOA5	- 1131T > C	rs662799	0.07 (C)	W	1596(SAPHIR)	-3.5 mg/dl per copy; p=0.00038	(Grallert et al. 2007)
APOA5	- 1131T > C	rs662799	0.23–0.30 (C)	C, Ma	2711 (C) 707 (M)	-2.3/- 5.4 mg/dl 1/2 copies; p<0.0001 - 1.2 / - 8.1 mg/dl 1/2 copies; p<0.0001	(Lai et al. 2003)

APOA5	- 1131T > C	rs662799	0.34 (C)	A	521 HoCo	-3.3 mg/dl per copy; p<0.001	(Yamada et al. 2007)
APOA5	-3A > G	rs651821	0.07	W	2056 (P)	M; p=0.30; F; p=0.26	(Klos et al. 2006a)
APOA5	-3A > G	rs651821	0.18 (G)	C	2711 (GP)	-2.3/-5.8 mg/dl 1/2 copies ; p<0.0001	(Lai et al. 2003)
APOA5	-3A > G	rs651821	0.34 (C)	A	5207 (Ho Co, P)	-2.7 mg/dl per copy; p<0.001	(Yamada et al. 2007)
APOA5	-3A > G	rs651821	0.36 (G)	A	2417 (Ho Co)	-3.9 / - 7.0 mg/dl 1/2 copies ; p<0.001	(Yamada et al. 2008)
APOA5	S19W	rs3135506	0.06 (W)	UK	1660 (P)	-1.9 / +1.2 mg/dl (1/2 copies); p=0.02	(Talmud et al. 2002a)
APOA5	56C>G	rs3135506	0.06 (G)	W	2347 (P)	-2.0 mg/dl for carriers; p=0.008	(Lai et al. 2004)
APOA5		rs2072560	0.16 (A)	C	2711 (GP)	-1.9 /-3.9 mg/dl (1/2 copies) ; p=0.003	(Lai et al. 2003)
APOA5	IVS3+476 G>A	rs2072560		Ma	707 (P)	-0.4 /9.3 mg/dl (1/2 copies) ; p=0.004	(Qi et al. 2007)
APOA5	V153M	rs3135507		W	2557	F:- 3.5 mg/dl for carriers; p<0.01	(Hubacek 2005)
APOA5	+553	rs2075291	0.07 (T)	A	5206 HoCo	-4.6 mg/dl per copy; p<0.001	(Yamada et al. 2007)
APOA5	Gly185Cys	rs2075291	0.08 (T)	A	2417 HoCo	-5.0 /-11.2 mg/dl (1/2 copies); p<0.001	(Yamada et al. 2008)
APOA5	1259T>C	rs2266788	0.18 (C)	C	2711 (GP)	-2.3 /-3.1 mg/dl 1/2 copies; p<0.0001	(Lai et al. 2003)
APOB		rs11902417	0.78 (G)	E	17723	p= 3.7x10^{-7}	(Waterworth et al. 2010)
APOC3	C455T	rs2854116	0.41 (C)	In	1308 (P)	-3.1/-5.4 mg/dl (1/2 copies) ; p<0.05	(Lahiry et al. 2007)
APOC3	PvuII	rs618354	0.49	A	F:291 (GP)	F: +0.1/-4.2 mg/dl 1/2 copies;p=0.029	(Kamboh et al. 1999)
APOC3	Sst1 RFLP	rs5128	0.09 (S2)	W	M:1219 (P)	M: -1.8 mg/dl for carriers; p=0.04.	(Russo et al. 2001)
APOC3	3′-utr/Sac I	rs5128	0.09 (+)	Hu	713 (P)	-5.0 mg/dl for heteroz.; p=0.0014	(Hegele et al. 1995)

APOC3	3238C > G	rs5128	0.07 (S2)	W	906 (GP)	+1.9 mg/dl for carriers; p=0.079	(Corella et al. 2002)
APOE	Cys112Arg	rs429358	0.16 (A)	N	3575	p=0.001	(Povel et al. 2011)
CETP	G2708A	rs12149545	0.30 (A)	W	2683 GP 556 Cvd	+1.9 mg/dl per copy; p<0.001	(McCaskie et al. 2007)
CETP	G2708A	rs12149545	0.31 (A)	W	709 (CVD)	+1.5 / +3.5 mg/dl (1/2 copies) ;p=0.0016	(Klerkx et al. 2003)
CETP		rs3764261	0.14 (T)	C	4192	+0.07 mg/dl; $p=4.3x10^{-14}$	(Liu et al. 2011)
CETP	G971A	rs4783961	0.49 (A)	W	709 (CVD)	+1.2/+1.9 mg/dl (1/2 copies) ; p=0.09	(Klerkx et al. 2003)
CETP	C629A	rs1800775	0.48 (A)	W	7083 (P)	+2.7 / +5.4 mg/dl (1/2 copies); p<0.001	(Borggreve et al. 2005a)
CETP	C629A	rs1800775	0.51 (A)	W	847 M, 873 F (P)	+4.2 mg/dl for homoz.; p<0.002	(Bernstein et al. 2003)
CETP	C629A	rs1800775	0.49 (A)	W	5287 (GP)	+3 / +5 mg/dl (1/2 copies) ; p= 2x10-29	(Kathiresan et al. 2008)
CETP	C629A	rs1800775	0.42 A	A	4050 (GP)	+2.2/+3.4 mg/dl 1/2 copies; p=3.28x10-9	(Tai et al. 2003b)
CETP	C629A	rs1800775	0.48 (A)	W	2683 GP 556 Cvd	+2.7 mg/dl per copy; p<0.001	(McCaskie et al. 2007)
CETP	C629A	rs1800775	0.40 (A)	W	1214 (CVD) 574 (Co)	CVD: +2.0/3.5mg/dl (1/2 copies) ; p=0.02 Co: +3.3/6.1 mg/dl (1/2 copies) ; p=0.05	(Blankenberg et al. 2004)
CETP	C629A	rs1800775	0.44 (A)	W	709 (CVD)	+0.8/3.9 mg/dl (1/2 copies) ; p<0.0001	(Klerkx et al. 2003)
CETP	C629A	rs1800775	0.50 (A)	W	309 (MI) 757 (Co)	+1.9/6.1 mg/dl (1/2 copies) ; p<0.0001	(Eiriksdottir et al. 2001)
CETP	C629A	rs1800775	0.48 (A)	W	498 (cvd) 1107(Co)	+2.9/4.4 mg/dl (1/2 copies) ; p<0.001	(Freeman et al. 2003)
CETP	Taq1B	rs708272	0.40 (B2)		13,677 (Meta)	+1.2 / +3.8 mg/dl 1/2 copies; p<0.0001	(Boekholdt et al. 2005)

CETP	Taq1B	rs708272			>10,000 (Meta)	+4.6 mg/dl for homoz.; p<0.00001	(Boekholdt & Thompson 2003)
CETP	Taq1B	rs708272	0.42 (B2)	W	7083 (P)	+2.7/5.0 mg/dl (1/2 copies) ; p<0.001	(Borggreve et al. 2005b)
CETP	Taq1B	rs708272	0.44 (B2)	W	2916 (P)	+2.5/4.7 mg/dl (1/2 copies) ; p<0.001	(Ordovas et al. 2000)
CETP	Taq1B	rs708272	0.43 0.26 (A)	W B	2056 1943 (P)	p<0.01; p<0.02	(Klos et al. 2006b)
CETP	Taq1B	rs708272	0.44 0.27 (A)	W B	8764 (P)	+2.3/5.8 mg/dl (1/2 copies) ; p<0.001 +3.8/9.8 mg/dl (1/2 copies) ; p<0.001	(Nettleton et al. 2007)
CETP	Taq1B	rs708272	0.41 (A)	W	1503 (P)	+2 /+5 mg/dl (1/2 copies) ; p<0.001	(Sandhofer et al. 2008)
CETP	Taq1B	rs708272	0.33 (A)	A	4207 (GP)	+2.5/4.4 mg/dl (1/2 copies ; p=1.25x10-10	(Tai et al. 2003b)
CETP	Taq1B	rs708272	0.40 (A)	A	1729 (GP)	M: +1.2/3.5 mg/dl (1/2 copies); p=0.096 F: +1.9/6.2 mg/dl (1/2 copies); p<0.001	(Tsujita et al. 2007)
CETP	Taq1B	rs708272	0.42 (A)	W	2683 GP 556 CVd	+2.7 mg/dl per copy; p<0.001	(McCaskie et al. 2007)
CETP	Taq1B	rs708272	0.42 (A)	W	2392 cvd 827 Co	+1.7/3.6 mg/dl (1/2 copies) ; p<0.001	(Whiting et al. 2005)
CETP	Taq1B	rs708272	0.40 (A)	W	1464 CVD	+2.1/3.0 mg/dl (1/2 copies) ; p=0.003	(Carlquist & Anderson 2007)
CETP	Taq1B	rs708272	0.41 (A)	W	1200 CV 571 (Co)	+2.6 /+4.3 mg/dl (1/2 copies) ; p<0.02	(Blankenberg et al. 2004)
CETP	Taq1B	rs708272	0.44 (A)	W	499 CVD 1105 Co	+2.1/3.6 mg/dl (1/2 copies) ; p<0.001	(Freeman et al. 2003)
CETP	+784CCC	rs34145065	0.39 (A)	W	709 (CVD)	+1.2/3.5 mg/dl (1/2 copies) ; p=0.0009	(Klerkx et al. 2003)

CETP	A373P	rs5880	0.05 (A)	W	8467 P 1636 CV	5.4 mg/dl for heteroz.; p<0.0001	(Agerholm-Larsen et al. 2000)
CETP	Ile405Val	rs5882			>10,000 (Meta)	+1.9 mg/dl for homoz. ; p<0.00001	(Boekholdt & Thompson 2003)
CETP	A + 16G/Ex.14	rs61212082	0.32 (A)	W	6421 (P)	M: +1.5/2.3 mg/dl (1/2 copies); p=0.002 F: +0.0/+2.3 mg/dl (1/2 copies); p=0.007	(Isaacs et al. 2007)
CETP		rs61212082	0.30 (A)	W	1208 (CVD) 572 (Co)	+1.4 /+3.1 mg/dl (1/2 copies) ; p=0.08 +0.3 /+8.4 mg/dl (1/2 copies); p=0.003	(Blankenberg et al. 2004)
CETP		rs61212082	0.30 (A)	W	498 (CVD) 1108 (Co)	+1.2 /+3.5 mg/dl (1/2 copies); p<0.05 +1.5 /+1.5 mg/dl (1/2 copies); p<0.05	(Freeman et al. 2003)
CETP	D442G	rs2303790b	0.03 (A)	A	3469 (He Ex)	+4.9 mg/dl for heteroz.; p<0.001	(Zhong et al. 1996)
CETP	R451Q	rs1800777	0.04 (A)	W	8467 (P) 1636 (CVD)	5.4 mg/dl for heterozygotes ; p<0.001	(Agerholm-Larsen et al. 2000)
CETP	G + 82A/Ex15	rs1800777	0.03 (A)	W	1071 CV 532 Co	3.6 /5.2 mg/dl for heteroz.; p=0.06/0.07	(Blankenberg et al. 2004)
CETP		rs12596776	0.90 (C)	EA	25,167	p=1.18E-05	(Dumitrescu et al. 2011)
CETP		rs9989419	0.39 (A)	EA	25,167	p=1.71E-53	(Dumitrescu et al. 2011)
LCAT	Gly230Arg			W	156 low 160 high	Variant sig. only in low HDL group	(Miettinen et al. 1998)
LCAT	608C/T	rs5922	.	A	203 (CVD)	Increase in HDL; p=0.015	(Zhang et al. 2003)
LCAT		rs5922		A	150 Str 122 Co	Lower HDL-C in heteroz.; p<0.05	(Zhu et al. 2006)
LCAT	P143L +511C>T			A	190 CVD 209 (Co)	Association with low HDLC; p<0.01	(Zhang et al. 2004)
LCAT		rs2292318	0.12 (A)	W	1442 CVD,Co	Increases HDLC; p=2 x 10 -5	(Pare et al. 2007)

LDLR	Exon 2	rs2228671		W	1543 (P)	+3.8 mg/dl for carriers; p=0.0056	(Costanza et al. 2005)
LDLR	1866C > T Asn591Asn	rs688 = rs57911429	0.12 (T)	A	2417 (Ho Co)	+1.5 / +8.5 mg/dl (1/2 copies) ; p=0.0155	(Yamada et al. 2008)
LDLR	Exon 12/HincII	rs688 = rs57911429	0.39 (+)	Hu	713 (P)	2.3 / 4.3 mg/dl (1/2 copies) ; p=0.047	(Hegele et al. 1995)
LDLR	2052T >C	rs5925 = rs57369606	0.17 (C)	A	2417 HoCo	+1.2/+5.4 (1/2 copies) ; p=0.043	(Yamada et al. 2008)
LIPC	T-710C	rs1077834	0.22 (C)	W	9121 (P)	+3–4% per copy; p<0.001	(Andersen et al. 2003)
LIPC	C-514Ta	rs1800588	0.25 (T)	Va	>24,000 (Meta)	+1.5 / +3.5 mg/dl (1/2 copies); p<0.001	(Isaacs et al. 2004)
LIPC	Pos.-480T	rs1800588	0.21 (T) 0.53 (T)	W B	8897 (P) 2909 (P)	W: +2.2/+3.8 mg/dl (1/2 copies); p<0.001 B: +1.6/+4.0 mg/dl (1/2 copies); p<0.001	(Nettleton et al. 2007)
LIPC		rs1800588	0.21 (T)	W	6239 (P)	+1.3/+4.3 mg/dl (1/2 copies); p<0.001	(Isaacs et al. 2007)
LIPC		rs1800588	0.38 (T)	A	2170 (P)	+2.3 / +2.7 mg/dl (1/2 copies); p=0.001	(Tai et al. 2003a)
LIPC		rs1800588	0.21 (T)	W	5287 (GP)	+1 / +4 mg/dl (1/2 copies) ; p=4x 10 -10	(Kathiresan et al. 2008)
LIPC		rs1800588	0.25 (T)	W	2773 (GP)	+1.5 mg/dl per copy; p=0.04	(Talmud et al. 2002b)
LIPC		rs1800588	0.24 (T)	W	3319 CV 1385 Co	+1.0 / +3.8 mg/dl (1/2 copies); p=0.001	(Whiting et al. 2005)
LIPC		rs1800588	0.51 (T)	A	5207 Ho Co	+2.5 mg/dl per copy; p<0.001	(Yamada et al. 2007)
LIPC		rs1800588	0.21 (T)	W	6412 (CVD)	+2.0–2.5 mg/dl per copy; p<0.001	(McCaskie et al. 2006)
LIPC	G -250A	rs2070895	0.22 (A)	W	9121 (P)	+3–4% per copy; p<0.001	(Andersen et al. 2003)
LIPC		rs2070895		W	1543 (P)	+1.5 mg/dl for carriers; p=0.020	(Costanza et al. 2005)
LIPC		rs2070895	0.32 (A)	W	514 (P)	M; p=0.001	(de Andrade et al. 2004)

LIPC		rs2070895	0.23 (A)	W	5585 (P)	+3.9/3.9 mg/dl (1/2 copies); p=8x10-10	(Grarup et al. 2008)
LIPC		rs2070895	0.51 (A)	A	5213 HoCo	+2.7 mg/dl per copy; p<0.001	(Yamada et al. 2007)
LIPC		rs2070895	0.39 (A)	A	716 HeEx	+2.1 mg/dl for carriers; p=0.026	(Ko et al. 2004)
LIPC		rs12594375	0.37 (A)	A	2970 (GP)	p=0.00003	(Iijima et al. 2008)
LIPC		rs8023503	0.38 (T)	A	2970 (GP)	p=0.0001	(Iijima et al. 2008)
LIPC	+1075C	rs3829462	0.05 (C)	A	823	+8.0 mg/dl for heterozygotes; p<0.05	(Fang & Liu 2002)
LIPC		rs4775041	0.29C	EA	25,167	p=1.03E-16	(Dumitrescu et al. 2011)
LIPC		rs261332	0.20 (A)	EA	25,167	p=1.99E-13	(Dumitrescu et al. 2011)
LPC		rs261334	0.20 (T)	E	17723	p= 4.9×10^{-22}	(Waterworth et al. 2010)
LIPG	-384A > C	rs3813082	0.12 (C)	A	541 (Co)	+1.3/+10.2 mg/dl (1/2 copies) ; p=0.021	(Hutter et al. 2006)
LIPG		rs3813082	0.12 (C)	A	340 (Kids)	+0.7/+9.8 (1/2 copies) ; p=0.0086	(Yamakawa-Kobayashi et al. 2003)
LIPG	584 C/T T111I	rs2000813	0.32 (I)	W	495 (GP)	M: 1.2 /+2.7 mg/dl (1/2 copies) ; p=0.82 F: 0.4 /+1.9 mg/dl (1/2 copies) ; p=0.09	(Paradis et al. 2003)
LIPG		rs2000813	0.24 (T)	A	541 (Co)	+0.5/+6.1 mg/dl (1/2 copies) ; p=0.048	(Hutter et al. 2006)
LIPG		rs2000813	0.30 (T)	A	265 CVD 265 Co	+3.7 for carries; p=<0.02	(Tang et al. 2008)
LIPG		rs2000813	0.29 (T)	W 90%	372 (CVD)	+1.6 /+6.0 mg/dl (1/2 copies) ; p=0.035	(Ma et al. 2003)
LIPG	C+42T/In 5	rs2276269	0.44 (T)	W	594 (HDL)	Decreases HDLC; p=0.007	(Mank-Seymour et al. 2004)

LIPG	T+2864C/In8	rs6507931	0.42 (C)	W	594 (HDL)	Decreases HDLC; p=0.004	(Mank-Seymour et al. 2004)
LIPG	2237G > A	rs3744841	0.36 (A)	A	340 (Kids)	4.0 mg/dl / -4.3 mg/dl (1/2 copies) ; p=0.011	(Yamakawa-Kobayashi et al. 2003)
LPL	D9N; Asp9Asn	rs1801177		-	5067 (Meta)	-3.1 mg/dl for heteroz.; p=0.002	(Wittrup et al. 1999)
LPL	Gly188Glu			-	10,434 (Meta)	- 9.7 mg/dl for heteroz.; p<0.001	(Wittrup et al. 1999)
LPL	N291S	rs268		-	14,912 (Meta)	-4.6 mg/dl for heteroz.; p<0.001	(Wittrup et al. 1999)
LPL	HindIll; Int8	rs320	0.30 (H)	W	520 (P)	+5.5 mg/dl in H - H- vs. H+H+; p=0.025	(Senti et al. 2001)
LPL	HindIll; Int8	rs320	0.26 (H1)	W	1361 (P)	M: +3.5 mg/dl for heteroz. ; p=0.0018 F : +4.2 mg/dl for heteroz. ; p=0.0212	(Holmer et al. 2000)
LPL	HindIll; Int8	rs320	0.32 (H)	W	906 (GP)	+1.9 mg/dl; p=0.003	(Corella et al. 2002)
LPL	HindIll; Int8	rs320		A	550 (NGT) 465 (DM)	NGT: +3.0 mg/dl for carriers; p<0.05 DM: +1.0 mg/dl for carriers; p<0.05	(Radha et al. 2006)
LPL	HindIll; Int8	rs320	0.27-0.31	NHW, H	615(W); 579(H)	p=0.005	(Ahn et al. 1993)
LPL		rs326	0.44	B	1943 (P)	M; p=0.013; F; p=0.004	(Klos et al. 2006a)
LPL	S447X Ser447Ter	rs328			4388 (Meta)	+1.5 mg/dl for heteroz.; p<0.001	(Wittrup et al. 1999)
LPL	S447X Ser447Ter	rs328	0.10 (G)	W	8968 (P)	+2.8 / +4.0 mg/dl (1/2 copies); p<0.001	(Nettleton et al. 2007)
LPL	S447X Ser447Ter	rs328	0.07 (G)	B	2677 (P)	+3.1 / +12.6 mg/dl (1/2 copies); p<0.001	
LPL	S447X	rs328	0.11 (X)	A	4058 (P)	+3.1 mg/dl; p<0.001	(Lee et al. 2004)
LPL		rs328		W	1543 (P)	+2.7 mg/dl; p=0.0017	(Costanza et al. 2005)
LPL		rs328			25,167	P=5.6E-22	(Dumitrescu et al. 2011)
LPL		rs328	0.09 (G)	W	5287 (GP)	+3 / +5 mg/dl (1/2 copies); p=3 x 10-12	(Kathiresan et al. 2008)

LPL		rs325	0.89 (T)	E	17723	p= 7.8×10-25	(Waterworth et al. 2010)
MLXIPL		rs17145738	0.12 (T)	EA	25,167	p=1.64E-05	(Dumitrescu et al. 2011)
PON1	Q192R	rs662 = rs60480675	0.30 (G)	W	1232 (P)	W: +0.1 / +2.3 mg/dl (1/2 copies) ; p=0.041	(Srinivasan et al. 2004)
PON1	Gln192Arg	rs662 = rs60480675	0.67	B	554	-5.4 / - 6.7 mg/dl (1/2 copies) ; p=0.008	"
PON1		rs662 = rs60480675	0.29 (R)	Hu	738 (P)	-3.1 mg/dl / - 3.1 mg/dl (1/2 copies) ; p=0.001	(Hegele et al. 1995)
PON1		rs662 = rs60480675	0.36 (R)	W-Bra	261 CVD, Co	M: +1.5 / +2.7 mg/dl (1/2 copies) ; p=0.035	(Rios et al. 2007)
PON1	C -107T	rs705379	0.48 (C)	W	710 (CVD)	-3.1/ - 2.3 mg/dl (1/2 copies) ; p=0.006	(Blatter Garin et al. 2006)
PON1	Leu55M	rs85456	0.20 (T)	MA	741	p=0.02	(Chang et al. 2010)
SCARB1	Exon 8 C>T	rs5888	0.44 (T)	W	865 (P)	+1.9/2.7 mg/dl 1/2 copies;p=0.006	(Morabia et al. 2004)
SCARB1	C1050T	rs5888	0.49 (T)	W	546 (CVD)	+2.3 / +1.9 mg/dl (1/2 copies); p=0.03	(Boekholdt et al. 2006)

Table 1. Genetic Polymorphisms Associated With HDL-C. MAF=Minor Allele Frequency; Ethn.: A=Asians; AA=African Americans; Am=Amish; A-I=Asian Indian; B=Blacks; C=Chinese; CH=Caribbean Hispanics; In=Inuit; Ma= Malays; N=Netherlands; NHW=Non-Hispanic Whites; H=Hispanics; Hu=Hutteries; Tu=Turks; UK=United Kingdom; W-Bra=Caucasian Brazilians; W= Whites; Va=Various; Non-DM C0=Non diabetic control subjects; MI=Myocardial infarction; NGT=Normal glucose tolerance; DM= Diabetes mellitus; Ho Sta= Hospital staff; HBP= Hypertensive patients; He Ex=Health examination; Cor Ang=coronary angiography; hyperCH=hypercholesterolemia patients; CVD= Cardiovascular Disease; Co=Controls; Ho Co=Hospital based controls; GP=General Population; Meta= Meta Analysis; P=Population based; M= Males; F= females; + =increase; - = decrease; n.s.=not significant; see text for full gene names. Adapted from Boes et al. (2009) with permission from Elsevier.

2.1 Genetic variation in enzymes involved in lipid metabolism and HDL-C levels

Perhaps, the most notable gene in the HDL-C synthesis and metabolism pathways, whose variants have been consistently associated with HDL-C, is the cholesterol ester transfer protein (CETP), which is a key plasma protein that mediates the transfer of esterfied cholesterol from HDL to APOB containing particles in exchange for TG. Although complete loss of CETP function is rare and can yield HDL-C levels up to five times higher than normal (Klos and Kullo, 2007), three common polymorphisms (Table 1: TaqIB (rs708272); -

629C>A (rs1800775); Ile405Val (rs5882)) can all modestly inhibit CETP activity and have been consistently associated with higher HDL-C levels (Bernstein et al., 2003; Blankenberg et al., 2004; Boekholdt et al., 2005; Boekholdt and Thompson, 2003; Borggreve et al., 2005; Eiriksdottir et al., 2001; Freeman et al., 2003; Kathiresan et al., 2008a; Klerkx et al., 2003; Tai et al., 2003b; Thompson et al., 2008). The CETP gene is located on chromosome 16 (16q21).

Lipoprotein lipase (LPL) is an enzyme involved in lipolysis of TG-containing lipoproteins such as VLDL and chlyomicrons (Miller and Zhan, 2004), which generate free fatty acids (FFA) that can be taken up by the liver, muscle and adipose tissues (Kwan et al., 2007). Thus, LPL affects LDL levels directly (see Section 3.2) may only affect HDL-C levels indirectly (Lewis and Rader, 2005). The human LPL gene is located on chromosome 8 (8p22). Several LPL SNPs have been associated with HDL-C (Table 1) (Ahn et al., 1993; Corella et al., 2002; Holmer et al., 2000; Klos and Kullo, 2007; Klos et al., 2006; Komurcu-Bayrak et al., 2007; Lee et al., 2004; Nettleton et al., 2007; Senti et al., 2001; Wittrup et al., 1999); however, many of them are in strong linkage disequilibrium with each other (e.g., rs320, rs326, rs13702, rs10105606) (Boes et al., 2009; Heid et al., 2008).

Hepatic lipase (HL; LIPC) is a glycoprotein that is synthesized by liver cells (hepatocytes) and catalyzes the hydrolysis of TG and phospholipids (Miller et al., 2003). For example, after hydrolysis of TG by LPL, VLDL particles are reduced to IDL particles and can be further hydrolyzed by HL/LIPC to LDL or taken up by the liver (Kwan et al., 2007). The human HL/LIPC gene is located on chromosome 15 (15q21). Several HL/LIPC SNPs have been associated with HDL-C levels (Table 1) (Andersen et al., 2003; Costanza et al., 2005; de Andrade et al., 2004; Fang and Liu, 2002; Grarup et al., 2008; Iijima et al., 2008; Isaacs et al., 2007; Kathiresan et al., 2008b; Ko et al., 2004; McCaskie et al., 2006; Nettleton et al., 2007; Tai et al., 2003a; Talmud et al., 2002b; Whiting et al., 2005; Yamada et al., 2007). However, the most consistent associations have been observed for rs1800588 and rs2070895 and, several SNPs in the promoter region are in strong LD (Boes et al., 2009).

Endothelial lipase (EL; LIPG) is an enzyme expressed in endothelial cells that, in the presence of HL/LIPC, metabolizes larger (HDL_3) to smaller (HDL_2) HDL-C particles and increases the catabolism of APOA-I (see Section 2.3) (Jaye and Krawiec, 2004). EL/LIPG plays a role in the dyslipidemia component and, possibly, the yet to be established, proinflammatrory component of MetSyn (Lamarche and Paradis, 2007) (see Section 5.0). The human EL/LIPG gene is located on chromosome 18 (18q21.1). Several polymorphisms in EL/LPIG have been associated with HDL-C levels (Table 1) (Hutter et al., 2006; Ma et al., 2003; Mank-Seymour et al., 2004; Paradis et al., 2003; Tang et al., 2008; Yamakawa-Kobayashi et al., 2003). However, most of these SNPs have not been as well studied as those in CETP, LPL and EL; and, only the nonsynonymous SNP, rs2000813, has been consistently associated with HDL-C levels in African American populations (Hutter et al., 2006; Tang et al., 2008; Yamakawa-Kobayashi et al., 2003).

In the presence of cofactor, APOA-I (see Section 2.3), lecithin-cholesteryl acyltransferase (LCAT), catalyzes the esterification of free cholesterol and, can metabolize larger HDL-C particles to smaller HDL-C particles (Klos and Kullo, 2007; Miller and Zhan, 2004). The human LCAT is located on chromosome 16 (16q22.1). Although mutations leading to complete loss of LCAT and marked (5-10%) reduction in HDL-C levels are rare and can cause cornea opacifications (fish eye disease) and renal disease (Garg and Simha, 2007), several common polymorphisms in LCAT have been associated, albeit inconsistently, with much more modest changes in HDL-C levels (Table 1) (Boekholdt et al., 2006; Miettinen et al., 1998; Pare et al., 2007; Zhang et al., 2004; Zhu et al., 2006).

Parroxanonase 1 (PON1), inhibits the oxidation of LDL (Mackness et al., 1991) and, therefore, may only indirectly affect antioxidant properties of HDL-C. The human PON1 gene is located on chromosome 7 (7q21.3). Several SNPs in PON1 have been associated with HDL-C levels, most notably, two nonsynonymous SNPs, rs662 and rs3202100, which are in strong LD, but results are inconsistent across studies (Table 1) (Blatter Garin et al., 2006; Hegele et al., 1995; Manresa et al., 2006; Rios et al., 2007; van Aalst-Cohen et al., 2005).

2.2 Genetic variation in receptors and transporters and HDL-C levels

Scavenger receptor class B, type 1 (SCARB1; SR-B1), which is highly expressed in liver and steroidogenic tissues (testes, ovaries, adrenal) (Cao et al., 1997), has been shown to participate in the uptake of HDL in animals by transferring cholesterol from the HDL-C particle and releasing the lipid-depleted HDL particle into the circulation (Acton et al., 1996; Miller et al., 2003). The human SCARB1 gene is located on chromosome 12 (12q24.31). Only a few studies have examined potential associations between SCARB1 polymorphisms and HDL-C levels (Table 1) (Boekholdt et al., 2006; Costanza et al., 2005; Hsu et al., 2003; Morabia et al., 2004; Osgood et al., 2003; Roberts et al., 2007). The most well studied polymorphism has been rs5888; however, the association with rs5888 and HDL-C levels was only significant among Caucasian (White, W) males in one study (Morabia et al., 2004), Amish females (Roberts et al., 2007) and Caucasian CVD patients (Boekholdt et al., 2006).

The LDL receptor (LDLR) and LDLR-related protein participate in the uptake of LDL and chylomicron remnants by hepatocytes (Kwan et al., 2007) and, therefore, may only indirectly affect HDL-C levels. The human LDLR is located on chromosome 19 (19p13.2). Although some common polymorphisms in LDLR have been associated with HDL-C levels (Table 1: (Costanza et al., 2005; Hegele et al., 1995; Yamada et al., 2008), their impact is likely greater on LDL-C levels (see Section 3.1).

The ATP-binding cassette transporter A1 (ABCA1), which is highly expressed in the liver, steroidogenic tissues and macrophages, plays a key role in 'reverse cholesterol transport' by mediating the efflux of cholesterol and phospholipids from macrophages to the nascent lipid-free, APOA-1 HDL particle (Cavelier et al., 2006; Miller et al., 2003). The human ABCA1 gene is located on chromosome 9 (9q31.1). Due to its functional importance, genetic variants in this gene have been well investigated but many of them are quite rare including the homozygous deletion that leads to Tangier's disease that is characterized by very low HDL-C levels (~5 mg/dl), orange colored tonsils, peripheral neuropathy and, sometimes, premature CHD (Garg and Simha, 2007). Several common polymorphisms have been fairly consistently associated with more modest changes in HDL-C levels but different variants appear to drive this association in different ethnic groups (Table 1) (Clee et al., 2001; Costanza et al., 2005; Frikke-Schmidt et al., 2004; Hodoglugil et al., 2005; Kathiresan et al., 2008b; Klos et al., 2006; Porchay et al., 2006; Shioji et al., 2004b; Whiting et al., 2005).

2.3 Genetic variation in apolipoproteins and HDL-C levels

Apolipoprotein A-1 (APOA1; APOA-I) is a ligand required for HDL-C binding to its receptors including SCARB1 and ABCA1 and, is an important cofactor in 'reverse cholesterol transport' (Miller et al., 2003; Remaley et al., 2001; Rigotti et al., 1997). The human APOA1 gene is located on chromosome 11 (11q23-24). APOA-I is a major constituent of HDL particles and deletions leading to complete APOA-I deficiency are rare but lead to HDL deficiency (HDL-C <10 mg/dl) and sometimes CHD (Garg and Simha, 2007). Several common polymorphisms in APOA-I have been associated with more modest reductions in HDL-C but results across studies are inconsistent (Table 1) (Brown et al., 2006; Kamboh et al., 1999b; Larson et al., 2002; Shioji et al., 2004a).

Apolipoprotein A-4 (APOA4; APOA-IV) is a potent activator of LCAT and modulates the activation of LPL and transfer of cholestryl esters from HDL to LDL (Kwan et al., 2007). The human APOA4 gene is located on chromosome 11 near APOA1 (11q23) and is part of what is known as the APOA1/C3/A4/A5 gene cluster. Polymorphisms in APOA4 have not been as well studied; however, the nonsynonymous SNP, rs5110 (Gln360His), has recently been associated with reduced HDL-C levels in Brazilian elderly (Ota et al., 2011) and coronary artery calcification (CAC) progression, a marker of subclinical atherosclerosis, in patients with Type I Diabetes Mellitus (T1DM) (Kretowski et al., 2006). The rs675 polymorphism has been associated with reduced HDL-C levels in females with T2DM (Qi et al., 2007).

Apolipoprotein A-5 (APOA5; APOA-V) is located predominantly on TG-rich chylomicrons and VLDL and activates LPL (Hubacek, 2005). The human APOA5 gene is located on chromosome 11 (11q23) in the APOA1/C3/A4/A5 gene cluster. Several APOA5 SNPs have been associated with reduced HDL-C levels; and, perhaps, the most well studied and consistent associations have been observed for rs651821 and rs662799 (Table 1) (Grallert et al., 2007; Hubacek, 2005; Klos et al., 2006; Lai et al., 2003; Qi et al., 2007; Talmud et al., 2002a; Yamada et al., 2008; Yamada et al., 2007).

Apolipoprotein C-3 (APOC3; APOC-III) is an inhibitor of LPL and is transferred to HDL during the hydrolysis of TG-rich lipoproteins (Kwan et al., 2007; Miller and Zhan, 2004). The human APOC3 gene is located on chromosome 11 (11q23) in the APOA1/C3/A4/A5 gene cluster. Although several APOC3 SNPs have been identified and investigated, associations between these SNPs and HDL-C levels have been quite inconsistent (Table 1) (Arai and Hirose, 2004; Brown et al., 2006; Corella et al., 2002; Hegele et al., 1995; Kamboh et al., 1999a; Lahiry et al., 2007; Pallaud et al., 2001; Qi et al., 2007; Russo et al., 2001).

Chylomicron remnants, VLDL and IDL particles are rich in apolipoprotein E (APOE) and APOE is a critical ligand for binding to hepatic receptors that remove these particles from the circulation (Kwan et al., 2007). Mutations in APOE are well known to modify LDL-C levels; however, their independent influence on HDL-C levels remains controversial (Sviridov and Nestel, 2007). Nevertheless, associations between APOE SNPs and HDL-C levels in large scale studies have been fairly consistent (Costanza et al., 2005; Frikke-Schmidt et al., 2000; Gronroos et al., 2008; Kataoka et al., 1996; Srinivasan et al., 1999; Volcik et al., 2006; Wilson et al., 1994; Wu et al., 2007).

2.4 GWAS and HDL-C Levels

Results from genomewide association studies (GWAS) have confirmed associations between polymorphisms in viable candidate genes including CETP, LPL, HL/LIPIC, EL/LIPG, ABCA1, LCAT and the APOA1/C3/A4/A5 gene cluster and HDL-C levels (Boes et al., 2009). GWAS have also identified several novel putative loci, which are discussed in detail in a recent review (Teslovich et al., 2010).

3. Genetic variants in lipid metabolism and LDL-C levels

3.1 Genetic variation in enzymes, receptors and transporters and LDL-C levels

LDL-C is a widely accepted risk factor for atherosclerotic cardiovascular diseases. The most marketed drugs for lowering LDL-C are statins, which inhibit hydroxy-3-methylglutaryl coenzyme A reductase (HMGCR), the rate limiting enzyme in cholesterol synthesis that is normally suppressed (Endo, 1992). The human HMGCR gene is located on chromosome 5 (5q13.3-14). Only a few common HMGCR polymorphisms have been associated with LDL-C levels including rs3846662, which was identified through GWAS (Table 2) (Burkhardt et al., 2008; Hiura et al., 2010; Polisecki et al., 2008; Teslovich et al., 2010).

As mentioned above, the LDL receptor (LDLR) regulates the uptake of LDL and chylomicron remnants by hepatocytes (Kwan et al., 2007) and, the human LDLR gene is located on chromosome 19 (19p13.2). Familial (or monogenic) hypercholesterolemia (FH: OMIM No. 143890), which is due to mutations in LDLR occurring at a frequency of approximately 1 in 500 (heterozygotes) to 1 in 1,000,000 (homozygotes), is one of the most common inherited metabolic diseases and results in a reduced number of LDL receptors and, in heterozygotes, a 2- to 3-fold increase in LDL-C levels and, in homozygotes, complete loss of LDLR function and a greater than 5-fold increase in LDL-C (Garg and Simha, 2007). A few common polymorphisms in LDLR have been identified and associated with more modest changes in LDL-C levels, most notably, rs6511720, which was highly significantly associated with LDL-C in a recent meta analysis (Table 2) (Teslovich et al., 2010; Willer et al., 2008).

ATP-binding cassette transporters G5 and G8 (ABCG5/8) regulate the efflux of cholesterol back into the intestinal lumen and, in hepatocytes, the efflux of cholesterol into bile (Graf et al., 2003). The human ABCG5/8 gene cluster is located on chromosome 2 (2p21). A rare autosomal recessive mutation in ABCG5/8 leads to sitosterolemia characterized by xanthomas, premature atherosclerosis and other features (Berge et al., 2000). Only a couple of common variants in ABCG5/8 have been associated with LDL-C levels and a recent meta-analysis failed to find associations between ABCG5/G8 polymorphisms including, ABCG8 rs6544718, and plasma lipid levels (Table 2) (Jakulj et al., 2010; Teslovich et al., 2010)

3.2 Genetic variation in lipoproteins and LDL-C levels

Apolipoprotein B (APOB; main isoform: ApoB-100) is responsible for the recognition and uptake of LDL by LDLR, which clears approximately 60-80% of the LDL in 'normal' individuals with the remaining taken up by LRP or SCARB1 (Kwan et al., 2007). The human APOB gene is located on chromosome 2 (2p23-24). Familial defective APOB (FDB: OMIM No. 144010) is an autosomal codominant disorder due to mutations in APOB that are a bit more rare than FH mutations at approximately 1 in 500 to 1 in 700 resulting in lower LDL-C levels than in FH patients (Garg and Simha, 2007). Common polymorphisms have also been identified and associated with more modest changes in LDL-C (Table 2) (Haas et al., 2011; Teslovich et al., 2010; Waterworth et al., 2010; Willer et al., 2008).

As mentioned above, APOE is a critical ligand for binding chylomicron remnants, VLDL and IDL particles to hepatic receptors to remove these particles from the circulation (Kwan et al., 2007). The human APOE gene is located on chromosome 19 (19q13.2). The structural APOE gene is polymorphic with three common alleles, designated as ε2, ε3 and ε4 which encode for E2, E3 and E4 proteins, respectively. Although several APOE polymorphisms have been identified, the APOE ε4 allele has been the most consistently associated with CHD and LDL-C levels (Table 2) (Anoop et al., 2010; Chang et al., 2010; Eichner et al., 2002; Teslovich et al., 2010; Willer et al., 2008).

Gene	Polym.	rs Number	MAF	Ethn.	Sample Size	Results (Effect Size, p-value)	Reference
ABCG8		rs4299376	0.30 (G)	E	95,454 (Meta)	+2.75 mg/dl; $p=2x10^{-8}$	(Teslovich et al. 2010)
ABCG8	A632V	rs6544718		Va	982	p=0.02	(Jakulјl et al. 2010)
APOB		rs562338	0.18 (A)	Va	10,849	+4.89 mg/dl; $p=3.6 X 10^{-12}$	(Willer et al. 2008)
APOB		rs754523	0.28 (A)	Va	6,542	+2.78 mg/dl; $p=1.3 X10^{-6}$	(Willer et al. 2008)
APOB		rs693	0.42 (G)	Va	3,222	+2.44 mg/dl; p=0.0034	(Willer et al. 2008)
APOB	Thr98Ile	rs1367117	0.30 (A)	E	95,454 (Meta)	+4.05 mg/dl; $p=4x10^{-114}$	(Teslovich et al. 2010)
APOB		rs7575840	0.28 (T)	F	5054	0.131 $p= 3.88x10^{-9}$	(Haas et al. 2011)
APOB		rs515135	0.19 (A)	Va	982	$p=2.4X10^{-20}$	Waterworth et al. (2010)
APOE		rs4420638	0.17 (G)	E	95,454 (Meta)	+7.14 mg/dl; $p=9x10^{-147}$	(Teslovich et al. 2010)
APOE	Arg176 Cys	rs7412	0.06 (T)	N-HB	683	-22.52mg/dl; p< 0.0001	(Chang et al. 2010)
APOE	Cys130 Arg	rs429358	0.076 (T)	M-A	739	10.54mg/dl; p< 0.0001	(Chang et al. 2010)
APOC1		rs4420638	0.82 (A)	Va	10,806	+6.61 mg/dl; $p = 4.9 X10^{-24}$	(Willer et al. 2008)
APOE/ C1/C4		rs10402271	0.67 (T)	Va	6,519	+2.62 mg/dl; $p =1.5 X 10^{-5}$	(Willer et al. 2008)
LDLR		rs6511720	0.11 (T)	E	95,454 (Meta)	-6.99 mg/dl; $p=4x10^{-117}$	(Teslovich et al. 2010)
LDLR		rs6511720	0.90 (T)	Va	7,442	+9.17 mg/dl; $p =3.3 X 10^{-19}$	(Willer et al. 2008)
PCSK9		rs11206510	0.81 (C)	Va	10,805	+3.04 mg/dl; $p=5.4 X 10^{-7}$	(Willer et al. 2008)
PCSK9		rs2479409	0.30 (G)	E	95,454 (Meta)	+2.01mg/dl; $p= 2x10^{-28}$	(Teslovich et al. 2010)
PCSK9	A443T Ala443Thr	rs28362263	0.06 (A)	B	1750	95.5 vs. 106.9 mg/dl;p<0.001	(Huang et al. 2009)
PCSK9	C679X	rs28362286		B	1750	81.5 vs. 106.9 mg/dl;p<0.001	(Huang et al. 2009)
PCSK9	E670G	rs505151	0.11 (G)	W	691	P=0.001	(Chen et al. 2005)
PCSK9		rs11206510	0.81 (T)	EA	21,986 (Meta)	p=1.44E-05	(Dumitrescu et al. 2011)
SORT1		rs629301	0.22 (G)	E	95,454 (Meta)	-5.65 mg/dl; $p=1 x 10^{-170}$	(Teslovich et al. 2010)

Table 2. Genetic Polymorphisms Associated with LDL-C. See Table 1 legend.

3.3 Genetic variation in proteases and LDL-C levels

Proprotein convertase subtilisin-like kexin type 9 (PCSK9) is a serine protease that degrades hepatic LDLR in endosomes (Maxwell et al., 2005). The human PCSK9 gene is located on chromosome 1 (1p32.3). A mutation in PCSK9 results in an autosomal dominant form of hypercholesterolemia (OMIM No. 607786) with clinical features similar to FH patients (Garg and Simha, 2007). Over 50 variants in PCSK9 have been shown to affect circulating levels of cholesterol; however, most of these are relatively rare (see Davignon et al., 2010) for a complete list). The number of common polymorphisms in PCSK9 is substantially less with only a few SNPs having been associated with changes in LDL-C levels (Table 2) (Chen et al., 2005; Evans and Beil, 2006; Huang et al., 2009; Teslovich et al., 2010; Willer et al., 2008).

3.4 GWAS and LDL-C Levels

GWAS have confirmed associations between polymorphisms in viable candidate genes including APOB, APOE, LDLR and PCSK9, and have identified novel SNPs associated with LDL-C levels with strong biological plausibility including an inhibitor of lipase (ANGPTL3), see Section 4.1 and a transcription factor activating triglyceride synthesis (MLXIPL) see Section 4.2 (Teslovich et al., 2010).

4. Genetic variants in lipid metabolism and TG levels

Plasma triglycerides (TG) integrate multiple TG-rich lipoprotein particles, predominantly, intestinally synthesized chylomicrons in the postprandial state and hepatically synthesized VLDL in the fasted state. Therefore, not surprisingly, there is considerable overlap between genetic variants associated with HDL-C and LDL-C levels as well as TG levels. For example, the Global Lipids Genetics Consortium (GLGC) found that 15 of the 32 loci associated with TG levels were also jointly associated with HDL-C levels, explaining 9.6% of the total variation in plasma TG, which corresponded to 25–30% of the total genetic contribution to TG variability (Teslovich et al., 2010). However, the joint associations reported do not appear additionally adjusted for the other lipid phenotype. Furthermore, certain loci appear to be more strongly associated with one lipid phenotype over the other while others have similar effect sizes; and, genetic heterogeneity between loci clearly exists between major ethnic groups.

4.1 Genetic variation in aolipoproteins and TG levels

As mentioned above (see Section 3.2), APOB is the backbone of atherogenic lipoproteins and is located on chromosome 2 (2p23-24). A rare monogenic autosomal recessive disorder called homozygous hypobetalipoproteinemia and rare autosomal codominant disorder called familial hypobetalipoproteinaemia (HHBL and FHBL, respectively: OMIM No. 107730), characterized by very low (<5th percentile of age- and sex-specific values) of plasma TG (and LDL-C) levels, which are caused by rare mutations in APOB (Burnett and Hooper, 2008; Di et al., 2009). Although common APOB polymorphisms have primarily been associated with LDL-C levels (Benn, 2009), GWAS has revealed that a common SNP in APOB, rs1042034, is associated with TG (Johansen and Hegele, 2011; Teslovich et al., 2010). Common polymorphisms in the APOA1/C3/A4/A5 gene cluster, located on chromosome 11 (11q23), have been associated with HDL-C levels (see Section 2.3) as well as TG levels (Teslovich et al., 2010; Willer et al., 2008). A SNP in the APOE gene, rs439401, has also been shown to be strongly associated with TG levels in a recent GWAS meta analyses (Johansen and Hegele, 2011; Teslovich et al., 2010).

z	Polym.	rs Number	MAF	Ethn.	Sample Size	Results (Effect Size, p-value)	Reference
ANGPTL3		rs2131925	0.32 (G)	E	96,598 (Meta)	-4.94mg/dl; $p=9x10^{-43}$	(Teslovich et al. 2010)
ANGPTL3		rs1748195	0.70 (G)	Va	9,559	7.12 mg/dl; $p=5.4x10^{-8}$	(Willer et al. 2008)
APOA5		rs964184	0.13 (G)	E	96,598 (Meta)	+16.95mg/dl; $p=7x10^{-240}$	(Teslovich et al. 2010)
APOA5/A 4/C3/A1		rs12286037	0.94 (C)	Va	9,738	25.82 mg/dl; $p=1.6x10^{-22}$	(Willer et al. 2008)
APOA5		rs662799	0.05 (A)	Va	3,248	16.88 mg/dl $p=2.7x10^{-10}$	(Willer et al. 2008)
APOA5/A 4/C3/A1		rs2000571	0.17 (G)	Va	3,209	6.93 mg/dl; $p=8.7x10^{-5}$	(Willer et al. 2008)
APOA5/A 4/C3/A1		rs486394	0.28 (A)	Va	3,597	1.50 mg/dl; p=0.0073	(Willer et al. 2008)
APOE		rs439401	0.40 (C)	C	4.192	$p=2.2\times10^{-5}$	(Liu et al. 2011)
APOE		rs439401	0.64 (C)	Va	Meta	$p=5.5x10^{-30}$	Johansen et al. (2010)
LIPC/HL		rs4775041	0.67 (G)	Va	8,462	3.62 mg/dl; $p=2.9x10^{-5}$	(Willer et al. 2008)
LIPC/HL		rs261342	0.22 (G)	Va	Meta	$p=2.0x10^{-13}$	Johansen et al. (2010)
LPL		rs12678919	0.12 (G)	E	96,598 (Meta)	-13.64 mg/dl $p=2x10^{-115}$	(Teslovich et al. 2010)
LPL		rs10503669	0.90 (A)	Va	9,711	11.57 mg/dl; $p=1.6x10^{-14}$	(Willer et al. 2008)
LPL		rs2197089	0.58 (A)	Va	3,202	3.38 mg/dl; p=0.0029	(Willer et al. 2008)
LPL		rs6586891	0.66 (A)	Va	3,622	4.60 mg/dl; $p=5x10^{-4}$	(Willer et al. 2008)
LPL	S447X	rs328	0.90 (C)	EA	24,258	p=4.16E-30	(Dumitrescu et al. 2011)
LPL	S447X	rs328	0.10 (X)	Va	43,242	-0.15 (-0.12- -0.19) mmol/l	(Sagoo et al. 2008)
LPL	D9N	rs1801177	0.03 (N)	Va	21,040	0.14 (0.08-0.20) mmol/l	(Sagoo et al. 2008)
LPL	N291S	rs368	0.03 (S)	Va	27,204	0.19 (0.12-0.26) mmol/l	(Sagoo et al. 2008)
LPL		rs326	0.18 (G)	C	4,192	$p=2.3\times10^{-6}$	(Liu et al. 2011)
LRP1		rs11613352	0.23 (T)	E	96,598 (Meta)	-2.70 mg/dl $p=4x10^{-10}$	(Teslovich et al. 2010)
MLXIPL		rs17145738	0.12 (T)	E	96,598 (Meta)	-9.32 mg/dl $p=6x10^{-58}$	(Teslovich et al. 2010)
MLXIPL		rs17145738	0.84 (T)	Va	9,741	8.21 mg/dl; $p=5x10^{-8}$	(Willer et al. 2008)
MLXIPL		rs7811265	0.81 (A)	Va	Meta	7.91 mg/dl $p=9.0\times10^{-59}$	(Johansen et al. 2011)

Table 3. Genetic Polymorphisms Associated With TG Levels. See Table 1 legend.

Angiopoietin-like 3 protein (ANGPTL3) inhibits LPL catalytic activity but this process is reversible (Shan et al., 2009; Shimizugawa et al., 2002). A monogenic autosomal recessive disorder called familial combined hypolipidemia (FCH: OMIM No. 605019), characterized by very low TG levels, is genetically complex and poorly understood; however, mutations in ANGPTL3 are believed to play a role. Common polymorphisms in ANGPTL3, most notably, rs2131925, have been associated with more modest changes in TG levels (Johansen and Hegele, 2011; Keebler et al., 2009; Lanktree et al., 2009; Teslovich et al., 2010; Willer et al., 2008). Sequencing individuals in the Dallas Heart Study has identified several additional nonsynonymous ANGPTL3 variants affecting TG levels (Musunuru et al., 2010); however, these SNPs require further investigation in other populations.

4.2 Genetic variation in enzymes and transcription factors and TG levels

As mentioned above (see Section 2.1), LPL is an enzyme that hydrolyzes TG-rich particles in peripheral tissues (muscle, macrophages, adipose) generating FFA and glycerol for energy metabolism and storage (Goldberg, 1996). More than 100 mutations in LPL have been identified (Murthy et al., 1996); however, only a few common nonsynonymous SNPs have been consistently associated with TG levels including rs1801177, rs328 and rs268 (Mailly et al., 1995; Rip et al., 2006; Sagoo et al., 2008; Teslovich et al., 2010; Willer et al., 2008). Two SNPs, rs1801177 and rs328, have also been consistently associated with CHD; however, there is fairly strong LD between these SNPs, at least in Caucasians (Sagoo et al., 2008).

MLX interacting protein like (MLXIPL) locus encodes a transcription factor of the Myc/Max/Mad superfamily which activates, in a glucose-dependent manner, carbohydrate response element binding protein (CREBP) that is expressed in lipogenic tissues coordinating the subsequent activation of lipogenic enzymes such as fatty acid synthase (FAS) to convert dietary carbohydrate to TG (Iizuka and Horikawa, 2008). The human MLXIPL gene is located on chromosome 7 (7q11.23). Although initially identified through GWAS, the rs1745738 polymorphism has been replicated in other studies (Johansen and Hegele, 2011; Teslovich et al., 2010; Wang et al., 2008; Willer et al., 2008).

5. Genetic variants in dyslipidemia and the Metabolic Syndrome (MetSyn)

As mentioned in the Introduction (see Section 1.0), MetSyn is a clustering of traits including dyslipidemia as well as obesity, hypertension and insulin resistance/dysglycemia. Undoubtedly, there is complex interplay between genetic determinants of each of these traits and 'environmental' factors including those related to lifestyle (diet, exercise, sleep) and those related to toxin exposure. Due to space limitations, we focus only on the genetic determinants of dyslipidemia that overlap with MetSyn defined as a single, unifying trait and refer the reader to other reviews for genetic determinants of the other traits involved in MetSyn (Joy et al., 2008; Monda et al., 2010; Pollex and Hegele, 2006; Sharma and McNeill, 2006) and their interactions with lifestyle factors (Adamo and Tesson, 2008; Garaulet et al., 2009; Ordovas and Shen, 2008; Phillips et al., 2008) and toxins (Andreassi, 2009).

Lipoprotein related genes with common SNPs associated with MetSyn (as defined by NCEP ATP III and AHA/NHLBI criteria) and HDL-C, LDL-C or TG levels include APOA5 and APOC3 (Table 4) (Grallert et al., 2007; Joy et al., 2008; Miller et al., 2007; Pollex et al., 2006; Pollex and Hegele, 2006; Yamada et al., 2008). Enzymes involved in lipid metabolism with genetic polymorphisms that have also been associated with MetSyn (using the NCEP ATPIII criteria) appear limited to the nonsynonymous SNP in LPL, rs328 (Table 4) (Joy et al., 2008;

Komurcu-Bayrak et al., 2007). Several SNPs in the LDLR have been associated with MetSyn (using AHA/NHLBI criteria) and LDL-C or HDL-C (Joy et al., 2008; Yamada et al., 2008).

Gene	Polymorphism	rs Number	Ethn.	Sample Size	Results (p-value)	Reference	Comments (definition)
APOA5	-1131T→C		J	1788	$p < 0.0009$	(Yamada et al. 2007)	NCEP ATP III
APOA5	c.56C→G		C	3124	$p=0.026$	(Grallert et al. 2007)	NCEP ATP III
APOA5	-3A→G		J	2417	$p < 0.0001$	(Yamada et al. 2008)	AHA/NHLBI
APOC3	-455T→C		O-C	515	$p=0.029$*	(Miller et al. 2007) (Pollex et al. 2006)	*Women only NCEP ATP III
LDLR	2052TmC		J	2417	$p=0.0005$	(Yamada et al. 2008)	AHA/NHLBI
LPL	S447X		Tu	1586	$p=0.04$	(Komurcu-Bayrak et al. 2007)	NCEP ATP III
LPL		rs295	Va	1407	OR= 0.7; $p=2.1 \times 10^{-3}$	(Grassi et al. 2011)	NCEP ATPIII

Table 4. Genetic Polymorphisms in Lipid Metabolism Associated with MetSyn. See Table 1 legend. WHO= World Health Organization; NCEP ATP III=National Cholesterol Education Program Adult Treatment Panel III, IDF=International Diabetes Federation; AHA=American Heart Association; NHLBI=National Heart, Lung, and Blood institute.

6. Genetic variants in dyslipidemia and MetSyn: Future directions

Given the polygenic nature and multi-level complexity of Dyslipidemia and MetSyn, a better understanding of the genetic determinants of each intermediate (lower level) phenotype as well as the collective integration of these traits as unifying syndromes (higher/hierarchical level) is needed, which will require more elegant statistical modeling methods and, perhaps, a paradigm shift in the way in which we think about dissecting genetic and environmental factors in complex traits. As stated throughout this chapter, there is considerable overlap between genetic variants associated with HDL-C, LDL-C and TG levels as well MetSyn as a unifying trait. As a result, there is great need to understand not only the aggregate effects of multiple variants in each of these genes but to also understand how the effects of variation in one gene are modified in the presence of other genes.

Aggregate effects of multiple variants in genes affecting dyslipidemia and MetSyn related traits have included calculation of 'risk scores', which simply add the number of 'risk alleles' in a weighted or unweighted manner. For example, unweighted risk scores were constructed by summing the number of 'TG-raising' alleles at 32 loci and placed in 'risk bins' (categories) to show that higher risk scores were significantly associated with patients with hypertriglyceridemia (HTG) compared to controls (Johansen and Hegele, 2011; Teslovich et al., 2010). Increasing genotype risk scores comprised by summing risk alleles in 9 common SNPs were associated with decreasing HDL-C levels (Kathiresan et al., 2008a).

We have used the multivariate statistical framework of structural equation modeling (SEM) to evaluate multiple genetic determinants of MetSyn and aggregate effects of individual genes by modeling MetSyn as a second-order factor together with multiple putative candidate genes represented by latent constructs, which we mathematically defined by multiple SNPs in each gene (Nock et al., 2009b). Using this approach with the Framingham Heart Study (Offspring Cohort, Exam 7; Affymetrix 50k Human Gene Panel) data, we found that the CETP gene had a very strong association with the Dyslipidemia factor but little effect on MetSyn directly. Furthermore, we found that the effects of the CSMD1 gene diminished when modeled simultaneously with six other candidate genes, most notably CETP and STARD13. Work to identify the genetic determinants of 'Syndrome Z', modeled as a higher-order, unifying syndrome defined by 5 first-order factors (dyslipidemia, insulin resistance, obesity, hypertension, sleep disturbance) (Nock et al., 2009a) using the latent gene construct SEM approach is underway.

The use of other forms of 'causal modeling' (edge/node; integrative genetics) has been proposed (Lusis et al., 2008), particularly, to improve our understanding of differential effects by gender as well as to better understand how maternal nutrition and epigenetics affect MetSyn. Furthermore, a complex model for the genetic determinants of MetSyn associated phenotypes was recently proposed and, using gene enrichment analysis and protein-protein interaction network approaches, the retinoid X receptor and farnesoid X receptor (FXR) were identified as key players in MetSyn given their multiple interactions with metabolism, cell proliferation and oxidative stress (Sookoian and Pirola, 2011). However, more elegant kinetic models may be required to understand the true influence of genetic variants on Dsylipidemia and MetSyn given the presence of multiple feedback loops and reversible reactions (Bakker et al., 2010; Gutierrez-Cirlos et al., 2011).

7. Acknowledgement

This work was supported, in part, by the National Institutes of Health/National Cancer Institute Grant [K07CA129162] awarded to NLN.

8. References

2001. Executive Summary of The Third Report of The National Cholesterol Education Program (NCEP) Expert Panel on Detection, Evaluation, And Treatment of High Blood Cholesterol In Adults (Adult Treatment Panel III). JAMA 285: 2486-2497.

Acton S, Rigotti A, Landschulz KT, Xu S, Hobbs HH, Krieger M. 1996. Identification of scavenger receptor SR-BI as a high density lipoprotein receptor. Science 271: 518-520.

Adamo KB, Tesson F. 2008. Gene-environment interaction and the metabolic syndrome. Novartis. Found. Symp. 293: 103-119.

Adiels M, Olofsson SO, Taskinen MR, Boren J. 2006. Diabetic dyslipidaemia. Curr. Opin. Lipidol. 17: 238-246.

Ahn YI, Kamboh MI, Hamman RF, Cole SA, Ferrell RE. 1993. Two DNA polymorphisms in the lipoprotein lipase gene and their associations with factors related to cardiovascular disease. J. Lipid Res. 34: 421-428.

Alberti KG, Eckel RH, Grundy SM, et al. 2009. Harmonizing the metabolic syndrome: a joint interim statement of the International Diabetes Federation Task Force on Epidemiology and Prevention; National Heart, Lung, and Blood Institute; American Heart Association; World Heart Federation; International Atherosclerosis Society; and International Association for the Study of Obesity. Circulation 120: 1640-1645.

Alberti KG, Zimmet P, Shaw J. 2005. The metabolic syndrome--a new worldwide definition. Lancet 366: 1059-1062.

Alberti KG, Zimmet PZ. 1998. Definition, diagnosis and classification of diabetes mellitus and its complications. Part 1: diagnosis and classification of diabetes mellitus provisional report of a WHO consultation. Diabet. Med. 15: 539-553.

Andersen RV, Wittrup HH, Tybjaerg-Hansen A, Steffensen R, Schnohr P, Nordestgaard BG. 2003. Hepatic lipase mutations,elevated high-density lipoprotein cholesterol, and increased risk of ischemic heart disease: the Copenhagen City Heart Study. J. Am. Coll. Cardiol. 41: 1972-1982.

Andreassi MG. 2009. Metabolic syndrome, diabetes and atherosclerosis: influence of gene-environment interaction. Mutat. Res. 667: 35-43.

Anoop S, Misra A, Meena K, Luthra K. 2010. Apolipoprotein E polymorphism in cerebrovascular & coronary heart diseases. Indian J. Med. Res. 132: 363-378.

Arai Y, Hirose N. 2004. Aging and HDL metabolism in elderly people more than 100 years old. J. Atheroscler. Thromb. 11: 246-252.

Athyros VG, Mikhailidis DP, Papageorgiou AA, et al. 2004. Prevalence of atherosclerotic vascular disease among subjects with the metabolic syndrome with or without diabetes mellitus: the METS-GREECE Multicentre Study. Curr. Med. Res. Opin. 20: 1691-1701.

Austin MA, King MC, Vranizan KM, Krauss RM. 1990. Atherogenic lipoprotein phenotype. A proposed genetic marker for coronary heart disease risk. Circulation 82: 495-506.

Bakker BM, van EK, Jeneson JA, van Riel NA, Bruggeman FJ, Teusink B. 2010. Systems biology from micro-organisms to human metabolic diseases: the role of detailed kinetic models. Biochem. Soc. Trans. 38: 1294-1301.

Balkau B, Charles MA. 1999. Comment on the provisional report from the WHO consultation. European Group for the Study of Insulin Resistance (EGIR). Diabet. Med. 16: 442-443.

Benn M. 2009. Apolipoprotein B levels, APOB alleles, and risk of ischemic cardiovascular disease in the general population, a review. Atherosclerosis 206: 17-30.

Berge KE, Tian H, Graf GA, Yu L, Grishin NV, Schultz J, Kwiterovich P, Shan B, Barnes R, Hobbs HH. 2000. Accumulation of dietary cholesterol in sitosterolemia caused by mutations in adjacent ABC transporters. Science 290: 1771-1775.

Bernstein MS, Costanza MC, James RW, Morris MA, Cambien F, Raoux S, Morabia A. 2003. No physical activity x CETP 1b.-629 interaction effects on lipid profile. Med. Sci. Sports Exerc. 35: 1124-1129.

Blankenberg S, Tiret L, Bickel C, et al. 2004. [Genetic variation of the cholesterol ester transfer protein gene and the prevalence of coronary artery disease. The AtheroGene case control study]. Z. Kardiol. 93 Suppl 4: IV16-IV23.

Blatter Garin MC, Moren X, James RW. 2006. Paraoxonase-1 and serum concentrations of HDL-cholesterol and apoA-I. J. Lipid Res. 47: 515-520.

Boekholdt SM, Sacks FM, Jukema JW, et al. 2005. Cholesteryl ester transfer protein TaqIB variant, high-density lipoprotein cholesterol levels, cardiovascular risk, and efficacy of pravastatin treatment: individual patient meta-analysis of 13,677 subjects. Circulation 111: 278-287.

Boekholdt SM, Souverein OW, Tanck MW, et al. 2006. Common variants of multiple genes that control reverse cholesterol transport together explain only a minor part of the variation of HDL cholesterol levels. Clin. Genet. 69: 263-270.

Boekholdt SM, Thompson JF. 2003. Natural genetic variation as a tool in understanding the role of CETP in lipid levels and disease. J. Lipid Res. 44: 1080-1093.

Boes E, Coassin S, Kollerits B, Heid IM, Kronenberg F. 2009. Genetic-epidemiological evidence on genes associated with HDL cholesterol levels: a systematic in-depth review. Exp Gerontol. 44: 136-160.

Borggreve SE, Hillege HL, Wolffenbuttel BH, de Jong PE, Bakker SJ, van der Steege G, van TA, Dullaart RP. 2005. The effect of cholesteryl ester transfer protein -629C->A promoter polymorphism on high-density lipoprotein cholesterol is dependent on serum triglycerides. J. Clin. Endocrinol. Metab 90: 4198-4204.

Brown CM, Rea TJ, Hamon SC, Hixson JE, Boerwinkle E, Clark AG, Sing CF. 2006. The contribution of individual and pairwise combinations of SNPs in the APOA1 and APOC3 genes to interindividual HDL-C variability. J. Mol. Med. (Berl) 84: 561-572.

Burkhardt R, Kenny EE, Lowe JK, et al.. 2008. Common SNPs in HMGCR in micronesians and whites associated with LDL-cholesterol levels affect alternative splicing of exon13. Arterioscler. Thromb. Vasc. Biol. 28: 2078-2084.

Burnett JR, Hooper AJ. 2008. Common and rare gene variants affecting plasma LDL cholesterol. Clin Biochem. Rev. 29: 11-26.

Cao G, Garcia CK, Wyne KL, Schultz RA, Parker KL, Hobbs HH. 1997. Structure and localization of the human gene encoding SR-BI/CLA-1. Evidence for transcriptional control by steroidogenic factor 1. J. Biol. Chem. 272: 33068-33076.

Cavelier C, Rohrer L, von EA. 2006. ATP-Binding cassette transporter A1 modulates apolipoprotein A-I transcytosis through aortic endothelial cells. Circ. Res. 99: 1060-1066.

Chang MH, Yesupriya A, Ned RM, Mueller PW, Dowling NF. 2010. Genetic variants associated with fasting blood lipids in the U.S. population: Third National Health and Nutrition Examination Survey. BMC. Med. Genet. 11: 62.

Chen SN, Ballantyne CM, Gotto AM, Jr., Tan Y, Willerson JT, Marian AJ. 2005. A common PCSK9 haplotype, encompassing the E670G coding single nucleotide polymorphism, is a novel genetic marker for plasma low-density lipoprotein cholesterol levels and severity of coronary atherosclerosis. J. Am. Coll. Cardiol. 45: 1611-1619.

Clee SM, Zwinderman AH, Engert JC, et al. 2001. Common genetic variation in ABCA1 is associated with altered lipoprotein levels and a modified risk for coronary artery disease. Circulation 103: 1198-1205.

Corella D, Guillen M, Saiz C, Portoles O, Sabater A, Folch J, Ordovas JM. 2002. Associations of LPL and APOC3 gene polymorphisms on plasma lipids in a Mediterranean population: interaction with tobacco smoking and the APOE locus. J. Lipid Res. 43: 416-427.

Costanza MC, Cayanis E, Ross BM, Flaherty MS, Alvin GB, Das K, Morabia A. 2005. Relative contributions of genes, environment, and interactions to blood lipid concentrations in a general adult population. Am. J. Epidemiol. 161: 714-724.

Davignon J, Dubuc G, Seidah NG. 2010. The influence of PCSK9 polymorphisms on serum low-density lipoprotein cholesterol and risk of atherosclerosis. Curr. Atheroscler. Rep. 12: 308-315.

de Andrade FM, Silveira FR, Arsand M, et al. 2004. Association between -250G/A polymorphism of the hepatic lipase gene promoter and coronary artery disease and HDL-C levels in a Southern Brazilian population. Clin. Genet. 65: 390-395.

Di LE, Magnolo L, Pinotti E, et al. 2009. Functional analysis of two novel splice site mutations of APOB gene in familial hypobetalipoproteinemia. Mol. Genet. Metab 96: 66-72.

Edwards KL, Newman B, Mayer E, Selby JV, Krauss RM, Austin MA. 1997. Heritability of factors of the insulin resistance syndrome in women twins. Genet. Epidemiol. 14: 241-253.

Eichner JE, Dunn ST, Perveen G, Thompson DM, Stewart KE, Stroehla BC. 2002. Apolipoprotein E polymorphism and cardiovascular disease: a HuGE review. Am. J. Epidemiol. 155: 487-495.

Einhorn D, Reaven GM, Cobin RH, et al. 2003. American College of Endocrinology position statement on the insulin resistance syndrome. Endocr. Pract. 9: 237-252.

Eiriksdottir G, Bolla MK, Thorsson B, Sigurdsson G, Humphries SE, Gudnason V. 2001. The -629C>A polymorphism in the CETP gene does not explain the association of TaqIB polymorphism with risk and age of myocardial infarction in Icelandic men. Atherosclerosis 159: 187-192.

Endo A. 1992. The discovery and development of HMG-CoA reductase inhibitors. J. Lipid Res. 33: 1569-1582.

Evans D, Beil FU. 2006. The E670G SNP in the PCSK9 gene is associated with polygenic hypercholesterolemia in men but not in women. BMC. Med. Genet. 7: 66.

Fang DZ, Liu BW. 2002. Polymorphism of HL +1075C, but not -480T, is associated with plasma high density lipoprotein cholesterol and apolipoprotein AI in men of a Chinese population. Atherosclerosis 161: 417-424.

Ford ES, Giles WH, Dietz WH. 2002. Prevalence of the metabolic syndrome among US adults: findings from the third National Health and Nutrition Examination Survey. JAMA 287: 356-359.

Freeman DJ, Samani NJ, Wilson V, et al. 2003. A polymorphism of the cholesteryl ester transfer protein gene predicts cardiovascular events in non-smokers in the West of Scotland Coronary Prevention Study. Eur. Heart J. 24: 1833-1842.

Frikke-Schmidt R, Nordestgaard BG, Jensen GB, Tybjaerg-Hansen A. 2004. Genetic variation in ABC transporter A1 contributes to HDL cholesterol in the general population. J. Clin. Invest 114: 1343-1353.

Frikke-Schmidt R, Tybjaerg-Hansen A, Steffensen R, Jensen G, Nordestgaard BG. 2000. Apolipoprotein E genotype: epsilon32 women are protected while epsilon43 and epsilon44 men are susceptible to ischemic heart disease: the Copenhagen City Heart Study. J. Am. Coll. Cardiol. 35: 1192-1199.

Garaulet M, Lee YC, Shen J, Parnell LD, Arnett DK, Tsai MY, Lai CQ, Ordovas JM. 2009. CLOCK genetic variation and metabolic syndrome risk: modulation by monounsaturated fatty acids. Am. J. Clin Nutr. 90: 1466-1475.

Garg A, Simha V. 2007. Update on dyslipidemia. J. Clin Endocrinol. Metab 92: 1581-1589.

Goldberg IJ. 1996. Lipoprotein lipase and lipolysis: central roles in lipoprotein metabolism and atherogenesis. J. Lipid Res. 37: 693-707.

Goode EL, Cherny SS, Christian JC, Jarvik GP, de AM. 2007. Heritability of longitudinal measures of body mass index and lipid and lipoprotein levels in aging twins. Twin. Res. Hum. Genet. 10: 703-711.

Graf GA, Yu L, Li WP, Gerard R, Tuma PL, Cohen JC, Hobbs HH. 2003. ABCG5 and ABCG8 are obligate heterodimers for protein trafficking and biliary cholesterol excretion. J. Biol. Chem. 278: 48275-48282.

Grallert H, Sedlmeier EM, Huth C, Kolz M, Heid IM, Meisinger C, Herder C, Strassburger K, Gehringer A, Haak M, Giani G, Kronenberg F, Wichmann HE, Adamski J, Paulweber B, Illig T, Rathmann W. 2007. APOA5 variants and metabolic syndrome in Caucasians. J. Lipid Res. 48: 2614-2621.

Grarup N, Andreasen CH, Andersen MK, et al. 2008. The -250G>A promoter variant in hepatic lipase associates with elevated fasting serum high-density lipoprotein cholesterol modulated by interaction with physical activity in a study of 16,156 Danish subjects. J. Clin. Endocrinol. Metab 93: 2294-2299.

Gronroos P, Raitakari OT, Kahonen M, et al.. 2008. Relation of apolipoprotein E polymorphism to markers of early atherosclerotic changes in young adults--the Cardiovascular Risk in Young Finns Study. Circ. J. 72: 29-34.

Grundy SM, Cleeman JI, Daniels SR, et al. 2006. Diagnosis and management of the metabolic syndrome: an American Heart Association/National Heart, Lung, and Blood Institute scientific statement. Curr. Opin. Cardiol. 21: 1-6.

Grundy SM, Cleeman JI, Merz CN, et al. 2004. Implications of recent clinical trials for the National Cholesterol Education Program Adult Treatment Panel III Guidelines. J. Am. Coll. Cardiol. 44: 720-732.

Gutierrez-Cirlos C, Ordonez-Sanchez ML, Tusie-Luna MT, Patterson BW, Schonfeld G, Aguilar-Salinas CA. 2011. Familial hypobetalipoproteinemia in a hospital survey: genetics, metabolism and non-alcoholic fatty liver disease. Ann. Hepatol. 10: 155-164.

Haas BE, Weissglas-Volkov D, Aguilar-Salinas CA, et al. 2011. Evidence of how rs7575840 influences apolipoprotein B-containing lipid particles. Arterioscler. Thromb. Vasc. Biol. 31: 1201-1207.

Halpern A, Mancini MC, Magalhaes ME, et al. 2010. Metabolic syndrome, dyslipidemia, hypertension and type 2 diabetes in youth: from diagnosis to treatment. Diabetol. Metab Syndr. 2: 55.

Hegele RA, Brunt JH, Connelly PW. 1995. Multiple genetic determinants of variation of plasma lipoproteins in Alberta Hutterites. Arterioscler. Thromb. Vasc. Biol. 15: 861-871.

Heid IM, Boes E, Muller M, Kollerits B, et al. 2008. Genome-wide association analysis of high-density lipoprotein cholesterol in the population-based KORA study sheds new light on intergenic regions. Circ. Cardiovasc. Genet. 1: 10-20.

Herbeth B, Samara A, Ndiaye C, Marteau JB, Berrahmoune H, Siest G, Visvikis-Siest S. 2010. Metabolic syndrome-related composite factors over 5 years in the STANISLAS family study: genetic heritability and common environmental influences. Clin Chim. Acta 411: 833-839.

Hiura Y, Tabara Y, Kokubo Y, Okamura T, Goto Y, Nonogi H, Miki T, Tomoike H, Iwai N. 2010. Association of the functional variant in the 3-hydroxy-3-methylglutaryl-coenzyme a reductase gene with low-density lipoprotein-cholesterol in Japanese. Circ. J. 74: 518-522.

Hodoglugil U, Williamson DW, Huang Y, Mahley RW. 2005. Common polymorphisms of ATP binding cassette transporter A1, including a functional promoter polymorphism, associated with plasma high density lipoprotein cholesterol levels in Turks. Atherosclerosis 183: 199-212.

Holmer SR, Hengstenberg C, Mayer B, Doring A, Lowel H, Engel S, Hense HW, Wolf M, Klein G, Riegger GA, Schunkert H. 2000. Lipoprotein lipase gene polymorphism, cholesterol subfractions and myocardial infarction in large samples of the general population. Cardiovasc. Res. 47: 806-812.

Hsu LA, Ko YL, Wu S, Teng MS, Peng TY, Chen CF, Chen CF, Lee YS. 2003. Association between a novel 11-base pair deletion mutation in the promoter region of the scavenger receptor class B type I gene and plasma HDL cholesterol levels in Taiwanese Chinese. Arterioscler. Thromb. Vasc. Biol. 23: 1869-1874.

Huang CC, Fornage M, Lloyd-Jones DM, Wei GS, Boerwinkle E, Liu K. 2009. Longitudinal association of PCSK9 sequence variations with low-density lipoprotein cholesterol levels: the Coronary Artery Risk Development in Young Adults Study. Circ. Cardiovasc. Genet. 2: 354-361.

Hubacek JA. 2005. Apolipoprotein A5 and triglyceridemia. Focus on the effects of the common variants. Clin. Chem. Lab Med. 43: 897-902.

Hutter CM, Austin MA, Farin FM, Viernes HM, Edwards KL, Leonetti DL, McNeely MJ, Fujimoto WY. 2006. Association of endothelial lipase gene (LIPG) haplotypes with high-density lipoprotein cholesterol subfractions and apolipoprotein AI plasma levels in Japanese Americans. Atherosclerosis 185: 78-86.

Iijima H, Emi M, Wada M, Daimon M, Toriyama S, Koyano S, Sato H, Hopkins PN, Hunt SC, Kubota I, Kawata S, Kato T. 2008. Association of an intronic haplotype of the LIPC gene with hyperalphalipoproteinemia in two independent populations. J. Hum. Genet. 53: 193-200.

Iizuka K, Horikawa Y. 2008. ChREBP: a glucose-activated transcription factor involved in the development of metabolic syndrome. Endocr. J. 55: 617-624.

Isaacs A, Aulchenko YS, Hofman A, et al. 2007. Epistatic effect of cholesteryl ester transfer protein and hepatic lipase on serum high-density lipoprotein cholesterol levels. J. Clin. Endocrinol. Metab 92: 2680-2687.

Jakulj L, Vissers MN, Tanck MW, Hutten BA, Stellaard F, Kastelein JJ, Dallinga-Thie GM. 2010. ABCG5/G8 polymorphisms and markers of cholesterol metabolism: systematic review and meta-analysis. J. Lipid Res. 51: 3016-3023.

Jaye M, Krawiec J. 2004. Endothelial lipase and HDL metabolism. Curr. Opin. Lipidol. 15: 183-189.

Johansen CT, Hegele RA. 2011. Genetic bases of hypertriglyceridemic phenotypes. Curr. Opin. Lipidol. 22: 247-253.

Joy T, Lahiry P, Pollex RL, Hegele RA. 2008. Genetics of metabolic syndrome. Curr. Diab. Rep. 8: 141-148.

Kahn R, Buse J, Ferrannini E, Stern M. 2005. The metabolic syndrome: time for a critical appraisal: joint statement from the American Diabetes Association and the European Association for the Study of Diabetes. Diabetes Care 28: 2289-2304.

Kamboh MI, Bunker CH, Aston CE, Nestlerode CS, McAllister AE, Ukoli FA. 1999a. Genetic association of five apolipoprotein polymorphisms with serum lipoprotein-lipid levels in African blacks. Genet. Epidemiol. 16: 205-222.

Kamboh MI, Manzi S, Mehdi H, Fitzgerald S, Sanghera DK, Kuller LH, Atson CE. 1999b. Genetic variation in apolipoprotein H (beta2-glycoprotein I) affects the occurrence of antiphospholipid antibodies and apolipoprotein H concentrations in systemic lupus erythematosus. Lupus 8: 742-750.

Kataoka S, Robbins DC, Cowan LD, Go O, Yeh JL, Devereux RB, Fabsitz RR, Lee ET, Welty TK, Howard BV. 1996. Apolipoprotein E polymorphism in American Indians and its relation to plasma lipoproteins and diabetes. The Strong Heart Study. Arterioscler. Thromb. Vasc. Biol. 16: 918-925.

Kathiresan S, Melander O, Anevski D, et al. 2008a. Polymorphisms associated with cholesterol and risk of cardiovascular events. N. Engl. J. Med. 358: 1240-1249.

Kathiresan S, Melander O, Guiducci C, et al. 2008b. Six new loci associated with blood low-density lipoprotein cholesterol, high-density lipoprotein cholesterol or triglycerides in humans. Nat. Genet. 40: 189-197.

Keebler ME, Sanders CL, Surti A, Guiducci C, Burtt NP, Kathiresan S. 2009. Association of blood lipids with common DNA sequence variants at 19 genetic loci in the multiethnic United States National Health and Nutrition Examination Survey III. Circ. Cardiovasc. Genet. 2: 238-243.

Klerkx AH, Tanck MW, Kastelein JJ, Molhuizen HO, Jukema JW, Zwinderman AH, Kuivenhoven JA. 2003. Haplotype analysis of the CETP gene: not TaqIB, but the closely linked -629C-->A polymorphism and a novel promoter variant are independently associated with CETP concentration. Hum. Mol. Genet. 12: 111-123.

Klos KL, Kullo IJ. 2007. Genetic determinants of HDL: monogenic disorders and contributions to variation. Curr. Opin. Cardiol. 22: 344-351.

Klos KL, Sing CF, Boerwinkle E, Hamon SC, Rea TJ, Clark A, Fornage M, Hixson JE. 2006. Consistent effects of genes involved in reverse cholesterol transport on plasma lipid and apolipoprotein levels in CARDIA participants. Arterioscler. Thromb. Vasc. Biol. 26: 1828-1836.

Ko YL, Hsu LA, Hsu KH, Ko YH, Lee YS. 2004. The interactive effects of hepatic lipase gene promoter polymorphisms with sex and obesity on high-density-lipoprotein cholesterol levels in Taiwanese-Chinese. Atherosclerosis 172: 135-142.

Komurcu-Bayrak E, Onat A, Poda M, Humphries SE, Acharya J, Hergenc G, Coban N, Can G, Erginel-Unaltuna N. 2007. The S447X variant of lipoprotein lipase gene is associated with metabolic syndrome and lipid levels among Turks. Clin. Chim. Acta 383: 110-115.

Kretowski A, Hokanson JE, McFann K, Kinney GL, Snell-Bergeon JK, Maahs DM, Wadwa RP, Eckel RH, Ogden LG, Garg SK, Li J, Cheng S, Erlich HA, Rewers M. 2006. The apolipoprotein A-IV Gln360His polymorphism predicts progression of coronary artery calcification in patients with type 1 diabetes. Diabetologia 49: 1946-1954.

Kronenberg F, Coon H, Ellison RC, Borecki I, Arnett DK, Province MA, Eckfeldt JH, Hopkins PN, Hunt SC. 2002. Segregation analysis of HDL cholesterol in the NHLBI Family Heart Study and in Utah pedigrees. Eur. J. Hum. Genet. 10: 367-374.

Kruit JK, Brunham LR, Verchere CB, Hayden MR. 2010. HDL and LDL cholesterol significantly influence beta-cell function in type 2 diabetes mellitus. Curr. Opin. Lipidol. 21: 178-185.

Kwan BC, Kronenberg F, Beddhu S, Cheung AK. 2007. Lipoprotein metabolism and lipid management in chronic kidney disease. J. Am. Soc. Nephrol. 18: 1246-1261.

Lahiry P, Ban MR, Pollex RL, et al. 2007. Common variants APOC3, APOA5, APOE and PON1 are associated with variation in plasma lipoprotein traits in Greenlanders. Int. J. Circumpolar. Health 66: 390-400.

Lai CQ, Tai ES, Tan CE, Cutter J, Chew SK, Zhu YP, Adiconis X, Ordovas JM. 2003. The APOA5 locus is a strong determinant of plasma triglyceride concentrations across ethnic groups in Singapore. J. Lipid Res. 44: 2365-2373.

Lamarche B, Paradis ME. 2007. Endothelial lipase and the metabolic syndrome. Curr. Opin. Lipidol. 18: 298-303.

Lanktree MB, Anand SS, Yusuf S, Hegele RA. 2009. Replication of genetic associations with plasma lipoprotein traits in a multiethnic sample. J. Lipid Res. 50: 1487-1496.

Larson IA, Ordovas JM, Barnard JR, Hoffmann MM, Feussner G, Lamon-Fava S, Schaefer EJ. 2002. Effects of apolipoprotein A-I genetic variations on plasma apolipoprotein, serum lipoprotein and glucose levels. Clin Genet. 61: 176-184.

Lee J, Tan CS, Chia KS, Tan CE, Chew SK, Ordovas JM, Tai ES. 2004. The lipoprotein lipase S447X polymorphism and plasma lipids: interactions with APOE polymorphisms, smoking, and alcohol consumption. J. Lipid Res. 45: 1132-1139.

Lewington S, Whitlock G, Clarke R, Sherliker P, Emberson J, Halsey J, Qizilbash N, Peto R, Collins R. 2007. Blood cholesterol and vascular mortality by age, sex, and blood pressure: a meta-analysis of individual data from 61 prospective studies with 55,000 vascular deaths. Lancet 370: 1829-1839.

Lewis GF, Rader DJ. 2005. New insights into the regulation of HDL metabolism and reverse cholesterol transport. Circ. Res. 96: 1221-1232.

Lin HF, Boden-Albala B, Juo SH, Park N, Rundek T, Sacco RL. 2005. Heritabilities of the metabolic syndrome and its components in the Northern Manhattan Family Study. Diabetologia 48: 2006-2012.

Linsel-Nitschke P, Tall AR. 2005. HDL as a target in the treatment of atherosclerotic cardiovascular disease. Nat. Rev. Drug Discov. 4: 193-205.

Littlewood TD, Bennett MR. 2003. Apoptotic cell death in atherosclerosis. Curr. Opin. Lipidol. 14: 469-475.

Lusis AJ, Attie AD, Reue K. 2008. Metabolic syndrome: from epidemiology to systems biology. Nat. Rev. Genet. 9: 819-830.

Ma K, Cilingiroglu M, Otvos JD, Ballantyne CM, Marian AJ, Chan L. 2003. Endothelial lipase is a major genetic determinant for high-density lipoprotein concentration, structure, and metabolism. Proc. Natl. Acad. Sci. U. S. A 100: 2748-2753.

Mackness MI, Arrol S, Durrington PN. 1991. Paraoxonase prevents accumulation of lipoperoxides in low-density lipoprotein. FEBS Lett. 286: 152-154.

Mailly F, Tugrul Y, Reymer PW, et al. 1995. A common variant in the gene for lipoprotein lipase (Asp9-->Asn). Functional implications and prevalence in normal and hyperlipidemic subjects. Arterioscler. Thromb. Vasc. Biol. 15: 468-478.
Mank-Seymour AR, Durham KL, Thompson JF, Seymour AB, Milos PM. 2004. Association between single-nucleotide polymorphisms in the endothelial lipase (LIPG) gene and high-density lipoprotein cholesterol levels. Biochim. Biophys. Acta 1636: 40-46.
Manresa JM, Zamora A, Tomas M, et al. 2006. Relationship of classical and non-classical risk factors with genetic variants relevant to coronary heart disease. Eur. J. Cardiovasc. Prev. Rehabil. 13: 738-744.
Maxwell KN, Fisher EA, Breslow JL. 2005. Overexpression of PCSK9 accelerates the degradation of the LDLR in a post-endoplasmic reticulum compartment. Proc. Natl. Acad. Sci. U. S. A 102: 2069-2074.
McCaskie PA, Cadby G, Hung J, McQuillan BM, Chapman CM, Carter KW, Thompson PL, Palmer LJ, Beilby JP. 2006. The C-480T hepatic lipase polymorphism is associated with HDL-C but not with risk of coronary heart disease. Clin. Genet. 70: 114-121.
Miettinen HE, Gylling H, Tenhunen J, et al. 1998. Molecular genetic study of Finns with hypoalphalipoproteinemia and hyperalphalipoproteinemia: a novel Gly230 Arg mutation (LCAT[Fin]) of lecithin:cholesterol acyltransferase (LCAT) accounts for 5% of cases with very low serum HDL cholesterol levels. Arterioscler. Thromb. Vasc. Biol. 18: 591-598.
Miller M, Rhyne J, Chen H, Beach V, Ericson R, Luthra K, Dwivedi M, Misra A. 2007. APOC3 promoter polymorphisms C-482T and T-455C are associated with the metabolic syndrome. Arch. Med. Res. 38: 444-451.
Miller M, Rhyne J, Hamlette S, Birnbaum J, Rodriguez A. 2003. Genetics of HDL regulation in humans. Curr. Opin. Lipidol. 14: 273-279.
Miller M, Zhan M. 2004. Genetic determinants of low high-density lipoprotein cholesterol. Curr. Opin. Cardiol. 19: 380-384.
Monda KL, North KE, Hunt SC, Rao DC, Province MA, Kraja AT. 2010. The genetics of obesity and the metabolic syndrome. Endocr. Metab Immune. Disord. Drug Targets. 10: 86-108.
Morabia A, Ross BM, Costanza MC, Cayanis E, Flaherty MS, Alvin GB, Das K, James R, Yang AS, Evagrafov O, Gilliam TC. 2004. Population-based study of SR-BI genetic variation and lipid profile. Atherosclerosis 175: 159-168.
Murthy V, Julien P, Gagne C. 1996. Molecular pathobiology of the human lipoprotein lipase gene. Pharmacol Ther. 70: 101-135.
Musunuru K, Pirruccello JP, Do R, et al. 2010. Exome sequencing, ANGPTL3 mutations, and familial combined hypolipidemia. N. Engl. J. Med. 363: 2220-2227.
Nettleton JA, Steffen LM, Ballantyne CM, Boerwinkle E, Folsom AR. 2007. Associations between HDL-cholesterol and polymorphisms in hepatic lipase and lipoprotein lipase genes are modified by dietary fat intake in African American and White adults. Atherosclerosis 194: e131-e140.
Nock NL, Li L, Larkin EK, Patel SR, Redline S. 2009a. Empirical evidence for "syndrome Z": a hierarchical 5-factor model of the metabolic syndrome incorporating sleep disturbance measures. Sleep 32: 615-622.

Nock NL, Wang X, Thompson CL, Song Y, Baechle D, Raska P, Stein CM, Gray-McGuire C. 2009b. Defining genetic determinants of the Metabolic Syndrome in the Framingham Heart Study using association and structural equation modeling methods. BMC. Proc. 3 Suppl 7: S50.

Ordovas JM, Shen J. 2008. Gene-environment interactions and susceptibility to metabolic syndrome and other chronic diseases. J. Periodontol. 79: 1508-1513.

Osgood D, Corella D, Demissie S, et al. 2003. Genetic variation at the scavenger receptor class B type I gene locus determines plasma lipoprotein concentrations and particle size and interacts with type 2 diabetes: the framingham study. J. Clin Endocrinol. Metab 88: 2869-2879.

Ota VK, Chen ES, Ejchel TF, Furuya TK, Mazzotti DR, Cendoroglo MS, Ramos LR, Araujo LQ, Burbano RR, Smith MD. 2011. APOA4 Polymorphism as a Risk Factor for Unfavorable Lipid Serum Profile and Depression: A Cross-Sectional Study. J. Investig. Med.

Pallaud C, Sass C, Zannad F, Siest G, Visvikis S. 2001. APOC3, CETP, fibrinogen, and MTHFR are genetic determinants of carotid intima-media thickness in healthy men (the Stanislas cohort). Clin Genet. 59: 316-324.

Paradis ME, Couture P, Bosse Y, Despres JP, Perusse L, Bouchard C, Vohl MC, Lamarche B. 2003. The T111I mutation in the EL gene modulates the impact of dietary fat on the HDL profile in women. J. Lipid Res. 44: 1902-1908.

Pare G, Serre D, Brisson D, Anand SS, Montpetit A, Tremblay G, Engert JC, Hudson TJ, Gaudet D. 2007. Genetic analysis of 103 candidate genes for coronary artery disease and associated phenotypes in a founder population reveals a new association between endothelin-1 and high-density lipoprotein cholesterol. Am. J. Hum. Genet. 80: 673-682.

Phillips CM, Tierney AC, Roche HM. 2008. Gene-nutrient interactions in the metabolic syndrome. J. Nutrigenet. Nutrigenomics. 1: 136-151.

Polisecki E, Muallem H, Maeda N, et al. 2008. Genetic variation at the LDL receptor and HMG-CoA reductase gene loci, lipid levels, statin response, and cardiovascular disease incidence in PROSPER. Atherosclerosis 200: 109-114.

Pollex RL, Hanley AJ, Zinman B, Harris SB, Khan HM, Hegele RA. 2006. Metabolic syndrome in aboriginal Canadians: prevalence and genetic associations. Atherosclerosis 184: 121-129.

Pollex RL, Hegele RA. 2006. Genetic determinants of the metabolic syndrome. Nat. Clin Pract. Cardiovasc. Med. 3: 482-489.

Porchay I, Pean F, Bellili N, et al. 2006. ABCA1 single nucleotide polymorphisms on high-density lipoprotein-cholesterol and overweight: the D.E.S.I.R. study. Obesity. (Silver. Spring) 14: 1874-1879.

Qi L, Liu S, Rifai N, Hunter D, Hu FB. 2007. Associations of the apolipoprotein A1/C3/A4/A5 gene cluster with triglyceride and HDL cholesterol levels in women with type 2 diabetes. Atherosclerosis 192: 204-210.

Remaley AT, Stonik JA, Demosky SJ, et al. 2001. Apolipoprotein specificity for lipid efflux by the human ABCAI transporter. Biochem. Biophys. Res. Commun. 280: 818-823.

Rigotti A, Trigatti B, Babitt J, Penman M, Xu S, Krieger M. 1997. Scavenger receptor BI--a cell surface receptor for high density lipoprotein. Curr. Opin. Lipidol. 8: 181-188.

Rios DL, D'Onofrio LO, Cerqueira CC, et al. 2007. Paraoxonase 1 gene polymorphisms in angiographically assessed coronary artery disease: evidence for gender interaction among Brazilians. Clin. Chem. Lab Med. 45: 874-878.

Rip J, Nierman MC, Ross CJ, Jukema JW, Hayden MR, Kastelein JJ, Stroes ES, Kuivenhoven JA. 2006. Lipoprotein lipase S447X: a naturally occurring gain-of-function mutation. Arterioscler. Thromb. Vasc. Biol. 26: 1236-1245.

Roberts CG, Shen H, Mitchell BD, Damcott CM, Shuldiner AR, Rodriguez A. 2007. Variants in scavenger receptor class B type I gene are associated with HDL cholesterol levels in younger women. Hum. Hered. 64: 107-113.

Roth GA, Fihn SD, Mokdad AH. 2010. High total serum cholesterol, medication coverage and therapeutic control: an analysis of national health examination survey data from eight countries. In: pp. 92-101.

Russo GT, Meigs JB, Cupples LA, et al. 2001. Association of the Sst-I polymorphism at the APOC3 gene locus with variations in lipid levels, lipoprotein subclass profiles and coronary heart disease risk: the Framingham offspring study. Atherosclerosis 158: 173-181.

Sagoo GS, Tatt I, Salanti G, Butterworth AS, Sarwar N, van MM, Jukema JW, Wiman B, Kastelein JJ, Bennet AM, de FU, Danesh J, Higgins JP. 2008. Seven lipoprotein lipase gene polymorphisms, lipid fractions, and coronary disease: a HuGE association review and meta-analysis. Am. J. Epidemiol. 168: 1233-1246.

Senti M, Elosua R, Tomas M, Sala J, Masia R, Ordovas JM, Shen H, Marrugat J. 2001. Physical activity modulates the combined effect of a common variant of the lipoprotein lipase gene and smoking on serum triglyceride levels and high-density lipoprotein cholesterol in men. Hum. Genet. 109: 385-392.

Shan L, Yu XC, Liu Z, Hu Y, Sturgis LT, Miranda ML, Liu Q. 2009. The angiopoietin-like proteins ANGPTL3 and ANGPTL4 inhibit lipoprotein lipase activity through distinct mechanisms. J. Biol. Chem. 284: 1419-1424.

Sharma V, McNeill JH. 2006. The etiology of hypertension in the metabolic syndrome part one: an introduction to the history, the concept and the models. Curr. Vasc. Pharmacol 4: 293-304.

Shimizugawa T, Ono M, Shimamura M, Yoshida K, Ando Y, Koishi R, Ueda K, Inaba T, Minekura H, Kohama T, Furukawa H. 2002. ANGPTL3 decreases very low density lipoprotein triglyceride clearance by inhibition of lipoprotein lipase. J. Biol. Chem. 277: 33742-33748.

Shioji K, Mannami T, Kokubo Y, Goto Y, Nonogi H, Iwai N. 2004a. An association analysis between ApoA1 polymorphisms and the high-density lipoprotein (HDL) cholesterol level and myocardial infarction (MI) in Japanese. J. Hum. Genet. 49: 433-439.

Shioji K, Nishioka J, Naraba H, et al. 2004b. A promoter variant of the ATP-binding cassette transporter A1 gene alters the HDL cholesterol level in the general Japanese population. J. Hum. Genet. 49: 141-147.

Sookoian S, Pirola CJ. 2011. Metabolic syndrome: from the genetics to the pathophysiology. Curr. Hypertens. Rep. 13: 149-157.

Srinivasan SR, Ehnholm C, Elkasabany A, Berenson G. 1999. Influence of apolipoprotein E polymorphism on serum lipids and lipoprotein changes from childhood to adulthood: the Bogalusa Heart Study. Atherosclerosis 143: 435-443.

Sung J, Lee K, Song YM. 2009. Heritabilities of the metabolic syndrome phenotypes and related factors in Korean twins. J. Clin Endocrinol. Metab 94: 4946-4952.

Sviridov D, Nestel PJ. 2007. Genetic factors affecting HDL levels, structure, metabolism and function. Curr. Opin. Lipidol. 18: 157-163.

Tai ES, Corella D, Deurenberg-Yap M, Cutter J, Chew SK, Tan CE, Ordovas JM. 2003a. Dietary fat interacts with the -514C>T polymorphism in the hepatic lipase gene promoter on plasma lipid profiles in a multiethnic Asian population: the 1998 Singapore National Health Survey. J. Nutr. 133: 3399-3408.

Tai ES, Ordovas JM, Corella D, Deurenberg-Yap M, Chan E, Adiconis X, Chew SK, Loh LM, Tan CE. 2003b. The TaqIB and -629C>A polymorphisms at the cholesteryl ester transfer protein locus: associations with lipid levels in a multiethnic population. The 1998 Singapore National Health Survey. Clin. Genet. 63: 19-30.

Talmud PJ, Hawe E, Martin S, Olivier M, Miller GJ, Rubin EM, Pennacchio LA, Humphries SE. 2002a. Relative contribution of variation within the APOC3/A4/A5 gene cluster in determining plasma triglycerides. Hum. Mol. Genet. 11: 3039-3046.

Talmud PJ, Hawe E, Robertson K, Miller GJ, Miller NE, Humphries SE. 2002b. Genetic and environmental determinants of plasma high density lipoprotein cholesterol and apolipoprotein AI concentrations in healthy middle-aged men. Ann. Hum. Genet. 66: 111-124.

Tang NP, Wang LS, Yang L, Zhou B, Gu HJ, Sun QM, Cong RH, Zhu HJ, Wang B. 2008. Protective effect of an endothelial lipase gene variant on coronary artery disease in a Chinese population. J. Lipid Res. 49: 369-375.

Teslovich TM, Musunuru K, Smith AV, Edmondson AC, et al. 2010. Biological, clinical and population relevance of 95 loci for blood lipids. Nature 466: 707-713.

Thompson A, Di AE, Sarwar N, Erqou S, Saleheen D, Dullaart RP, Keavney B, Ye Z, Danesh J. 2008. Association of cholesteryl ester transfer protein genotypes with CETP mass and activity, lipid levels, and coronary risk. JAMA 299: 2777-2788.

van Aalst-Cohen ES, Jansen AC, Boekholdt SM, Tanck MW, Fontecha MR, Cheng S, Li J, Defesche JC, Kuivenhoven JA, Kastelein JJ. 2005. Genetic determinants of plasma HDL-cholesterol levels in familial hypercholesterolemia. Eur. J. Hum. Genet. 13: 1137-1142.

Volcik KA, Barkley RA, Hutchinson RG, Mosley TH, Heiss G, Sharrett AR, Ballantyne CM, Boerwinkle E. 2006. Apolipoprotein E polymorphisms predict low density lipoprotein cholesterol levels and carotid artery wall thickness but not incident coronary heart disease in 12,491 ARIC study participants. Am. J. Epidemiol. 164: 342-348.

Wang J, Ban MR, Zou GY, Cao H, Lin T, Kennedy BA, Anand S, Yusuf S, Huff MW, Pollex RL, Hegele RA. 2008. Polygenic determinants of severe hypertriglyceridemia. Hum. Mol. Genet. 17: 2894-2899.

Wang X, Paigen B. 2005. Genetics of variation in HDL cholesterol in humans and mice. Circ. Res. 96: 27-42.

Waterworth DM, Ricketts SL, Song K, et al. 2010. Genetic variants influencing circulating lipid levels and risk of coronary artery disease. Arterioscler. Thromb. Vasc. Biol. 30: 2264-2276.

Whiting BM, Anderson JL, Muhlestein JB, Horne BD, Bair TL, Pearson RR, Carlquist JF. 2005. Candidate gene susceptibility variants predict intermediate end points but not angiographic coronary artery disease. Am. Heart J. 150: 243-250.

Willer CJ, Sanna S, Jackson AU, et al. 2008. Newly identified loci that influence lipid concentrations and risk of coronary artery disease. Nat. Genet. 40: 161-169.

Wilson PW, Myers RH, Larson MG, Ordovas JM, Wolf PA, Schaefer EJ. 1994. Apolipoprotein E alleles, dyslipidemia, and coronary heart disease. The Framingham Offspring Study. JAMA 272: 1666-1671.

Wittrup HH, Tybjaerg-Hansen A, Nordestgaard BG. 1999. Lipoprotein lipase mutations, plasma lipids and lipoproteins, and risk of ischemic heart disease. A meta-analysis. Circulation 99: 2901-2907.

Wu K, Bowman R, Welch AA, Luben RN, Wareham N, Khaw KT, Bingham SA. 2007. Apolipoprotein E polymorphisms, dietary fat and fibre, and serum lipids: the EPIC Norfolk study. Eur. Heart J. 28: 2930-2936.

Yamada Y, Ichihara S, Kato K, et al. 2008. Genetic risk for metabolic syndrome: examination of candidate gene polymorphisms related to lipid metabolism in Japanese people. J. Med. Genet. 45: 22-28.

Yamada Y, Matsuo H, Warita S, et al. 2007. Prediction of genetic risk for dyslipidemia. Genomics 90: 551-558.

Yamakawa-Kobayashi K, Yanagi H, Endo K, Arinami T, Hamaguchi H. 2003. Relationship between serum HDL-C levels and common genetic variants of the endothelial lipase gene in Japanese school-aged children. Hum. Genet. 113: 311-315.

Zhang K, Zhang S, Zheng K, Hou Y, Liao L, He Y, Zhang L, Nebert DW, Shi J, Su Z, Xiao C. 2004. Novel P143L polymorphism of the LCAT gene is associated with dyslipidemia in Chinese patients who have coronary atherosclerotic heart disease. Biochem. Biophys. Res. Commun. 318: 4-10.

Zhu XY, Xu HW, Hou RY, Liu HF, Xiao B, Yang XS, Yang QD, Tang BS. 2006. [Lecithin-cholesterol acyltransferase gene 608C/T polymorphism associated with atherosclerotic cerebral infarction]. Zhonghua Yi. Xue. Yi. Chuan Xue. Za Zhi. 23: 419-422.

7

Functions of OSBP/ORP Family Proteins and Their Relation to Dyslipidemia

Hiroshi Koriyama, Hironori Nakagami,
Tomohiro Katsuya and Ryuichi Morishita
Osaka University
Japan

1. Introduction

The pathway of intracellular cholesterol synthesis, uptake and efflux is much affected by both the positive and the negative feedbacks from direct interaction between cholesterol and its oxygenated derivatives (oxysterols) as well as the regulatory factors such as the sterol-regulatory-element-binding protein (SREBP)– cleavage-activating protein–Insig complex (Radhakrishnan, Ikeda et al. 2007), 3-hydroxy-3-methylglutaryl-CoA (HMG-CoA) reductase (Sever, Song et al. 2003) and liver X receptors (LXRs) (Chen, Chen et al. 2007). Since these regulatory factors are located in the compartments with comparatively low cholesterol density, they can react promptly on acute changes in local cholesterol or oxysterol density. While much is known about the interaction between these regulatory factors and cholesterol, only little has been studied about the mechanism to deliver the cholesterol or oxysterol to its appropriate compartments.

Therefore, there arises a possibility that oxysterol-binding protein/oxysterol-binding protein-related protein (OSBP/ORP) family may regulate such processes by binding oxyterol and/or cholesterol and by functioning as a cholesterol sensor or cholesterol transporter. According to the study about the family members, it is now becoming clear that they affect the regulation such as the cholesterol or triglyceride level.

For comprehensive information on OSBP/ORP family, please refer to several good reviews already published (Fairn and McMaster 2008; Ngo, Colbourne et al. 2010; Raychaudhuri and Prinz 2010; Vihervaara, Jansen et al. 2011). This review focuses more on the family's association with dyslipidemia from a perspective of the individual features of the structure, the expression, the cellular localization, the molecular functions, and the epidemiologial study-based information of each member.

2. Overview of functions of OSBP/ORP family proteins and their relation to dyslipidemia

It has become widely known that each member of OSBP/ORP family respectively affects diverse processes considered to have an association with dyslipidemia, such as intracellular trafficking of cholesterol or neutral lipid. The first presented is a brief overview of the members as a whole before the individual explanation of each member.

OSBP negatively regulates ATP-binding cassette transporter A1 (ABCA1) protein stability (Bowden and Ridgway 2008). OSBP induces upregulation of SREBP-1c and enhances hepatic lipogenesis (Yan, Lehto et al. 2007).

ORP1L forms a RILP-Rab7-ORP1L complex (Johansson, Rocha et al. 2007) and is involved in both protein and lipid transport functions of the late endocytic compartments (Vihervaara, Uronen et al. 2011).

ORP1S and ORP2 enhance plasma membrane (PM)-to-lipid droplet (LD) sterol transport (Jansen, Ohsaki et al. 2011). ORP2 presents on LD and has a functional role in the regulation of neutral lipid metabolism, possibly as a factor that integrates the cellular metabolism of triglycerides (TG) with that of cholesterol (Hynynen, Suchanek et al. 2009).

ORP3 may play an important role in efficient directed membrane trafficking (Lehto, Mayranpaa et al. 2008). But the direct evidence that ORP3 functions to regulate dyslipidemia is yet to be reported.

ORP4 in an interaction with intermediate filaments inhibits an intracellular cholesterol-transport pathway mediated by vimentin (Wang, JeBailey et al. 2002).

ORP5 may cooperate with Niemann-Pick C1 (NPC1) to mediate the exit of cholesterol from endosomes/lysosomes (Du, Kumar et al. 2011).

ORP6 is identified as one of the candidate genes that are possibly involved in the regulation of high-density lipoprotein (HDL) cholesterol levels (North, Martin et al. 2003).

SNPs near ORP7 gene show a genome-wide significant association with low-density lipoprotein (LDL) cholesterol (Teslovich, Musunuru et al. 2010).

ORP8 negatively regulates ABCA1 expression and macrophage cholesterol efflux (Yan, Mayranpaa et al. 2008). ORP8 has the capacity to modulate lipid homeostasis and SREBP activity, probably through an indirect mechanism required Nup62 (Zhou, Li et al. 2011). The OSBPL8-ZDHHC17 region (chr12) is detected for HDL cholesterol identified by one new SNP with genome-wide significance (Ma, Yang et al. 2010).

ORP9 and ORP11 are dimerized and may act as an intracellular lipid sensor or transporter (Zhou, Li et al. 2010).

ORP10 suppresses hepatic lipogenesis and very-low-density lipoprotein production (Perttila, Merikanto et al. 2009). ORP10 is genetically associated with both TG (Perttila, Merikanto et al. 2009) and LDL cholesterol level (Koriyama, Nakagami et al. 2010).

SNPs in the ORP11 gene is associated with LDL cholesterol levels, hyperglycemia /diabetes as well as with metabolic syndrome per se (Bouchard, Faucher et al. 2009).

2.1 Phylogenetic distribution and molecular structure of OSBP/ORP family

As a result of differential promoter usage and splicing, there are 16 major OSBP/ORP family members. The human ORP family is divided into six subfamilies based on the gene structure and amino acid sequence homology (Fig. 1). Some of the proteins, for example ORP1 and ORP4, have both short (S) and long (L) variants.

A feature in common for all ORPs is a conserved C-terminal OSBP-related domain (ORD), which contains the highly conserved "OSBP-fingerprint (OF)" sequence EQVSHHPP (Fig. 1). Most of the human ORPs belong to the long subtype have a pleckstrin homology domain (PH domain), which bind phosphoinositides (PIPs). This interaction controls the subcellular localization of the proteins. 12 out of the 16 major mammalian OSBP/ORP family members contain a FFAT motif, which is a short sequence that binds VAMP associated proteins (VAPs), integral membrane proteins of the ER. Instead of an ER targeting FFAT motif, ORP5 and ORP8 contain a putative C-terminal transmembrane segment, which anchors these proteins in the ER. The human ORP1L have at their N-terminus ankyrin repeats, which interacts with the active GTP-bound form of Rab7 on late endosomes, and thus mediates targeting of the protein to late endosomes.

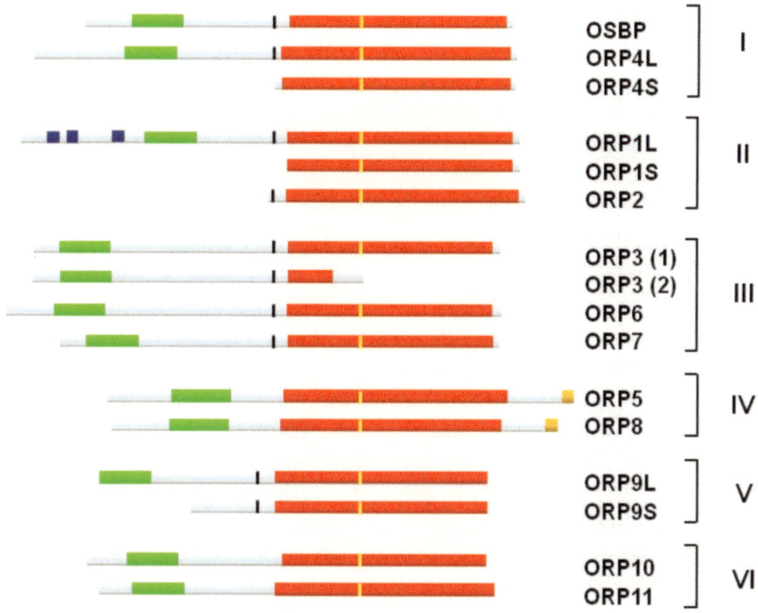

Fig. 1. Domain organization of the humam OSBP/ORP family.

Human OSBP/ORP family members are arranged into subfamilies I-VI. The color codes are: red, OSBP-related domain (ORD); yellow, OSBP-fingerprint (OF) motif; green, pleckstrin homology (PH) domain; Blue, ankirin repeats; black, VAP targeting motif (FFAT motif); Orange, transmembrane domain. L and S in the protein names indicate long and short variants, respectively.

2.2 OSBP

Structure, Tissue distribution and Intracellular localization: OSBP belongs to the subfamily I of OSBP/ORP homologues. OSBP has an ORD, a PH domain and an FFAT motif. OSBP shares the highest degree of similarity with ORP4 and dimerizes with ORP4. In the transfected cells, some of the OSBP was distributed diffusely in the cytoplasm, and some was bound to small vesicles near the nucleus. Upon addition of 25-hydroxycholesterol, most of the OSBP became concentrated in the Golgi apparatus (Ridgway, Dawson et al. 1992).

Molecular functions related to dyslipidemia: OSBP is the founding member of the OSBP/ORP family. Human OSBP was cloned in 1990 (Levanon, Hsieh et al. 1990) and was studied intensively (Ridgway, Dawson et al. 1992; Lagace, Byers et al. 1997; Ridgway, Badiani et al. 1998; Ridgway, Lagace et al. 1998; Storey, Byers et al. 1998; Lagace, Byers et al. 1999; Mohammadi, Perry et al. 2001; Levine and Munro 2002).

Yan et al. reported that adenovirus-mediated hepatic overexpression of OSBP induced a marked increase of VLDL TG. Also, the liver tissue TG were elevated in the AdOSBP-injected mice, and their TG secretion rate was increased by 70%. The messenger RNAs for enzymes of fatty acid synthesis and their transcriptional regulator, SREBP-1c, as well as the

Insig-1 mRNA, were upregulated two-fold in the OSBP expressing livers. Silencing of OSBP in hepatocytes suppressed the induction of SREBP1-c by insulin and resulted in a reduction of TG synthesis. These results demonstrate that OSBP regulates hepatic TG metabolism and suggest the involvement of OSBP in the insulin signaling pathways that control hepatic lipogenesis (Yan, Lehto et al. 2007).

Bowden et al. revealed that suppression of OSBP in Chinese hamster ovary cells by RNA interference resulted in increased ABCA1 protein expression and cholesterol efflux activity following induction with oxysterols or the synthetic LXR agonist TO901317. OSBP knockdown in J774 macrophages also increased ABCA1 expression in the presence and absence of LXR agonists. Their results demonstrate that OSBP opposes the activity of LXR by negatively regulating ABCA1 activity in the cytoplasm by sterol-binding domain-dependent protein destabilization (Bowden and Ridgway 2008).

Cephalostatin 1, OSW-1, ritterazine B and schweinfurthin A are natural products that potently, and in some cases selectively, inhibit the growth of cultured human cancer cell lines. Recently, Burgett et al. have discovered that these molecules target OSBP and its closest paralog, ORP4L, and have named these natural products ORPphilins (Burgett, Poulsen et al. 2011). By uncovering the cellular targets of the ORPphilins, they have revealed that OSBP and ORP4L are involved in cancer cell survival.

They also show that ORPphilins perturb the cellular localization of OSBP and affect sphingomyelin biosynthesis. The ORPphilins are powerful probes of OSBP and ORP4L that will be useful in uncovering their cellular functions and their roles in human diseases.

Epidemiological study: Epidemiological study of OSBP is not reported yet.

2.3 OSBPL1B (ORP1L)

Structure, Tissue distribution and Intracellular localization: ORP1L belongs to the subfamily II of OSBP/ORP homologues. ORP1L has an ORD, an FFAT motif, a PH domain and three ankyrin repeats.

While macrophages, brain, and lung are the areas where ORP1L is expressed most predominantly, it is also found in colon, kidney, and liver (Johansson, Bocher et al. 2003). ORP1L localizes to late endosomes.

Molecular functions related to dyslipidemia: Johansson et al. reported that ORP1L binds to Rab7, modifies its functional cycle, and can interfere with LE/lysosome organization and endocytic membrane trafficking (Johansson, Lehto et al. 2005).

They show that the GTPase Rab7, when bound to GTP, simultaneously binds to ORP1L and RILP to form a RILP-Rab7-ORP1L complex, which is required for the perinuclear localization of late endosomes/lysosomes (Johansson, Rocha et al. 2007). The later study of Rocha et al., went deeper in examining these processes more in detail. They found that the cholesterol levels in late endosomes are sensed by ORP1L and are lower in peripheral vesicles. Under low cholesterol conditions, ORP1L conformation induces the formation of endoplasmic reticulum (ER)- late endosome membrane contact sites. At these sites, the ER protein VAP (VAMP [vesicle-associated membrane protein]-associated ER protein) can interact in trans with the Rab7-RILP complex to remove p150 (Glued) and associated motors. late endosomes then move to the microtubule plus end. Under high cholesterol conditions, as in Niemann-Pick type C disease, this process is prevented, and late endosomes accumulate at the microtubule minus end as the result of dynein motor activity. These data explain how the ER and cholesterol control the association of late endosomes with motor proteins and their positioning in cells (Rocha, Kuijl et al. 2009).

Recently, Vihervaara et al. have shown that ORP1L silencing in macrophage foam cells inhibits the efflux of lipoprotein-derived endocytosed cholesterol to apolipoprotein A-I, providing evidence for the involvement of ORP1L in both protein and lipid transport functions of the late endocytic compartments (Vihervaara, Uronen et al. 2011).

The multivesicular body(MVB) sorting pathway is known to be involved in many processes, including growth factor receptor down-regulation, exosome secretion, antigen presentation, the budding of enveloped viruses, and cytokinesis. Recently, Kobuna et al. have shown that knockdown of ORP1L induces the formation of enlarged MVBs in HeLa cells. They suggest that the proper cholesterol level of late endosomes/lysosomes generated by ORPs is required for normal MVB formation and MVB-mediated membrane protein degradation (Kobuna, Inoue et al. 2010).

Epidemiological study: Epidemiological study of ORP1L is not reported yet.

2.4 OSBPL1A (ORP1S) and OSBPL2 (ORP2)

Structure, Tissue distribution and Intracellular localization: ORP1S and ORP2 belong to the subfamily II of OSBP/ORP homologues. ORP1S and ORP2 have an ORD and an FFAT motif but lack PH domain.

ORP1S is expressed predominantly in skeletal muscle and heart (Johansson, Bocher et al. 2003). ORP2 is expressed ubiquitously in mammalian tissues. Highest mRNA levels of ORP2 are present in specific parts of the central nervous system (cerebellum, pituitary gland, pons, and putamen) as well as in leukocytes, placenta, and pancreas (Laitinen, Lehto et al. 2002).

ORP1S has been reported to be largely cytosolic (Johansson, Bocher et al. 2003) and ORP2 localizes, in addition to a cytosolic fraction, on the surface of lipid droplets (LDs) and also the plasma membrane (PM) (Hynynen, Suchanek et al. 2009).

Molecular functions related to dyslipidemia: In the earlier study of Hynynen et al., overexpression of ORP2 induces enhancement of [14C]cholesterol efflux to all extracellular acceptors, which results in a reduction of cellular free cholesterol. They also show that ORP2 binds PtdIns(3,4,5)P(3) and enhances endocytosis.

In their recent study, Hynynen et al. discover that ORP2 localizes not only cytosolic fraction but also on cytoplasmic LDs and reveal its function in neutral lipid metabolism. They show that the ORP2 LD association depends on sterol binding: Treatment with 5 mM 22(R)OHC inhibits the LD association, while a mutant defective in sterol binding is constitutively LD bound. Silencing of ORP2 using RNA interference slows down cellular TG hydrolysis. Furthermore, ORP2 silencing increases the amount of [14C]cholesteryl esters but only under conditions in which lipogenesis and LD formation are enhanced by treatment with oleic acid (Hynynen, Suchanek et al. 2009). These results identify ORP2 as a sterol receptor present on LD and provide an evidence for its role in the regulation of neutral lipid metabolism, possibly as a factor that integrates the cellular metabolism of TG with that of cholesterol.

By overexpressing all mammalian ORPs, Jansen et al. found that especially ORP1S and ORP2 enhanced PM-to-LD sterol transport. This reflected the stimulation of transport from the PM to the ER, rather than from the ER to LDs. Double knockdown of ORP1S and ORP2 inhibited sterol transport from the PM to the ER and LDs, suggesting a physiological role for these ORPs in the process (Jansen, Ohsaki et al. 2011). These findings suggest that ORP1S and ORP2 are essential in controlling cellular neutral lipid and cholesterol and has a strong association with the pathophysiology of dyslipidemia.

Epidemiological study: Epidemiological studies of ORP1S or ORP2 are not reported yet.

2.5 OSBPL3 (ORP3)

Structure, Tissue distribution and Intracellular localization: ORP3 belongs to the subfamily III of OSBP/ORP homologues. ORP3 has an ORD, a PH domain and an FFAT motif. A total of eight isoforms of ORP3 were demonstrated with alternative splicing (Collier, Gregorio-King et al. 2003). In human tissues there was specific isoform distribution, with most tissues expressing varied levels of isoforms with the complete ORD; while only whole brain, kidney, spleen, thymus, and thyroid expressed high levels of the isoforms associated with the truncated ORD. The expression in cerebellum, heart, and liver of most isoforms was negligible. Lehto et al described that ORP3 was expressed at high levels in kidney tubule epithelia and in the human embryonic kidney cell line HEK293 (Lehto, Mayranpaa et al. 2008).

They also described that the endogenous ORP3 protein in HEK293 cells localized at the ER and the PM, especially thin filopodial cell-surface projections.

Molecular functions related to dyslipidemia: The direct evidence that ORP3 functions to regulate Dyslipidemia is yet to be reported.

ORP3 interacts with R-Ras, a small GTPase regulating cell adhesion, spreading and migration (Lehto, Mayranpaa et al. 2008). Gene silencing of ORP3 and overexpression of ORP3 in HEK293 cells or primary macrophages demonstrate the function of ORP3 as part of the machinery that controls the actin cytoskeleton, cell polarity and cell adhesion. These functional evidences, together with the abundant expression of ORP3 in polarized cell types, suggest that ORP3 may play an important role in efficient directed membrane trafficking.

Epidemiological study: Epidemiological study of ORP3 is not reported yet.

2.6 OSBPL4 (ORP4, OSBP2, HLM)

Structure, Tissue distribution and Intracellular localization: ORP4 belongs to the subfamily I of OSBP/ORP homologues. ORP4 has an ORD, a PH domain and an FFAT motif. ORP4 shares the highest degree of similarity with OSBP and dimerizes with OSBP.

Two ORP4 cDNAs were identified: a full-length ORP4 containing a PH domain and an ORD (designated ORP4-L), and a splice variant in which the PH domain and part of the ORD were deleted (designated ORP4-S). ORP4 mRNA and protein expression overlapped partially with OSBP and were restricted to brain, heart, muscle and kidney(Wang, JeBailey et al. 2002).

Immunofluorescence localization in stably transfected Chinese hamster ovary cells showed that ORP4-S co-localized with vimentin and caused the intermediate filament network to bundle or aggregate. ORP4-L displayed a diffuse staining pattern that did not overlap with vimentin except when the microtubule network was disrupted with nocodazole.

Molecular functions related to dyslipidemia: Cells overexpressing ORP4S had a 40% reduction in the esterification of low-density-lipoprotein-derived cholesterol, demonstrating that ORP4 in an interaction with intermediate filaments inhibits an intracellular cholesterol-transport pathway mediated by vimentin (Wang, JeBailey et al. 2002).

ORP4L bound [3H]25-hydroxycholesterol with high affinity and specificity. However, sterol-binding or a mutation that ablated sterol-binding did not influence the interaction of GST-ORP4 with vimentin (Wyles, Perry et al. 2007). Thus the precise mechanism about what ORP4L senses to regulate intracellular cholesterol-transport pathway still remains unidentified.

Epidemiological study: Epidemiological study of ORP4 is not reported yet.

2.7 OSBPL5 (ORP5)

Structure, Tissue distribution and Intracellular localization: ORP5 belongs to the subfamily IV of OSBP/ORP homologues. ORP5 has an ORD, a PH domain and a transmembrane domain. ORP5 localizes to the ER.

Molecular functions related to dyslipidemia: Knocking down ORP5 causes cholesterol accumulation in late endosomes and lysosomes, which is reminiscent of the cholesterol trafficking defect in Niemann Pick C (NPC) fibroblasts (Du, Kumar et al. 2011). Cholesterol appears to accumulate in the limiting membranes of endosomal compartments in ORP5-depleted cells, whereas depletion of NPC1 or both ORP5 and NPC1 results in luminal accumulation of cholesterol. Moreover, trans-Golgi resident proteins mislocalize to endosomal compartments upon ORP5 depletion, which depends on a functional NPC1.

Niemann-Pick type C (NPC) disease is most often caused by mutations in the NPC1 gene, whose protein product is believed to facilitate the egress of cholesterol and other lipids from late endosomes and lysosomes to other cellular compartments (Boadu and Francis 2006).

The results of the research by Du et al. establish the first link between NPC1 and a cytoplasmic sterol carrier, and suggest that ORP5 may cooperate with NPC1 to mediate the exit of cholesterol from endosomes/lysosomes.

Epidemiological study: Epidemiological study of ORP5 is not reported yet.

2.8 OSBPL6 (ORP6)

Structure, Tissue distribution and Intracellular localization: ORP6 belongs to the subfamily III of OSBP/ORP homologues. ORP6 has an ORD, a PH domain and an FFAT motif. ORP6 shows the highest expression in brain and skeletal muscle (Lehto, Tienari et al. 2004). Endogenous ORP6 associated predominantly with the nuclear envelope. When expressed from the cDNA in cultured cells, ORP6 was distributed between the cytosol and ER membranes, with a minor portion found at the PM.

Molecular functions related to dyslipidemia: The direct evidence that ORP6 functions to regulate Dyslipidemia is yet to be reported.

Epidemiological study: Using the Framingham Heart Study data set, a quantitative trait locus in the chromosome 2q was found to be significantly involved in variations of HDL cholesterol levels. ORP6 is identified as one of the candidate genes that are possibly involved in the regulation of HDL cholesterol levels in this region (North, Martin et al. 2003).

2.9 OSBPL7 (ORP7)

Structure, Tissue distribution and Intracellular localization: ORP7 belongs to the subfamily III of OSBP/ORP homologues. ORP7 has an ORD, a PH domain and a an FFAT motif. ORP7 shows the highest expression in the gastrointestinal tract (Lehto, Tienari et al. 2004). When expressed from the cDNA in cultured cells, ORP7 was distributed between the cytosol and ER membranes, with a minor portion found at the PM. The N-terminal portion of the proteins, containing a PH domain, has markedly strong PM targeting specificity, while the C-terminal half remains largely cytosolic. The dual targeting of the proteins indicates a putative role in communication between the ER and the PM.

Molecular functions related to dyslipidemia: Recently, Zhong et al. identified by yeast two-hybrid screening an interaction partner of ORP7, GATE-16, which (i) regulates the function and stability of Golgi SNARE of 28kDa (GS28), and (ii) plays a role in autophagosome biogenesis (Zhong, Zhou et al. 2011).

GATE-16 is a ubiquitin-like low molecular weight peripheral membrane protein which was initially reported to localize at the Golgi complex and to regulate docking/fusing reactions in intra-Golgi traffic and Golgi assembly from mitotic fragments via interactions with NSF and the Golgi v-SNARE GS28 (Sagiv, Legesse-Miller et al. 2000). GS28 was identified as a SNARE protein, the majority of which is associated with the cis-Golgi, and is implicated in both ER-Golgi and intra-Golgi transport (Subramaniam, Peter et al. 1996). In the presence of NSF, SNAP and ATP, GATE-16 interacts with GS28, apparently maintaining GS28 in a transport competent form and protecting it from proteolysis.

Zhong et al. revealed that ORP7 knockdown in 293A cells resulted in a 40% increase of GS28 protein while ORP7 overexpression had the opposite effect. Similar to ORP7 overexpression, treatment of cells with 25-hydroxycholesterol (25-OH) resulted in GS28 destabilization, which was potentiated by excess ORP7 and inhibited by ORP7 silencing. Their results suggest that ORP7 negatively regulates GS28 protein stability via sequestration of GATE-16, and may mediate the effect of 25-OH on GS28 and Golgi function.

Epidemiological study: It is reported that SNPs near ORP7 gene show genome-wide significant association with LDL cholesterol (Teslovich, Musunuru et al. 2010).

2.10 OSBPL8 (ORP8)

Structure, Tissue distribution and Intracellular localization: ORP8 belongs to the subfamily IV of OSBP/ORP homologues. ORP8 has an ORD, a PH domain and a transmembrane domain. ORP8 is expressed at the highest levels in macrophages, liver, spleen, kidney, and brain (Yan, Mayranpaa et al. 2008). ORP8 is localized in the ER via its C-terminal transmembrane domain.

Molecular functions related to dyslipidemia: It is reported that silencing of ORP8 by RNA interference in THP-1 macrophages increased the expression of ABCA1 and concomitantly cholesterol efflux to lipid-free apolipoprotein A-I. Experiments employing an ABCA1 promoter-luciferase reporter confirmed that ORP8 silencing enhances ABCA1 transcription. These data identify ORP8 as a negative regulator of ABCA1 expression and macrophage cholesterol efflux. But the precise mechanism to regulate the expression of ABCA1 has not been revealed.

Recently, Zhou et al. investigated the action of ORP8 in hepatic cells in vivo and in vitro. They found that adenoviral overexpression of ORP8 in mouse liver induced a decrease of cholesterol, phospholipids, and triglycerides in serum (-34%, -26%, -37%, respectively) and liver tissue (-40%, -12%, -24%), coinciding with reduction of nuclear (n)SREBP-1 and -2 and mRNA levels of their target genes. Consistently, excess ORP8 reduced nSREBPs in HuH7 cells, and ORP8 overexpression or silencing by RNA interference moderately suppressed or induced the expression of SREBP-1 and SREBP-2 target genes, respectively. In accordance, cholesterol biosynthesis was reduced by ORP8 overexpression and enhanced by ORP8 silencing in [(3)H]acetate pulse-labeling experiments.

They also performed yeast two-hybrid, bimolecular fluorescence complementation (BiFC), and co-immunoprecipitation analyses, and revealed the nuclear pore component Nup62 as an interaction partner of ORP8. They showed that the impact of overexpressed ORP8 on nSREBPs and their target mRNAs was inhibited in cells depleted of Nup62.

These results reveal that ORP8 has the capacity to modulate lipid homeostasis and SREBP activity, probably through an indirect mechanism required Nup62.

Epidemiological study: Ma et al. performed a genome-wide association analysis of total cholesterol and HDL cholesterol levels using the Framingham heart study data. In that study, single-locus effects and pairwise epistasis effects of 432,096 SNP markers were tested for their significance on log-transformed total cholesterol and HDL cholesterol levels.
As a result, the OSBPL8-ZDHHC17 region (chr12) was detected for HDL cholesterol identified by one new SNP with genome-wide significance (Ma, Yang et al. 2010).

2.11 OSBPL9 (ORP9)

Structure, Tissue distribution and Intracellular localization: ORP9 belongs to the subfamily V of OSBP/ORP homologues. ORP9 has an ORD, a PH domain and an FFAT motif. VAP binding FFAT motif and PH domains target ORP9 to the ER and a Golgi-COPII compartment, respectively (Wyles and Ridgway 2004).
Molecular functions related to dyslipidemia: Ngo et al. demonstrate that ORP9L partitioning between the trans-Golgi/trans-Golgi network (TGN), and the ER is mediated by a phosphatidylinositol 4-phosphate (PI-4P)-specific PH domain and VAP, respectively (Ngo and Ridgway 2009). In vitro, ORP9L mediates PI-4P-dependent cholesterol transport between liposomes, suggesting that its primary function in vivo is sterol transfer between the Golgi and ER. Depletion of ORP9L by RNAi caused Golgi fragmentation, inhibition of vesicular somatitus virus glycoprotein transport from the ER and accumulation of cholesterol in endosomes/lysosomes. These findings indicate that ORP9 maintains the integrity of the early secretory pathway by mediating transport of sterols between the ER and trans-Golgi/TGN.
It is also reported that ORP9, in interaction with ORP11, may act as an intracellular lipid sensor or transporter (Zhou, Li et al. 2010). (see also ORP11.)
Epidemiological study: Epidemiological study of ORP9 is not reported yet.

2.12 OSBPL10 (ORP10)

Structure, Tissue distribution and Intracellular localization: ORP10 belongs to the subfamily VI of OSBP/ORP homologues. ORP10 has an ORD and a PH domain but does not have an FFAT motif or a transmembrane domain.
ORP10 was shown to associate dynamically with microtubules, being consistent with its involvement in intracellular transport or organelle positioning (Perttila, Merikanto et al. 2009).
Immunofluorescence localization in transiently transfected bovine aorta endothelial cells showed that EGFP-ORP10 co-localized with alpha-tubulin (Fig. 2 c, g) and not with actin (Fig. 2 a, e) or vimentin (Fig. 2 b, f). The microtubules co-localize with EGFP-ORP10 show the aberrant bundled structures. These structures were disrupted by treatment with nocodazol (Fig. 2 d, h).
Molecular functions related to dyslipidemia: Silencing of ORP10 increased the incorporation of [(3)H]acetate into cholesterol and both [(3)H]acetate and [(3)H]oleate into triglycerides and enhanced the accumulation of secreted apolipoprotein B100 in growth medium, suggesting that ORP10 suppresses hepatic lipogenesis and very-low-density lipoprotein production.
Epidemiological study: We examined the association between polymorphisms in the ORP10 gene and risk factors for the metabolic syndrome in the Tanno and Sobetsu Study in Japan (Koriyama, Nakagami et al. 2010).

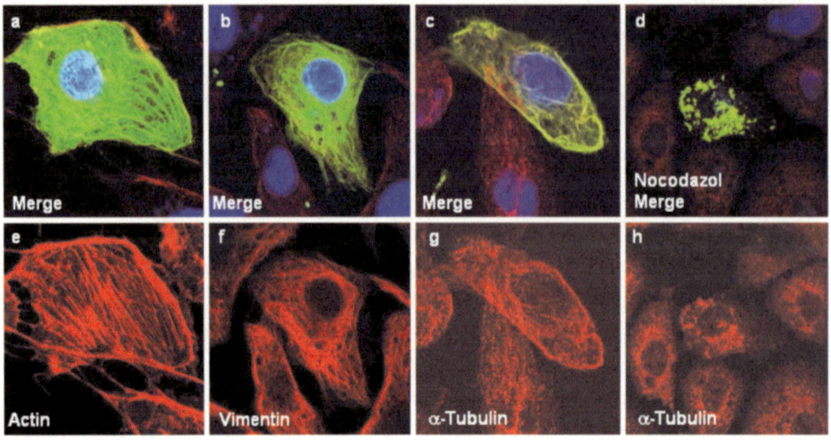

Fig. 2. Intracellular localization of ORP10.

As a result, we found that the LDL cholesterol of individuals with the rs2290532 (D254N) polymorphism was significantly greater in subjects with the CC+CT genotype than in subjects with the TT genotype (124.3+/-1.3 vs. 111.6+/-4.1 mg per 100 ml, P=0.009) (Fig. 3). Comparison of the genotype frequency in both groups indicated that the genotype associated with low risk (TT) reduced the risk of hyper-LDL cholesterolemia significantly (P=0.003), with an odds ratio of 0.35 (95% confidence interval=0.17-0.76). These findings suggest that the rs2290532 (D254N) polymorphism in OSBPL10 may predispose individuals with this SNP to hyper-LDL cholesterolemia.

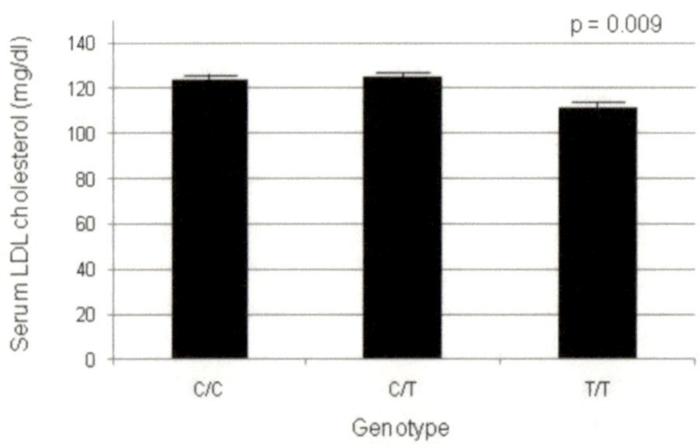

Fig. 3. Relation of rs2290532 of ORP10 with serum LDL cholesterol.

Perttila et al. also reported that the analysis of variants in ORP10 gene revealed suggestive linkage of ORP10 single-nucleotide polymorphisms (SNPs) with extreme end high TG (>90th percentile) trait. They carried out an association analysis in a metabolic syndrome subcohort (Genmets) of Health2000 examination survey (N = 2,138), revealing an association of multiple ORP10 SNPs with high serum TG levels (>95th percentile).

The result proves that ORP10 is genetically associated with both TG and LDL cholesterol levels. Though it is estimated that microtubule dependent intracellular transport of vesicles plays an important role in that process, the mechanism to control TG and LDL cholesterol levels is yet to be explained. A further analysis is highly expected.

2.13 OSBPL11 (ORP11)

Structure, Tissue distribution and Intracellular localization: ORP11 belongs to the subfamily VI of OSBP/ORP homologues. ORP11 has an ORD and a PH domain but does not have an FFAT motif or a transmembrane domain. ORP11 is present at the highest levels in human ovary, testis, kidney, liver, stomach, brain, and adipose tissue. Immunohistochemistry demonstrates abundant ORP11 in the epithelial cells of kidney tubules, testicular tubules, caecum, and skin. ORP11 dimerizes with ORP9 and localizes at the Golgi-late endosome interface (Zhou, Li et al. 2010).

Molecular functions related to dyslipidemia: Cells overexpressing ORP11 displayed lamellar lipid bodies associated with vacuolar structures or the Golgi complex, indicating a disturbance of lipid trafficking. Similar multilamellar membranes arise in endo-lysosomal compartments in phospholipidosis occurring, for instance, upon incubation of macrophage with oxidized low-density lipoprotein, or associated with inheritable lysosomal storage disorders, situations in which normal lipid transport is disturbed. These findings indicate that ORP11, in interaction with ORP9, may act as an intracellular lipid sensor or transporter.

Epidemiological study: it is reported that ORP11 is significantly overexpressed in the visceral adipose tissue of obese men with metabolic syndrome (Bouchard, Faucher et al. 2009). Furthermore, they found SNPs in the ORP11 gene to be associated with several cardiovascular risk factors in obese individuals. IVS12+95 T>C, a newly discovered SNP of the study, was associated with LDL cholesterol levels (OR = 1.63; $P < 0.001$), hyperglycemia/diabetes (OR = 1.48; $P < 0.004$) as well as with metabolic syndrome per se (OR = 1.56; $P < 0.01$). These results suggest that ORP11 is involved in cholesterol and glucose metabolism in obese individuals.

3. Conclusion

Since OSBP/ORP family involves functional redundancy as well as overlap tissue expression and intracellular localization, the function of each family member has been mostly left unrevealed. Various studies including the genome-wide association study, however, have succeeded to prove the direct association between the individual members and dyslipidemia. Analyses on the individual members have also made it clear that the members affect the regulation of cholesterol and triglyceride level in interaction with diverse molecules.

Nevertheless, the precise molecular mechanism of the process still remains unascertained. The recent findings such as the identification of the small molecule which associates with OSBP are expected to act as a convenient tool to clarify the more detailed functions of OSBP/ORP family in future.

4. Acknowledgment

Work in the authors' group is supported by a Grant-in-Aid for Scientific Research from Japan Society for the Promotion of Science and research grants from Takeda Science Foundation.

5. References

Boadu, E. and G. A. Francis (2006). "The role of vesicular transport in ABCA1-dependent lipid efflux and its connection with NPC pathways." J Mol Med (Berl) 84(4): 266-275.

Bouchard, L., G. Faucher, et al. (2009). "Association of OSBPL11 gene polymorphisms with cardiovascular disease risk factors in obesity." Obesity (Silver Spring) 17(7): 1466-1472.

Bowden, K. and N. D. Ridgway (2008). "OSBP negatively regulates ABCA1 protein stability." J Biol Chem 283(26): 18210-18217.

Burgett, A. W., T. B. Poulsen, et al. (2011). "Natural products reveal cancer cell dependence on oxysterol-binding proteins." Nat Chem Biol.

Chen, W., G. Chen, et al. (2007). "Enzymatic reduction of oxysterols impairs LXR signaling in cultured cells and the livers of mice." Cell Metab 5(1): 73-79.

Collier, F. M., C. C. Gregorio-King, et al. (2003). "ORP3 splice variants and their expression in human tissues and hematopoietic cells." DNA Cell Biol 22(1): 1-9.

Du, X., J. Kumar, et al. (2011). "A role for oxysterol-binding protein-related protein 5 in endosomal cholesterol trafficking." J Cell Biol 192(1): 121-135.

Fairn, G. D. and C. R. McMaster (2008). "Emerging roles of the oxysterol-binding protein family in metabolism, transport, and signaling." Cell Mol Life Sci 65(2): 228-236.

Hynynen, R., M. Suchanek, et al. (2009). "OSBP-related protein 2 is a sterol receptor on lipid droplets that regulates the metabolism of neutral lipids." J Lipid Res 50(7): 1305-1315.

Jansen, M., Y. Ohsaki, et al. (2011). "Role of ORPs in sterol transport from plasma membrane to ER and lipid droplets in mammalian cells." Traffic 12(2): 218-231.

Johansson, M., V. Bocher, et al. (2003). "The two variants of oxysterol binding protein-related protein-1 display different tissue expression patterns, have different intracellular localization, and are functionally distinct." Mol Biol Cell 14(3): 903-915.

Johansson, M., M. Lehto, et al. (2005). "The oxysterol-binding protein homologue ORP1L interacts with Rab7 and alters functional properties of late endocytic compartments." Mol Biol Cell 16(12): 5480-5492.

Johansson, M., N. Rocha, et al. (2007). "Activation of endosomal dynein motors by stepwise assembly of Rab7-RILP-p150Glued, ORP1L, and the receptor betalll spectrin." J Cell Biol 176(4): 459-471.

Kobuna, H., T. Inoue, et al. (2010). "Multivesicular body formation requires OSBP-related proteins and cholesterol." PLoS Genet 6(8).

Koriyama, H., H. Nakagami, et al. (2010). "Variation in OSBPL10 is associated with dyslipidemia." Hypertens Res 33(5): 511-514.

Lagace, T. A., D. M. Byers, et al. (1997). "Altered regulation of cholesterol and cholesteryl ester synthesis in Chinese-hamster ovary cells overexpressing the oxysterol-binding protein is dependent on the pleckstrin homology domain." Biochem J 326 (Pt 1): 205-213.

Lagace, T. A., D. M. Byers, et al. (1999). "Chinese hamster ovary cells overexpressing the oxysterol binding protein (OSBP) display enhanced synthesis of sphingomyelin in response to 25-hydroxycholesterol." J Lipid Res 40(1): 109-116.

Laitinen, S., M. Lehto, et al. (2002). "ORP2, a homolog of oxysterol binding protein, regulates cellular cholesterol metabolism." J Lipid Res 43(2): 245-255.

Lehto, M., M. I. Mayranpaa, et al. (2008). "The R-Ras interaction partner ORP3 regulates cell adhesion." J Cell Sci 121(Pt 5): 695-705.

Lehto, M., J. Tienari, et al. (2004). "Subfamily III of mammalian oxysterol-binding protein (OSBP) homologues: the expression and intracellular localization of ORP3, ORP6, and ORP7." Cell Tissue Res 315(1): 39-57.

Levanon, D., C. L. Hsieh, et al. (1990). "cDNA cloning of human oxysterol-binding protein and localization of the gene to human chromosome 11 and mouse chromosome 19." Genomics 7(1): 65-74.

Levine, T. P. and S. Munro (2002). "Targeting of Golgi-specific pleckstrin homology domains involves both PtdIns 4-kinase-dependent and -independent components." Curr Biol 12(9): 695-704.

Ma, L., J. Yang, et al. (2010). "Genome-wide association analysis of total cholesterol and high-density lipoprotein cholesterol levels using the Framingham heart study data." BMC Med Genet 11: 55.

Mohammadi, A., R. J. Perry, et al. (2001). "Golgi localization and phosphorylation of oxysterol binding protein in Niemann-Pick C and U18666A-treated cells." J Lipid Res 42(7): 1062-1071.

Ngo, M. and N. D. Ridgway (2009). "Oxysterol binding protein-related Protein 9 (ORP9) is a cholesterol transfer protein that regulates Golgi structure and function." Mol Biol Cell 20(5): 1388-1399.

Ngo, M. H., T. R. Colbourne, et al. (2010). "Functional implications of sterol transport by the oxysterol-binding protein gene family." Biochem J 429(1): 13-24.

North, K. E., L. J. Martin, et al. (2003). "HDL cholesterol in females in the Framingham Heart Study is linked to a region of chromosome 2q." BMC Genet 4 Suppl 1: S98.

Perttila, J., K. Merikanto, et al. (2009). "OSBPL10, a novel candidate gene for high triglyceride trait in dyslipidemic Finnish subjects, regulates cellular lipid metabolism." J Mol Med (Berl) 87(8): 825-835.

Radhakrishnan, A., Y. Ikeda, et al. (2007). "Sterol-regulated transport of SREBPs from endoplasmic reticulum to Golgi: oxysterols block transport by binding to Insig." Proc Natl Acad Sci U S A 104(16): 6511-6518.

Raychaudhuri, S. and W. A. Prinz (2010). "The diverse functions of oxysterol-binding proteins." Annu Rev Cell Dev Biol 26: 157-177.

Ridgway, N. D., K. Badiani, et al. (1998). "Inhibition of phosphorylation of the oxysterol binding protein by brefeldin A." Biochim Biophys Acta 1390(1): 37-51.

Ridgway, N. D., P. A. Dawson, et al. (1992). "Translocation of oxysterol binding protein to Golgi apparatus triggered by ligand binding." J Cell Biol 116(2): 307-319.

Ridgway, N. D., T. A. Lagace, et al. (1998). "Differential effects of sphingomyelin hydrolysis and cholesterol transport on oxysterol-binding protein phosphorylation and Golgi localization." J Biol Chem 273(47): 31621-31628.

Rocha, N., C. Kuijl, et al. (2009). "Cholesterol sensor ORP1L contacts the ER protein VAP to control Rab7-RILP-p150 Glued and late endosome positioning." J Cell Biol 185(7): 1209-1225.

Sagiv, Y., A. Legesse-Miller, et al. (2000). "GATE-16, a membrane transport modulator, interacts with NSF and the Golgi v-SNARE GOS-28." EMBO J 19(7): 1494-1504.

Sever, N., B. L. Song, et al. (2003). "Insig-dependent ubiquitination and degradation of mammalian 3-hydroxy-3-methylglutaryl-CoA reductase stimulated by sterols and geranylgeraniol." J Biol Chem 278(52): 52479-52490.

Storey, M. K., D. M. Byers, et al. (1998). "Cholesterol regulates oxysterol binding protein (OSBP) phosphorylation and Golgi localization in Chinese hamster ovary cells: correlation with stimulation of sphingomyelin synthesis by 25-hydroxycholesterol." Biochem J 336 (Pt 1): 247-256.

Subramaniam, V. N., F. Peter, et al. (1996). "GS28, a 28-kilodalton Golgi SNARE that participates in ER-Golgi transport." Science 272(5265): 1161-1163.

Teslovich, T. M., K. Musunuru, et al. (2010). "Biological, clinical and population relevance of 95 loci for blood lipids." Nature 466(7307): 707-713.

Vihervaara, T., M. Jansen, et al. (2011). "Cytoplasmic oxysterol-binding proteins: sterol sensors or transporters?" Chem Phys Lipids 164(6): 443-450.

Vihervaara, T., R. L. Uronen, et al. (2011). "Sterol binding by OSBP-related protein 1L regulates late endosome motility and function." Cell Mol Life Sci 68(3): 537-551.

Wang, C., L. JeBailey, et al. (2002). "Oxysterol-binding-protein (OSBP)-related protein 4 binds 25-hydroxycholesterol and interacts with vimentin intermediate filaments." Biochem J 361(Pt 3): 461-472.

Wyles, J. P., R. J. Perry, et al. (2007). "Characterization of the sterol-binding domain of oxysterol-binding protein (OSBP)-related protein 4 reveals a novel role in vimentin organization." Exp Cell Res 313(7): 1426-1437.

Wyles, J. P. and N. D. Ridgway (2004). "VAMP-associated protein-A regulates partitioning of oxysterol-binding protein-related protein-9 between the endoplasmic reticulum and Golgi apparatus." Exp Cell Res 297(2): 533-547.

Yan, D., M. Lehto, et al. (2007). "Oxysterol binding protein induces upregulation of SREBP-1c and enhances hepatic lipogenesis." Arterioscler Thromb Vasc Biol 27(5): 1108-1114.

Yan, D., M. I. Mayranpaa, et al. (2008). "OSBP-related protein 8 (ORP8) suppresses ABCA1 expression and cholesterol efflux from macrophages." J Biol Chem 283(1): 332-340.

Zhong, W., Y. Zhou, et al. (2011). "OSBP-related protein 7 interacts with GATE-16 and negatively regulates GS28 protein stability." Exp Cell Res.

Zhou, T., S. Li, et al. (2011). "OSBP-related protein 8 (ORP8) regulates plasma and liver tissue lipid levels and interacts with the nucleoporin Nup62." PLoS One 6(6): e21078.

Zhou, Y., S. Li, et al. (2010). "OSBP-related protein 11 (ORP11) dimerizes with ORP9 and localizes at the Golgi-late endosome interface." Exp Cell Res 316(19): 3304-3316.

8

Adipose Tissue and Skeletal Muscle Plasticity in Obesity and Metabolic Disease

Jozef Ukropec[1] and Barbara Ukropcova[1,2]
[1]*Institute of Experimental Endocrinology Slovak Academy of Sciences,*
[2]*Institute of Pathological Physiology, Faculty of Medicine Comenius University, Slovakia*

1. Introduction

Obesity and lack of physical activity are two major factors contributing considerably to the pathogenesis of many chronic diseases so prevalent in contemporary human population. Adipose tissue and skeletal muscle are therefore the primary organs one would immediately suggest to target in an attempt to battle metabolic disease progression. Fine tuning of the physiological processes within the two organs have a large potential to modulate (i) energy balance, (ii) lipid storage-utilization efficiency as well as (iii) central and peripheral actions in the brain, gastrointestinal system or liver which are integrated by the endocrine activity of the two energy balance maintaining tissues.

2. Adipose tissue in metabolic health and disease

Despite the fact that the primary role of adipose tissue is an effective lipid storage and timely regulation of its release and that these processes could, in a simplified adipocentric view, be the primary determinants of the dyslipidemia and metabolic disease progression, adipose tissue has a broad range of other regulatory functions exerted *via* its autocrine, paracrine and endocrine actions. Adipose tissue secretory products, "adipokines", could modulate food intake, energy expenditure, or tissue oxidative capacity (Trayhurn et al. 1998; Ukropec et al. 2001; Ahima & Lazar 2008; Henry & Clarke 2008; Friedman 2011). In addition, adipose tissue dynamically changes its structure (*tissue remodeling, lipid composition*), function (*lipid storage & lipolysis*) as well as endocrine action in response to different physiological (*fasting / refeeding, exercise, microgravity*) and pathophysiological (*obesity, prediabetes, diabetes, cachexia, lipodystrophy, growth hormone deficiency*) conditions (Ukropec et al. 2008; Itoh et al. 2011; Pietilainen et al. 2011). It is important to understand that adipose tissue is a mixture of very different cell-types. Apart from approximately 50% of mature lipid-laden adipocytes it contains various stromal cells including preadipocytes, endothelial cells, fibroblasts, pluripotent stem cells and immune cells which substantially influence its function (Bjorntorp 1974; Sethi & Vidal-Puig 2007; Divoux & Clement 2011). Extreme enlargement of the fat cell size, such as we have recently observed in individuals with growth hormone deficiency, is perhaps the best early marker of the obesity related - metabolic disease development (Ukropec et al. 2008a) (Fig. 1.). Adipose tissue with enlarged adipocytes, expressing markers of the local tissue microhypoxia but not responding to it properly and attracting large amount of activated immunocompetent cells, has recently been termed "pathogenic adipose tissue" (Bays et al. 2008; Ukropec et al. 2008b).

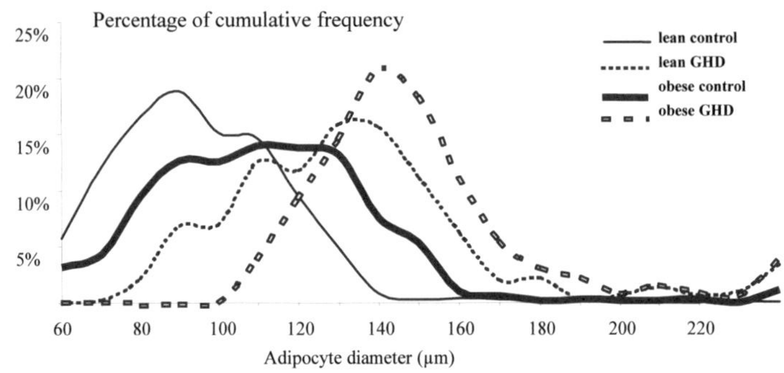

Fig. 1. Fat cell size in obesity and in growth hormone deficiency (GHD), percentage of cumulative frequency (Y axis), (Ukropec et al. 2008a).

The tissue damage due to overwhelming adipocytes with lipids, largely exceeding their lipid storage capacity, changes the adipokine secretory profile and leads to uncontrolled release of a large amount of lipids into circulation while the capacity of the adipose tissue adaptive remodeling is compromised. This is followed by the accumulation of lipids in tissues not designed for the lipid storage such as liver, skeletal muscle, pancreatic beta cells or lung which largely interferes with their physiological functions and accelerates the development of metabolic disease (Bays et al. 2008; Foster et al. 2010; Unger et al. 2010). Limited expandability of the adipose tissue seems to determine individual propensity to the development of metabolic disease (Arner, P. et al. 2011). Adaptive expansion of the adipose tissue is enabled by combination of adipocyte hypertrophy and hyperplasia. Expansion of adipose tissue requires quite extensive tissue remodeling, in order to maintain adequate energy and oxygen supply, active neuronal network as well as integrity and functional properties of cellular membranes (Itoh et al. 2011; Pietilainen et al. 2011). Broader knowledge of the fat cell life-cycle dynamics is critical for our understanding the pathophysiological mechanisms limiting adipose tissue hyperplastic expansion. In 2008, Arner's group analyzed the adipocyte turnover by detecting the genomic DNA incorporation of atmospheric ^{14}C derived from above-ground nuclear bomb tests in period between 1955 and 1963. This work revealed that approximately 10% of fat cells are renewed per year at all adult ages and levels of BMI and that neither adipocyte death nor generation rate is altered in early onset obesity. It seemed that the steady production of adipocytes in adults results in a stable size of the constantly turning over adipocyte population (Spalding et al. 2008). More recent work by these authors examining morphology of the subcutaneous adipose tissue from 764 individuals with broad range of BMI (18-60 $kg.m^2$) defines hyperplasia and hypertrophy as a difference between measured adipocyte volume and volume predicted by the curve-like fit, for adipocyte volume and body fat mass (Fig. 2.). In this analysis occurrence of hyperplasia or hypertrophy correlated with fasting plasma insulin and insulin sensitivity. In addition, total adipocyte number was greatest in individuals with pronounced hyperplasia, and smallest in those with pronounced hypertrophy. The absolute number of new adipocytes generated each year was 70% lower in patients with hypertrophy than with hyperplasia. Whereas the relative death rate (~ 10% per year) or mean age of adipocytes (~ 10 years) was not correlated with adipocyte morphology (Arner, E. et al. 2010).

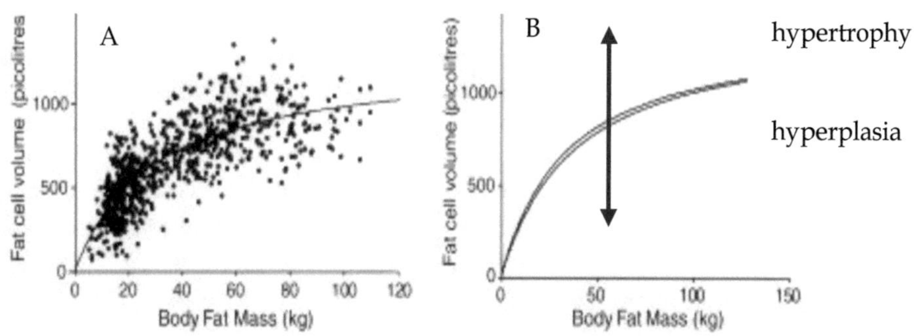

Fig. 2. (A) Graph depicts large variability in adipose tissue morphology in individuals with identical body fat mass (764 subjects). (B) Level of hyperplasia is represented by adequately lowered morphology value while hypertrophy is associated with parallel increase in morphology value defined as a difference between measured and expected adipocyte volume given by the curve-like fit , for given body fat mass (Arner, E. et al. 2010).

Insulin sensitivity could therefore govern adipose tissue morphology towards beneficial hyperplastic state at the population level. Conversely, defects in insulin action are interconnected with the hypertrophic adipocytes, and higher risk of lipid flooding the nonadipose tissues. Absolute numbers of adipocytes as well as their capacity to expand and store lipids are quite difficult to modulate. Morbid obesity and lipodystrophy represent the two medical conditions associated with excessive hypertriglyceridemia, hepatic steatosis, and disordered muscle glucose metabolism, due to defected ability of adipose tissue to store lipids or the selective loss of adipose tissue respectively. Activation of adipogenic programme by PPARγ agonists or chronic leptin treatment improves insulin-stimulated hepatic and peripheral glucose metabolism in obese and lipodystrophic patients respectively (Petersen et al. 2002; Rieusset et al. 2002; Van Gaal et al. 2003). Adipogenesis is necessary to increase the adipose tissue cellularity (hyperplastic adaptive change) and lipid storage capacity; it is largely dependent on the signal transducers and activators of transcription (STAT) pathway. In brief, transcription factors C/EBPα, C/EBPβ, and PPARγ control adipogenesis by regulating STAT5B and STAT5A. Regulation of PPARγ-STAT5 by C/EBPβ signaling seems to be the crucial adipogenesis - initiating cascade of the various adipogenic genes (Jung et al. 2011). Activation of adipogenic program should be paralleled with the extracellular matrix remodeling. As mentioned above, adipocytes are embedded in a unique extracellular matrix which main function is to provide mechanical support, in addition to participating in a variety of signaling events. Extracellular matrix requires remodeling to accommodate growing adipocytes in the expanding adipose tissue. We have recently participated in the research by Christian Wolfrum's laboratory investigating regulatory processes related to adipose tissue hyperplasia. In this work, the transcription factor retinoid-related orphan receptor γ (RORγ) was identified as an important regulator of adipocyte development through regulation of its newly identified target gene matrix metallopeptidase-3. RORγ might serve as a novel predictor for the risk of metabolic complications in obesity as well as a pharmaceutical target for the treatment of obesity-associated diseases (Meissburger et al. 2011).

Khan et al., recently proposed that "adipose tissue fibrosis" is a hallmark of metabolically challenged adipocytes. Authors observed that the absence of collagen VI, the highly enriched extracellular matrix component of adipose tissue, results in the uninhibited expansion of individual adipocytes, which is paradoxically associated with substantial improvements in whole-body energy homeostasis, both with high-fat diet exposure and in the ob/ob background. Weakening the extracellular scaffold of adipocytes seems to enable their stress-free expansion during states of positive energy balance, which is consequently associated with an improved inflammatory profile (Khan et al. 2009). Further support to the notion that metabolic deregulation is rather due to lipid-leakage than the adipocyte hypertrophy *per se* comes from the experiment where mice lacking leptin were made to overexpress adiponectin. This led to the modest increase in circulating levels of full-length adiponectin and to subsequent normalization of glucose and insulin levels, dramatic improvement of glucose tolerance and positive effect on serum triglyceride levels. Adiponectin in fact completely rescued the diabetic phenotype in ob/ob mice. These mice displayed increased expression of PPARγ target genes and a reduction in macrophage infiltration in adipose tissue and systemic inflammation. Adiponectin expressing ob/ob mice, however, were morbidly obese, with significantly higher levels of adiposity and adipocyte hypertrophy than their ob/ob littermates. Adiponectin seems to act as a peripheral "starvation" signal promoting the storage of triglycerides preferentially in adipose tissue. As a consequence, reduced triglyceride levels in the liver and muscle convey improved systemic insulin sensitivity despite adipocyte hypertrophy (Kim et al. 2007).

2.1 Specificities of subcutaneous and visceral adipose tissue

In contrast to visceral adipose tissue, which is often blamed from inducing detrimental metabolic effects, subcutaneous adipose tissue has the potential to benefit lipid and glucose metabolism. It has been repeatedly shown that differences in regional body fat distribution determine the propensity for the development of obesity related metabolic complications (Tchernof 2007). Accumulation of fat in the visceral region (mesentery, omentum, retroperitoneum), that in fact corresponds to central obesity (determined by increased waist circumference) is associated with cardiovascular disease and type 2 diabetes, independently on overall obesity (Wajchenberg 2000; Hamdy et al. 2006; Pischon et al. 2008). The amount of visceral fat increases with age in both genders but man in general have greater visceral adiposity than women (Wajchenberg 2000). Consistent with this notion, removal of visceral adipose tissue (omentectomy) decreases glucose and insulin levels in humans (Thorne et al. 2002). By contrast peripheral obesity – increased subcutaneous adipose tissue mass, mainly in the region of buttock and thighs seem to be associated with improved insulin sensitivity and lower risk for type 2 diabetes mellitus (Snijder et al. 2003; Koska et al. 2008). One possible explanation for the detrimental effect of visceral fat accumulation comes from its unfortunate anatomical location (Arner, P. 1998; Bergman et al. 2006), but second theory based on adipose tissue transplantation experiments blames rather the tissue internal properties such as unfavorable secretory profile (Matsuzawa et al. 1999).

Adipose tissue transplantation experiments have been primarily used as a tool to study physiology for human reconstructive surgery, but they provide important information on differences between visceral and subcutaneous adipose tissue which opens the vision of the adipose tissue or adipose tissue derived stem cells transplantation for the treatment of obesity and metabolic disorders.

2.2 Brown adipose tissue in human physiology

Humans and other mammals have two types of adipose tissue that contribute to control of the whole body energy metabolism. The above discussed white adipose tissue, "the bad guy" associated with obesity, is necessary for energy storage. Brown adipose, "the good guy", contains a lots of mitochondria and is ready to burn energy to generate heat in response to cold or dietary intake, keeping the body warm and slim (Cannon & Nedergaard 2004). Until recently, physiologically relevant amount of brown fat was only found in newborns. However, accumulating evidence indicates that adult humans - or at least significant portion of us retain physiologically relevant amount of brown fat (van Marken Lichtenbelt et al. 2009; Vijgen et al. 2011; Virtanen & Nuutila 2011). This provides an exciting possibility to precisely regulate the adaptive thermogenic process in humans, which could dissipate energy and lower the obesity related metabolic burden. Brown adipose tissue activity in humans was determined with the aid of ^{18}F-fluorodeoxyglucose positron-emission tomography and computing tomography mainly in the supraclavicular region of cold-exposed individuals. Importantly, specimens of the adipose tissue from the supraclavicular region of adult humans with active brown adipose tissue were positive for UCP1 protein (Fig. 3.) (van Marken Lichtenbelt et al. 2009; Zingaretti et al. 2009). Vision of translating this knowledge into the clinical practice is quite reachable (Nedergaard & Cannon 2010; Tseng et al. 2010). Clinical importance could be significant, despite the fact that the volume of active brown adipose tissue tends to be lower in the overweight or obese than in the lean individuals (van Marken Lichtenbelt et al. 2009), and that it decreases with age (Cypess et al. 2009). Interestingly, applying the personalized cooling protocol for maximal nonshivering conditions to morbidly obese individuals could still increase brown adipose tissue activity (Vijgen et al. 2011).

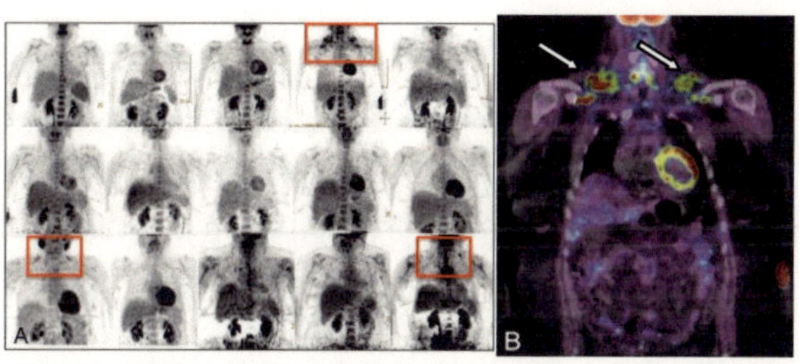

Fig. 3. Metabolically activated brown adipose tissue in supraclavicular region (arrows, B) in morbidly obese individuals after personalized cooling protocol (Vijgen et al. 2011).

2.3 Metabolic activation of the white adipose tissue

It has recently been shown that brown adipocytes and muscle cells share the common origin and in this respect they are quite distinct from white adipocytes (Tseng et al. 2008; Seale & Lazar 2009). The question remains, what is the origin of "brown fat-like white (brite) " adipocytes containing UCP1 which could be induced in white fat depots under certain pohysiological (cold exposure) (Fig. 4.) or pharmacological (activation of SNS, agonists of PPARγ) conditions (Granneman et al. 2005; Li et al. 2005; Ukropec et al. 2006). Nedegaard`s laboratory had recently reported that chronic treatment with the PPARγ agonist rosiglitazone promotes not only the expression of PGC1α and mitochondriogenesis but also a catecholamine - inducible UCP1 gene expression in a significant subset of the white adipocytes, giving them the genuine, thermogenic capacity.

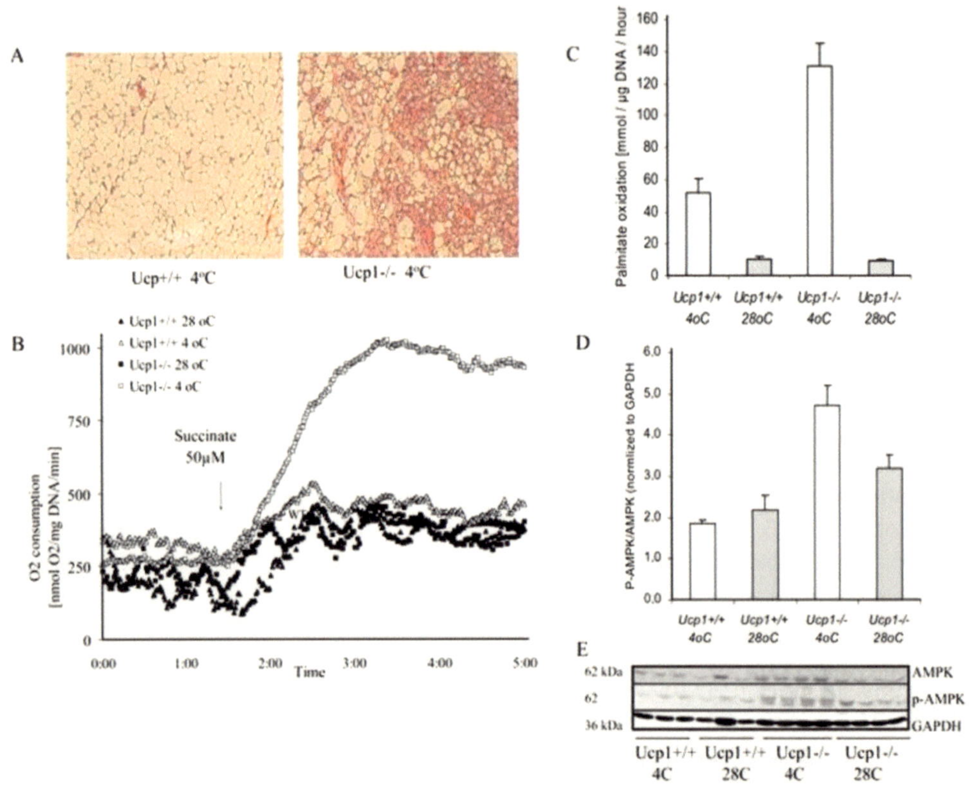

Fig. 4. Metabolically activated "brite adipocytes" as found in inguinal white adipose tissue of mice lacking the UCP1-thermogenesis after gradual exposure to cold.
(**A**) histomorphology, (**B**) O_2 consumption by oxymetry, (**C**) adipose tissue *ex vivo* palmitate oxidation, (**D&E**) evidence for AMPK activation (Ukropec et al. 2006).

In collaboration with laboratory of dr. Kvatnansky we have recently observed that catecholamines, important regulators of lipolysis in adipose tissue, could be produced within adipocytes. Adipocytes isolated from mesenteric adipose tissue expressed genes encoding the catecholamine biosynthetic enzymes and produced catecholamines *de novo*. Administration of tyrosine hydroxylase inhibitor, alpha-methyl-p-tyrosine, significantly reduced concentration of catecholamines in isolated adipocytes *in vitro* (Fig. 5.). We therefore hypothesized that the sympathetic innervation of adipose tissue is not the only source of catecholamines and that adipocyte-derived catecholamines could dynamically modulate metabolic or thermogenic properties of the white adipose tissue perhaps by enhancing "brite adipocyte" function (Vargovic et al. 2011).

3. Adipocentric view on the pathophysiology of metabolic disease

The prevalence of obesity and its consequent pathologies in modern society is of serious health concern. Although the expansion of adipose tissue mass during pathological obesity is in itself not a grave problem, rather it is the ensuing pathologies resultant of this state, including development of hypertension, type 2 diabetes and cardiac myopathies, that impacts peoples lives and health services worldwide.

Clearly not all obese individuals develop metabolic and cardiovascular complications; here we discuss several regulatory mechanisms representing a base for the strategies to prevent metabolic disease development.

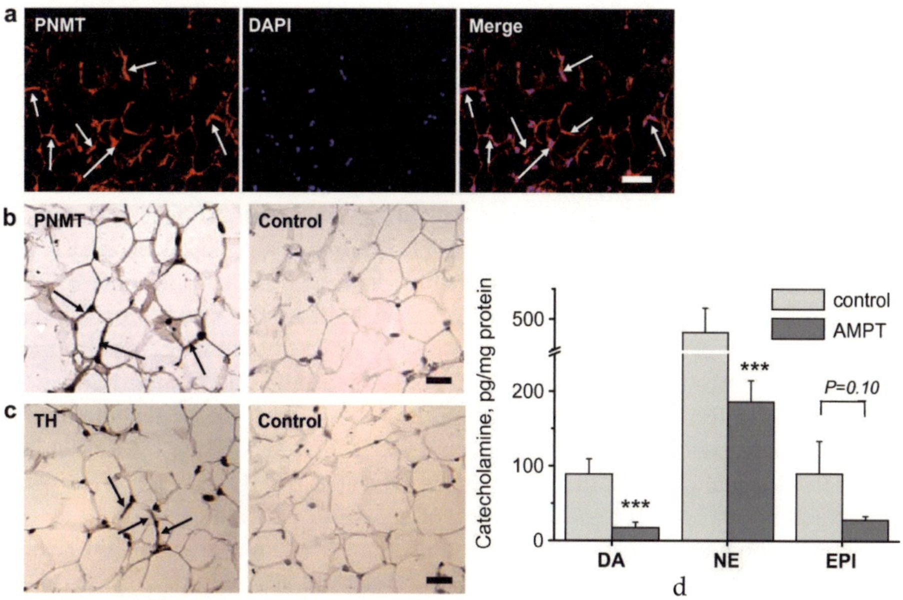

Fig. 5. Adipocytes have internal catecholamine production capacity. Adipose tissue contains mRNA and proteins specific for tyrosine hydroxylase (TH) and phenylethanolamine N-methyltransferase PNMT as shown on histological sections probed with specific PNMT (**a**,**b**) and TH (**c**) antibodies, scale bar: 20 µm. (**d**) Adipocytes freshly isolated from mesenteric adipose tissue produce dopamine (DA), norepinephrine (NE) and epinephrine (EPI) into the media. Production of catecholamines is largely inhibited by addition of alpha-methyl-p-tyrosine (AMPT) - competitive inhibitor of TH activity (Vargovic et al. 2011).

3.1 Hypoxia

Hypothesis that adipose tissue populated by large adipocytes contains the local microhypoxia suffering areas, which has a profound effect on the tissue metabolic and inflammatory phenotype, has been largely accepted. Hypoxia is one of the major triggers strongly inhibiting adipocyte differentiation. Tissue hypoxia in obesity is associated with the defects in the nutrient and oxygen supply into the tissue, related to a defective blood flow regulation which might be perpetuated by the increased fat cell size (Yun et al. 2002). This is happening in spite of the almost unlimited capacity of adipose tissue to expand in a non-transformed form, which is a very unique property of adipose tissue that cannot be seen in any other organ. To accomplish this adipose tissue requires potent mechanisms to remodel, acutely and chronically, as it can rapidly reach the diffusional limit of oxygen; molecular response to hypoxia is therefore an early determinant that limits healthy adipose tissue expansion. Proper expansion requires a highly coordinated response among many different cell types, including endothelial precursor cells, immune cells, and preadipocytes (Sun et al. 2011). It has also been demonstrated that mitochondrial oxidative apparatus is essential for the white fat adipocyte differentiation (De Pauw et al. 2009). Beside their key role in ATP

production, mitochondria constitute the primary source of reactive oxygen species (ROS), which have a great potential to influence the tissue plasticity.
ROS are not only considered a negative factors contributing to degenerative processes and ageing, but also a physiological signal molecules participating in the oxygen sensing mechanisms (Chandel & Budinger 2007). Mitochondrial ROS production influences the size of the white adipocytes, and ROS are in fact antiadipogenic signaling molecules triggering the hypoxia-dependent inhibition of adipocyte differentiation (Carriere et al. 2004). In addition, decreased oxygen availability stimulates the programming of cellular metabolism towards increased glycolysis and fatty acid and triacylglyceride synthesis (Halperin et al. 1969; Kinnula et al. 1978). Hypoxia-inducible factor (HIF), dimers composed of HIF1α, HIF2α or HIF3α (collectively HIFα) and HIF1β/ARNT subunits, play a key role in the coordination of these metabolic adaptations (Trayhurn et al. 2008; Krishnan et al. 2009). HIFα subunits are constitutively expressed but degraded under normoxia due to prolyl hydroxylase activity, which marks them for recognition by the von Hippel-Lindau (VHL) tumor suppressor protein pVHL, that acts as part of an E3 ubiquitin ligase complex to target HIFα subunit for proteasomal degradation. Loss of pVHL function or hypoxia leads to accumulation of HIFα, dimerization with HIFα/ARNT and the activation of numerous hypoxia-inducible genes (Krek 2000; Semenza 2001). Previous work by Krek`s laboratory provided the seminal observation that hypoxia activated pVHL and HIF1α oxygen sensing system affects normal physiological function of heart and pancreatic beta cells by triggering the changes in the glucose and fatty acid metabolism (Zehetner et al. 2008; Krishnan et al. 2009). Interestingly, hypoxia present in atherosclerotic lesions contributes to the pro-inflammatory lipid-loaded foam cells formation, as it decreases expression of enzymes involved in β-oxidation and increases expression of enzymes related to fatty acid synthesis and lipid droplet formation. The aforementioned processes possibly stimulate progression of the atherosclerotic plaque formation (Bostrom et al. 2007). Finally, tissue hypoxia largely modulates adipocytokine production and possibly contributes to the adipose tissue inflammation in obesity (Hosogai et al. 2007; Wang et al. 2007; Ukropec et al. 2008).

3.2 Inflammation – Macrophage, adipocyte and preadipocyte plasticity

Chronic low level of inflammation present in the "pathogenic" adipose tissue has been found to have adverse effects on the adipose tissue physiological functions contributing thus to the metabolic disease. It has been shown that increase in both body fat mass and adipocyte cell size are directly related to the number of macrophages found in the adipose tissue (Wellen & Hotamisligil 2005; Weisberg et al. 2006; Goossens 2008). A net pro-inflammatory response of the adipose tissue may result from adipose tissue secretion of pro-inflammatory factors; adipose tissue secretion of factors that stimulate other tissues to produce inflammatory factors; and decreased production of anti-inflammatory factors. Although the contribution of specific cell types to inflammation is uncertain, evidence is mounting that implicates adipose tissue macrophages as the significant contributor to inflammation in insulin resistant adipose tissue (Kanda et al. 2006; Neels & Olefsky 2006). There are controversial reports related to the importance of the CC chemokine ligand 2 (CCL2, monocyte chemoattractant protein-1) for the macrophage-recruitment and activation in obesity (Kamei et al. 2006; Inouye et al. 2007). Interestingly CCL2 has also been proposed to affect metabolism independently of its macrophage-recruiting capabilities (Inouye et al. 2007). There is also preliminary data indicating that the tissue infiltration by macrophages depends upon the expression of osteopontin, an extracellular matrix protein and pro-inflammatory cytokine which promotes the monocyte chemotaxis and cell motility. Mice exposed to a high-fat diet exhibited increased plasma osteopontin level, and elevated expression of osteopontin in macrophages recruited into adipose tissue. In addition, obese mice lacking osteopontin displayed improved insulin sensitivity in the absence of an effect on the diet-induced obesity, body composition or energy expenditure. These mice further demonstrated decreased macrophage infiltration into adipose tissue, which may reflect both impaired macrophage motility and attenuated monocyte recruitment by stromal vascular cells. Finally, obese osteopontin-deficient mice exhibited decreased markers of inflammation, both in adipose tissue and systemically (Nomiyama et al. 2007).

Adipose tissue resident macrophages show significant heterogeneity in their properties and activation state, reflecting the local metabolic and immune microenvironment (Gordon & Taylor 2005). Different stimuli activate macrophages to express distinct patterns of chemokines, surface markers and enzymes that ultimately generate the diversity of macrophage function seen in inflammatory and non-inflammatory settings. It has recently been proposed that adipose tissue macrophages, which accumulate with obesity and are implicated in insulin resistance switch their phenotype from one of an alternatively activated (M2) to pro-inflammatory (M1) cells (Lumeng et al. 2007). Characteristic features of the IFN-γ induced pro-inflammatory (M1) macrophages include enhanced MHC class II expression, but distinctive up-regulation of i-NOS. Alternative activation of macrophages (M2) is strongly associated with extracellular parasitic infections, allergy, humoral immunity, and fibrosis. It is characterized by up-regulation of the endocytic lecithin-like receptors and arginase rather than i-NOS (Gordon 2007). Therefore, the alternatively activated (M2) macrophages seem to have high capacity for the tissue remodeling and repair.

It had been recently proposed that PPARγ is required for maturation of alternatively activated macrophages (M2), which could also participate to its insulin sensitizing effect (Odegaard et al. 2007). Disruption of PPARγ in myeloid cells impaired alternative macrophage activation and predisposed to the development of diet-induced obesity, insulin resistance, and glucose intolerance. This might be related to the concomitant down-regulation of oxidative phosphorylation gene expression in skeletal muscle and liver (Odegaard et al. 2007). Phenotype of macrophages in the pathogenic-hypoxic adipose tissue might also be regulated by HIF-1 since the functional loss of HIF-1α resulted in a dramatic reduction of the intracellular ATP stores in macrophages to approximately 15-20%, most likely due to the inhibition of the HIF-1α regulated glycolytic energy generation (Cramer & Johnson 2003; Cramer et al. 2003). It could be hypothesized that resident alternatively activated macrophages have a beneficial role in regulating nutrient homeostasis and suggest that macrophage polarization towards the alternative state might be a useful strategy for treating type 2 diabetes, by modulating adipose tissue phenotype.

Fatty acid binding proteins (FABPs), which are common to adipocytes and macrophages, could also play an important role in metabolic and inflammatory disease, and might therefore represent desirable therapeutic targets for metabolic syndrome (Erbay et al. 2007). Macrophage-derived foam cells express the adipocyte fatty acid-binding protein (FABP) aP2 that plays an important role in regulating the development of insulin resistance in obesity. It has been shown that macrophages deficient in aP2 display alterations in the inflammatory cytokine production. Through its distinct actions in adipocytes and macrophages, aP2 links together the features of the metabolic syndrome including insulin resistance, obesity, inflammation, and atherosclerosis (Linton & Fazio 2003).

3.3 Phospholipid membrane composition

In the last decades, free radical processes delineated an interdisciplinary field linking chemistry to biology and medicine. Free radical mechanisms became of importance as molecular basis of physiological and pathological conditions. Lipids, in particular unsaturated fatty acids, are susceptible to free radical attack. The reactivity of the double bond toward free radicals is well known; in particular the reversible addition of radical species to this functionality determines the cis-trans double bond isomerization. Since the prevalent geometry displayed by unsaturated fatty acids in eukaryotes is cis, the occurrence of the cis-trans isomerization by free radicals corresponds to the loss of an important structural information linked to biological activity (Ferreri & Chatgilialoglu 2009). Formation of trans isomers of unsaturated fatty acid in biological membranes can have important meaning and consequences connected to radical stress associated with nutritional overload and mitochondrial defects. It might, together with changes in membrane lipid composition (Pietilainen et al. 2011), substantially modulate lipid membrane biophysical characteristics such as thickness, fluidity, protein lateral diffusion capacity, permeability to small molecules in expanding adipocytes and contribute thus to the development of metabolic disease in obesity.

3.4 Pollutants and metabolic health

Physical inactivity and unhealthy diet are well recognized environmental influences largely increasing the risk for metabolic disease development. Recent advances in detecting the presence of various persistent organic pollutants in the surrounding world as well as within our bodies, prompted us to evaluate its possible role in pathogenesis of different endocrine and metabolic pathological states (Langer et al. 2003; Langer et al. 2007; Langer 2010; Langer et al. 2010; Ukropec et al. 2010; Langer et al. 2011).

A heavily polluted area of Eastern Slovakia was targeted by the PCBrisk cross-sectional survey to search for possible links between environmental pollution and both prediabetes and diabetes. Associations of serum levels of five persistent organic pollutants (POPs), namely polychlorinated biphenyls (PCBs), 2,2'-bis(4-chlorophenyl)-1,1-dichloroethylene (p,p'-DDE), 2,2'-bis(4-chlorophenyl)-1,1,1-trichloro-ethane (p,p'-DDT), hexachlorobenzene (HCB) and beta-hexachlorocyclohexane (β-HCH), with prediabetes and diabetes were investigated in 2,047 adults. Prevalence of prediabetes and diabetes increased in a dose-dependent manner, with individuals in upper quintiles of individual POPs showing striking increases in prevalence of prediabetes (Fig. 6.) Interestingly, unlike PCBs, DDT and DDE, increased levels of HCB and β-HCH seemed not to be associated with increased prevalence of diabetes (Ukropec et al. 2010). Cumulative effect of all five persistent organic pollutants (sum of orders) more than tripled the prevalence of prediabetes while that of diabetes was increased more than six times as compared to the referent quintile composed of individuals with lowest levels of pollutants in serum. We as well as the others have clearly shown that increasing serum concentrations of individual persistent organic pollutants considerably increased prevalence of prediabetes and diabetes in a dose-dependent manner. Interaction of industrial and agricultural pollutants in increasing prevalence of prediabetes or diabetes is likely (Hong et al. 2010; Ukropec et al. 2010; Howard & Lee 2011; Lee, D. H. et al. 2011; Lee, D. H. et al. 2011; Lee, H. K. 2011).

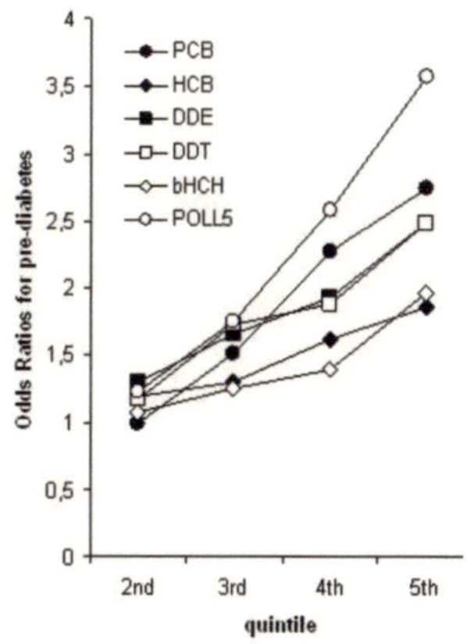

Fig. 6. The prevalence of prediabetes increases with increased circulating levels of PCBs (sum 15 congeners of polychlorinated biphenyls); DDE (2,2'-bis(4-chlorophenyl)-1,1-dichloroethylene); DDT (2,2'-bis(4-chlorophenyl)-1,1,1-trichloro-ethane); HCB (hexachlorobenzene) and b-HCH (beta-hexachlorocyclohexane); POLL5 represents the sum of orders for all 5 pollutants. Odds ratios were adjusted for age, gender and BMI.

4. Skeletal muscle in metabolic health and disease

Skeletal muscle represents a large mass of tissue, and its primary function is to use energy, though quite inefficiently, to enable us the 3D life, voluntary positioning and moving our bodies in a surrounding space. This makes an active muscle to be the most effective energy burner. In addition to obvious metabolic consequences, regular exercise activates central reward mechanisms and makes us happy (Figure 7.) (Sher 1998; Boecker et al. 2008).

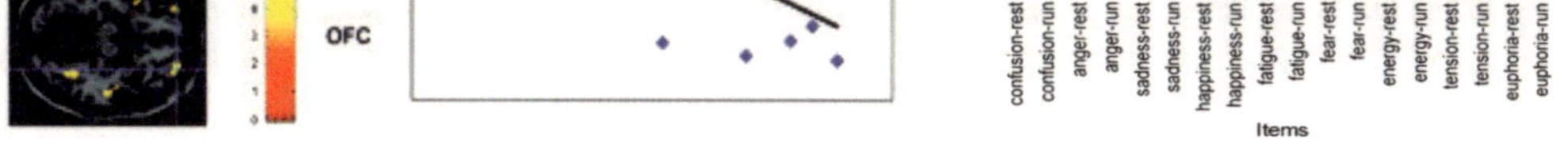

Fig. 7. Correlation of opidergic ligand 6-O-(2-[18F]fluoroethyl)-6-O-desmethyldiprenorphine binding in right orbitofrontal cortex (OFC) with the visual analog mood scale (for euphoria) in runners (**A**) and effect of exercise on the individual's mood expressed in the visual analog mood scale (**B**) (Boecker et al. 2008).

More importantly, inadequate physical activity, associated with defects in mitochondrial function and changes in ultrastructure as well as muscle endocrine properties, largely contributes to the imbalance between energy intake and energy expenditure and is tightly associated with many chronic metabolic and cardiovascular diseases (Bluher & Zimmer 2010; Pedersen 2011). Physical activity is a key factor to bring individuals living in a modern society with plenty of palatable food choices to energy balance. The mechanisms that tie muscle activity to health are unclear. Generation of "exercise pill" targeting organ systems involved in facultative thermogenesis had been envisaged (Himms-Hagen 2004). And results of studies aimed at identifying the endocrine properties of exercising muscle are encouraging our thinking in this respect. In our recent study we observed on the sample of 71 individuals with a broad range of BMI that overweight and obesity is associated with decreased physical activity. This might be not so surprising. But low physical activity level was also associated with decreased insulin sensitivity, increased fat cell size and expanded visceral adiposity all independent on BMI (Fig. 8.). In addition, the basic metabolic rate was positively and respiratory quotient negatively associated with the duration of the daily physical activity representing thus a direct link between physical activity and major determinants of energy homeostasis (Ukropcova et al., unpublished observations).

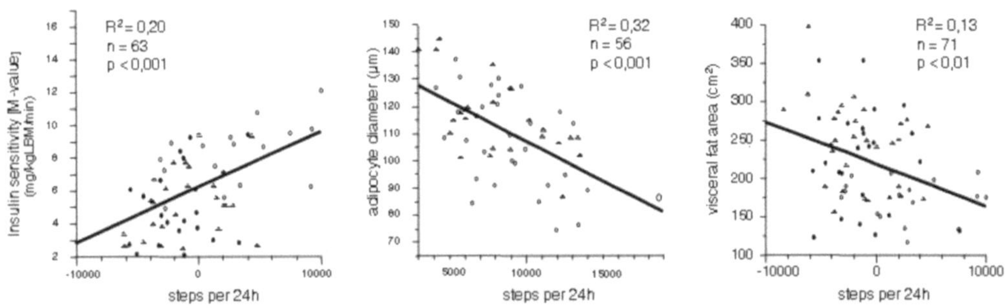

Fig. 8. Free-living ambulatory activity (number of steps in 24h) correlates with insulin sensitivity, modulates adipocyte diameter as well as visceral adiposity (Ukropcova et al., unpublished observations).

This complements the previous observations by others indicating that inactivity initiates unique cellular processes that are qualitatively different from the exercise responses. Inactivity physiology studies are beginning to raise a new concern with potentially major clinical and public health significance. Sedentary lifestyle threatens our society. The average nonexercising person may become even more metabolically unfit in the coming years if they sit too much and thereby lower the normally high volume of intermittent nonexercise physical activity in everyday life (Fig. 8) (Hamilton et al. 2007; Levine et al. 2008). Dynamic interrelations of skeletal muscle and adipose tissue during exercise are necessary to support muscle performance. This requires precise spacio-temporal management of the adipose tissue metabolic flux. The transcriptional coactivator PGC1α has recently been shown to regulate several exercise-associated aspects of muscle function. There is mounting evidence suggesting that this transcription factor controls muscle plasticity, suppresses a broad inflammatory response and integrates many beneficial effects of exercise on metabolic health (Handschin & Spiegelman 2008).

4.1 Exercise and skeletal muscle endocrinology

The recent identification of skeletal muscle as an endocrine organ that produces and releases biologically active substances, "myokines", expands our knowledge on how the endocrine, immune and nervous systems contribute to the maintenance of homeostasis, especially when energy demands are increased (Pedersen & Febbraio 2008). To date, only a few muscle cell-secreted proteins with auto-, para-, or endocrine functions have been identified. It could be hypothesized that skeletal muscle releases a large number of biologically active substances which participate to cell-to-cell and organ-to-organ cross-talk. It also has to be noted that specific biological functions of known myokines are very incompletely understood.

Certain myokines, such as calprotectin (Mortensen et al. 2008), IL15 (Nielsen & Pedersen 2007) and IL6 (Jonsdottir et al. 2000), are acutely induced by muscle contraction but might not necessarily be increased in response to muscle training (Pedersen & Febbraio 2008; Haugen et al. 2010). Exercise training involves multiple adaptations including increased pre-exercise skeletal muscle glycogen content (Kirwan et al. 1990), enhanced activity of key enzymes involved in β-oxidation (Schantz 1986), increased sensitivity of adipose tissue to epinephrine-induced lipolysis (Crampes et al. 1986), and increased muscle capacity to oxidize fat (Holloszy & Booth 1976; Phillips et al. 1996). It could therefore be hypothesized that secretory activity of muscle subjected to inadequate physical activity would be qualitatively and quantitatively distinct from that of the trained athlete, and that it could simply be regulated by e.g. the glycogen level (Keller et al. 2001; Steensberg et al. 2001), reactive oxygen species production (Kosmidou et al. 2002; Steensberg et al. 2007) or by modulating biological availability of various forms of lipids (Peter et al. 2009), such as found in obesity.

Previous reports indicate that calprotectin, IL6 and IL15 might contribute to homeostatic control of glucose and lipid metabolism (Van Hall et al. 2003; Febbraio et al. 2004). In addition, fibroblast growth factor-21 (FGF-21), the potent metabolic regulator, shown to improve glucose metabolism and insulin sensitivity in animal models, had recently been found to be expressed and secreted *in vitro* from murine muscle cells and *in vivo* from human muscle in response to insulin stimulation (hyperinsulinemic-euglycemic clamp) (Hojman et al. 2009). Follistatin-like 1 (Fstl-1) is another myokine whose functional significance in physiological and pathological processes is incompletely understood. Preliminary evidence indicates that Fstl-1 promotes endothelial cell function and stimulates revascularization in response to ischemic insult through its ability to activate Akt-eNOS signaling in muscle (Ouchi et al. 2008). Interleukin-8 is a CXC family chemokine increased in human muscle in response to concentric exercise (Akerstrom et al. 2005), which has also been shown to have angiogenic actions associated with activation of CXCR2 receptors in the human microvascular endothelial cells (Bek et al. 2002; Frydelund-Larsen et al. 2007). Recent report by Drevon's laboratory describes interleukin-7 as a novel myokine affecting myogenesis *in vitro* in human primary muscle cells. Interleukin-7 is up-regulated by exercise training in male individuals undergoing a strength training program (Haugen et al. 2010).

4.2 Mitochondrial biogenesis in skeletal muscle – Energetic remodeling of muscle phenotype in obesity, insulin resistance and exercise

Mitochondria are energy power plants of the cells, believed to have evolved over billions of years from invading prokaryotic oxygen utilizing "quite energizing" eubacterium to early eucaryotic cells, giving the life on earth new energy spark (Lanza & Nair 2010). Their structure and function is orchestrated by a strict coordination of nuclear and mitochondrial genome. Of ~1.000 mitochondrial proteins, only 13 are encoded by the mitochondrial genome, remaining proteins are translated from nuclear genome and transported across the inner mitochondrial membrane (Lanza & Nair 2010). Mitochondria cover majority of energetic needs of cells by coupling substrate oxidation with ATP formation, the process known as oxidative phosphorylation. This process also generates reactive oxygen species (ROS). It has been estimated that 0.2 - 2% of oxygen taken up by the cell is converted into ROS (Harper et al. 2004). Mechanisms for detoxifying the ROS are quite well developed in a eukaryotic cell which is another reason for their long lasting partnership with "dangerous" mitochondria. Sustained excessive production may accumulate amount of ROS exceeding the antioxidant capacity of the specific cell, eventually leading to cell damage and death (Harman 1956). During recent years, mitochondria , though not only those found in skeletal muscle, were put on the spot as organelles involved in aging and associated chronic civilization diseases such as Alzheimer's disease (Reddy 2009), some forms of cancer, obesity and type 2 diabetes (Johannsen & Ravussin 2009).

4.2.1 Mitochondria in obesity, insulin resistance and type 2 diabetes

Recent evidence indicates that insulin resistance in skeletal muscle might develop due to the reduced capacity of mitochondria to oxidize lipids (Bjorntorp et al. 1967; Kelley et al. 2002; Petersen et al. 2004; Ukropcova et al. 2007) and reduced capacity for insulin-stimulated ATP-synthesis (Petersen et al. 2005). Obese individuals and subjects with type 2 diabetes are characterized also by reduced adiponectin signaling (Kern et al. 2003; Civitarese et al. 2004; Rasmussen et al. 2006), lower rates of fasting lipid utilization and impaired switch to carbohydrate oxidation in response to insulin (Kelley et al. 1999; Kelley & Mandarino 2000; Ukropcova et al. 2005; Ukropcova et al. 2007). Recent studies using microarray expression analysis reported a decrease in the expression of genes involved in mitochondrial biogenesis in skeletal muscle of individuals with insulin resistance (Patti et al. 2003) and T2D (Mootha et al. 2003). Further studies in insulin resistant subjects and individuals with type 2 diabetes have shown reduced mitochondrial content, lower electron transport chain activity in total mitochondria and in intramyofibrilar and subsarcolemal mitochondrial fractions (Kelley et al. 2002; Ritov et al. 2005). Taken together, these data support the hypothesis that insulin resistance in human skeletal muscle arises from lowering mitochondrial number and functional capacity. Another hypothesis challenges this paradigm; it is supported by observations that increased fatty acid availability is associated with increased mitochondrial fat oxidation. However, mitochondrial overload with energy rich substrates highlights the pathophysiological role of ROS and that of products of incomplete mitochondrial oxidation rather than simple lowering of mitochondrial functional capacity (Koves et al. 2008; Holloszy 2009). The importance of mitochondria for energy homeostasis makes this organelle an exciting target for investigation and better understanding to regulation of mitochondrial biogenesis and function would help us to understand its putative role in the pathogenesis of obesity and insulin resistance.

4.2.2 Exercise and ageing keep constant battle for healthy mitochondria

Exercise is one of the two physiological stimuli known to increase production of new mitochondria and to improve mitochondrial efficiency. In our work, we have shown that caloric restriction, the only officially acknowledged physiological stimulus demonstrated to prolong lifespan, is also inducing mitochondrial biogenesis in human skeletal muscle (Civitarese et al. 2007). Many scientists are on a quest, pursuing the vision of exercise mimicking pill, capable of induction of mitochondrial biogenesis *in vivo*. „Exercise in a pill" (another option would be a pill mimicking caloric restriction) is by many considered a putatively great tool to combat obesity and civilization diseases. However, healthy lifestyle intervention, with sufficient physical activity and matching caloric intake still proves to be the most natural and effective way how to stay fit, healthy and with increased chances to live up to be a hundred.

4.2.3 Adipose tissue and skeletal muscle interplay

Our organism can be viewed as a very complex society of tissues that need to communicate with one another in order to maintain metabolic health. Tissue cross-talk plays the central role in the regulation of food intake, energy expenditure, oxidative capacity, adaptation to changes in physical activity, nutritional status etc. As mentioned above, adipose tissue (as well as many other tissues in our body) is (are) a (the) source of many biologically active substances with autocrine, paracrine and endocrine activities, exerting effects over many different neighboring as well as distant tissues and organs.

Adiponectin is the most studied adipocytokine which is in relatively high quantities secreted from adipose tissue into the bloodstream. Adiponectin has very positive effects on our metabolic health as it activates glucose and fatty acid metabolism and improves insulin sensitivity. Adiponectin levels are inversely correlated with body fat mass and positively with insulin sensitivity (Hara et al. 2005) and it also displays anti-atherogenic and anti-inflammatory effects (Antoniades et al. 2009). This hormone was first characterized in mice as a transcript overexpressed in preadipocytes (precursors of fat cells) differentiating into adipocytes. The human homologue was identified as the most abundant transcript in adipose tissue. Contrary to expectations and despite being produced in adipose tissue, adiponectin was found to be decreased in obesity. The gene was localized to chromosome 3p27, a region highlighted as affecting genetic susceptibility to T2D and obesity. Supplementation by differing forms of adiponectin was able to improve insulin control, blood glucose and triglyceride levels in mouse models. The question remains what are the mechanisms underlying positive effects of adiponectin on metabolism?

The molecular mechanisms leading to mitochondrial dysfunction in obesity and T2D remain largely unknown. Bergeron et al (Bergeron et al. 2001) demonstrated that activation of cAMP-activated protein kinase (AMPK) increases both mitochondrial biogenesis and oxidative capacity in skeletal muscle of rodents. In animal models of T2D, the activation of AMPK by adiponectin increases muscle and hepatic fat oxidation and improves insulin sensitivity (Yamauchi et al. 2001). Studies in obese and diabetic rhesus monkey demonstrate that plasma adiponectin level declines in the early phases of obesity and in parallel to the progressive development of insulin resistance (Hotta et al. 2001). Furthermore, circulating plasma adiponectin levels and the expression of both adiponectin receptors are reduced in subjects with a family history of diabetes (Civitarese et al. 2004), while prospective studies in Pima Indians show that high concentrations of adiponectin is protective against the development of T2D (Lindsay et al. 2002). Collectively, these data define a pathway in skeletal muscle by which adiponectin contributes to energy homeostasis by modulating mitochondrial number and function (Civitarese et al. 2006). Early defects in the secretion of adiponectin or in adiponectin signaling might contribute to the lower mitochondrial content and/or function in the prediabetic state. Interestingly and in accordance with our results, it has been recently demonstrated that an adiponectin-like molecule, a recombinant globular domain of adiponectin (rgAd110-244), has a significant therapeutic potential to treat insulin resistance in mice fed a high fat diet for 3 months (Sulpice et al. 2009). This makes adiponectin derivatives a promising new treatment for T2D.

It appears that adiponectin is also produced by skeletal muscle and that globular adiponectin is capable of inducing the differentiation and fusion of muscle cells in vitro (Fiaschi et al. 2009). Mimicking of pro-inflammatory settings or exposure to oxidative stress strongly increases the production of adiponectin from differentiating primary muscle cells. These data suggest a novel function of adiponectin, coordinating the myogenic differentiation program.

4.2.4 Mitochondrial biogenesis in muscle cells – Lipids and exercise

Fatty acids are known to be the ligands of various transcription factors involved in the regulation of metabolism and mitochondrial biogenesis (Gilde & Van Bilsen 2003). It has been shown previously that fatty acids as well as a diet with an increased fat content is capable of inducing mitochondrial biogenesis both in vitro and in vivo (Watt et al. 2006; Hancock et al. 2008). In our work, we have tested the effect of chronic, 4-day long exposure to palmitate on metabolic phenotypes of human primary skeletal muscle cells. We observed an increase in number of active mitochondria as measured by incorporation of mitotracker (fluorescencent dye selectively activated within respiring mitochondria) as well as increased expression of genes involved in mitochondrial biogenesis, increase in the capacity for fatty acid oxidation (Ukropcova et al. 2005, Ukropcova et al, unpublished observation). At this moment we can only speculate on the mechanisms behind this oxidation boosting effect of palmitate. However, it has been shown that fatty acids are capable of activating AMP activated protein kinase (AMPK) in skeletal muscle (Watt et al. 2006). AMPK signaling is activated in energy deficit states and it primarily saves the cell by inducing *de novo* mitochondrial biogenesis. It cooperates with transcription factor PGC1α, overexpression of which has been demonstrated to enhance both lipid oxidation and synthesis (Espinoza et al. 2010). Another possibility is that palmitate is a ligand for the transcription factors involved in the regulation of cell´s oxidative capacity, such as PPARδ (Gilde & Van Bilsen 2003). Animal (Hancock et al. 2008) as well as clinical studies (Bajaj et al. 2007) also support the role of fatty acids for PGC1α regulation at the level of gene expression. We and others have indicated that saturated fatty acids (e.g. palmitate) contribute to the regulation of metabolism by self-promoting their utilization *via* increased oxidative capacity of the skeletal muscle cell.

In addition, dynamic interrelations of skeletal muscle and adipose tissue during exercise are necessary to support muscle performance and adipose tissue energy fluxes management. The transcriptional coactivator PGC1α has also been shown to regulate several exercise-associated aspects of muscle function. It could be hypothesized that this protein controls muscle plasticity, suppresses a broad inflammatory response and mediates the beneficial effects of exercise on metabolic health (Handschin and Spiegelman 2008).

4.2.5 Caloric restriction induces mitochondrial biogenesis in skeletal muscle

Caloric restriction is a non-genetic manipulation that results in the lifespan extension of many different species, from yeasts to dogs, and even primates, and it is accompanied by delayed onset of chronic civilization diseases (Ball et al. 1947; Anderson et al. 2009). There are also hints that people who eat a calorie-restricted diet might live longer than those who overeat. People living in Okinawa, Japan, have a lower energy intake than the rest of the Japanese population and an extremely long life span (Willcox et al. 2007). In addition, calorie-restricted diets beneficially affect several biomarkers of aging, including decreased insulin sensitivity. Based on combined favorable changes in lipid and blood pressure, caloric restriction with or without exercise induces weight loss and favorably reduces risk for cardiovascular disease even in healthy non-obese individuals (Lefevre et al. 2009) and ameliorates the age-related loss of muscle mass, sarcopenia, in a variety a species (Marzetti et al. 2009). But how might caloric restriction slow aging? Some of the theories behind the lifespan extending effect of caloric restriction include (i) decreased oxidative damage, (ii) altered glucose utilization, (iii) increased insulin sensitivity, (iv) neuroendocrine changes and (v) enhanced stress responsiveness (Allard et al. 2009). Reduction of oxidative damage to proteins, lipids, and DNA is one of the leading theories, although the underlying mechanisms of this process are unclear. Cellular nutrient sensing systems seem to mediate many of the metabolic responses to caloric restriction, including the regulation of free radical production and oxidative stress. Mitochondria are the major consumers of cellular oxygen (~85%) and the predominant production site of free radicals, a by-product of oxidative phosphorylation. Studies in mammals have shown that caloric restriction reduces the generation of free radicals by mitochondria, in parallel to reductions in mitochondrial proton leak and whole-body energy expenditure. Paradoxically, caloric restriction induces mitochondrial proliferation in rodents (Lanza & Nair 2010), and either lowers (Handschin & Spiegelman 2008) or does not affect mitochondrial oxygen consumption (Lanza & Nair 2010). Low mitochondrial content seems to contribute to increased ROS production. When mitochondrial mass is reduced, mitochondria have increased "workload," leading to higher membrane potential and increased ROS production (Handschin & Spiegelman 2008; Lanza & Nair 2009; Lanza & Nair 2010). It has also been demonstrated that caloric restriction is strongly associated with an increased level and activation of sirtuins, namely the Sir2 histone deacetylase and its mammalian ortholog Sirt1. Sirtuins are members of the silent information regulator 2 (Sir2) family, a family of Class III histone/protein deacetylases. The enzymatic activity of most sirtuins has been shown to be dependent on nicotinamide dinucleotide, suggesting that the activity of these enzymes is dependent on the nutritive state of the organism (Allard et al. 2009). Specific Sirt1 activation mimics low energy levels and protects against diet-induced metabolic disorders by enhancing fat oxidation (Feige et al. 2008). PGC1α is a transcriptional coactivator playing a pivotal role in the regulation of mitochondrial biogenesis, which is known to be induced in response to exercise and caloric restriction (Fig. 8.). Research strongly supports the health benefits of exercise in humans of all ages. Increased exercise in the absence of other behavioral changes prevents the onset of many chronic diseases (Elbekai & El-Kadi 2005).

In our study we showed that short-term caloric deficit (caloric restriction with or without exercise) coordinately up-regulated the expression of genes involved in mitochondrial biogenesis in skeletal muscle resulting in increased mitochondrial content, improved whole body energy efficiency, and decreased DNA fragmentation in non-obese humans (Civitarese et al. 2007). Our results suggest that caloric restriction induces biogenesis of "efficient" mitochondria as an adaptive mechanism, which in turn lowers oxidative stress.

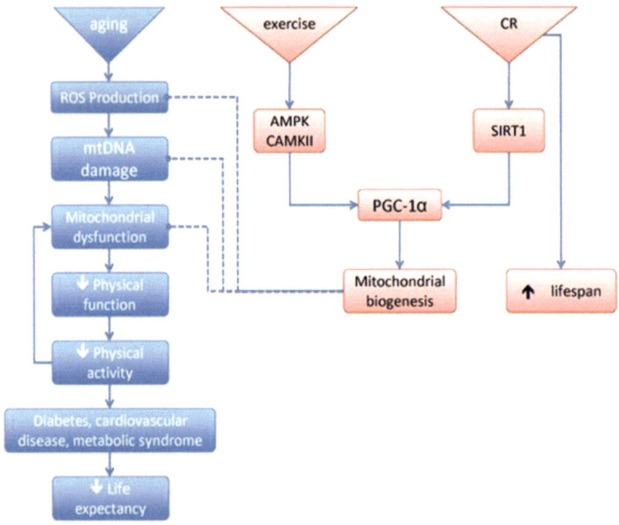

Fig. 9. The free radical theory of aging posits that a senescent phenotype is induced by accumulation of oxidative damage resulting from reactive oxygen species. Exercise and caloric restriction (CR) are two interventions that induce mitochondrial biogenesis through PGC-1α. Although exercise and CR increase average life expectancy by protecting against age-related comorbidities, only CR has been shown to increase maximal life span; an effect that seems to require the activation of sirtuins (Lanza & Nair 2010).

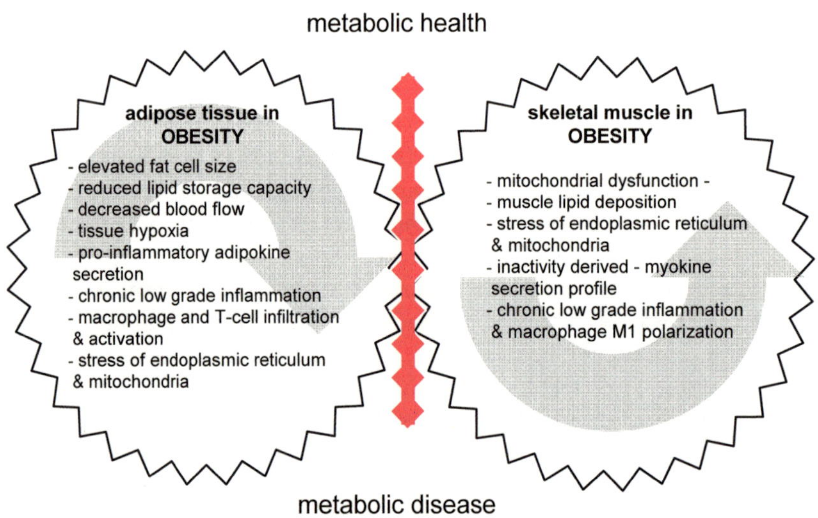

Fig. 10. Determinants of metabolic health and disease (Ukropec et al. 2008)

5. Conclusion

Ability of tissues to adapt morphologically and functionally to different physiological situations determines the overall metabolic health. Increased adipose tissue mass but mainly adipocyte lipid overload is responsible for the "pathogenic" adipose tissue phenotype. This phenotype, characteristic by extra-large unilocular adipocytes, further promotes tissue hypoxia and development of chronic persistent inflammation and metabolic stress. Pathogenic modification of the adipocyte modulates its metabolic, secretory and immunologic function leading to the development of metabolic disease (Fig. 10.). Inactive skeletal muscle, overloaded with fat could also contribute to metabolic imbalance by switching the fiber type towards less oxidative (less insulin sensitive) fibers, by lack of anti-inflammatory and insulin-sensitizing myokine production as well as by chronic inflammation associated with mitochondrial stress and stress of endoplasmic reticulum (Fig. 10.). Our environment greatly modifies our metabolic health by means of dietary influences and exercise activity which together with pathologies associated with hyperlipidemia, chronic systemic hypoxia and tissue inflammation determines adipose tissue and skeletal muscle metabolic and secretory phenotype and subsequently our metabolic health.

It is generally accepted that regular physical activity prevents metabolic and cardiovascular disease development, and supports healthy aging. Skeletal muscle has been shown to produce and secrete several bioactive factors (hormones) termed "myokines". Different spectra of myokines originating from either active "trained" or inactive "sedentary" skeletal muscles elicit distinct adaptive changes in immune system, metabolic balance and processes of cellular growth and differentiation in order to maintain the whole body homeostasis. This requires extensive communication of skeletal muscle with many different cells and organs but the nature of mechanisms that tie muscle activity to metabolic health is not completely understood. It seems to be essential (i) to identify myokines differentially expressed and secreted from muscle cells derived from healthy and obese individuals, and individuals with type 2 diabetes; to (ii) determine basic principles of the muscle cross-communication with adipocytes (differentiation) and endothelial cells (angiogenesis) in fostering tissue plasticity necessary for adaptation to obesity and type 2 diabetes; and (iii) to discover novel myokines and to investigate their physiological significance in cell culture models and *in vivo* in genetically modified animal models as well as in humans. Myokines may be involved in mediating the health beneficial effects of exercise and play important roles in the protection against chronic diseases associated with low-grade inflammation, insulin resistance, hyperlipidemia, such as cardiovascular disease, type-2-diabetes, and cancer. Extension of the knowledge on the mechanisms whereby regular exercise offers protection against chronic diseases in combination with clinical research serves as a foundation for the development of public health guidelines with regard to exercise. Moreover, identification of new myokines and understanding basic principles and mechanisms of their action will potentially provide pharmacological targets for the treatment of metabolic and cardiovascular disorders.

6. Acknowledgement

We would like to express our cordial gratitude to everybody who contributed to this work. There is too many people to thank. Above all we would like to acknowledge our parents and our wonderfull children Kiki and Jakub, our inspiration in everyday life. We would also like to thank the funding agencies: APVV grant agency (APVV 0122-06), European Foundation to Study Diabetes (EFSD New Horizons Collaborative Research Grant) and the 7th FP EC 2007-2.1.1-6. grant entitled „LipidomicNET" for their generous support.

7. References

Ahima, R.S. & Lazar, M.A. (2008). Adipokines and the peripheral and neural control of energy balance, *Mol Endocrinol,* vol.22, No.5, pp. 1023-1031, issn 0888-8809 (Print)

Akerstrom, T.; Steensberg, A.; Keller, P.; Keller, C.; Penkowa, M. & Pedersen, B.K. (2005). Exercise induces interleukin-8 expression in human skeletal muscle, *J Physiol,* vol.563, No.Pt 2, pp. 507-516, issn 0022-3751 (Print)

Allard, J.S.; Perez, E.; Zou, S. & De Cabo, R. (2009). Dietary activators of sirt1, *Mol Cell Endocrinol,* vol.299, No.1, pp. 58-63, issn 0303-7207 (Print)

Anderson, R.M.; Shanmuganayagam, D. & Weindruch, R. (2009). Caloric restriction and aging: Studies in mice and monkeys, *Toxicol Pathol,* vol.37, No.1, pp. 47-51, issn 1533-1601 (Electronic)

Antoniades, C.; Antonopoulos, A.S.; Tousoulis, D. & Stefanadis, C. (2009). Adiponectin: From obesity to cardiovascular disease, *Obes Rev,* vol.10, No.3, pp. 269-279, issn 1467-789X (Electronic)

Arner, E.; Westermark, P.O.; Spalding, K.L.; Britton, T.; Ryden, M.; Frisen, J.; Bernard, S. & Arner, P. (2010). Adipocyte turnover: Relevance to human adipose tissue morphology, *Diabetes,* vol.59, No.1, pp. 105-109, issn 1939-327X (Electronic)

Arner, P. (1998). Not all fat is alike, *Lancet,* vol.351, No.9112, pp. 1301-1302, issn 0140-6736 (Print)

Arner, P.; Arner, E.; Hammarstedt, A. & Smith, U. (2011). Genetic predisposition for type 2 diabetes, but not for overweight/obesity, is associated with a restricted adipogenesis, *PLoS One,* vol.6, No.4, p. e18284, issn 1932-6203 (Electronic)

Bajaj, M.; Medina-Navarro, R.; Suraamornkul, S.; Meyer, C.; Defronzo, R.A. & Mandarino, L.J. (2007). Paradoxical changes in muscle gene expression in insulin-resistant subjects after sustained reduction in plasma free fatty acid concentration, *Diabetes,* vol.56, No.3, pp. 743-752, issn 0012-1797 (Print)

Ball, Z.B.; Barnes, R.H. & Visscher, M.B. (1947). The effects of dietary caloric restriction on maturity and senescence, with particular reference to fertility and longevity, *Am J Physiol,* vol.150, No.3, pp. 511-519, issn 0002-9513 (Print)

Bays, H.E.; Gonzalez-Campoy, J.M.; Bray, G.A.; Kitabchi, A.E.; Bergman, D.A.; Schorr, A.B.; Rodbard, H.W. & Henry, R.R. (2008). Pathogenic potential of adipose tissue and metabolic consequences of adipocyte hypertrophy and increased visceral adiposity, *Expert Rev Cardiovasc Ther,* vol.6, No.3, pp. 343-368, issn 1744-8344 (Electronic)

Bek, E.L.; Mcmillen, M.A.; Scott, P.; Angus, L.D. & Shaftan, G.W. (2002). The effect of diabetes on endothelin, interleukin-8 and vascular endothelial growth factor-mediated angiogenesis in rats, *Clin Sci (Lond),* vol.103 Suppl 48, pp. 424S-429S, issn 0143-5221 (Print)

Bergeron, R.; Ren, J.M.; Cadman, K.S.; Moore, I.K.; Perret, P.; Pypaert, M.; Young, L.H.; Semenkovich, C.F. & Shulman, G.I. (2001). Chronic activation of amp kinase results in nrf-1 activation and mitochondrial biogenesis, *Am J Physiol Endocrinol Metab,* vol.281, No.6, pp. E1340-1346, issn 0193-1849 (Print)

Bergman, R.N.; Kim, S.P.; Catalano, K.J.; Hsu, I.R.; Chiu, J.D.; Kabir, M.; Hucking, K. & Ader, M. (2006). Why visceral fat is bad: Mechanisms of the metabolic syndrome, *Obesity (Silver Spring),* vol.14 Suppl 1, pp. 16S-19S, issn 1930-7381 (Print)

Bjorntorp, P.; Schersten, T. & Fagerberg, S.E. (1967). Respiration and phosphorylation of mitochondria isolated from the skeletal muscle of diabetic and normal subjects, *Diabetologia,* vol.3, No.3, pp. 346-352, issn 0012-186X (Print)

Bjorntorp, P. (1974). Size, number and function of adipose tissue cells in human obesity, *Horm Metab Res,* vol.Suppl 4, pp. 77-83, issn 0018-5043 (Print)

Bluher, M. & Zimmer, P. (2010). [metabolic and cardiovascular effects of physical activity, exercise and fitness in patients with type 2 diabetes], *Dtsch Med Wochenschr,* vol.135, No.18, pp. 930-934, issn 1439-4413 (Electronic)

Boecker, H.; Sprenger, T.; Spilker, M.E.; Henriksen, G.; Koppenhoefer, M.; Wagner, K.J.; Valet, M.; Berthele, A. & Tolle, T.R. (2008). The runner's high: Opioidergic mechanisms in the human brain, *Cereb Cortex,* vol.18, No.11, pp. 2523-2531, issn 1460-2199 (Electronic)

Bostrom, M.A.; Boyanovsky, B.B.; Jordan, C.T.; Wadsworth, M.P.; Taatjes, D.J.; De Beer, F.C. & Webb, N.R. (2007). Group v secretory phospholipase a2 promotes atherosclerosis: Evidence from genetically altered mice, *Arterioscler Thromb Vasc Biol,* vol.27, No.3, pp. 600-606, issn 1524-4636 (Electronic)

Cannon, B. & Nedergaard, J. (2004). Brown adipose tissue: Function and physiological significance, *Physiol Rev,* vol.84, No.1, pp. 277-359, issn 0031-9333 (Print)

Carriere, A.; Carmona, M.C.; Fernandez, Y.; Rigoulet, M.; Wenger, R.H.; Penicaud, L. & Casteilla, L. (2004). Mitochondrial reactive oxygen species control the transcription factor chop-10/gadd153 and adipocyte differentiation: A mechanism for hypoxia-dependent effect, *J Biol Chem,* vol.279, No.39, pp. 40462-40469, issn 0021-9258 (Print)

Civitarese, A.E.; Jenkinson, C.P.; Richardson, D.; Bajaj, M.; Cusi, K.; Kashyap, S.; Berria, R.; Belfort, R.; Defronzo, R.A.; Mandarino, L.J. & Ravussin, E. (2004). Adiponectin receptors gene expression and insulin sensitivity in non-diabetic mexican americans with or without a family history of type 2 diabetes, *Diabetologia,* vol.47, No.5, pp. 816-820, issn 0012-186X (Print)

Civitarese, A.E.; Ukropcova, B.; Carling, S.; Hulver, M.; Defronzo, R.A.; Mandarino, L.; Ravussin, E. & Smith, S.R. (2006). Role of adiponectin in human skeletal muscle bioenergetics, *Cell Metab,* vol.4, No.1, pp. 75-87, issn 1550-4131 (Print)

Civitarese, A.E.; Carling, S.; Heilbronn, L.K.; Hulver, M.H.; Ukropcova, B.; Deutsch, W.A.; Smith, S.R. & Ravussin, E. (2007). Calorie restriction increases muscle mitochondrial biogenesis in healthy humans, *PLoS Med,* vol.4, No.3, p. e76, issn 1549-1676

Cramer, T. & Johnson, R.S. (2003). A novel role for the hypoxia inducible transcription factor hif-1alpha: Critical regulation of inflammatory cell function, *Cell Cycle,* vol.2, No.3, pp. 192-193, issn 1538-4101 (Print)

Cramer, T.; Yamanishi, Y.; Clausen, B.E.; Forster, I.; Pawlinski, R.; Mackman, N.; Haase, V.H.; Jaenisch, R.; Corr, M.; Nizet, V.; Firestein, G.S.; Gerber, H.P.; Ferrara, N. & Johnson, R.S. (2003). Hif-1alpha is essential for myeloid cell-mediated inflammation, *Cell,* vol.112, No.5, pp. 645-657, issn 0092-8674 (Print)

Crampes, F.; Beauville, M.; Riviere, D. & Garrigues, M. (1986). Effect of physical training in humans on the response of isolated fat cells to epinephrine, *J Appl Physiol,* vol.61, No.1, pp. 25-29, issn 8750-7587 (Print)

Cypess, A.M.; Lehman, S.; Williams, G.; Tal, I.; Rodman, D.; Goldfine, A.B.; Kuo, F.C.; Palmer, E.L.; Tseng, Y.H.; Doria, A.; Kolodny, G.M. & Kahn, C.R. (2009). Identification and importance of brown adipose tissue in adult humans, *N Engl J Med,* vol.360, No.15, pp. 1509-1517, issn 1533-4406 (Electronic)

De Pauw, A.; Tejerina, S.; Raes, M.; Keijer, J. & Arnould, T. (2009). Mitochondrial (dys)function in adipocyte (de)differentiation and systemic metabolic alterations, *Am J Pathol,* vol.175, No.3, pp. 927-939, issn 1525-2191 (Electronic)

Divoux, A. & Clement, K. (2011). Architecture and the extracellular matrix: The still unappreciated components of the adipose tissue, *Obes Rev,* vol.12, No.5, pp. e494-503, issn 1467-789X (Electronic)

Elbekai, R.H. & El-Kadi, A.O. (2005). The role of oxidative stress in the modulation of aryl hydrocarbon receptor-regulated genes by as3+, cd2+, and cr6+, *Free Radic Biol Med,* vol.39, No.11, pp. 1499-1511, issn 0891-5849 (Print)

Erbay, E.; Cao, H. & Hotamisligil, G.S. (2007). Adipocyte/macrophage fatty acid binding proteins in metabolic syndrome, *Curr Atheroscler Rep,* vol.9, No.3, pp. 222-229, issn 1523-3804 (Print)

Espinoza, D.O.; Boros, L.G.; Crunkhorn, S.; Gami, H. & Patti, M.E. (2010). Dual modulation of both lipid oxidation and synthesis by peroxisome proliferator-activated receptor-gamma coactivator-1alpha and -1beta in cultured myotubes, *FASEB J,* vol.24, No.4, pp. 1003-1014, issn 1530-6860 (Electronic)

Febbraio, M.A.; Hiscock, N.; Sacchetti, M.; Fischer, C.P. & Pedersen, B.K. (2004). Interleukin-6 is a novel factor mediating glucose homeostasis during skeletal muscle contraction, *Diabetes,* vol.53, No.7, pp. 1643-1648, issn 0012-1797 (Print)

Feige, J.N.; Lagouge, M.; Canto, C.; Strehle, A.; Houten, S.M.; Milne, J.C.; Lambert, P.D.; Mataki, C.; Elliott, P.J. & Auwerx, J. (2008). Specific sirt1 activation mimics low energy levels and protects against diet-induced metabolic disorders by enhancing fat oxidation, *Cell Metab,* vol.8, No.5, pp. 347-358, issn 1932-7420 (Electronic)

Ferreri, C. & Chatgilialoglu, C. (2009). Membrane lipidomics and the geometry of unsaturated fatty acids from biomimetic models to biological consequences, *Methods Mol Biol,* vol.579, pp. 391-411, issn 1940-6029 (Electronic)

Fiaschi, T.; Cirelli, D.; Comito, G.; Gelmini, S.; Ramponi, G.; Serio, M. & Chiarugi, P. (2009). Globular adiponectin induces differentiation and fusion of skeletal muscle cells, *Cell Res,* vol.19, No.5, pp. 584-597, issn 1748-7838 (Electronic)

Foster, D.J.; Ravikumar, P.; Bellotto, D.J.; Unger, R.H. & Hsia, C.C. (2010). Fatty diabetic lung: Altered alveolar structure and surfactant protein expression, *Am J Physiol Lung Cell Mol Physiol,* vol.298, No.3, pp. L392-403, issn 1522-1504 (Electronic)

Friedman, J.M. (2011). Leptin and the regulation of body weigh, *Keio J Med,* vol.60, No.1, pp. 1-9, issn 1880-1293 (Electronic)

Frydelund-Larsen, L.; Penkowa, M.; Akerstrom, T.; Zankari, A.; Nielsen, S. & Pedersen, B.K. (2007). Exercise induces interleukin-8 receptor (cxcr2) expression in human skeletal muscle, *Exp Physiol,* vol.92, No.1, pp. 233-240, issn 0958-0670 (Print)

Gilde, A.J. & Van Bilsen, M. (2003). Peroxisome proliferator-activated receptors (ppars): Regulators of gene expression in heart and skeletal muscle, *Acta Physiol Scand,* vol.178, No.4, pp. 425-434, issn 0001-6772 (Print)

Goossens, G.H. (2008). The role of adipose tissue dysfunction in the pathogenesis of obesity-related insulin resistance, *Physiol Behav,* vol.94, No.2, pp. 206-218, issn 0031-9384

Gordon, S. & Taylor, P.R. (2005). Monocyte and macrophage heterogeneity, *Nat Rev Immunol,* vol.5, No.12, pp. 953-964, issn 1474-1733 (Print)

Gordon, S. (2007). The macrophage: Past, present and future, *Eur J Immunol,* vol.37 Suppl 1, pp. S9-17, issn 0014-2980 (Print)

Granneman, J.G.; Li, P.; Zhu, Z. & Lu, Y. (2005). Metabolic and cellular plasticity in white adipose tissue i: Effects of beta3-adrenergic receptor activation, *Am J Physiol Endocrinol Metab,* vol.289, No.4, pp. E608-616, issn 0193-1849 (Print)

Halperin, M.L.; Connors, H.P.; Relman, A.S. & Karnovsky, M.L. (1969). Factors that control the effect of ph on glycolysis in leukocytes, *J Biol Chem,* vol.244, No.2, pp. 384-390, issn 0021-9258 (Print)

Hamdy, O.; Porramatikul, S. & Al-Ozairi, E. (2006). Metabolic obesity: The paradox between visceral and subcutaneous fat, *Curr Diabetes Rev,* vol.2, No.4, pp. 367-373, issn 1573-3998 (Print)

Hamilton, M.T.; Hamilton, D.G. & Zderic, T.W. (2007). Role of low energy expenditure and sitting in obesity, metabolic syndrome, type 2 diabetes, and cardiovascular disease, *Diabetes,* vol.56, No.11, pp. 2655-2667, issn 1939-327X (Electronic)

Hancock, C.R.; Han, D.H.; Chen, M.; Terada, S.; Yasuda, T.; Wright, D.C. & Holloszy, J.O. (2008). High-fat diets cause insulin resistance despite an increase in muscle mitochondria, *Proc Natl Acad Sci U S A,* vol.105, No.22, pp. 7815-7820, issn 1091-6490 (Electronic)

Handschin, C. & Spiegelman, B.M. (2008). The role of exercise and pgc1alpha in inflammation and chronic disease, *Nature,* vol.454, No.7203, pp. 463-469, issn 1476-4687 (Electronic)

Hara, K.; Yamauchi, T. & Kadowaki, T. (2005). Adiponectin: An adipokine linking adipocytes and type 2 diabetes in humans, *Curr Diab Rep,* vol.5, No.2, pp. 136-140, issn 1534-4827 (Print)

Harman, D. (1956). Aging: A theory based on free radical and radiation chemistry, *J Gerontol,* vol.11, No.3, pp. 298-300, issn 0022-1422 (Print)

Harper, M.E.; Bevilacqua, L.; Hagopian, K.; Weindruch, R. & Ramsey, J.J. (2004). Ageing, oxidative stress, and mitochondrial uncoupling, *Acta Physiol Scand,* vol.182, No.4, pp. 321-331, issn 0001-6772 (Print)

Haugen, F.; Norheim, F.; Lian, H.; Wensaas, A.J.; Dueland, S.; Berg, O.; Funderud, A.; Skalhegg, B.S.; Raastad, T. & Drevon, C.A. (2010). Il-7 is expressed and secreted by human skeletal muscle cells, *Am J Physiol Cell Physiol,* vol.298, No.4, pp. C807-816, issn 1522-1563 (Electronic)

Henry, B.A. & Clarke, I.J. (2008). Adipose tissue hormones and the regulation of food intake, *J Neuroendocrinol,* vol.20, No.6, pp. 842-849, issn 1365-2826 (Electronic)

Himms-Hagen, J. (2004). Exercise in a pill: Feasibility of energy expenditure targets, *Curr Drug Targets CNS Neurol Disord,* vol.3, No.5, pp. 389-409, issn 1568-007X (Print)

Hojman, P.; Pedersen, M.; Nielsen, A.R.; Krogh-Madsen, R.; Yfanti, C.; Akerstrom, T.; Nielsen, S. & Pedersen, B.K. (2009). Fibroblast growth factor-21 is induced in human skeletal muscles by hyperinsulinemia, *Diabetes,* vol.58, No.12, pp. 2797-2801, issn 1939-327X (Electronic)

Holloszy, J.O. & Booth, F.W. (1976). Biochemical adaptations to endurance exercise in muscle, *Annu Rev Physiol,* vol.38, pp. 273-291, issn 0066-4278 (Print)

Holloszy, J.O. (2009). Skeletal muscle "Mitochondrial deficiency" Does not mediate insulin resistance, *Am J Clin Nutr,* vol.89, No.1, pp. 463S-466S, issn 1938-3207 (Electronic)

Hong, S.; Lee, H.J.; Kim, S.J. & Hahm, K.B. (2010). Connection between inflammation and carcinogenesis in gastrointestinal tract: Focus on tgf-beta signaling, *World J Gastroenterol,* vol.16, No.17, pp. 2080-2093, issn 1007-9327 (Print)

Hosogai, N.; Fukuhara, A.; Oshima, K.; Miyata, Y.; Tanaka, S.; Segawa, K.; Furukawa, S.; Tochino, Y.; Komuro, R.; Matsuda, M. & Shimomura, I. (2007). Adipose tissue hypoxia in obesity and its impact on adipocytokine dysregulation, *Diabetes,* vol.56, No.4, pp. 901-911, issn 0012-1797 (Print)

Hotta, K.; Funahashi, T.; Bodkin, N.L.; Ortmeyer, H.K.; Arita, Y.; Hansen, B.C. & Matsuzawa, Y. (2001). Circulating concentrations of the adipocyte protein adiponectin are decreased in parallel with reduced insulin sensitivity during the progression to type 2 diabetes in rhesus monkeys, *Diabetes,* vol.50, No.5, pp. 1126-1133, issn 0012-1797 (Print)

Howard, S.G. & Lee, D.H. (2011). What is the role of human contamination by environmental chemicals in the development of type 1 diabetes?, *J Epidemiol Community Health,* issn 1470-2738 (Electronic)

Chandel, N.S. & Budinger, G.R. (2007). The cellular basis for diverse responses to oxygen, *Free Radic Biol Med,* vol.42, No.2, pp. 165-174, issn 0891-5849 (Print)

Inouye, K.E.; Shi, H.; Howard, J.K.; Daly, C.H.; Lord, G.M.; Rollins, B.J. & Flier, J.S. (2007). Absence of cc chemokine ligand 2 does not limit obesity-associated infiltration of macrophages into adipose tissue, *Diabetes,* vol.56, No.9, pp. 2242-2250, issn 1939-327X (Electronic)

Itoh, M.; Suganami, T.; Hachiya, R. & Ogawa, Y. (2011). Adipose tissue remodeling as homeostatic inflammation, *Int J Inflam,* vol.2011, p. 720926, issn 2042-0099 (Electronic)

Johannsen, D.L. & Ravussin, E. (2009). The role of mitochondria in health and disease, *Curr Opin Pharmacol,* vol.9, No.6, pp. 780-786, issn 1471-4973 (Electronic)

Jonsdottir, I.H.; Schjerling, P.; Ostrowski, K.; Asp, S.; Richter, E.A. & Pedersen, B.K. (2000). Muscle contractions induce interleukin-6 mrna production in rat skeletal muscles, *J Physiol,* vol.528 Pt 1, pp. 157-163, issn 0022-3751 (Print)

Jung, H.S.; Lee, Y.J.; Kim, Y.H.; Paik, S.; Kim, J.W. & Lee, J.W. (2011). Peroxisome proliferator-activated receptor gamma/signal transducers and activators of transcription 5a pathway plays a key factor in adipogenesis of human bone marrow-derived stromal cells and 3t3-l1 preadipocytes, *Stem Cells Dev,* issn 1557-8534 (Electronic)

Kamei, N.; Tobe, K.; Suzuki, R.; Ohsugi, M.; Watanabe, T.; Kubota, N.; Ohtsuka-Kowatari, N.; Kumagai, K.; Sakamoto, K.; Kobayashi, M.; Yamauchi, T.; Ueki, K.; Oishi, Y.; Nishimura, S.; Manabe, I.; Hashimoto, H.; Ohnishi, Y.; Ogata, H.; Tokuyama, K.; Tsunoda, M.; Ide, T.; Murakami, K.; Nagai, R. & Kadowaki, T. (2006). Overexpression of monocyte chemoattractant protein-1 in adipose tissues causes macrophage recruitment and insulin resistance, *J Biol Chem,* vol.281, No.36, pp. 26602-26614, issn 0021-9258 (Print)

Kanda, H.; Tateya, S.; Tamori, Y.; Kotani, K.; Hiasa, K.; Kitazawa, R.; Kitazawa, S.; Miyachi, H.; Maeda, S.; Egashira, K. & Kasuga, M. (2006). Mcp-1 contributes to macrophage infiltration into adipose tissue, insulin resistance, and hepatic steatosis in obesity, *J Clin Invest,* vol.116, No.6, pp. 1494-1505, issn 0021-9738 (Print)

Keller, C.; Steensberg, A.; Pilegaard, H.; Osada, T.; Saltin, B.; Pedersen, B.K. & Neufer, P.D. (2001). Transcriptional activation of the il-6 gene in human contracting skeletal muscle: Influence of muscle glycogen content, *FASEB J*, vol.15, No.14, pp. 2748-2750, issn 1530-6860 (Electronic)

Kelley, D.E.; Goodpaster, B.; Wing, R.R. & Simoneau, J.A. (1999). Skeletal muscle fatty acid metabolism in association with insulin resistance, obesity, and weight loss, *Am J Physiol*, vol.277, No.6 Pt 1, pp. E1130-1141, issn 0002-9513 (Print)

Kelley, D.E. & Mandarino, L.J. (2000). Fuel selection in human skeletal muscle in insulin resistance: A reexamination, *Diabetes*, vol.49, No.5, pp. 677-683, issn 0012-1797

Kelley, D.E.; He, J.; Menshikova, E.V. & Ritov, V.B. (2002). Dysfunction of mitochondria in human skeletal muscle in type 2 diabetes, *Diabetes*, vol.51, No.10, pp. 2944-2950, issn 0012-1797 (Print)

Kern, P.A.; Di Gregorio, G.B.; Lu, T.; Rassouli, N. & Ranganathan, G. (2003). Adiponectin expression from human adipose tissue: Relation to obesity, insulin resistance, and tumor necrosis factor-alpha expression, *Diabetes*, vol.52, No.7, pp. 1779-1785, issn 0012-1797 (Print)

Khan, T.; Muise, E.S.; Iyengar, P.; Wang, Z.V.; Chandalia, M.; Abate, N.; Zhang, B.B.; Bonaldo, P.; Chua, S. & Scherer, P.E. (2009). Metabolic dysregulation and adipose tissue fibrosis: Role of collagen vi, *Mol Cell Biol*, vol.29, No.6, pp. 1575-1591, issn 1098-5549 (Electronic)

Kim, J.Y.; Van De Wall, E.; Laplante, M.; Azzara, A.; Trujillo, M.E.; Hofmann, S.M.; Schraw, T.; Durand, J.L.; Li, H.; Li, G.; Jelicks, L.A.; Mehler, M.F.; Hui, D.Y.; Deshaies, Y.; Shulman, G.I.; Schwartz, G.J. & Scherer, P.E. (2007). Obesity-associated improvements in metabolic profile through expansion of adipose tissue, *J Clin Invest*, vol.117, No.9, pp. 2621-2637, issn 0021-9738 (Print)

Kinnula, V.L.; Savolainen, M.J. & Hassinen, I. (1978). Hepatic triacylglycerol and fatty-acid biosynthesis during hypoxia in vivo, *Acta Physiol Scand*, vol.104, No.2, pp. 148-155, issn 0001-6772 (Print)

Kirwan, J.P.; Costill, D.L.; Flynn, M.G.; Neufer, P.D.; Fink, W.J. & Morse, W.M. (1990). Effects of increased training volume on the oxidative capacity, glycogen content and tension development of rat skeletal muscle, *Int J Sports Med*, vol.11, No.6, pp. 479-483, issn 0172-4622 (Print)

Koska, J.; Stefan, N.; Votruba, S.B.; Smith, S.R.; Krakoff, J. & Bunt, J.C. (2008). Distribution of subcutaneous fat predicts insulin action in obesity in sex-specific manner, *Obesity (Silver Spring)*, vol.16, No.9, pp. 2003-2009, issn 1930-7381 (Print)

Kosmidou, I.; Vassilakopoulos, T.; Xagorari, A.; Zakynthinos, S.; Papapetropoulos, A. & Roussos, C. (2002). Production of interleukin-6 by skeletal myotubes: Role of reactive oxygen species, *Am J Respir Cell Mol Biol*, vol.26, No.5, pp. 587-593, issn 1044-1549 (Print)

Koves, T.R.; Ussher, J.R.; Noland, R.C.; Slentz, D.; Mosedale, M.; Ilkayeva, O.; Bain, J.; Stevens, R.; Dyck, J.R.; Newgard, C.B.; Lopaschuk, G.D. & Muoio, D.M. (2008). Mitochondrial overload and incomplete fatty acid oxidation contribute to skeletal muscle insulin resistance, *Cell Metab*, vol.7, No.1, pp. 45-56, issn 1550-4131 (Print)

Krek, W. (2000). Vhl takes hif's breath away, *Nat Cell Biol*, vol.2, No.7, pp. E121-123, issn 1465-7392 (Print)

Krishnan, J.; Suter, M.; Windak, R.; Krebs, T.; Felley, A.; Montessuit, C.; Tokarska-Schlattner, M.; Aasum, E.; Bogdanova, A.; Perriard, E.; Perriard, J.C.; Larsen, T.; Pedrazzini, T. & Krek, W. (2009). Activation of a hif1alpha-ppargamma axis underlies the integration of glycolytic and lipid anabolic pathways in pathologic cardiac hypertrophy, *Cell Metab,* vol.9, No.6, pp. 512-524, issn 1932-7420 (Electronic)

Langer, P.; Kocan, A.; Tajtakova, M.; Petrik, J.; Chovancova, J.; Drobna, B.; Jursa, S.; Pavuk, M.; Koska, J.; Trnovec, T.; Sebokova, E. & Klimes, I. (2003). Possible effects of polychlorinated biphenyls and organochlorinated pesticides on the thyroid after long-term exposure to heavy environmental pollution, *J Occup Environ Med,* vol.45, No.5, pp. 526-532, issn 1076-2752 (Print)

Langer, P.; Kocan, A.; Tajtakova, M.; Petrik, J.; Chovancova, J.; Drobna, B.; Jursa, S.; Radikova, Z.; Koska, J.; Ksinantova, L.; Huckova, M.; Imrich, R.; Wimmerova, S.; Gasperikova, D.; Shishiba, Y.; Trnovec, T.; Sebokova, E. & Klimes, I. (2007). Fish from industrially polluted freshwater as the main source of organochlorinated pollutants and increased frequency of thyroid disorders and dysglycemia, *Chemosphere,* vol.67, No.9, pp. S379-385, issn 0045-6535 (Print)

Langer, P. (2010). The impacts of organochlorines and other persistent pollutants on thyroid and metabolic health, *Front Neuroendocrinol,* vol.31, No.4, pp. 497-518, issn 1095-6808 (Electronic)

Langer, P.; Kocan, A.; Drobna, B.; Susienkova, K.; Radikova, Z.; Huckova, M.; Imrich, R.; Ksinantova, L. & Klimes, I. (2010). Polychlorinated biphenyls and testosterone: Age and congener related correlation approach in heavily exposed males, *Endocr Regul,* vol.44, No.3, pp. 109-114, issn 1210-0668 (Print)

Langer, P.; Kocan, A.; Drobna, B.; Huckova, M.; Radikova, Z.; Susienkova, K.; Imrich, R. & Ukropec, J. (2011). Alpha-fetoprotein, carcinoembryonic antigen and beta2-microglobulin in adult population highly exposed to organochlorinated pollutants (pcb, dde and hcb), *Endocr Regul,* vol.45, No.3, pp. 149-155, issn 1210-0668 (Print)

Lanza, I.R. & Nair, K.S. (2009). Muscle mitochondrial changes with aging and exercise, *Am J Clin Nutr,* vol.89, No.1, pp. 467S-471S, issn 1938-3207 (Electronic)

Lanza, I.R. & Nair, K.S. (2010). Mitochondrial function as a determinant of life span, *Pflugers Arch,* vol.459, No.2, pp. 277-289, issn 1432-2013 (Electronic)

Lee, D.H.; Lind, L.; Jacobs, D.R., Jr.; Salihovic, S.; Van Bavel, B. & Lind, P.M. (2011). Associations of persistent organic pollutants with abdominal obesity in the elderly: The prospective investigation of the vasculature in uppsala seniors (pivus) study, *Environ Int,* issn 1873-6750 (Electronic)

Lee, D.H.; Lind, P.M.; Jacobs, D.R., Jr.; Salihovic, S.; Van Bavel, B. & Lind, L. (2011). Polychlorinated biphenyls and organochlorine pesticides in plasma predict development of type 2 diabetes in the elderly: The prospective investigation of the vasculature in uppsala seniors (pivus) study, *Diabetes Care,* vol.34, No.8, pp. 1778-1784, issn 1935-5548 (Electronic)

Lee, H.K. (2011). Mitochondrial dysfunction and insulin resistance: The contribution of dioxin-like substances, *Diabetes Metab J,* vol.35, No.3, pp. 207-215, issn 2233-6087

Lefevre, M.; Redman, L.M.; Heilbronn, L.K.; Smith, J.V.; Martin, C.K.; Rood, J.C.; Greenway, F.L.; Williamson, D.A.; Smith, S.R. & Ravussin, E. (2009). Caloric restriction alone and with exercise improves cvd risk in healthy non-obese individuals, *Atherosclerosis,* vol.203, No.1, pp. 206-213, issn 1879-1484 (Electronic)

Levine, J.A.; Mccrady, S.K.; Lanningham-Foster, L.M.; Kane, P.H.; Foster, R.C. & Manohar, C.U. (2008). The role of free-living daily walking in human weight gain and obesity, *Diabetes,* vol.57, No.3, pp. 548-554, issn 1939-327X (Electronic)

Li, P.; Zhu, Z.; Lu, Y. & Granneman, J.G. (2005). Metabolic and cellular plasticity in white adipose tissue ii: Role of peroxisome proliferator-activated receptor-alpha, *Am J Physiol Endocrinol Metab,* vol.289, No.4, pp. E617-626, issn 0193-1849 (Print)

Lindsay, R.S.; Funahashi, T.; Hanson, R.L.; Matsuzawa, Y.; Tanaka, S.; Tataranni, P.A.; Knowler, W.C. & Krakoff, J. (2002). Adiponectin and development of type 2 diabetes in the pima indian population, *Lancet,* vol.360, No.9326, pp. 57-58, issn 0140-6736 (Print)

Linton, M.F. & Fazio, S. (2003). Macrophages, inflammation, and atherosclerosis, *Int J Obes Relat Metab Disord,* vol.27 Suppl 3, pp. S35-40, issn 0307-0565 (Print)

Lumeng, C.N.; Bodzin, J.L. & Saltiel, A.R. (2007). Obesity induces a phenotypic switch in adipose tissue macrophage polarization, *J Clin Invest,* vol.117, No.1, pp. 175-184, issn 0021-9738 (Print)

Marzetti, E.; Lees, H.A.; Wohlgemuth, S.E. & Leeuwenburgh, C. (2009). Sarcopenia of aging: Underlying cellular mechanisms and protection by calorie restriction, *Biofactors,* vol.35, No.1, pp. 28-35, issn 0951-6433 (Print)

Matsuzawa, Y.; Funahashi, T. & Nakamura, T. (1999). Molecular mechanism of metabolic syndrome x: Contribution of adipocytokines adipocyte-derived bioactive substances, *Ann N Y Acad Sci,* vol.892, pp. 146-154, issn 0077-8923 (Print)

Meissburger, B.; Ukropec, J.; Roeder, E.; Beaton, N.; Geiger, M.; Teupser, D.; Civan, B.; Langhans, W.; Nawroth, P.P.; Gasperikova, D.; Rudofsky, G. & Wolfrum, C. (2011). Adipogenesis and insulin sensitivity in obesity are regulated by retinoid-related orphan receptor gamma, *EMBO Mol Med,* issn 1757-4684 (Electronic)

Mootha, V.K.; Lindgren, C.M.; Eriksson, K.F.; Subramanian, A.; Sihag, S.; Lehar, J.; Puigserver, P.; Carlsson, E.; Ridderstrale, M.; Laurila, E.; Houstis, N.; Daly, M.J.; Patterson, N.; Mesirov, J.P.; Golub, T.R.; Tamayo, P.; Spiegelman, B.; Lander, E.S.; Hirschhorn, J.N.; Altshuler, D. & Groop, L.C. (2003). Pgc-1alpha-responsive genes involved in oxidative phosphorylation are coordinately downregulated in human diabetes, *Nat Genet,* vol.34, No.3, pp. 267-273, issn 1061-4036 (Print)

Mortensen, O.H.; Andersen, K.; Fischer, C.; Nielsen, A.R.; Nielsen, S.; Akerstrom, T.; Aastrom, M.B.; Borup, R. & Pedersen, B.K. (2008). Calprotectin is released from human skeletal muscle tissue during exercise, *J Physiol,* vol.586, No.14, pp. 3551-3562, issn 1469-7793 (Electronic)

Nedergaard, J. & Cannon, B. (2010). The changed metabolic world with human brown adipose tissue: Therapeutic visions, *Cell Metab,* vol.11, No.4, pp. 268-272, issn 1932-7420

Neels, J.G. & Olefsky, J.M. (2006). Inflamed fat: What starts the fire?, *J Clin Invest,* vol.116, No.1, pp. 33-35, issn 0021-9738 (Print)

Nielsen, A.R. & Pedersen, B.K. (2007). The biological roles of exercise-induced cytokines: Il-6, il-8, and il-15, *Appl Physiol Nutr Metab,* vol.32, No.5, pp. 833-839, issn 1715-5312

Nomiyama, T.; Perez-Tilve, D.; Ogawa, D.; Gizard, F.; Zhao, Y.; Heywood, E.B.; Jones, K.L.; Kawamori, R.; Cassis, L.A.; Tschop, M.H. & Bruemmer, D. (2007). Osteopontin mediates obesity-induced adipose tissue macrophage infiltration and insulin resistance in mice, *J Clin Invest,* vol.117, No.10, pp. 2877-2888, issn 0021-9738 (Print)

Odegaard, J.I.; Ricardo-Gonzalez, R.R.; Goforth, M.H.; Morel, C.R.; Subramanian, V.; Mukundan, L.; Red Eagle, A.; Vats, D.; Brombacher, F.; Ferrante, A.W. & Chawla, A. (2007). Macrophage-specific ppargamma controls alternative activation and improves insulin resistance, *Nature,* vol.447, No.7148, pp. 1116-1120, issn 1476-4687

Ouchi, N.; Oshima, Y.; Ohashi, K.; Higuchi, A.; Ikegami, C.; Izumiya, Y. & Walsh, K. (2008). Follistatin-like 1, a secreted muscle protein, promotes endothelial cell function and revascularization in ischemic tissue through a nitric-oxide synthase-dependent mechanism, *J Biol Chem,* vol.283, No.47, pp. 32802-32811, issn 0021-9258 (Print)

Patti, M.E.; Butte, A.J.; Crunkhorn, S.; Cusi, K.; Berria, R.; Kashyap, S.; Miyazaki, Y.; Kohane, I.; Costello, M.; Saccone, R.; Landaker, E.J.; Goldfine, A.B.; Mun, E.; Defronzo, R.; Finlayson, J.; Kahn, C.R. & Mandarino, L.J. (2003). Coordinated reduction of genes of oxidative metabolism in humans with insulin resistance and diabetes: Potential role of pgc1 and nrf1, *Proc Natl Acad Sci U S A,* vol.100, No.14, pp. 8466-8471, issn 0027-8424 (Print)

Pedersen, B.K. & Febbraio, M.A. (2008). Muscle as an endocrine organ: Focus on muscle-derived interleukin-6, *Physiol Rev,* vol.88, No.4, pp. 1379-1406, issn 0031-9333 (Print)

Pedersen, B.K. (2011). Muscles and their myokines, *J Exp Biol,* vol.214, No.Pt 2, pp. 337-346, issn 1477-9145 (Electronic)

Peter, A.; Weigert, C.; Staiger, H.; Machicao, F.; Schick, F.; Machann, J.; Stefan, N.; Thamer, C.; Haring, H.U. & Schleicher, E. (2009). Individual stearoyl-coa desaturase 1 expression modulates endoplasmic reticulum stress and inflammation in human myotubes and is associated with skeletal muscle lipid storage and insulin sensitivity in vivo, *Diabetes,* vol.58, No.8, pp. 1757-1765, issn 1939-327X (Electronic)

Petersen, K.F.; Oral, E.A.; Dufour, S.; Befroy, D.; Ariyan, C.; Yu, C.; Cline, G.W.; Depaoli, A.M.; Taylor, S.I.; Gorden, P. & Shulman, G.I. (2002). Leptin reverses insulin resistance and hepatic steatosis in patients with severe lipodystrophy, *J Clin Invest,* vol.109, No.10, pp. 1345-1350, issn 0021-9738 (Print)

Petersen, K.F.; Dufour, S.; Befroy, D.; Garcia, R. & Shulman, G.I. (2004). Impaired mitochondrial activity in the insulin-resistant offspring of patients with type 2 diabetes, *N Engl J Med,* vol.350, No.7, pp. 664-671, issn 1533-4406 (Electronic)

Petersen, K.F.; Dufour, S. & Shulman, G.I. (2005). Decreased insulin-stimulated atp synthesis and phosphate transport in muscle of insulin-resistant offspring of type 2 diabetic parents, *PLoS Med,* vol.2, No.9, p. e233, issn 1549-1676 (Electronic)

Phillips, S.M.; Green, H.J.; Tarnopolsky, M.A.; Heigenhauser, G.F.; Hill, R.E. & Grant, S.M. (1996). Effects of training duration on substrate turnover and oxidation during exercise, *J Appl Physiol,* vol.81, No.5, pp. 2182-2191, issn 8750-7587 (Print)

Pietilainen, K.H.; Rog, T.; Seppanen-Laakso, T.; Virtue, S.; Gopalacharyulu, P.; Tang, J.; Rodriguez-Cuenca, S.; Maciejewski, A.; Naukkarinen, J.; Ruskeepaa, A.L.; Niemela, P.S.; Yetukuri, L.; Tan, C.Y.; Velagapudi, V.; Castillo, S.; Nygren, H.; Hyotylainen, T.; Rissanen, A.; Kaprio, J.; Yki-Jarvinen, H.; Vattulainen, I.; Vidal-Puig, A. & Oresic, M. (2011). Association of lipidome remodeling in the adipocyte membrane with acquired obesity in humans, *PLoS Biol,* vol.9, No.6, p. e1000623, issn 1545-7885

Pischon, T.; Boeing, H.; Hoffmann, K.; Bergmann, M.; Schulze, M.B.; Overvad, K.; Van Der Schouw, Y.T.; Spencer, E.; Moons, K.G.; Tjonneland, A.; Halkjaer, J.; Jensen, M.K.; Stegger, J.; Clavel-Chapelon, F.; Boutron-Ruault, M.C.; Chajes, V.; Linseisen, J.; Kaaks, R.; Trichopoulou, A.; Trichopoulos, D.; Bamia, C.; Sieri, S.; Palli, D.; Tumino, R.; Vineis, P.; Panico, S.; Peeters, P.H.; May, A.M.; Bueno-De-Mesquita, H.B.; Van Duijnhoven, F.J.; Hallmans, G.; Weinehall, L.; Manjer, J.; Hedblad, B.; Lund, E.; Agudo, A.; Arriola, L.; Barricarte, A.; Navarro, C.; Martinez, C.; Quiros, J.R.; Key, T.; Bingham, S.; Khaw, K.T.; Boffetta, P.; Jenab, M.; Ferrari, P. & Riboli, E. (2008). General and abdominal adiposity and risk of death in europe, *N Engl J Med,* vol.359, No.20, pp. 2105-2120, issn 1533-4406 (Electronic)

Rasmussen, M.S.; Lihn, A.S.; Pedersen, S.B.; Bruun, J.M.; Rasmussen, M. & Richelsen, B. (2006). Adiponectin receptors in human adipose tissue: Effects of obesity, weight loss, and fat depots, *Obesity (Silver Spring),* vol.14, No.1, pp. 28-35, issn 1930-7381

Reddy, P.H. (2009). Role of mitochondria in neurodegenerative diseases: Mitochondria as a therapeutic target in alzheimer's disease, *CNS Spectr,* vol.14, No.8 Suppl 7, pp. 8-13; discussion 16-18, issn 1092-8529 (Print)

Rieusset, J.; Touri, F.; Michalik, L.; Escher, P.; Desvergne, B.; Niesor, E. & Wahli, W. (2002). A new selective peroxisome proliferator-activated receptor gamma antagonist with antiobesity and antidiabetic activity, *Mol Endocrinol,* vol.16, No.11, pp. 2628-2644, issn 0888-8809 (Print)

Ritov, V.B.; Menshikova, E.V.; He, J.; Ferrell, R.E.; Goodpaster, B.H. & Kelley, D.E. (2005). Deficiency of subsarcolemmal mitochondria in obesity and type 2 diabetes, *Diabetes,* vol.54, No.1, pp. 8-14, issn 0012-1797 (Print)

Seale, P. & Lazar, M.A. (2009). Brown fat in humans: Turning up the heat on obesity, *Diabetes,* vol.58, No.7, pp. 1482-1484, issn 1939-327X (Electronic)

Semenza, G.L. (2001). Hif-1 and mechanisms of hypoxia sensing, *Curr Opin Cell Biol,* vol.13, No.2, pp. 167-171, issn 0955-0674 (Print)

Sethi, J.K. & Vidal-Puig, A.J. (2007). Thematic review series: Adipocyte biology. Adipose tissue function and plasticity orchestrate nutritional adaptation, *J Lipid Res,* vol.48, No.6, pp. 1253-1262, issn 0022-2275 (Print)

Sher, L. (1998). The endogenous euphoric reward system that reinforces physical training: A mechanism for mankind's survival, *Med Hypotheses,* vol.51, No.6, pp. 449-450, issn 0306-9877 (Print)

Schantz, P.G. (1986). Plasticity of human skeletal muscle with special reference to effects of physical training on enzyme levels of the nadh shuttles and phenotypic expression of slow and fast myofibrillar proteins, *Acta Physiol Scand Suppl,* vol.558, pp. 1-62, issn 0302-2994 (Print)

Snijder, M.B.; Dekker, J.M.; Visser, M.; Yudkin, J.S.; Stehouwer, C.D.; Bouter, L.M.; Heine, R.J.; Nijpels, G. & Seidell, J.C. (2003). Larger thigh and hip circumferences are associated with better glucose tolerance: The hoorn study, *Obes Res,* vol.11, No.1, pp. 104-111, issn 1071-7323 (Print)

Spalding, K.L.; Arner, E.; Westermark, P.O.; Bernard, S.; Buchholz, B.A.; Bergmann, O.; Blomqvist, L.; Hoffstedt, J.; Naslund, E.; Britton, T.; Concha, H.; Hassan, M.; Ryden, M.; Frisen, J. & Arner, P. (2008). Dynamics of fat cell turnover in humans, *Nature,* vol.453, No.7196, pp. 783-787, issn 1476-4687 (Electronic)

Steensberg, A.; Febbraio, M.A.; Osada, T.; Schjerling, P.; Van Hall, G.; Saltin, B. & Pedersen, B.K. (2001). Interleukin-6 production in contracting human skeletal muscle is influenced by pre-exercise muscle glycogen content, *J Physiol,* vol.537, No.Pt 2, pp. 633-639, issn 0022-3751 (Print)

Steensberg, A.; Keller, C.; Hillig, T.; Frosig, C.; Wojtaszewski, J.F.; Pedersen, B.K.; Pilegaard, H. & Sander, M. (2007). Nitric oxide production is a proximal signaling event controlling exercise-induced mrna expression in human skeletal muscle, *FASEB J,* vol.21, No.11, pp. 2683-2694, issn 1530-6860 (Electronic)

Sulpice, T.; Prunet-Marcassus, B.; Molveaux, C.; Cani, P.D.; Vitte, P.A.; Graber, P.; Dreano, M. & Burcelin, R. (2009). An adiponectin-like molecule with antidiabetic properties, *Endocrinology,* vol.150, No.10, pp. 4493-4501, issn 1945-7170 (Electronic)

Sun, K.; Kusminski, C.M. & Scherer, P.E. (2011). Adipose tissue remodeling and obesity, *J Clin Invest,* vol.121, No.6, pp. 2094-2101, issn 1558-8238 (Electronic)

Thorne, A.; Lonnqvist, F.; Apelman, J.; Hellers, G. & Arner, P. (2002). A pilot study of long-term effects of a novel obesity treatment: Omentectomy in connection with adjustable gastric banding, *Int J Obes Relat Metab Disord,* vol.26, No.2, pp. 193-199, issn 0307-0565 (Print)

Tchernof, A. (2007). Visceral adipocytes and the metabolic syndrome, *Nutr Rev,* vol.65, No.6 Pt 2, pp. S24-29, issn 0029-6643 (Print)

Trayhurn, P.; Hoggard, N.; Mercer, J.G. & Rayner, D.V. (1998). Hormonal and neuroendocrine regulation of energy balance--the role of leptin, *Arch Tierernahr,* vol.51, No.2-3, pp. 177-185, issn 0003-942X (Print)

Trayhurn, P.; Wang, B. & Wood, I.S. (2008). Hif-1alpha protein rather than mrna as a marker of hypoxia in adipose tissue in obesity: Focus on "Inflammation is associated with a decrease of lipogenic factors in omental fat in women," By poulain-godefroy et al, *Am J Physiol Regul Integr Comp Physiol,* vol.295, No.4, p. R1097; author reply R1098, issn 0363-6119 (Print)

Tseng, Y.H.; Kokkotou, E.; Schulz, T.J.; Huang, T.L.; Winnay, J.N.; Taniguchi, C.M.; Tran, T.T.; Suzuki, R.; Espinoza, D.O.; Yamamoto, Y.; Ahrens, M.J.; Dudley, A.T.; Norris, A.W.; Kulkarni, R.N. & Kahn, C.R. (2008). New role of bone morphogenetic protein 7 in brown adipogenesis and energy expenditure, *Nature,* vol.454, No.7207, pp. 1000-1004, issn 1476-4687 (Electronic)

Tseng, Y.H.; Cypess, A.M. & Kahn, C.R. (2010). Cellular bioenergetics as a target for obesity therapy, *Nat Rev Drug Discov,* vol.9, No.6, pp. 465-482, issn 1474-1784 (Electronic)

Ukropcova, B.; Mcneil, M.; Sereda, O.; De Jonge, L.; Xie, H.; Bray, G.A. & Smith, S.R. (2005). Dynamic changes in fat oxidation in human primary myocytes mirror metabolic characteristics of the donor, *J Clin Invest,* vol.115, No.7, pp. 1934-1941, issn 0021-9738

Ukropcova, B.; Sereda, O.; De Jonge, L.; Bogacka, I.; Nguyen, T.; Xie, H.; Bray, G.A. & Smith, S.R. (2007). Family history of diabetes links impaired substrate switching and reduced mitochondrial content in skeletal muscle, *Diabetes,* vol.56, No.3, pp. 720-727, issn 0012-1797 (Print)

Ukropec, J.; Sebokova, E. & Klimes, I. (2001). Nutrient sensing, leptin and insulin action, *Arch Physiol Biochem,* vol.109, No.1, pp. 38-51, issn 1381-3455 (Print)

Ukropec, J.; Anunciado, R.P.; Ravussin, Y.; Hulver, M.W. & Kozak, L.P. (2006). Ucp1-independent thermogenesis in white adipose tissue of cold-acclimated ucp1-/-mice, *J Biol Chem,* vol.281, No.42, pp. 31894-31908, issn 0021-9258 (Print)

Ukropec, J.; Penesova, A.; Skopkova, M.; Pura, M.; Vlcek, M.; Radikova, Z.; Imrich, R.; Ukropcova, B.; Tajtakova, M.; Koska, J.; Zorad, S.; Belan, V.; Vanuga, P.; Payer, J.; Eckel, J.; Klimes, I. & Gasperikova, D. (2008a). Adipokine protein expression pattern in growth hormone deficiency predisposes to the increased fat cell size and the whole body metabolic derangements, *J Clin Endocrinol Metab,* vol.93, No.6, pp. 2255-2262, issn 0021-972X (Print)

Ukropec, J.; Ukropcova, B.; Kurdiova, T.; Gasperikova, D. & Klimes, I. (2008b). Adipose tissue and skeletal muscle plasticity modulates metabolic health, *Arch Physiol Biochem,* vol.114, No.5, pp. 357-368, issn 1744-4160 (Electronic)

Ukropec, J.; Radikova, Z.; Huckova, M.; Koska, J.; Kocan, A.; Sebokova, E.; Drobna, B.; Trnovec, T.; Susienkova, K.; Labudova, V.; Gasperikova, D.; Langer, P. & Klimes, I. (2010). High prevalence of prediabetes and diabetes in a population exposed to high levels of an organochlorine cocktail, *Diabetologia,* vol.53, No.5, pp. 899-906, issn 1432-0428 (Electronic)

Unger, R.H.; Clark, G.O.; Scherer, P.E. & Orci, L. (2010). Lipid homeostasis, lipotoxicity and the metabolic syndrome, *Biochim Biophys Acta,* vol.1801, No.3, pp. 209-214, issn 0006-3002 (Print)

Van Gaal, L.F.; Mertens, I.L. & Abrams, P.J. (2003). Health risks of lipodystrophy and abdominal fat accumulation: Therapeutic possibilities with leptin and human growth hormone, *Growth Horm IGF Res,* vol.13 Suppl A, pp. S4-9, issn 1096-6374

Van Hall, G.; Jensen-Urstad, M.; Rosdahl, H.; Holmberg, H.C.; Saltin, B. & Calbet, J.A. (2003). Leg and arm lactate and substrate kinetics during exercise, *Am J Physiol Endocrinol Metab,* vol.284, No.1, pp. E193-205, issn 0193-1849 (Print)

Van Marken Lichtenbelt, W.D.; Vanhommerig, J.W.; Smulders, N.M.; Drossaerts, J.M.; Kemerink, G.J.; Bouvy, N.D.; Schrauwen, P. & Teule, G.J. (2009). Cold-activated brown adipose tissue in healthy men, *N Engl J Med,* vol.360, No.15, pp. 1500-1508, issn 1533-4406 (Electronic)

Vargovic, P.; Ukropec, J.; Laukova, M.; Cleary, S.; Manz, B.; Pacak, K. & Kvetnansky, R. (2011). Adipocytes as a new source of catecholamine production, *FEBS Lett,* vol.585, No.14, pp. 2279-2284, issn 1873-3468 (Electronic)

Vijgen, G.H.; Bouvy, N.D.; Teule, G.J.; Brans, B.; Schrauwen, P. & Van Marken Lichtenbelt, W.D. (2011). Brown adipose tissue in morbidly obese subjects, *PLoS One,* vol.6, No.2, p. e17247, issn 1932-6203 (Electronic)

Virtanen, K.A. & Nuutila, P. (2011). Brown adipose tissue in humans, *Curr Opin Lipidol,* vol.22, No.1, pp. 49-54, issn 1473-6535 (Electronic)

Wajchenberg, B.L. (2000). Subcutaneous and visceral adipose tissue: Their relation to the metabolic syndrome, *Endocr Rev,* vol.21, No.6, pp. 697-738, issn 0163-769X (Print)

Wang, B.; Wood, I.S. & Trayhurn, P. (2007). Dysregulation of the expression and secretion of inflammation-related adipokines by hypoxia in human adipocytes, *Pflugers Arch,* vol.455, No.3, pp. 479-492, issn 0031-6768 (Print)

Watt, M.J.; Steinberg, G.R.; Chen, Z.P.; Kemp, B.E. & Febbraio, M.A. (2006). Fatty acids stimulate amp-activated protein kinase and enhance fatty acid oxidation in l6 myotubes, *J Physiol,* vol.574, No.Pt 1, pp. 139-147, issn 0022-3751 (Print)

Weisberg, S.P.; Hunter, D.; Huber, R.; Lemieux, J.; Slaymaker, S.; Vaddi, K.; Charo, I.; Leibel, R.L. & Ferrante, A.W., Jr. (2006). Ccr2 modulates inflammatory and metabolic effects of high-fat feeding, *J Clin Invest*, vol.116, No.1, pp. 115-124, issn 0021-9738

Wellen, K.E. & Hotamisligil, G.S. (2005). Inflammation, stress, and diabetes, *J Clin Invest*, vol.115, No.5, pp. 1111-1119, issn 0021-9738 (Print)

Willcox, B.J.; Willcox, D.C.; Todoriki, H.; Fujiyoshi, A.; Yano, K.; He, Q.; Curb, J.D. & Suzuki, M. (2007). Caloric restriction, the traditional okinawan diet, and healthy aging: The diet of the world's longest-lived people and its potential impact on morbidity and life span, *Ann N Y Acad Sci*, vol.1114, pp. 434-455, issn 0077-8923 (Print)

Yamauchi, T.; Kamon, J.; Waki, H.; Terauchi, Y.; Kubota, N.; Hara, K.; Mori, Y.; Ide, T.; Murakami, K.; Tsuboyama-Kasaoka, N.; Ezaki, O.; Akanuma, Y.; Gavrilova, O.; Vinson, C.; Reitman, M.L.; Kagechika, H.; Shudo, K.; Yoda, M.; Nakano, Y.; Tobe, K.; Nagai, R.; Kimura, S.; Tomita, M.; Froguel, P. & Kadowaki, T. (2001). The fat-derived hormone adiponectin reverses insulin resistance associated with both lipoatrophy and obesity, *Nat Med*, vol.7, No.8, pp. 941-946, issn 1078-8956 (Print)

Yun, Z.; Maecker, H.L.; Johnson, R.S. & Giaccia, A.J. (2002). Inhibition of ppar gamma 2 gene expression by the hif-1-regulated gene dec1/stra13: A mechanism for regulation of adipogenesis by hypoxia, *Dev Cell*, vol.2, No.3, pp. 331-341, issn 1534-5807 (Print)

Zehetner, J.; Danzer, C.; Collins, S.; Eckhardt, K.; Gerber, P.A.; Ballschmieter, P.; Galvanovskis, J.; Shimomura, K.; Ashcroft, F.M.; Thorens, B.; Rorsman, P. & Krek, W. (2008). Pvhl is a regulator of glucose metabolism and insulin secretion in pancreatic beta cells, *Genes Dev*, vol.22, No.22, pp. 3135-3146, issn 0890-9369 (Print)

Zingaretti, M.C.; Crosta, F.; Vitali, A.; Guerrieri, M.; Frontini, A.; Cannon, B.; Nedergaard, J. & Cinti, S. (2009). The presence of ucp1 demonstrates that metabolically active adipose tissue in the neck of adult humans truly represents brown adipose tissue, *FASEB J*, vol.23, No.9, pp. 3113-3120, issn 1530-6860 (Electronic)

9

Pleiotropic Functions of HDL Lead to Protection from Atherosclerosis and Other Diseases

Vassilis Zannis[1,2], Andreas Kateifides[1,2], Panagiotis Fotakis[1,2], Eleni Zanni[1] and Dimitris Kardassis[2]
[1]Molecular Genetics, Boston University School of Medicine Boston, MA,
[2]University of Crete Medical School, Greece,
[1]USA
[2]Greece

1. Introduction

High density lipoprotein (HDL) is a macromolecular complex of proteins and lipids that is produced primarily by the liver through a complex pathway that requires initially the functions of apolipoprotein A-I (apoA-I), ATP binding cassette transporter A1 (ABCA1) and lecithin:cholesterol acetyl transferase (LCAT) (Zannis et al., 2006b). Following synthesis, HDL affects the functions of the arterial wall cells through signaling mechanisms mediated by scavenger receptor class B type-I (SR-BI) and other cell surface proteins. The impetus for studying HDL has been the inverse correlation that exists between plasma HDL levels and the risk for coronary artery disease (CAD) (Gordon et al., 1989). HDL promotes cholesterol efflux (Gu et al., 2000; Nakamura et al., 2004), prevents oxidation of low density lipoprotein (LDL) (Navab et al., 2000a; Navab et al., 2000b), inhibits expression of proinflammatory cytokines by macrophages (Okura et al., 2010) as well as expression of adhesion molecules by endothelial cells (Cockerill et al., 1995; Nicholls et al,. 2005b). HDL inhibits cell apoptosis (Nofer et al., 2001) and promotes endothelial cell proliferation and migration (Seetharam et al., 2006). HDL stimulates release of nitric oxide (NO) from endothelial cells thus promoting vasodilation (Mineo et al., 2003). HDL also inhibits platelet aggregation and thrombosis (Dole et al., 2008) and has antibacterial, antiparasitic and antiviral activities (Parker et al., 1995; Singh et al., 1999; Vanhollebeke and Pays, 2010). Due to these properties HDL is thought to protect the endothelium and inhibit several steps in the cascade of events that lead to the pathogenesis of atherosclerosis and various other human diseases.

This review focuses on two important aspects of contemporary HDL research. The first part considers briefly the structure of apoA-I and HDL and the key proteins that participate in the pathway of the biogenesis of HDL as well as clinical phenotypes associated with HDL abnormalities. The second part considers various physiological functions of HDL and apoA-I and the protective role of HDL against atherosclerosis and other diseases.

2. Biogenesis of HDL

HDL is synthesized through a complex pathway (Zannis et al., 2004a). The first step involves an ABCA1 mediated transfer of cellular phospholipids and cholesterol to lipid poor apoA-I extracellularly. The lipidated apoA-I is gradually converted to discoidal particles that are remodelled in the plasma compartment by the esterification of cholesterol by the enzyme LCAT (Zannis et al., 2006a) and are converted to spherical HDL particles. The cholesteryl esters formed are transferred to very low-density lipoproteins/intermediate-density lipoproteins/low density lipoproteins (VLDL/IDL/LDL) by the cholesteryl ester transfer protein (CETP) (Barter et al., 2003). Additional remodelling of HDL involves transfer of phospholipids from VLDL/LDL to HDL by the phospholipid transfer protein (PLTP) (Lusa et al., 1996), cholesterol efflux from cells or delivery of cholesteryl esters to cells mediated by the SR-BI (Krieger, 2001) as well as cholesterol efflux mediated by the cell surface transporter ATP binding cassette transporter G1 (ABCG1) (Wang et al., 2004). Finally hydrolysis of lipids of HDL is mediated by various lipases [lipoprotein lipase (LpL), hepatic lipase (HL), endothelial lipase (EL)] (Breckenridge et al., 1982; Brunzell and Deeb, 2001; Ishida et al., 2003; Krauss et al., 1974). Mutations in any of these proteins may affect the biogenesis, maturation and the functions of HDL (Fig. 1).

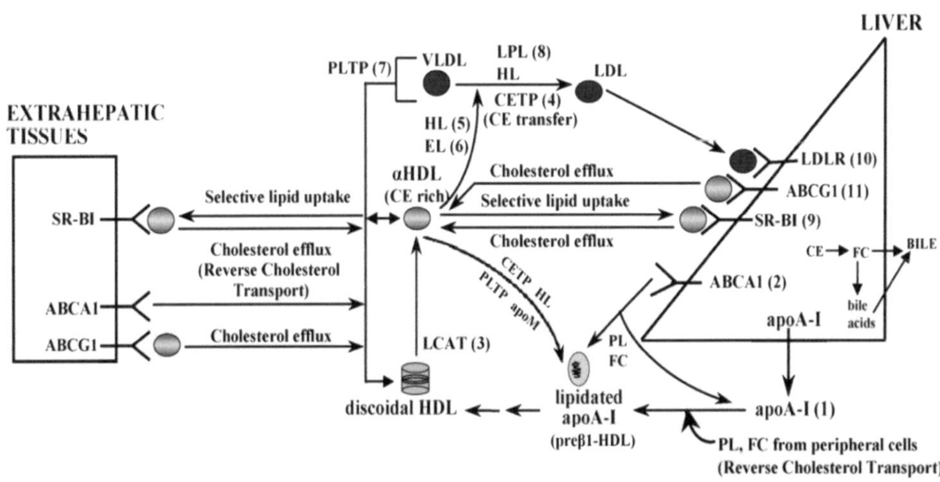

Fig. 1. Schematic representation of the pathway of the biogenesis and catabolism of HDL Numbers 1-11 indicate key cell membrane or plasma proteins shown to influence HDL levels or composition as follows: 1) apoA-I; 2) ABCA1; 3) LCAT; 4) CETP; 5) HL; 6) EL; 7) PLTP; 8) lipoproteins lipase; 9) SR-BI; 10) LDL receptor; 11) ABCG1. The figure is modified from ref. (Zannis et al., 2004b; Zannis et al., 2006b).

3. Proteins involved in the biogenesis, remodeling and signaling of HDL

3.1 Apolipoprotein A-I and its structure in solution and in discoidal and spherical HDL

ApoA-I is synthesized by the liver and the intestine in humans (Williamson et al., 1992) and it is the major protein component of the HDL. ApoA-I along with several other proteins participate in the biogenesis and remodeling of HDL as well as in signaling pathways induced by apoA-I and HDL (Yuhanna et al., 2001; Zannis et al., 2004a). ApoA-I contains 22 or 11 amino acid repeats which are organized in amphipathic a-helices (Nolte and Atkinson, 1992). Based on the crystal structure of apoA-I in solution (Borhani et al., 1997) a belt model was proposed to explain the structure of apoA-I on discoidal HDL particles. In this model, two antiparallel molecules of apoA-I are wrapped like a belt around a discoidal bilayer containing 160 phospholipid molecules and shields the hydrophobic fatty acid chains of the phospholipids. Analysis of the 93 Å spherical HDL in solution by small angle neutron scattering (SANS) showed that three molecules of apoA-I fold around a central lipid core that has 88.4 Å x 62.8 Å dimensions to form a spheroidal HDL (sHDL) particle (Wu et al., 2011).

3.2 Interactions of ApoA-I with ABCA1 are the first step in the biogenesis of HDL

ABCA1 is a ubiquitous protein that belongs to the ABC family of transporters and is expressed abundantly in the liver, macrophages, brain and various other tissues (Kielar et al., 2001). ABCA1 was shown to promote the efflux of cellular phospholipids and cholesterol to lipid free or minimally lipidated apoA-I and other apolipoproteins and amphipathic peptides, but it does not promote efflux to spherical HDL particles (Remaley et al., 2001; Wang et al., 2000). The functional interactions between apoA-I and ABCA-1 are important for the biogenesis of HDL. In the abscence of either apoA-I (Matsunaga et al., 1991) or ABCA-1 (Brunham et al., 2006) HDL is not formed. Adenovirus mediated gene transfer of apoA-I mutants in apoA-I$^{-/-}$ mice showed that deletion of the C-terminal region of apoA-I prevented the formation of HDL (Chroni et al., 2007). The ability of ABCA1 to promote cholesterol efflux from macrophages is very important for the prevention of formation of foam cells in the atherosclerotic lesions (Van Eck et al., 2002). Mutations resulting in inactivation of ABCA1 are present in patients with Tangier disease (Brunham et al., 2006). The deficiency is associated with very low levels of total plasma and HDL cholesterol and abnormal lipid deposition in various tissues (Christiansen-Weber et al., 2000; McNeish et al., 2000). The ABCA1 deficiency in humans or experimental animals may contribute to accelerated atherosclerosis (Joyce et al., 2002; Singaraja et al., 2003). Inactivation of the ABCA1 gene in macrophages increases the susceptibility to atherosclerosis (Van Eck et al., 2002; Van Eck et al., 2006). Specific amino acid substitutions found in the Danish general population were predictors of ischemic heart disease and reduced life expectancy (Frikke-Schmidt et al., 2008).

3.3 Interactions of lipid-bound ApoA-I with LCAT stabilize the nascent HDL

Plasma LCAT is a 416 amino acid long enzyme that is synthesized and secreted by the liver and esterifies the free cholesterol of HDL and LDL. ApoA-I is a potent activator of LCAT (Fielding et al., 1972). Following esterification, the cholesteryl esters formed become part of the lipid core and the discoidal HDL is converted to mature spherical HDL (Chroni et al., 2005a).

Mutations in LCAT are associated with two phenotypes in humans. The familiar LCAT deficiency (FLD) is characterized by the inability of the mutant LCAT to esterify cholesterol on HDL and LDL and causes accumulation of discoidal HDL in the plasma. The fish eye disease (FED) is characterized by the inability of mutant LCAT to esterify cholesterol on HDL only. Both diseases are characterized by low HDL levels due to the inability of LCAT to convert the nascent immature pre-β and discoidal particles to mature spherical HDL (Santamarina-Fojo et al., 2001).

3.4 Interactions of lipid-bound ApoA-I with SR-BI

SR-BI is an 82 kDa membrane glycoprotein primarily expressed in the liver, steroidogenic tissues and endothelial cells but is also found in other tissues. The most important property of SR-BI is considered to be its ability to act as the HDL receptor (Acton et al., 1996). SR-BI mediates both selective uptake of cholesteryl esters and other lipids from HDL to cells (Acton et al., 1996; Stangl et al., 1999; Thuahnai et al., 2001), as well as efflux of unesterified cholesterol (Gu et al., 2000). Transgenic mice expressing SR-BI in the liver had greatly decreased apoA-I and HDL levels as well as increased clearance of VLDL and LDL (Ueda et al., 1999) and were protected from atherosclerosis (Arai et al., 1999). SR-BI deficient mice had decreased HDL cholesterol clearance (Out et al., 2004), two fold increased plasma cholesterol and presence of large size abnormal apolipoprotein E (apoE) enriched particles that were distributed in the HDL/IDL/LDL region (Rigotti et al., 1997). The SR-BI deficiency in the background of LDL receptor (LDLr) deficient or apoE deficient mice accelerated dramatically the development of atherosclerosis (Huszar et al., 2000; Trigatti et al., 1999). The double deficient mice for apoE and SR-BI developed occlusive coronary atherosclerosis, cardiac hypertrophy, myocardial infarctions, cardiac dysfunction and died prematurely (mean age of death ~6 weeks) (Braun et al., 2002; Trigatti et al., 1999). The SR-BI deficiency reduced greatly cholesteryl ester levels in the steroidogenic tissues that utilize HDL cholesterol for synthesis of steroid hormones (Ji et al., 1999). It also decreased secretion of biliary cholesterol by approximately 50% (Mardones et al., 2001; Rigotti et al., 1997). The SR-BI deficiency also caused defective maturation of oocytes and red blood cells due to accumulation of cholesterol in the plasma membrane of progenitor cells (Holm et al., 2002; Trigatti et al., 1999) and caused infertility in the female but not the male mice (Trigatti et al., 1999; Yesilaltay et al., 2006). Interactions of HDL with SR-BI in endothelial cells triggers signaling mechanisms discussed below that involve activation of endothelial nitric oxide synthase (eNOS) and release of NO that causes vasodilation (Mineo et al., 2003; Yuhanna et al., 2001). Human subjects have been identified with a P297S substitution in SR-BI. Heterozygote carriers for this mutation had increased HDL levels, decreased adrenal stereoidogenesis and dysfunctional platelets but did not develop atherosclerosis (Vergeer et al., 2011).

A [Gly2Ser]SR-BI substitution in humans is associated with decreased follicular progesterone levels in Caucasian women and non viable fetuses 42 days post embryo transfer. Another single nucleotide polymorphism (SNP) (rs10846744) was associated with gestational sacs and fetal heart beats and with poor fetal viability in African-American women (Yates et al., 2011).

3.5 Interactions of HDL with ABCG1

ABCG1 is a 67 kDa protein which is a member of ABC family of half transporters. ABCG1 is expressed in the spleen, thymus, lung, brain, endothelial cells and other tissues (Savary et al., 1996) and promotes cholesterol efflux from cells to HDL but not to lipid free apoA-I (Nakamura et al., 2004; Vaughan and Oram, 2005). The absence of ABCG1 in mice causes cholesterol accumulation in various tissues (Kennedy et al., 2005) and selective deletion of both ABCA1 and ABCG1 genes in macrophages further increases cholesterol accumulation and results in severe atherosclerosis (Out et al., 2008; Yvan-Charvet et al., 2007).

4. Phenotypes of humans and experimental animals having apoA-I mutations

4.1 Natural apoA-I mutations

Several apoA-I mutations have been described in the general population that are associated with low plasma HDL levels. Most of the mutations affect the interaction of apoA-I with LCAT. Eight mutations between residues 26 and 107 and one on residue 173, have been associated with amyloidosis and low HDL levels (Sorci-Thomas and Thomas, 2002; Zannis et al., 1993) and one mutation on residue 164 is associated with increased risk for ischemic heart disease and reduced life expectancy (Haase et al., 2011). The in vivo interactions of representative naturally occurring apoA-I mutants with LCAT were studied by adenovirus-mediated gene transfer in apoA-I deficient mice. The mutants apoA-I(Leu141Arg)$_{Pisa}$ and apoA-I(Leu159Arg)$_{FIN}$ produced only small amounts of HDL that formed mostly preβ1 and small size α4 HDL particles. The apoA-I(Arg151Cys)$_{Paris}$ and apoA-I(arg160Leu)$_{Oslo}$ formed discoidal HDL particles. These studies indicated that apoA-I(Leu141Arg)$_{Pisa}$ and apoA-I(Leu159Arg)$_{FIN}$ mutation may inhibit an early step in the biogenesis of HDL due to insufficient esterification of the cholesterol of the preβ1-HDL particles by the endogenous LCAT. The LCAT insufficiency appears to result from depletion of the plasma LCAT mass (Koukos et al., 2007). A remarkable finding of these studies was that all the aberrant phenotypes were corrected by treatment with exogenous LCAT. This indicates that LCAT administration could be a potential therapeutic intervention to correct low-HDL conditions in humans that are caused by these and other unidentified mutations (Amar et al., 2009).

4.2 Specific bioengineered mutations in ApoA-I may cause dyslipidemia

Four bioengineered mutations in apoA-I have been studied by adenovirus-mediated gene transfer in apoA-I deficient mice. Mutants apoA-I[Δ(62-78)], apoA-I [Glu110Ala/Glu111Ala] and apoA-I[Asp89Ala/Glu90Ala/Glu92Ala], caused combined hyperlipidemia, characterized by elevated plasma cholesterol and severe hypertriglyceridemia (Chroni et al., 2004; Chroni et al., 2005b; Kateifides et al., 2011). An apoA-I[Δ89-99] mutant induced high plasma cholesterol, but did not affect plasma triglyceride levels (Chroni et al., 2005b).

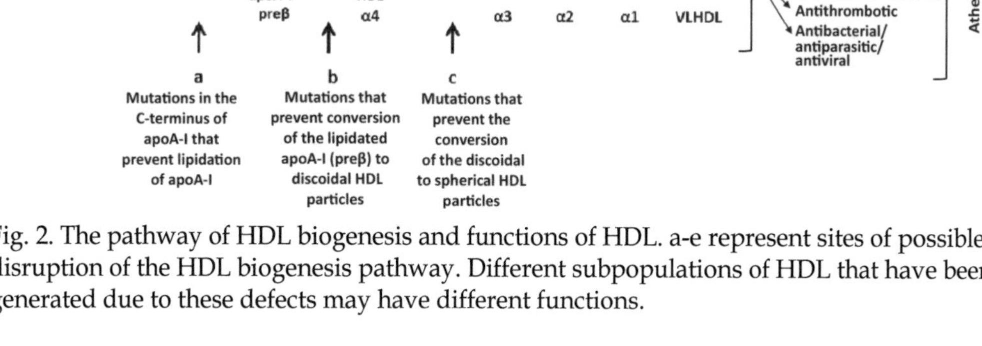

Fig. 2. The pathway of HDL biogenesis and functions of HDL. a-e represent sites of possible disruption of the HDL biogenesis pathway. Different subpopulations of HDL that have been generated due to these defects may have different functions.

The systematic study of the functions of apoA-I by adenovirus mediated gene transfer as well as the phenotypes of naturally occurring apoA-I mutants identified the following five steps where the pathway of biogenesis and/or catabolism of HDL can be disrupted: a) Lack of synthesis of HDL due to mutations in ABCA1 or mutations in apoA-I that affect the ABCA1/apoA-I interaction, b) Failure to convert efficiently the lipidated pre-β HDL to discoidal HDL. This defect most likely results from fast catabolism of apoA-I following its lipidation by ABCA1, c) Accumulation of discoidal HDL. This phenotype has been generated by the mutations in the 149-160 region of apoA-I that affect LCAT activation, d) Accumulation of discoidal HDL and induction of hypercholesterolemia. This condition has been observed in the case of the apoA-I[Δ(89-99)] mutant, e) Induction of hypertriglyceridemia. This defect has been observed in the case of apoA-I[Δ(62-78)], apoA-I[Glu110Ala/Glu111Ala] and apoA-I[Asp89Ala/Glu90Ala/Glu92Ala] mutants (Fig. 2).

5. Physiological functions of ApoA-I and HDL that may be relevant to its atheroprotective properties

5.1 Cell signaling pathways mediated by HDL and apoA-I

Various studies have shown that increased HDL levels are associated with greater vasodilator effects in humans and this effect is impaired in patients with coronary heart disease (CHD) (Li et al., 2000; Zeiher et al., 1994). Treatment with HDL increased eNOS protein levels in cultured human aortic endothelial cells (HAECs) (Ramet et al., 2003). Other studies in endothelial cells and Chinese hamster ovary (CHO) cells that express SR-BI, showed that SR-BI-HDL interactions lead to the phosphorylation and activation of eNOS. The HDL-induced eNOS activation occurs in the caveolae. The HDL-mediated NO-dependent relaxation is lost in aortic rings of SR-BI$^{-/-}$ mice (Yuhanna et al., 2001). Experiments in cultures of endothelial cells and COS M6 cells transfected with eNOS and SR-BI showed that interaction of HDL with SR-BI triggered signalling mechanisms which led to phosphorylation of eNOS at Ser1179 and increased its activity. On the other hand phosphorylation of Thr 497 of eNOS attenuated its activity. The signalling cascade initially involves the nonreceptor tyrosine kinase Src which phosphorylated PI3 kinase (PI3K). Inhibition of Src by specific inhibitors prevented eNOS phosphorylation. PI3K activation led to phosphorylation of Akt and mitogen-activated protein kinase (MAPK) which independently phosphorylated eNOS. Inhibitors of MAPK did not affect HDL-mediated Akt activation and a dominant negative Akt did not affect HDL-mediated MAPK activation and eNOS phosphorylation (Mineo et al., 2003) (figure 3A).

The mechanism of the SR-BI mediated activation of eNOS was studied in detail (Assanasen et al., 2005). HDL and cholesterol-free reconstituted HDL (rHDL) particles containing apoA-I and phosphatidylocholine (Lp2A-I) as well as cyclodextrin stimulated eNOS activity whereas rHDL particles that contain cholesterol did not. Blocking of cholesterol efflux with a monoclonal antibody to SR-BI abolished the activation of eNOS. Experiments were performed using SR-BII, a splice variant of SR-BI as well as a SR-BI mutant that lacks the carboxyterminal amino acid 509 [SR-BI(Δ509)] and chimeric receptors where the transmembrane and the C-terminal domains of SR-BI were replaced by the corresponding domains of CD36. These studies established that the C-terminal cytoplasmic PDZ-interacting domain and the C-terminal transmembrane domain of SR-BI were both required for eNOS activation (Assanasen et al., 2005). The cytoplasmic PDZK1 interacting domain of SR-BI binds adaptor proteins such as PDZK1 that may participate in cell signalling (Kocher et al., 2003). A photoactive derivative of cholesterol binds in the transmembrane region of SR-BI indicating that this region serves as a cholesterol sensor on the plasma membrane (Assanasen et al., 2005). HDL and lysophospholipids that are components of HDL including sphingosylphosphorylcholine, sphingosine-1-phospate (S1P) and lysosulphatide cause eNOS dependent relaxation of mouse aortic rings via intracellular Ca^{2+} mobilization and eNOS phosphorylation mediated by Akt (Nofer et al., 2004). Another study however, indicated that interactions of HDL with SR-BI stimulate eNOS by increasing intracellular ceramide levels without affecting intracellular calcium levels and Akt phosphorylation (Li et al., 2002). The proposed role of HDL-associated estradiol in the stimulation of eNOS activity is unclear (Gong et al., 2003). 5′ AMP-activated protein kinase (AMPK) may also play a role in the HDL-mediated phosphorylation of eNOS at multiple sites (Ser116, Ser635, and Ser1179) (Drew et al., 2004). It was suggested that activation by AMPK may involve physical interactions between the apoA-I component of HDL and eNOS. Such interactions may be possible following SR-BI mediated endocytosis of HDL (Silver et al., 2001). HDL also affected the signaling in endothelial cells by the bone morphogenetic protein 4 (BMP4) and increased expression of the activin-like kinase receptor 1 and 2 (Yao et al., 2008). This resulted in increased expression of vascular endothelial growth factor (VEGF) and matrix gla protein (MGP). VEGF promotes endothelial cell survival and MGP prevents vascular calcification and thus contribute to the maintenance, the integrity and the preservation of the functions of the endothelium (Yao et al., 2008).

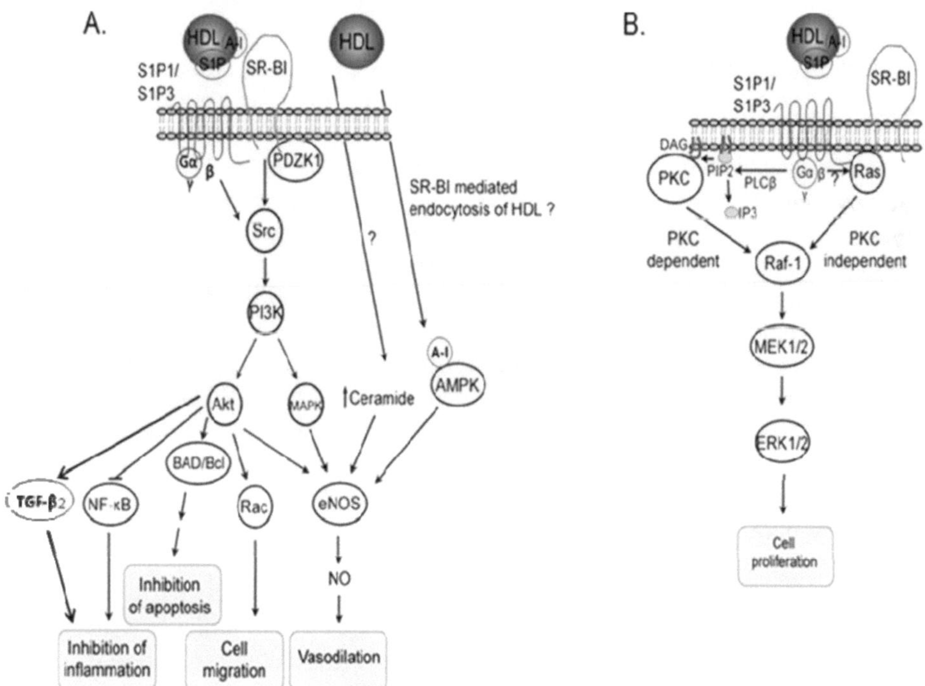

Fig. 3. A) Schematic representation of SR-BI signaling that can lead to vasodilation, cell migration and inhibition of inflammation and apoptosis. B) Schematic representation of PKC-dependent SR-BI-dependent signalling pathway that promote cell proliferation (Drew et al., 2004; Grewal et al., 2003; Kimura et al., 2003; Mineo et al., 2003).

5.2 Effect of HDL and apoA-I on inflammation

An initial step in the pathogenesis of atherosclerosis is the association of the monocytes to adhesion molecules of the endothelial cells that facilitates their entry in the sub-endothelial space (Zannis et al., 2004b). Induction of adhesion molecules is promoted by pro-inflammatory stimuli (Cybulsky and Gimbrone, Jr., 1991). Recruitment and migration of monocytes into sub-endothelial space is promoted by the monocyte chemoattractant factor (MCP-1) as well as by oxidized LDL (Peters and Charo, 2001). HDL has anti-oxidant properties and can prevent the oxidation of LDL (Navab et al., 2000a; Navab et al., 2000b). Interactions of HDL or apoA-I with cells of the vascular wall were shown to prevent the expression of pro-inflammatory cytokines and chemokines that induce the expression of adhesion molecules (Bursill et al., 2010; Cockerill et al., 1995; Nobecourt et al., 2010). The anti-inflammatory functions of HDL were manifested in several ways. HDL binds via its apoA-I moiety to progranulin produced by macrophages. This prevents conversion of progranulin to inflammatory granulins which were shown to induce expression of tumor necrosis factor α (TNFα) and interleukin (IL) 1β in monocyte macrophages (Okura et al., 2010). HDL and rHDL were shown to inhibit the cytokine induced expression of vascular cell adhesion molecule-1 (VCAM-1) and inter-cellular adhesion molecule-1 (ICAM-1) by endothelial cells (Cockerill et al., 1995). In addition, HDL promoted the expression of anti-inflammatory cytokines in endothelial cells. Thus treatment of endothelial cells (HUVEC) with HDL and lysosphingolipids present in HDL, increased the expression of TGF-β_2 through mechanisms that involve the activation of Akt and extracellular signal regulated kinases (ERK) 1/2. Consistent with cell culture studies, the expression of transforming growth factor-β_2 (TGF-β_2) and the phosphorylation of ERK1/2, Akt and Smad2/3 were increased in apoA-I transgenic mice and diminished in apoA-I deficient mice (Norata et al., 2005). In vivo studies also showed that infusion of rHDL inhibited the pro-oxidant and pro-inflammatory events that occurred following implantation of non occlusive periarteral collars in rabbits that induce acute arterial inflammation. In these studies the rHDL inhibited neutrofil infiltration, production of reactive oxygen species (ROS) and the expression of VCAM-1, ICAM-1, MCP-1 and E-selectin (Nicholls et al., 2005b). The carotid vascular inflammation and neutrofil infiltration could be inhibited by rHDL containing normal apoA-I but not by apoA-I obtained from diabetic patients (Nobecourt et al., 2010). The beneficial effects of rHDL containing apoA-I in vivo and in cell cultures could be duplicated using synthetic apoA-I mimetics such as 5A, L37pA and D37pA (Gomaraschi et al., 2008; Tabet et al., 2010). The 5A/PLPC complexes reduced the vascular inflammation that is associated with collar insertion in a rabbit model by reducing the ICAM-1 and VCAM-1 expression, the infiltration of neutrofils and the Nox4 activity. In cultures of human carotid endothelial cells (HCEC) 5A/PLPC and rHDL containing apoA-I inhibited the TNF-α induced VCAM-1 and ICAM-1 expression as well as the activation of nuclear factor κB (NF-κB) pathway and these effects were abolished by ABCA1 silencing (Tabet et al., 2010). Complexes of L37pA or D37pA with β-oleoyl-γ-palmitoyl-L-α-phosphatidylcholine reduced the postischemic cardiac contractile dysfunction in a rat heart model of ischemia/reperfusion. They also reduced TNF-α levels and increased prostacyclin levels in the perfusate and inhibited the TNF-α mediated VCAM-1 expression in endothelial cell cultures (Gomaraschi et al., 2008). In monocyte and endothelial cell cultures HDL also suppressed expression of chemokines CCL2, CCL5 and CX3CL1 and chemokine receptors CCR2, CCR5 and CX3CR1 (Bursill et al., 2010). This effect was mediated by inhibition of Iκ-

Bα phosphorylation and NF-κB(p65) expression and in some cases by peroxisome proliferator-activated receptor γ (PPARγ) activation. Consistent with cell culture studies, in vivo infusion of apoA-I in cholesterol fed apoE deficient mice reduced expression of chemokines and chemokine receptors (Bursill et al., 2010). HDL and its protein moiety apoA-I have been shown to inhibit the expression of CD11b of human monocytes that is induced by phorbol myristate acetate (PMA) and promote cell adhesion. Inhibition of the ABCA1-mediated and to a lesser extent SR-BI mediated cholesterol efflux by monoclonal antibodies attenuated the inhibitory effect of apoA-I and HDL respectively. Expression of CD11b was also affected by depletion of the membrane cholesterol by treatment of the cells with cyclodextrin (Murphy et al., 2008), pointing out to a potential role of cholesterol efflux in the inhibition of inflammation. Consistent with the ex vivo studies infusion of rHDL in patients with type 2 diabetes mellitus, reduced the expression of CD11b of the peripheral monocytes and reduced the adhesion of the patients' neutrophils to a fibrinogen matrix. Plasma HDL isolated 4 to 72 hours post rHDL infusion suppressed the expression of VCAM-1 in cultures of HAECs and had increased ability to promote cholesterol efflux from THP-1 macrophages (Patel et al., 2009). In cultures of smooth muscle cells, HDL downregulated the NADPH-oxidase mediated generation of reactive oxygen species (ROS) and inhibited production of MCP-1. The inhibitory effect was attenuated by antagonists of $S1P_1$ and $S1P_3$ receptors. The data showed that free S1P or S3P alone or as components of HDL could attenuate production of MCP-1. Consistent with these findings, MCP-1 production and ROS generation in the aortas of $S1P_3^{-/-}$ receptor and SR-BI$^{-/-}$ mice were not affected by treatment with HDL, S1P and sphingosylphosphorylcholine (SPC) (Tolle et al., 2008). ApoA-I induced the expression of the adhesion molecule CD31, and changed the morphology and size distribution of lineage negative bone marrow cells. The treatment also increased the ability of the cells to bind to fibronectin and to cultured endothelial cells. Deletion of the C-terminal helix 10 of apoA-I abolished the effects of apoA-I on bone marrow cells (Mythreye et al., 2008).

5.3 Effect of HDL and apoA-I on endothelial cell apoptosis

Exposure of endothelial cells to inflammatory stimuli may disturb the endothelial monolayer integrity (Dimmeler et al., 2002). Numerous factors that promote endothelial apoptosis have been described and include OxLDL (Li et al., 1998), TNF-a (Dimmeler et al., 1999), homocysteine (Welch and Loscalzo, 1998), and angiotensin II (Strawn and Ferrario, 2002). HDL also can reverse the TNF-a induced and growth deprivation induced endothelial cell apoptosis (Nofer et al., 2001; Sugano et al., 2000). OxLDL increased intracellular calcium and resulted in apoptosis that could be inhibited by HDL and apoA-I (Suc et al., 1997). ApoA-I interacts with ABCA1 and F1-ATPase (Chroni et al., 2003; Vantourout et al., 2010), whereas HDL interacts with SR-BI and ABCG1 (Liadaki et al., 2000; Wang et al., 2004) respectively and the sphingolipid components of HDL interact with the S1P receptors (Kimura et al., 2003; Okajima et al., 2009). HDL protected endothelial cells from apoptosis induced by oxLDL by preventing the generation of intracellular ROS. The anti-apoptotic activity was highest for HDL_3 and diminished as the size of HDL increased. It was suggested that approximately 70% of the anti-apoptotic activity of HDL was attributed to apoA-I which has the capacity to accept through its methionine residues the phospholipid hydroperoxides (PLOOH) of oxLDL (de Souza et al., 2010). The anti-apoptotic functions of small size HDL_3 was reduced by 35% in subjects with metabolic syndrome and this reduction was correlated with the clinical phenotype of the human subjects. Compared to normal HDL the HDL_3 fractions of the diabetic subjects had increased total triglyceride levels and decreased cholesteryl esters/triglycerides ratio suggesting that the lipid core of HDL_3 was enriched with triglycerides (de Souza et al., 2008). HDL_3 also inhibited apoptotic cell death induced by oxLDL and preserved lysosomal integrity of an osteoblastic cell line (Brodeur et al., 2008). The anti-apoptotic effects were attributed to the increased expression of SR-BI that is mediated by HDL_3, combined with the ability of HDL to compete for the binding of oxLDL to osteoblasts as well as increased selective uptake of the cholesterol of the oxLDL by these cells (Brodeur et al., 2008).

Interactions of apoA-I with cell surface F1-ATPase inhibited apoptosis of HUVEC and stimulated cell proliferation (Radojkovic et al., 2009). In the absence of apoA-I, specific inhibitors for F1-ATPase (IF_1-H49K) and angiostatin or specific antibodies to F1-ATPase promoted apoptosis and inhibited cell proliferation. In the presence of apoA-I, F1-ATPase inhibitors and antibodies diminished its anti-apoptotic and anti-proliferative effects. Down-regulation of the ABCA1 by siRNA did not affect the anti-apoptotic and proliferative functions of apoA-I whereas inhibition of SR-BI by a specific antibody diminished the anti-apoptotic and proliferative functions of HDL_3 (Radojkovic et al., 2009). The findings suggest that interactions of lipid free apoA-I with F1-ATPase and of HDL with SR-BI contribute to their anti-apoptotic and proliferative effects on endothelial cells. The antiapoptotic effects of HDL on endothelial cells could be mimicked by the lysosphingolipid components of HDL (Nofer et al., 2001). The SR-BI mediated signalling that leads to activation of eNOS, also promotes cell growth and migration and protects cells from apoptosis (Mineo et al., 2006; Noor et al., 2007). Activation of eNOS required its localization in the caveolae, where caveolin SR-BI and CD36 are also found (Uittenbogaard et al., 2000). It has been proposed that oxLDL acting through CD36 depletes the cholesterol content of caveolae and leads to eNOS redistribution to intracellular sites thus resulting in decreased eNOS activity (Blair et al., 1999; Uittenbogaard et al., 2000). HDL acting through SR-BI maintains the concentration of caveolae-associated cholesterol, inhibits the actions of oxLDL and maintains eNOS in the caveolae (Uittenbogaard et al., 2000). This interpretation implies that strong interactions between eNOS and caveolin-1 (Cav-1) stimulate eNOS activity. Other studies provided the opposite mechanism of modulation of eNOS activity by interactions of eNOS with Cav-1 (Terasaka et al., 2010). It was shown that these interactions were enhanced by loading cells with cholesterol or oxysterols and decreased by cholesterol depletion in endothelial cells as a result of ABCG1-mediated cholesterol efflux. Studies in murine lung endothelial cells (MLEC) also showed that HDL could reverse the inhibition of eNOS activity caused by cholesterol loading in the normal but not the Cav-1 deficient cells (Terasaka et al., 2010). It was proposed that diminished interactions between eNOS and Cav-1 caused by ABCG1-mediated efflux stimulated eNOS activity. It has been shown that oxidized phospholipids uncouple eNOS activity and lead to the generation of oxygen radicals which induces the expression of sterol regulatory element binding protein (SREBP) and IL-8 (Gharavi et al., 2006; Yeh et al., 2004). ApoA-I mimetic peptides also prevent LDL from uncoupling eNOS activity to favour O_2^{-} anion production as opposed to normal production of NO (Ou et al., 2003). Finally it has been shown that SR-BI via a highly conserved redox motif CXXS between residues 323-326 can promote a ligant independent apoptosis via a caspase 8 pathway and this effect could be reversed by HDL and eNOS (Li et al., 2005). It was proposed that at low HDL levels oxitative stress causes relocation of eNOS away from the caveolae and this results in SR-BI induced apoptosis (Li et al., 2005). The picture that emerges from these studies is that HDL promotes survival and migration of endothelial cells by signalling mechanisms that originate from the interactions of HDL with SR-BI, the interactions of S1P with S1P1 and S1P3 receptors and the interactions of lipid-free apoA-I with F1-ATPase.

5.4 Effect of HDL on endothelial cell proliferation and migration

Damage of the endothelium is associated with vascular disease which can be blunted by re-endothelialization (Werner et al., 2003). HDL promoted proliferation of HUVEC via mechanisms that increased intracellular Ca^{2+} and upregulated the production of prostacyclin (Tamagaki et al., 1996). HDL also promoted endothelial cell migration (Murugesan et al., 1994). Migration was promoted by signalling cascades mediated by interaction of S1P with S1P1 and S1P3 receptors that led to the activation of PI3 kinase, p38MAP kinase and Rho kinases (Kimura et al., 2003). Other studies showed that HDL can activate the MAPK pathway either through processes that involve protein kinase C (PKC), Raf-1, MEK and ERK1/2 or PKC independent pathways. This latter pathway leads to the activation of Ras and can be inhibited by pertussis toxin and neutralizing antibodies against SR-BI (Grewal et al., 2003). The data suggest that interactions of HDL with SR-BI activate Ras in a PKC independent manner and this leads to subsequent activation of MAPK signalling cascade (Grewal et al., 2003) (Fig.3B). Another beneficial effect of HDL is its capacity to promote capillary tube formation in vitro. This function is pertussis toxin sensitive and requires p44/42MAP kinase which is downstream of Ras (Miura et al., 2003). Other studies showed that interaction of SR-BI with HDL or rHDL, activated Src kinases and Rac GTPases and stimulated endothelial cell migration. In vivo experiments have also shown that re-endothelialization of carotid artery following injury is promoted by apoA-I expression and is inhibited in apoA-I deficient in mice (Seetharam et al., 2006).

5.5 Effect of HDL on thrombosis

Increased HDL cholesterol levels are associated with decreased risk of venous thrombosis (Doggen et al., 2004). In contrast low HDL levels are associated with increased risk of venous thrombosis (Deguchi et al., 2005). The ability of HDL to inhibit endothelial cell apoptosis (Dimmeler et al., 2002; Mineo et al., 2006) prevents vessel denudation and formation of microparticles that may contribute to thrombosis (Durand et al., 2004). It has been shown that thrombogenic membrane microparticles that may originate from apoptotic endothelial cells are increased in the plasma of patients with acute coronary syndrome (ACS) (Mallat et al., 2000). Infusion of rHDL in volunteers that received low levels of endotoxin limited the prothrombotic and procoagulant effect of endotoxin (Pajkrt et al., 1997). Furthermore infusion of apoA-I_{MILANO} in a rat model of acute arterial thrombosis increased the time of thrombus formation and decreased the weight of the thrombus (Li et al., 1999). HDL may affect thrombosis via a variety of mechanisms: Early studies showed that HDL causes increased synthesis of prostacyclin in cultured endothelial cells (Fleisher et al., 1983; Tamagaki et al., 1996). Prostacyclin in combination with NO promote smooth muscle cells relaxation, inhibit platelet activation and local smooth muscle cell proliferation (Vane and Botting, 1995). It has been reported that HDL_3 induced expression of cyclooxygenase-2 (Cox-2) by smooth muscle cells and promoted release of prostacyclin (PGI2) via a signalling pathway that involves p38MAP kinase and c-Jun N terminal kinase

(JNK-1) (Escudero et al., 2003; Vinals et al., 1997). PGI2 synthesis was enhanced by HMGCoA reductase inhibitors (Martinez-Gonzalez et al., 2004). It has been shown that there is a positive correlation between plasma HDL levels and anticoagulant response to activated protein C (APC)/protein S in vitro (Griffin et al., 1999) and negative correlation with the plasma thrombin activation markers such as prothrombin fragments F1.2 and D-dimer (MacCallum et al., 2000). APC inactivates, by proteolysis, factors Va and VIIIa in plasma and thus it can downregulate thrombin formation. Administration of HDL to cholesterol-fed rabbits also increased endothelial cell thrombomodulin levels, promoted generation of APC and inhibited formation of thrombin (Nicholls et al., 2005a). Glucosylceramide and glycosphingolipids which are present in HDL are lipid cofactors for the anticoagulant activity of APC and in a significant number of patients with venous thrombosis the levels of glucosylceramides are low (Deguchi et al., 2002; Deguchi et al., 2001). Shpingosine, another molecule present in HDL, has been shown to inhibit prothrombin activation on platelets' surface by disrupting procoagulant interactions between factors Xa and Va (Deguchi et al., 2004). HDL also downregulated expression of plasminogen activator inhibitor-1 (PAI-1) and upregulated tissue plasminogen activator (t-PA) in endothelial cell cultures (Eren et al., 2002). Transgenic mice expressing the human PAI-1 developed age-dependent coronary arterial thrombosis (Eren et al., 2002). In contrast oxidized HDL_3 induced the expression of PAI-1 in endothelial cells through signalling mechanisms that involve activation of ERK1/2 and p38MAPK and mRNA stabilization (Norata et al., 2004).

5.6 Effects of HDL on diabetes mellitus

In vivo and in vitro studies have provided evidence that HDL may have beneficial effects on glucose metabolism (Koseki et al., 2009; Rutti et al., 2009). Ex vivo studies showed that HDL and delipidated apoA-I or S1P decreased IL-1β and glucose-mediated apoptosis and thus increased the survival of human and murine islets. HDL treatment down-regulated the expression of iNOS and its downstream target Fas which is pro-apoptotic and up-regulated the expression of FLICE-like inhibitory protein (FLIP) which is anti-apoptotic (Rutti et al., 2009). HDL also reversed the toxic effects of oxidized LDL on beta cells that are associated with apoptosis and cJNK mediated transcriptional repression of the insulin gene caused cJNK mediated (Abderrahmani et al., 2007).
Oral glucose tolerance test in a limited number of patients with Tangier disease (that lack or have dysfunctional ABCA1) showed that they had glucose intolerance as compared to controls (Koseki et al., 2009), thus implicating ABCA1, apoA-I and HDL in glucose metabolism. Cell culture studies using primary pancreatic islets cells and a pancreatic β-cell line (Min6), showed that lipid free apoA-I or apoA-II or reconstituted HDL increased insulin secretion up to 5-fold in a Ca^{2+} dependant manner (Fryirs et al., 2010). The free apolipoproteins also increased insulin mRNA levels. HDL mediated insulin secretion has also been observed in cultures of mouse pancreatic β-cells (MIN6N8) (Drew et al., 2009). The increase in insulin secretion mediated by lipid-free apoproteins and rHDL required the functions of ABCA1 and SRBI or ABCG1 respectively. These functions may be different from those involved in cholesterol efflux. For high glucose concentrations enhanced insulin secretion required the action of K_{ATP} channel and glucose catabolism in the pancreatic cell, but this did not occur for low glucose concentrations (Fryirs et al., 2010).
Further insight on the role of ABCA1 in diabetes was obtained by studies in mice with selective deficiency of ABCA1 in the pancreas ($ABCA1^{-P/-P}$). These mice accumulated

cholesterol in their islets and were characterized by impaired acute phase insulin secretion and glucose intolerance. The ABCA1$^{-P/-P}$ mice exhibited normal insulin sensitivity indicating normal response of the peripheral tissues to insulin. The impairment in insulin secretion was verified in cell culture experiments using islets isolated from the ABCA1$^{-P/-P}$ mice. In contrast, whole ABCA1 deficient mice had normal glucose tolerance and displayed only small impairment in the islet function and did not accumulate significant amount of cholesterol in the islets (Brunham et al., 2007). Pancreatic islets isolated from apoE deficient mice had increased cholesterol content and reduced insulin secretion as compared to islets obtained from WT mice. The reduced insulin secretion in the pancreatic islets or cultures of β-cells could be restored by depletion of the cellular cholesterol using mevastatin or methyl-β-cyclodextrin (MβCD) (Hao et al., 2007). Experiments in cell lines of pancreatic β-cell origin indicated that cholesterol loading or cholesterol depletion affect the activity of glucokinase (GK) which is known to regulate insulin secretion (Rizzo and Piston, 2003). The experiments showed that under normal cholesterol levels GK is associated with a dimeric form of nNOS on insulin containing granules in the cytoplasm and is inactive (Rizzo and Piston, 2003). Increase in plasma cholesterol enhanced dimerization of nNOS and its association with GK whereas reduction in the cholesterol levels or increase in the extracellular glucose levels promoted monomerization of nNOS and release of active GK in the cytoplasm (Hao et al., 2007). The role of the increase in the cholesterol content of β-cells in insulin secretion was tested in transgenic mice expressing SREBP-2 in β-cells under the control of insulin promoter. These mice had normal plasma cholesterol levels but developed severe diabetes characterized by 5-fold increase in gluco-hemoglobin and defects in glucose and potassium-stimulated insulin secretion and were characterized by glucose intolerance. The islets were fewer, smaller and deformed and had increased levels of total and esterified cholesterol (Ishikawa et al., 2008). It was proposed that the loss of β-cell mass could be related to the down regulation of genes such as PDX-1 and BETA2 that are involved in β-cell differentiation.

A recent comprehensive study has measured the properties of HDL isolated from patients with type 2 diabetes mellitus and their functions on endothelial cells in vitro and in vivo. HDL isolated from patients with low HDL and type 2 diabetes mellitus contained increased levels of lipid peroxides and increased myeloperoxidase activity. In endothelial cell cultures diabetic HDL had reduced production of NO and increased NADPH oxidase activity that resulted in increased oxidant stress. Diabetic HDL had diminished endothelium dependent relaxation of aortic rings and endothelial progenitor cells obtained from diabetic subjects had diminished capacity to promote reendothelialization in vivo. A remarkable finding in this study was that extended release niacin treatment of the diabetic patients restored the properties and functions of HDL. The HDL obtained after treatment had normal levels of peroxides and normal myeloperoxidase (MPO) activity. Studies with endothelial cultures showed that following treatment of the diabetic patients their HDL could induce normal NO production and NADPH oxidase activity and could promote normal relaxation of aortic rings. Endothelial progenitor cells obtained from diabetic patients following niacin treatment had normal ability to promote reendothelialization in vivo (Sorrentino et al., 2010). In another study intravenous infusion of rHDL (80 mg/kg over 4 hours) in type 2 diabetic human subjects decreased plasma glucose level, increased plasma insulin level and increased β-cell functions as compared to patients receiving placebo (Drew et al., 2009). HDL and apoA-I increased glucose uptake of primary human skeletal muscle cultures established from patients with type 2 diabetes mellitus. HDL induced glucose uptake and fatty acid oxidation and increased AMPKα2 activity and phosphorylation. These effects were modulated through a Ca^{2+} dependent pathway. Subsequent in vitro and in vivo studies showed that rHDL inhibited lipolysis in 3T3-L1 adipocytes partially via activation of AMPK pathway (Drew et al., 2011). Infusion of rHDL also inhibited fasting induced lipolysis and fatty acid oxidation but increased the circulating non essential fatty acids possibly due to the action of phospholipase on the rHDL phospholipids (Drew et al., 2011). The HDL dependent glucose uptake by the skeletal muscle cells was abrogated by inhibition of ABCA1 with a blocking antibody suggesting that ABCA1 functions not related to cholesterol efflux, may contribute to the increased glucose uptake and β-oxidation by skeletal muscle cells obtained from patients with type 2 diabetic mellitus (Drew et al., 2011). The effect of apoA-I on glucose metabolism was also studied in C2C12 myocytes and apoA-I deficient mice. Consistent with the studies with primary human skeletal muscle cultures, apoA-I stimulated AMPK and acetyl-CoA carboxylase (ACC) phosphorylation and glucose uptake and endocytosis into C2C12 cells. The apoA-I deficient mice had increased fat content decreased glucose tolerance and increased expression of gluconeogenic enzymes in the liver and decreased AMPK-dependent phosphorylation in skeletal muscle and the liver (Han et al., 2007).

5.7 Role of apoA-I and HDL in atheroprotection

Atherosclerosis is associated with lipid and lipoprotein abnormalities (Zannis et al., 2004b). Low HDL levels (Gordon et al., 1989) and decreased concentration of the largest size HDL subpopulations (Asztalos et al., 2004) are associated with increased risk of CAD. The anti-atherogenic functions of HDL and apoA-I have been, to a large extent, attributed to the beneficial effects that HDL exerts on cells of the arterial wall as well as their ability to promote efflux from macrophages and other cells of the arterial wall via ABCA1, ABCG1 and SR-BI (Wang et al., 2007). Hepatic overexpression of apoA-I gene in the background of apoE or LDL_r deficient mice reduced the atherosclerosis burden of these mice following an atherogenic diet (Tangirala et al., 1999). These findings demonstrate the importance of apoA-I and HDL for atheroprotection. In contrast, double deficient mice for apoA-I and the LDL_r fed an atherogenic diet developed atherosclerosis and had increased concentration of circulating auto-anibodies, increased population of T, B, dendritic cells and macrophages, as well as increased T cell proliferation and activation. The abnormal phenotype was corrected by adenovirus mediated gene expression of apoA-I (Wilhelm et al., 2010). Similarly apoA-I transgenic rabbits were resistant to diet induced atherosclerosis (Duverger et al., 1996). Two clinical trials showed that intravenous administration of 15 mg/kg of apoA-I_{MILANO}/phospholipid complexes in five weekly doses in patients with acute coronary syndrome resulted in significant regression of atherosclerosis as it was shown by intravascular ultrasound (Nicholls et al., 2006; Nissen et al., 2003). The epidemiological studies (Gordon et al., 1989), combined with studies of experimental animals (Duverger et al., 1996; Tangirala et al., 1999) and clinical intervention studies (Barter et al., 2007; Sorrentino et al., 2010) highlight the importance of increased HDL levels for atheroprotection. However, human subjects have been identified with high HDL levels and CAD (Ansell et al., 2003). In addition, increased HDL levels in humans treated with the CETP inhibitor torcetrapib, increased cardiovascular, and non-cardiovascular deaths (Barter et al., 2007). These findings suggest that high HDL levels are not always synonymous with atheroprotection. The concept that emerges from all the studies is that the most important factor for atheroprotection is the functionality of HDL. Understanding of the structure-function and the cell signaling associated with HDL and apoA-I will provide molecular explanations for their beneficial effects for atherosclerosis and other human diseases and apoA-I.

6. Conclusion

Numerous prospective epidemiological studies have established an inverse correlation between HDL cholesterol levels and the risk for CAD. However, the discovery of human subjects with high HDL cholesterol levels and CAD, combined with clinical intervention studies designed to raise HDL levels and studies of animal models, led to the realization that high levels of HDL cholesterol alone are not sufficient to prevent atherosclerosis. HDL via its protein and/or lipid components participates in numerous interactions with the endothelium, other cells of the vascular wall, as well as with β pancreatic cells, and has a protective effect against atherothrombosis and other diseases. The key proteins that participate in the biogenesis, remodeling and signaling of HDL are of great importance for the functionality of HDL. Mutations in apoA-I, ABCA1 and LCAT affect the biogenesis of HDL and either prevent formation of HDL or generate aberrant HDL subpopulations which may have altered functions. The ability of HDL to inhibit the oxidation of LDL, prevents the induction of pro-inflammatory and pro-apoptotic pathways that are detrimental to the endothelium. HDL interacts directly with the endothelial cells via SR-BI and the ABCG1. These interactions lead to NO release and vasodilatation, promote reendothelialization and suppress expression of adhesion molecules on endothelial cells in response to pro-inflammatory cytokines. As a result of these and other interactions of the sphingolipid components of HDL with S1P receptors, HDL protects from apoptosis and inflammation and promotes endothelial cell growth and migration. Understanding the complexity and the functions of HDL may facilitate in the near future the development of new HDL-based therapies to prevent or treat atherosclerosis and other human diseases.

7. Acknowledgments

This work was supported by National Institutes of Health Grants HL-48739 and HL-68216. A.K. Kateifides and P. Fotakis are students of the graduate program "The Molecular Basis of Human Disease" of the University of Crete, Medical School and were supported by the Greek Ministry of Education, General Secretariat for Research and Technology Grants PENED 03-780 and HRAKLEITOS II.

8. References

Abderrahmani, A., G. Niederhauser, D. Favre et al., 2007, Human high-density lipoprotein particles prevent activation of the JNK pathway induced by human oxidised low-density lipoprotein particles in pancreatic beta cells: Diabetologia, v. 50, no. 6, p. 1304-1314.

Acton, S., A. Rigotti, K. T. Landschulz et al., 1996, Identification of scavenger receptor SR-BI as a high density lipoprotein receptor: Science, v. 271, no. 5248, p. 518-520.

Amar, M. J., R. D. Shamburek, B. Vaisman et al., 2009, Adenoviral expression of human lecithin-cholesterol acyltransferase in nonhuman primates leads to an antiatherogenic lipoprotein phenotype by increasing high-density lipoprotein and lowering low-density lipoprotein: Metabolism, v. 58, no. 4, p. 568-575.

Ansell, B. J., M. Navab, S. Hama et al., 2003, Inflammatory/antiinflammatory properties of high-density lipoprotein distinguish patients from control subjects better than high-density lipoprotein cholesterol levels and are favorably affected by simvastatin treatment: Circulation, v. 108, no. 22, p. 2751-2756.

Arai, T., N. Wang, M. Bezouevski et al., 1999, Decreased atherosclerosis in heterozygous low density lipoprotein receptor-deficient mice expressing the scavenger receptor BI transgene: J.Biol.Chem., v. 274, no. 4, p. 2366-2371.

Assanasen, C., C. Mineo, D. Seetharam et al., 2005, Cholesterol binding, efflux, and a PDZ-interacting domain of scavenger receptor-BI mediate HDL-initiated signaling: J.Clin.Invest, v. 115, no. 4, p. 969-977.

Asztalos, B. F., L. A. Cupples, S. Demissie et al., 2004, High-density lipoprotein subpopulation profile and coronary heart disease prevalence in male participants of the Framingham Offspring Study: Arterioscler.Thromb.Vasc.Biol., v. 24, no. 11, p. 2181-2187.

Barter, P. J., H. B. Brewer, Jr., M. J. Chapman et al., 2003, Cholesteryl ester transfer protein: a novel target for raising HDL and inhibiting atherosclerosis: Arterioscler.Thromb.Vasc.Biol., v. 23, no. 2, p. 160-167.

Barter, P. J., M. Caulfield, M. Eriksson et al., 2007, Effects of torcetrapib in patients at high risk for coronary events: N.Engl.J.Med., v. 357, no. 21, p. 2109-2122.

Blair, A., P. W. Shaul, I. S. Yuhanna et al., 1999, Oxidized low density lipoprotein displaces endothelial nitric-oxide synthase (eNOS) from plasmalemmal caveolae and impairs eNOS activation: J.Biol.Chem., v. 274, no. 45, p. 32512-32519.

Borhani, D. W., D. P. Rogers, J. A. Engler et al., 1997, Crystal structure of truncated human apolipoprotein A-I suggests a lipid-bound conformation: Proc.Natl.Acad.Sci.U.S.A, v. 94, no. 23, p. 12291-12296.

Braun, A., B. L. Trigatti, M. J. Post et al., 2002, Loss of SR-BI expression leads to the early onset of occlusive atherosclerotic coronary artery disease, spontaneous myocardial infarctions, severe cardiac dysfunction, and premature death in apolipoprotein E-deficient mice: Circ.Res., v. 90, no. 3, p. 270-276.

Breckenridge, W. C., J. A. Little, P. Alaupovic et al., 1982, Lipoprotein abnormalities associated with a familial deficiency of hepatic lipase: Atherosclerosis, v. 45, no. 2, p. 161-179.

Brodeur, M. R., L. Brissette, L. Falstrault et al., 2008, HDL3 reduces the association and modulates the metabolism of oxidized LDL by osteoblastic cells: a protection against cell death: J.Cell Biochem., v. 105, no. 6, p. 1374-1385.

Brunham, L. R., J. K. Kruit, T. D. Pape et al., 2007, Beta-cell ABCA1 influences insulin secretion, glucose homeostasis and response to thiazolidinedione treatment: Nat.Med., v. 13, no. 3, p. 340-347.

Brunham, L. R., R. R. Singaraja, and M. R. Hayden, 2006, Variations on a gene: rare and common variants in ABCA1 and their impact on HDL cholesterol levels and atherosclerosis: Annu.Rev.Nutr., v. 26, p. 105-129.

Brunzell, J. D., and S. S. Deeb, 2001, Familial lipoprotein lipase deficiency, apoC-II deficiency, and hepatic lipase deficiency, in CR Scriver, AL Beaudet, D Valle, and WS Sly eds., The Metabolic & Molecular Bases of Inherited Disease: New York, McGraw-Hill, p. 2789-2816.

Bursill, C. A., M. L. Castro, D. T. Beattie et al., 2010, High-density lipoproteins suppress chemokines and chemokine receptors in vitro and in vivo: Arterioscler.Thromb.Vasc.Biol., v. 30, no. 9, p. 1773-1778.

Christiansen-Weber, T. A., J. R. Voland, Y. Wu et al., 2000, Functional loss of ABCA1 in mice causes severe placental malformation, aberrant lipid distribution, and kidney glomerulonephritis as well as high-density lipoprotein cholesterol deficiency: Am.J.Pathol., v. 157, no. 3, p. 1017-1029.

Chroni, A., A. Duka, H. Y. Kan et al., 2005a, Point mutations in apolipoprotein a-I mimic the phenotype observed in patients with classical lecithin:cholesterol acyltransferase deficiency: Biochemistry, v. 44, no. 43, p. 14353-14366.

Chroni, A., H. Y. Kan, K. E. Kypreos et al., 2004, Substitutions of glutamate 110 and 111 in the middle helix 4 of human apolipoprotein A-I (apoA-I) by alanine affect the structure and in vitro functions of apoA-I and induce severe hypertriglyceridemia in apoA-I-deficient mice: Biochemistry, v. 43, no. 32, p. 10442-10457.

Chroni, A., H. Y. Kan, A. Shkodrani et al., 2005b, Deletions of helices 2 and 3 of human apoA-I are associated with severe dyslipidemia following adenovirus-mediated gene transfer in apoA-I-deficient mice: Biochemistry, v. 44, no. 10, p. 4108-4117.

Chroni, A., G. Koukos, A. Duka et al., 2007, The carboxy-terminal region of apoA-I is required for the ABCA1-dependent formation of alpha-HDL but not prebeta-HDL particles in vivo: Biochemistry, v. 46, no. 19, p. 5697-5708.

Chroni, A., T. Liu, I. Gorshkova et al., 2003, The central helices of apoA-I can promote ATP-binding cassette transporter A1 (ABCA1)-mediated lipid efflux. Amino acid residues 220-231 of the wild-type apoA-I are required for lipid efflux in vitro and high density lipoprotein formation in vivo: J.Biol.Chem., v. 278, no. 9, p. 6719-6730.

Cockerill, G. W., K. A. Rye, J. R. Gamble et al., 1995, High-density lipoproteins inhibit cytokine-induced expression of endothelial cell adhesion molecules: Arterioscler.Thromb.Vasc.Biol., v. 15, no. 11, p. 1987-1994.

Cybulsky, M. I., and M. A. Gimbrone, Jr., 1991, Endothelial expression of a mononuclear leukocyte adhesion molecule during atherogenesis: Science, v. 251, no. 4995, p. 788-791.

de Souza, J. A., C. Vindis, B. Hansel et al., 2008, Metabolic syndrome features small, apolipoprotein A-I-poor, triglyceride-rich HDL3 particles with defective anti-apoptotic activity: Atherosclerosis, v. 197, no. 1, p. 84-94.

de Souza, J. A., C. Vindis, A. Negre-Salvayre et al., 2010, Small, dense HDL 3 particles attenuate apoptosis in endothelial cells: pivotal role of apolipoprotein A-I: J.Cell Mol.Med., v. 14, no. 3, p. 608-620.

Deguchi, H., J. A. Fernandez, and J. H. Griffin, 2002, Neutral glycosphingolipid-dependent inactivation of coagulation factor Va by activated protein C and protein S: Journal of Biological Chemistry, v. 277, no. 11, p. 8861-8865.

Deguchi, H., J. A. Fernandez, I. Pabinger et al., 2001, Plasma glucosylceramide deficiency as potential risk factor for venous thrombosis and modulator of anticoagulant protein C pathway: Blood, v. 97, no. 7, p. 1907-1914.

Deguchi, H., N. M. Pecheniuk, D. J. Elias et al., 2005, High-density lipoprotein deficiency and dyslipoproteinemia associated with venous thrombosis in men: Circulation, v. 112, no. 6, p. 893-899.

Deguchi, H., S. Yegneswaran, and J. H. Griffin, 2004, Sphingolipids as bioactive regulators of thrombin generation: Journal of Biological Chemistry, v. 279, no. 13, p. 12036-12042.

Dimmeler, S., K. Breitschopf, J. Haendeler et al., 1999, Dephosphorylation targets Bcl-2 for ubiquitin-dependent degradation: a link between the apoptosome and the proteasome pathway: J.Exp.Med., v. 189, no. 11, p. 1815-1822.

Dimmeler, S., J. Haendeler, and A. M. Zeiher, 2002, Regulation of endothelial cell apoptosis in atherothrombosis: Curr.Opin.Lipidol., v. 13, no. 5, p. 531-536.

Doggen, C. J. M., N. L. Smith, R. N. Lemaitre et al., 2004, Serum lipid levels and the risk of venous thrombosis: Arteriosclerosis Thrombosis and Vascular Biology, v. 24, no. 10, p. 1970-1975.

Dole, V. S., J. Matuskova, E. Vasile et al., 2008, Thrombocytopenia and platelet abnormalities in high-density lipoprotein receptor-deficient mice: Arterioscler.Thromb.Vasc.Biol., v. 28, no. 6, p. 1111-1116.

Drew, B. G., A. L. Carey, A. K. Natoli et al., 2011, Reconstituted high-density lipoprotein infusion modulates fatty acid metabolism in patients with type 2 diabetes mellitus: Journal of Lipid Research, v. 52, no. 3, p. 572-581.

Drew, B. G., S. J. Duffy, M. F. Formosa et al., 2009, High-Density Lipoprotein Modulates Glucose Metabolism in Patients With Type 2 Diabetes Mellitus: Circulation, v. 119, no. 15, p. 2103-U134.

Drew, B. G., N. H. Fidge, G. Gallon-Beaumier et al., 2004, High-density lipoprotein and apolipoprotein AI increase endothelial NO synthase activity by protein association and multisite phosphorylation: Proc.Natl.Acad.Sci.U.S.A, v. 101, no. 18, p. 6999-7004.

Durand, E., A. Scoazec, A. Lafont et al., 2004, In vivo induction of endothelial apoptosis leads to vessel thrombosis and endothelial denudation - A clue to the understanding of the mechanisms of thrombotic plaque erosion: Circulation, v. 109, no. 21, p. 2503-2506.

Duverger, N., H. Kruth, F. Emmanuel et al., 1996, Inhibition of atherosclerosis development in cholesterol-fed human apolipoprotein A-I-transgenic rabbits: Circulation, v. 94, no. 4, p. 713-717.

Eren, M., C. A. Painter, J. B. Atkinson et al., 2002, Age-dependent spontaneous coronary arterial thrombosis in transgenic mice that express a stable form of human plasminogen activator inhibitor-1: Circulation, v. 106, no. 4, p. 491-496.

Escudero, I., J. Martinez-Gonzalez, R. Alonso et al., 2003, Experimental and interventional dietary study in humans on the role of HDL fatty acid composition in PGI(2) release and Cox-2 expression by VSMC: European Journal of Clinical Investigation, v. 33, no. 9, p. 779-786.

Fielding, C. J., V. G. Shore, and P. E. Fielding, 1972, A protein cofactor of lecithin:cholesterol acyltransferase: Biochem.Biophys.Res.Commun., v. 46, no. 4, p. 1493-1498.

Fleisher, L. N., A. R. Tall, L. D. Witte et al., 1983, Effects of high-density lipoprotein and the apoprotein of high-density lipoprotein on Prostacyclin synthesis by endothelial cells: Advances in Prostaglandin Thromboxane and Leukotriene Research, v. 11, p. 475-480.

Frikke-Schmidt, R., B. G. Nordestgaard, G. B. Jensen et al., 2008, Genetic variation in ABCA1 predicts ischemic heart disease in the general population: Arterioscler.Thromb.Vasc.Biol., v. 28, no. 1, p. 180-186.

Fryirs, M. A., P. J. Barter, M. Appavoo et al., 2010, Effects of High-Density Lipoproteins on Pancreatic beta-Cell Insulin Secretion: Arteriosclerosis Thrombosis and Vascular Biology, v. 30, no. 8, p. 1642-U296.

Gharavi, N. M., N. A. Baker, K. P. Mouillesseaux et al., 2006, Role of endothelial nitric oxide synthase in the regulation of SREBP activation by oxidized phospholipids: Circ.Res., v. 98, no. 6, p. 768-776.

Gomaraschi, M., L. Calabresi, G. Rossoni et al., 2008, Anti-inflammatory and cardioprotective activities of synthetic high-density lipoprotein containing apolipoprotein A-I mimetic peptides: J.Pharmacol.Exp.Ther., v. 324, no. 2, p. 776-783.

Gong, M., M. Wilson, T. Kelly et al., 2003, HDL-associated estradiol stimulates endothelial NO synthase and vasodilation in an SR-BI-dependent manner: J.Clin.Invest, v. 111, no. 10, p. 1579-1587.

Gordon, D. J., J. L. Probstfield, R. J. Garrison et al., 1989, High-density lipoprotein cholesterol and cardiovascular disease. Four prospective American studies: Circulation, v. 79, no. 1, p. 8-15.

Grewal, T., D. de, I, M. F. Kirchhoff et al., 2003, High density lipoprotein-induced signaling of the MAPK pathway involves scavenger receptor type BI-mediated activation of Ras: J.Biol.Chem., v. 278, no. 19, p. 16478-16481.

Griffin, J. H., K. Kojima, C. L. Banka et al., 1999, High-density lipoprotein enhancement of anticoagulant activities of plasma protein S and activated protein C: Journal of Clinical Investigation, v. 103, no. 2, p. 219-227.

Gu, X., K. Kozarsky, and M. Krieger, 2000, Scavenger receptor class B, type I-mediated [3H]cholesterol efflux to high and low density lipoproteins is dependent on lipoprotein binding to the receptor: J.Biol.Chem., v. 275, no. 39, p. 29993-30001.

Haase, C. L., R. Frikke-Schmidt, B. G. Nordestgaard et al., 2011, Mutation in APOA1 predicts increased risk of ischaemic heart disease and total mortality without low HDL cholesterol levels: J.Intern.Med..

Han, R., R. Lai, Q. Ding et al., 2007, Apolipoprotein A-I stimulates AMP-activated protein kinase and improves glucose metabolism: Diabetologia, v. 50, no. 9, p. 1960-1968.

Hao, M., W. S. Head, S. C. Gunawardana et al., 2007, Direct effect of cholesterol on insulin secretion - A novel mechanism for pancreatic beta-cell dysfunction: Diabetes, v. 56, no. 9, p. 2328-2338.

Holm, T. M., A. Braun, B. L. Trigatti et al., 2002, Failure of red blood cell maturation in mice with defects in the high-density lipoprotein receptor SR-BI: Blood, v. 99, no. 5, p. 1817-1824.

Huszar, D., M. L. Varban, F. Rinninger et al., 2000, Increased LDL cholesterol and atherosclerosis in LDL receptor-deficient mice with attenuated expression of scavenger receptor B1: Arterioscler.Thromb.Vasc.Biol., v. 20, no. 4, p. 1068-1073.

Ishida, T., S. Choi, R. K. Kundu et al., 2003, Endothelial lipase is a major determinant of HDL level: J.Clin.Invest, v. 111, no. 3, p. 347-355.

Ishikawa, M., Y. Iwasaki, S. Yatoh et al., 2008, Cholesterol accumulation and diabetes in pancreatic beta-cell-specific SREBP-2 transgenic mice: a new model for lipotoxicity: Journal of Lipid Research, v. 49, no. 12, p. 2524-2534.

Ji, Y., N. Wang, R. Ramakrishnan et al., 1999, Hepatic scavenger receptor BI promotes rapid clearance of high density lipoprotein free cholesterol and its transport into bile: J.Biol.Chem., v. 274, no. 47, p. 33398-33402.

Joyce, C. W., M. J. Amar, G. Lambert et al., 2002, The ATP binding cassette transporter A1 (ABCA1) modulates the development of aortic atherosclerosis in C57BL/6 and apoE-knockout mice: Proc.Natl.Acad.Sci.U.S.A, v. 99, no. 1, p. 407-412.

Kateifides, A. K., I. N. Gorshkova, A. Duka et al., 2011, Alteration of negatively charged residues in the 89 to 99 domain of apoA-I affects lipid homeostasis and maturation of HDL: J.Lipid Res., v. 52, no. 7, p. 1363-1372.

Kennedy, M. A., G. C. Barrera, K. Nakamura et al., 2005, ABCG1 has a critical role in mediating cholesterol efflux to HDL and preventing cellular lipid accumulation: Cell Metab, v. 1, no. 2, p. 121-131.

Kielar, D., W. Dietmaier, T. Langmann et al., 2001, Rapid quantification of human ABCA1 mRNA in various cell types and tissues by real-time reverse transcription-PCR: Clin.Chem., v. 47, no. 12, p. 2089-2097.

Kimura, T., K. Sato, E. Malchinkhuu et al., 2003, High-density lipoprotein stimulates endothelial cell migration and survival through sphingosine 1-phosphate and its receptors: Arterioscler.Thromb.Vasc.Biol., v. 23, no. 7, p. 1283-1288.

Kocher, O., A. Yesilaltay, C. Cirovic et al., 2003, Targeted disruption of the PDZK1 gene in mice causes tissue-specific depletion of the HDL Receptor SR-BI and altered lipoprotein metabolism: J.Biol.Chem., v. 278, p. 52820-52825.

Koseki, M., A. Matsuyama, K. Nakatani et al., 2009, Impaired Insulin Secretion in Four Tangier Disease Patients with ABCA1 Mutations: Journal of Atherosclerosis and Thrombosis, v. 16, no. 3, p. 292-296.

Koukos, G., A. Chroni, A. Duka et al., 2007, LCAT can rescue the abnormal phenotype produced by the natural ApoA-I mutations (Leu141Arg)Pisa and (Leu159Arg)FIN: Biochemistry, v. 46, no. 37, p. 10713-10721.

Krauss, R. M., R. I. Levy, and D. S. Fredrickson, 1974, Selective measurement of two lipase activities in postheparin plasma from normal subjects and patients with hyperlipoproteinemia: J.Clin.Invest, v. 54, no. 5, p. 1107-1124.

Krieger, M., 2001, Scavenger receptor class B type I is a multiligand HDL receptor that influences diverse physiologic systems: J.Clin.Invest, v. 108, no. 6, p. 793-797.

Li, D., B. Yang, and J. L. Mehta, 1998, Ox-LDL induces apoptosis in human coronary artery endothelial cells: role of PKC, PTK, bcl-2, and Fas: Am.J.Physiol, v. 275, no. 2 Pt 2, p. H568-H576.

Li, D. Y., S. Weng, B. C. Yang et al., 1999, Inhibition of arterial thrombus formation by apoA1 Milano: Arteriosclerosis Thrombosis and Vascular Biology, v. 19, no. 2, p. 378-383.

Li, X. A., L. Guo, J. L. Dressman et al., 2005, A novel ligand-independent apoptotic pathway induced by SR-BI and suppressed by eNOS and HDL: J.Biol.Chem., v. 280, p. 19087-19096.

Li, X. A., W. B. Titlow, B. A. Jackson et al., 2002, High density lipoprotein binding to scavenger receptor, Class B, type I activates endothelial nitric-oxide synthase in a ceramide-dependent manner: J.Biol.Chem., v. 277, no. 13, p. 11058-11063.

Li, X. P., S. P. Zhao, X. Y. Zhang et al., 2000, Protective effect of high density lipoprotein on endothelium-dependent vasodilatation: Int.J.Cardiol., v. 73, no. 3, p. 231-236.

Liadaki, K. N., T. Liu, S. Xu et al., 2000, Binding of high density lipoprotein (HDL) and discoidal reconstituted HDL to the HDL receptor scavenger receptor class B type I. Effect of lipid association and APOA-I mutations on receptor binding: J.Biol.Chem., v. 275, no. 28, p. 21262-21271.

Lusa, S., M. Jauhiainen, J. Metso et al., 1996, The mechanism of human plasma phospholipid transfer protein-induced enlargement of high-density lipoprotein particles: evidence for particle fusion: Biochem.J., v. 313 (Pt 1), p. 275-282.

MacCallum, P. K., J. A. Cooper, J. Martin et al., 2000, Haemostatic and lipid determinants of prothrombin fragment F1.2 and D-dimer in plasma: Thrombosis and Haemostasis, v. 83, no. 3, p. 421-426.

Mallat, Z., H. Benamer, B. Hugel et al., 2000, Elevated levels of shed membrane microparticles with procoagulant potential in the peripheral circulating blood of patients with acute coronary syndromes: Circulation, v. 101, no. 8, p. 841-843.

Mardones, P., V. Quinones, L. Amigo et al., 2001, Hepatic cholesterol and bile acid metabolism and intestinal cholesterol absorption in scavenger receptor class B type I-deficient mice: J.Lipid Res., v. 42, no. 2, p. 170-180.

Martinez-Gonzalez, J., I. Escudero, and L. Badimon, 2004, Simvastatin potenciates PGI(2) release induced by HDL in human VSMC: effect on Cox-2 up-regulation and MAPK signalling pathways activated by HDL: Atherosclerosis, v. 174, no. 2, p. 305-313.

Matsunaga, T., Y. Hiasa, H. Yanagi et al., 1991, Apolipoprotein A-I deficiency due to a codon 84 nonsense mutation of the apolipoprotein A-I gene: Proc.Natl.Acad.Sci.U.S.A, v. 88, no. 7, p. 2793-2797.

McNeish, J., R. J. Aiello, D. Guyot et al., 2000, High density lipoprotein deficiency and foam cell accumulation in mice with targeted disruption of ATP-binding cassette transporter-1: Proc.Natl.Acad.Sci.U.S.A, v. 97, no. 8, p. 4245-4250.

Mineo, C., H. Deguchi, J. H. Griffin et al., 2006, Endothelial and antithrombotic actions of HDL: Circ.Res., v. 98, no. 11, p. 1352-1364.

Mineo, C., I. S. Yuhanna, M. J. Quon et al., 2003, High density lipoprotein-induced endothelial nitric-oxide synthase activation is mediated by Akt and MAP kinases: J.Biol.Chem., v. 278, no. 11, p. 9142-9149.

Miura, S., M. Fujino, Y. Matsuo et al., 2003, High density lipoprotein-induced angiogenesis requires the activation of Ras/MAP kinase in human coronary artery endothelial cells: Arterioscler.Thromb.Vasc.Biol., v. 23, no. 5, p. 802-808.

Murphy, A. J., K. J. Woollard, A. Hoang et al., 2008, High-density lipoprotein reduces the human monocyte inflammatory response: Arterioscler.Thromb.Vasc.Biol., v. 28, no. 11, p. 2071-2077.

Murugesan, G., G. Sa, and P. L. Fox, 1994, High-density lipoprotein stimulates endothelial cell movement by a mechanism distinct from basic fibroblast growth factor: Circ.Res., v. 74, no. 6, p. 1149-1156.

Mythreye, K., L. L. Satterwhite, W. S. Davidson et al., 2008, ApoA-I induced CD31 in bone marrow-derived vascular progenitor cells increases adhesion: implications for vascular repair: Biochim.Biophys.Acta, v. 1781, no. 11-12, p. 703-709.

Nakamura, K., M. A. Kennedy, A. Baldan et al., 2004, Expression and regulation of multiple murine ATP-binding cassette transporter G1 mRNAs/isoforms that stimulate cellular cholesterol efflux to high density lipoprotein: J.Biol.Chem., v. 279, no. 44, p. 45980-45989.

Navab, M., S. Y. Hama, G. M. Anantharamaiah et al., 2000a, Normal high density lipoprotein inhibits three steps in the formation of mildly oxidized low density lipoprotein: steps 2 and 3: J.Lipid Res., v. 41, no. 9, p. 1495-1508.

Navab, M., S. Y. Hama, C. J. Cooke et al., 2000b, Normal high density lipoprotein inhibits three steps in the formation of mildly oxidized low density lipoprotein: step 1: J.Lipid Res., v. 41, no. 9, p. 1481-1494.

Nicholls, S. J., B. Cutri, S. G. Worthley et al., 2005a, Impact of short-term administration of high-density lipoproteins and atorvastatin on atherosclerosis in rabbits: Arteriosclerosis Thrombosis and Vascular Biology, v. 25, no. 11, p. 2416-2421.

Nicholls, S. J., G. J. Dusting, B. Cutri et al., 2005b, Reconstituted high-density lipoproteins inhibit the acute pro-oxidant and proinflammatory vascular changes induced by a periarterial collar in normocholesterolemic rabbits: Circulation, v. 111, no. 12, p. 1543-1550.

Nicholls, S. J., E. M. Tuzcu, I. Sipahi et al., 2006, Relationship between atheroma regression and change in lumen size after infusion of apolipoprotein A-I Milano: J.Am.Coll.Cardiol., v. 47, no. 5, p. 992-997.

Nissen, S. E., T. Tsunoda, E. M. Tuzcu et al., 2003, Effect of recombinant ApoA-I Milano on coronary atherosclerosis in patients with acute coronary syndromes: a randomized controlled trial: JAMA, v. 290, no. 17, p. 2292-2300.

Nobecourt, E., F. Tabet, G. Lambert et al., 2010, Nonenzymatic glycation impairs the antiinflammatory properties of apolipoprotein A-I: Arterioscler.Thromb.Vasc.Biol., v. 30, no. 4, p. 766-772.

Nofer, J. R., B. Levkau, I. Wolinska et al., 2001, Suppression of endothelial cell apoptosis by high density lipoproteins (HDL) and HDL-associated lysosphingolipids: J.Biol.Chem., v. 276, no. 37, p. 34480-34485.

Nofer, J. R., G. M. van der, M. Tolle et al., 2004, HDL induces NO-dependent vasorelaxation via the lysophospholipid receptor S1P3: J.Clin.Invest, v. 113, no. 4, p. 569-581.

Nolte, R. T., and D. Atkinson, 1992, Conformational analysis of apolipoprotein A-I and E-3 based on primary sequence and circular dichroism: Biophys.J., v. 63, no. 5, p. 1221-1239.

Noor, R., U. Shuaib, C. X. Wang et al., 2007, High-density lipoprotein cholesterol regulates endothelial progenitor cells by increasing eNOS and preventing apoptosis: Atherosclerosis, v. 192, no. 1, p. 92-99.

Norata, G. D., C. Banfi, A. Pirillo et al., 2004, Oxidised-HDL3 induces the expression of PAI-1 in human endothelial cells. Role of p38MAPK activation and mRNA stabilization: British Journal of Haematology, v. 127, no. 1, p. 97-104.

Norata, G. D., E. Callegari, M. Marchesi et al., 2005, High density lipoproteins induce transforming growth factor-beta2 expression in endothelial cells: Circulation, v. 111, no. 21, p. 2805-2811.

Okajima, F., K. Sato, and T. Kimura, 2009, Anti-atherogenic actions of high-density lipoprotein through sphingosine 1-phosphate receptors and scavenger receptor class B type I: Endocr.J., v. 56, no. 3, p. 317-334.

Okura, H., S. Yamashita, T. Ohama et al., 2010, HDL/Apolipoprotein A-I Binds to Macrophage-Derived Progranulin and Suppresses its Conversion into Proinflammatory Granulins: Journal of Atherosclerosis and Thrombosis, v. 17, no. 6, p. 568-577.

Ou, Z., J. Ou, A. W. Ackerman et al., 2003, L-4F, an apolipoprotein A-1 mimetic, restores nitric oxide and superoxide anion balance in low-density lipoprotein-treated endothelial cells: Circulation, v. 107, no. 11, p. 1520-1524.

Out, R., M. Hoekstra, J. A. Spijkers et al., 2004, Scavenger receptor class B type I is solely responsible for the selective uptake of cholesteryl esters from HDL by the liver and the adrenals in mice: J.Lipid Res., v. 45, no. 11, p. 2088-2095.

Out, R., W. Jessup, W. Le Goff et al., 2008, Coexistence of foam cells and hypocholesterolemia in mice lacking the ABC transporters A1 and G1: Circ.Res., v. 102, no. 1, p. 113-120.

Pajkrt, D., P. G. Lerch, T. vanderPoll et al., 1997, Differential effects of reconstituted high-density lipoprotein on coagulation, fibrinolysis and platelet activation during human endotoxemia: Thrombosis and Haemostasis, v. 77, no. 2, p. 303-307.

Parker, T. S., D. M. Levine, J. C. C. Chang et al., 1995, Reconstituted High-Density-Lipoprotein Neutralizes Gram-Negative Bacterial Lipopolysaccharides in Human Whole-Blood: Infection and Immunity, v. 63, no. 1, p. 253-258.

Patel, S., B. G. Drew, S. Nakhla et al., 2009, Reconstituted high-density lipoprotein increases plasma high-density lipoprotein anti-inflammatory properties and cholesterol efflux capacity in patients with type 2 diabetes: J.Am.Coll.Cardiol., v. 53, no. 11, p. 962-971.

Peters, W., and I. F. Charo, 2001, Involvement of chemokine receptor 2 and its ligand, monocyte chemoattractant protein-1, in the development of atherosclerosis: lessons from knockout mice: Curr Opin Lipidol., v. 12, no. 2, p. 175-180.

Radojkovic, C., A. Genoux, V. Pons et al., 2009, Stimulation of Cell Surface F-1-ATPase Activity by Apolipoprotein A-I Inhibits Endothelial Cell Apoptosis and Promotes Proliferation: Arteriosclerosis Thrombosis and Vascular Biology, v. 29, no. 7, p. 1125-U214.

Ramet, M. E., M. Ramet, Q. Lu et al., 2003, High-density lipoprotein increases the abundance of eNOS protein in human vascular endothelial cells by increasing its half-life: Journal of the American College of Cardiology, v. 41, no. 12, p. 2288-2297.

Remaley, A. T., J. A. Stonik, S. J. Demosky et al., 2001, Apolipoprotein specificity for lipid efflux by the human ABCAI transporter: Biochem.Biophys.Res.Commun., v. 280, no. 3, p. 818-823.

Rigotti, A., B. L. Trigatti, M. Penman et al., 1997, A targeted mutation in the murine gene encoding the high density lipoprotein (HDL) receptor scavenger receptor class B type I reveals its key role in HDL metabolism: Proc.Natl.Acad.Sci.U.S.A, v. 94, no. 23, p. 12610-12615.

Rizzo, M. A., and D. W. Piston, 2003, Regulation of beta cell glucokinase by S-nitrosylation and association with nitric oxide synthase: Journal of Cell Biology, v. 161, no. 2, p. 243-248.

Rutti, S., J. A. Ehses, R. A. Sibler et al., 2009, Low- and high-density lipoproteins modulate function, apoptosis, and proliferation of primary human and murine pancreatic beta-cells: Endocrinology, v. 150, no. 10, p. 4521-4530.

Santamarina-Fojo, S., J. M. Hoeg, G. Assmann, and H. B. Brewer, Jr., 2001, Lecithin cholesterol acyltransferase deficiency and fish eye disease, in CR Scriver, AL Beaudet, WS Sly, and D Valle eds., The Metabolic & Molecular Bases of Inherited Disease: New York, McGraw-Hill, p. 2817-2834.

Savary, S., F. Denizot, M. Luciani et al., 1996, Molecular cloning of a mammalian ABC transporter homologous to Drosophila white gene: Mamm.Genome, v. 7, no. 9, p. 673-676.

Seetharam, D., C. Mineo, A. K. Gormley et al., 2006, High-density lipoprotein promotes endothelial cell migration and reendothelialization via scavenger receptor-B type I: Circulation Research, v. 98, no. 1, p. 63-72.

Silver, D. L., N. Wang, X. Xiao et al., 2001, High density lipoprotein (HDL) particle uptake mediated by scavenger receptor class B type 1 results in selective sorting of HDL cholesterol from protein and polarized cholesterol secretion: J.Biol.Chem., v. 276, no. 27, p. 25287-25293.

Singaraja, R. R., L. R. Brunham, H. Visscher et al., 2003, Efflux and atherosclerosis: the clinical and biochemical impact of variations in the ABCA1 gene: Arterioscler.Thromb.Vasc.Biol., v. 23, no. 8, p. 1322-1332.

Singh, I. P., A. K. Chopra, D. H. Coppenhaver et al., 1999, Lipoproteins account for part of the broad non-specific antiviral activity of human serum: Antiviral Research, v. 42, no. 3, p. 211-218.

Sorci-Thomas, M. G., and M. J. Thomas, 2002, The effects of altered apolipoprotein A-I structure on plasma HDL concentration: Trends Cardiovasc.Med., v. 12, no. 3, p. 121-128.

Sorrentino, S. A., C. Besler, L. Rohrer et al., 2010, Endothelial-vasoprotective effects of high-density lipoprotein are impaired in patients with type 2 diabetes mellitus but are improved after extended-release niacin therapy: Circulation, v. 121, no. 1, p. 110-122.

Stangl, H., M. Hyatt, and H. H. Hobbs, 1999, Transport of lipids from high and low density lipoproteins via scavenger receptor-BI: J.Biol.Chem., v. 274, no. 46, p. 32692-32698.

Strawn, W. B., and C. M. Ferrario, 2002, Mechanisms linking angiotensin II and atherogenesis: Curr.Opin.Lipidol., v. 13, no. 5, p. 505-512.

Suc, I., I. Escargueil-Blanc, M. Troly et al., 1997, HDL and ApoA prevent cell death of endothelial cells induced by oxidized LDL: Arterioscler.Thromb.Vasc.Biol., v. 17, no. 10, p. 2158-2166.

Sugano, M., K. Tsuchida, and N. Makino, 2000, High-density lipoproteins protect endothelial cells from tumor necrosis factor-alpha-induced apoptosis: Biochem.Biophys.Res.Commun., v. 272, no. 3, p. 872-876.

Tabet, F., A. T. Remaley, A. I. Segaliny et al., 2010, The 5A apolipoprotein A-I mimetic peptide displays antiinflammatory and antioxidant properties in vivo and in vitro: Arterioscler.Thromb.Vasc.Biol., v. 30, no. 2, p. 246-252.

Tamagaki, T., S. Sawada, H. Imamura et al., 1996, Effects of high-density lipoproteins on intracellular pH and proliferation of human vascular endothelial cells: Atherosclerosis, v. 123, no. 1-2, p. 73-82.

Tangirala, R. K., K. Tsukamoto, S. H. Chun et al., 1999, Regression of atherosclerosis induced by liver-directed gene transfer of apolipoprotein A-I in mice: Circulation, v. 100, no. 17, p. 1816-1822.

Terasaka, N., M. Westerterp, J. Koetsveld et al., 2010, ATP-binding cassette transporter G1 and high-density lipoprotein promote endothelial NO synthesis through a decrease in the interaction of caveolin-1 and endothelial NO synthase: Arterioscler.Thromb.Vasc.Biol., v. 30, no. 11, p. 2219-2225.

Thuahnai, S. T., S. Lund-Katz, D. L. Williams et al., 2001, Scavenger receptor class B, type I-mediated uptake of various lipids into cells. Influence of the nature of the donor particle interaction with the receptor: J.Biol.Chem., v. 276, no. 47, p. 43801-43808.

Tolle, M., A. Pawlak, M. Schuchardt et al., 2008, HDL-associated lysosphingolipids inhibit NAD(P)H oxidase-dependent monocyte chemoattractant protein-1 production: Arteriosclerosis Thrombosis and Vascular Biology, v. 28, no. 8, p. 1542-1548.

Trigatti, B., H. Rayburn, M. Vinals et al., 1999, Influence of the high density lipoprotein receptor SR-BI on reproductive and cardiovascular pathophysiology: Proc.Natl.Acad.Sci.U.S.A, v. 96, no. 16, p. 9322-9327.

Ueda, Y., L. Royer, E. Gong et al., 1999, Lower plasma levels and accelerated clearance of high density lipoprotein (HDL) and non-HDL cholesterol in scavenger receptor class B type I transgenic mice: J.Biol.Chem., v. 274, no. 11, p. 7165-7171.

Uittenbogaard, A., P. W. Shaul, I. S. Yuhanna et al., 2000, High density lipoprotein prevents oxidized low density lipoprotein-induced inhibition of endothelial nitric-oxide synthase localization and activation in caveolae: Journal of Biological Chemistry, v. 275, no. 15, p. 11278-11283.

Van Eck, M., I. S. Bos, W. E. Kaminski et al., 2002, Leukocyte ABCA1 controls susceptibility to atherosclerosis and macrophage recruitment into tissues: Proc.Natl.Acad.Sci. U.S.A, v. 99, no. 9, p. 6298-6303.

Van Eck, M., R. R. Singaraja, D. Ye et al., 2006, Macrophage ATP-binding cassette transporter A1 overexpression inhibits atherosclerotic lesion progression in low-density lipoprotein receptor knockout mice: Arterioscler.Thromb.Vasc.Biol., v. 26, no. 4, p. 929-934.

Vane, J. R., and R. M. Botting, 1995, Pharmacodynamic Profile of Prostacyclin: American Journal of Cardiology, v. 75, no. 3, p. A3-A10.

Vanhollebeke, B., and E. Pays, 2010, The trypanolytic factor of human serum: many ways to enter the parasite, a single way to kill: Molecular Microbiology, v. 76, no. 4, p. 806-814.

Vantourout, P., C. Radojkovic, L. Lichtenstein et al., 2010, Ecto-F-ATPase: a moonlighting protein complex and an unexpected apoA-I receptor: World J.Gastroenterol., v. 16, no. 47, p. 5925-5935.

Vaughan, A. M., and J. F. Oram, 2005, ABCG1 redistributes cell cholesterol to domains removable by HDL but not by lipid-depleted apolipoproteins: J.Biol.Chem., v. 280, p. 30150-30157.

Vergeer, M., S. J. A. Korporaal, R. Franssen et al., 2011, Genetic Variant of the Scavenger Receptor BI in Humans: New England Journal of Medicine, v. 364, no. 2, p. 136-145.

Vinals, M., J. Martinez-Gonzalez, J. J. Badimon et al., 1997, HDL-induced prostacyclin release in smooth muscle cells is dependent on cyclooxygenase-2 (Cox-2): Arteriosclerosis Thrombosis and Vascular Biology, v. 17, no. 12, p. 3481-3488.

Wang, N., D. Lan, W. Chen et al., 2004, ATP-binding cassette transporters G1 and G4 mediate cellular cholesterol efflux to high-density lipoproteins: Proc.Natl.Acad.Sci. U.S.A, v. 101, no. 26, p. 9774-9779.

Wang, N., D. L. Silver, P. Costet et al., 2000, Specific binding of ApoA-I, enhanced cholesterol efflux, and altered plasma membrane morphology in cells expressing ABC1: J.Biol.Chem., v. 275, no. 42, p. 33053-33058.

Wang, X., H. L. Collins, M. Ranalletta et al., 2007, Macrophage ABCA1 and ABCG1, but not SR-BI, promote macrophage reverse cholesterol transport in vivo: J.Clin.Invest, v. 117, no. 8, p. 2216-2224.

Welch, G. N., and J. Loscalzo, 1998, Homocysteine and atherothrombosis: N.Engl.J.Med., v. 338, no. 15, p. 1042-1050.

Werner, N., S. Junk, U. Laufs et al., 2003, Intravenous transfusion of endothelial progenitor cells reduces neointima formation after vascular injury: Circ.Res., v. 93, p. e17-e24.

Wilhelm, A. J., M. Zabalawi, J. S. Owen et al., 2010, Apolipoprotein A-I modulates regulatory T cells in autoimmune LDLr-/-, ApoA-I-/- mice: J.Biol.Chem., v. 285, no. 46, p. 36158-36169.

Williamson, R., D. Lee, J. Hagaman et al., 1992, Marked reduction of high density lipoprotein cholesterol in mice genetically modified to lack apolipoprotein A-I: Proc.Natl.Acad.Sci.U.S.A, v. 89, no. 15, p. 7134-7138.

Wu, Z., V. Gogonea, X. Lee et al., 2011, The low resolution structure of ApoA1 in spherical high density lipoprotein revealed by small angle neutron scattering: J.Biol.Chem.

Yao, Y., E. S. Shao, M. Jumabay et al., 2008, High-density lipoproteins affect endothelial BMP-signaling by modulating expression of the activin-like kinase receptor 1 and 2: Arterioscler.Thromb.Vasc.Biol., v. 28, no. 12, p. 2266-2274.

Yates, M., A. Kolmakova, Y. Zhao et al., 2011, Clinical impact of scavenger receptor class B type I gene polymorphisms on human female fertility: Hum.Reprod..

Yeh, M., A. L. Cole, J. Choi et al., 2004, Role for sterol regulatory element-binding protein in activation of endothelial cells by phospholipid oxidation products: Circ.Res., v. 95, no. 8, p. 780-788.

Yesilaltay, A., M. G. Morales, L. Amigo et al., 2006, Effects of hepatic expression of the high-density lipoprotein receptor SR-BI on lipoprotein metabolism and female fertility: Endocrinology, v. 147, no. 4, p. 1577-1588.

Yuhanna, I. S., Y. Zhu, B. E. Cox et al., 2001, High-density lipoprotein binding to scavenger receptor-BI activates endothelial nitric oxide synthase: Nat.Med., v. 7, no. 7, p. 853-857.

Yvan-Charvet, L., M. Ranalletta, N. Wang et al., 2007, Combined deficiency of ABCA1 and ABCG1 promotes foam cell accumulation and accelerates atherosclerosis in mice: J.Clin.Invest, v. 117, no. 12, p. 3900-3908.

Zannis, V. I., A. Chroni, and M. Krieger, 2006a, Role of apoA-I, ABCA1, LCAT, and SR-BI in the biogenesis of HDL: J.Mol.Med., v. 84, no. 4, p. 276-294.

Zannis, V. I., A. Chroni, K. E. Kypreos et al., 2004a, Probing the pathways of chylomicron and HDL metabolism using adenovirus-mediated gene transfer: Curr Opin Lipidol., v. 15, no. 2, p. 151-166.

Zannis, V. I., D. Kardassis, and E. E. Zanni, 1993, Genetic mutations affecting human lipoproteins, their receptors, and their enzymes: Adv.Hum.Genet., v. 21, p. 145-319.

Zannis, V. I., K. E. Kypreos, A. Chroni, D. Kardassis, and E. E. Zanni, 2004b, Lipoproteins and atherogenesis, in J Loscalzo ed., Molecular Mechanisms of Atherosclerosis: New York, NY, Taylor & Francis, p. 111-174.

Zannis, V. I., E. E. Zanni, A. Papapanagiotou, D. Kardassis, and A. Chroni, 2006b, ApoA-I functions and synthesis of HDL: Insights from mouse models of human HDL metabolism, High-Density Lipoproteins. From Basic Biology to Clinical Aspects: Weinheim, Wiley-VCH, p. 237-265.

Zeiher, A. M., V. Schachlinger, S. H. Hohnloser et al., 1994, Coronary atherosclerotic wall thickening and vascular reactivity in humans. Elevated high-density lipoprotein levels ameliorate abnormal vasoconstriction in early atherosclerosis: Circulation, v. 89, no. 6, p. 2525-2532.

10

Disrupted VLDL Features and Lipoprotein Metabolism in Sepsis

Patricia Aspichueta, Nerea Bartolomé, Xabier Buqué,
María José Martínez, Begoña Ochoa and Yolanda Chico
Department of Physiology, Faculty of Medicine, University of the Basque Country
Spain

1. Introduction

Gram-negative sepsis is an increasingly clinical syndrome triggered by exposure to bacterial lipopolysaccharide (LPS) or endotoxin. It is associated with a plethora of physiological and biochemical changes, known as acute-phase response (APR), including disturbances in serum lipid and lipoprotein levels (Khovidhunkit et al., 2004). Within the blood, LPS is extracted by the acute phase reactant LPS-binding protein (LBP) and transferred to CD14 receptor on monocytes and macrophages. The CD14 associates with Toll like receptor 4, myeloid differentiation-2 and other proteins forming a receptor cluster that leads to LPS-induced activation (Triantafilou & Triantafilou, 2005), resulting in the release of soluble mediators, such as proinflammatory cytokines.

Kupffer cells (KC), the resident machrophages in the liver, secrete cytokines, particularly tumor necrosis factor α (TNF-α) and the interleukins (IL) IL-6 and IL-1β, that act as paracrine factors on neighboring hepatocytes and promote many of the metabolic changes that accompany the acute-phase response. One of the most striking changes associated to sepsis is the accumulation of triglycerides (TG) within very low density lipoprotein (VLDL) in the plasma, partly ascribed to an increased hepatic VLDL production and a decreased peripheral metabolism driven by pro-inflammatory cytokines. These metabolic alterations, clinically termed as the "lipemia of sepsis", have been postulated to be components of the innate defensive reaction against infection (Harris et al., 2000).

In this chapter we summarize the actual knowledge on sepsis induced alterations in VLDL metabolism, lipids and apoB availability and the involvement of inflammatory mediators.

2. Hiperlipemia of sepsis

Elevation of plasma lipid levels is an early hallmark of sepsis, clinically defined as lipemia of sepsis. The rise in circulating lipids is mainly caused by a rapid accumulation of triglycerides within very low density lipoproteins (Esteve et al., 2005; Khovidhunkit et al., 2004), although other lipids such as non-esterified fatty acids coming from peripheral tissue lipolysis (Khovidhunkit et al., 2004), or cholesterol, in the case of rodents, can also be elevated (Feingold et al., 1993). However, decreases in cholesterol associated to high density lipoproteins (HDL) have been reported as a characteristic associated to sepsis in primates and rodents (Khovidhunkit et al., 2004).

The accumulation of VLDL particles in plasma is attributable to complex disturbances in their metabolism, including increased hepatic production (Feingold et al., 1992; Khovidhunkit et al., 2004; Lanza-Jacoby et al., 1998) and depressed peripheral clearance in the bloodstream by lipoprotein lipase (LPL) depending upon the dose (Feingold et al., 1992; Khovidhunkit et al., 2004; Lanza-Jacoby et al., 1998). Initially, the sepsis-induced hypertriglyceridemia was thought to constitute a mechanism for supplying high-energy substrates to cells involved in host defence (Hardardottir et al., 1994). However, it is increasingly believed that TG-rich lipoproteins are also components of an innate, non-adaptive host immune reaction against infection in humans and animal models (Barcia & Harris, 2005; Harris et al., 2000; Harris et al., 2002).

Both in vitro (Levels et al., 2001; Van Lenten et al., 1986) and in vivo (Kitchens et al., 2003) studies have demonstrated that all lipoprotein classes are able to bind LPS, through their phospholipid (Kitchens et al., 2003) or apolipoprotein (Levels et al., 2001; Vreugdenhil et al., 2001) components, in such a way that lipoprotein-bound LPS is subsequently cleared from the circulation by hepatic parenchymal cells (Harris et al., 2002). Most of the LPS-binding ability corresponds to HDL particles (Levels et al., 2001); however, when levels of VLDL are increased and HDL diminished, as may occur in endotoxemia, the binding appears to shift towards VLDL (Kitchens & Thompson, 2003; Vreugdenhil et al., 2001) and partially depends on interacting with apolipoprotein B (apoB) (Vreugdenhil et al., 2001). Therefore, higher secretion levels of VLDL may be regarded as a protective mechanism against infection. We have shown in LPS-treated rats that plasma VLDL-apoB is rapidly elevated, and this can represent a defence mechanism to neutralize and remove LPS from the circulation (Fig. 1).

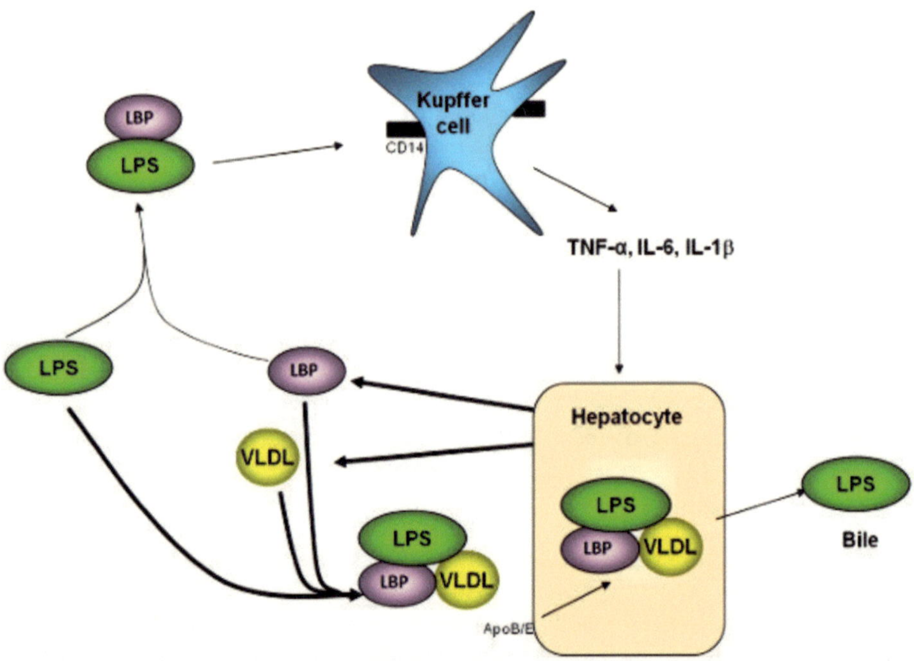

Fig. 1. Proposed role of VLDL in the host inflammatory response. Inflammatory mediators released from Kupffer cells act on hepatocytes inducing the production of VLDL and the synthesis of APR proteins, among them LBP. LBP mediates the binding of LPS to VLDL, the complex is taken up by the hepatocyte and LPS is eliminated through the bile.

Notwithstanding the beneficial role of VLDL, many of the sepsis-associated changes in lipoprotein characteristics and metabolism are similar to those promoting atherogenesis, and has been proposed that the APR associated changes in lipoproteins can be one possible link between infection/inflammation and atherosclerosis. During acute phase reaction, apart from changes in HDL-cholesterol, alterations in HDL associated proteins have been reported. These changes alter cholesterol reverse transport, leading to diminished HDL-cholesterol, and reduce their antioxidant properties (Esteve et al., 2005; Khovidhunkit et al., 2004). In fact, following acute infection low density lipoproteins (LDL) become more susceptible to oxidation (Memon et al., 2000).

One factor that may influence lipoprotein metabolism and is known to be altered during sepsis is food intake (Grunfeld et al., 1996). In order to avoid this variability, animals are food-deprived from the time of administration of endotoxin.

We have shown that endotoxin administration to fasted rats induced hipertriglyceridemia in a time-dependent pattern, related to different systemic fuels (Bartolome et al., 2010). Metabolic background is an important factor contributing to the sepsis-promoted VLDL abundance. We have demonstrated a biphasic response to endotoxin in systemic fuels of fasted rats, with two 12 h differentiated phases. We found that during the first phase serum fatty acids were markedly increased and glucose levels decreased, whereas in the second period hyperglycemia was recorded and fatty acid levels were bellow controls. Impaired glucose metabolism has been reported (McGuinness, 2005). During the second phase of the response we detected increased levels of insulin, that together with the high glucose levels indicate the reported sepsis induced insulin resistance (Andersen et al., 2004). It is well known that overproduction of VLDL is a characteristic of insulin-resistant states (Adeli et al., 2001).

	mean diamenter (nm)	Triglycerides		Cholesterol	
		8 h	18 h	8 h	18 h
VLDL	31,3-64	8,21**	3,16**	3,29***	2,24*
large	44,5-64	9,21***	2,74*	4,69***	2,37*
medium	36,8	6,62***	4,26**	2,89***	2,27*
small	31,3	5,83**	4,18**	1,76	2,00
LDL	16,7-28,6	3,66**	2,88**	0,97	1,36
large	28,6	4,37**	3,49*	1,37	1,78
medium	26,5	3,35**	2,87*	1,19	1,63
small	23	3,08**	2,61*	1,05	1,48
very small	16,7-20,7	3,82**	2,42**	0,83	1,21
HDL	7,6-15	4,64**	1,53*	0,98	0,72*
very large	13,5-15	7,28**	1,93**	1,11	0,72
large	12,1	5,78**	1,80**	1,03	0,69**
medium	10,9	4,15**	1,50**	0,79*	0,75**
small	9,8	4,84***	2,13**	0,83	0,76**
very small	7,6-8,8	4,12**	1,24	0,93	0,79*

Table 1. Fold-changes induced by LPS administration in triglyceride and cholesterol concentration in lipoprotein classes. Rats were injected with LPS and blood collected for lipoprotein triglyceride and total cholesterol measurements.

We analyzed the lipoprotein lipid profile in serum of rats after 8 or 18 h of LPS treatment (Table 1). We found that hypertriglyceridemia was associated with different VLDL, LDL and HDL subclasses depending on the metabolic background of the APR. Although TG increased in all lipoprotein classes, VLDL particles were the major contributors. We did find transient proatherogenic changes in VLDL particles. During the first phase of the APR hypertriglyceridemia was predominantly associated to large VLDL, which were increased 8 fold after 8 h (Bartolome et al., 2010). These large TG-rich VLDL particles, more than normal VLDL, are able to cross the endothelial barrier and interact with lipoprotein receptors in macrophages, initiating a sequence of events that result in the atherosclerotic lesion and, in addition they give rise to small-dense atherogenic LDL (Gianturco et al., 1998; Ginsberg, 2002; Taskinen, 2003). In addition, large TG-rich VLDL were also enriched in cholesterol, making them more proatherogenic.

In the second phase, the rise in serum VLDL-TG corresponded mainly to medium and small VLDL particles. Endotoxin did not affected serum total cholesterol, however changes occurs in lipoprotein subclasses. Total cholesterol increased in large and medium VLDL and HDL-cholesterol levels fell in all HDL subclasses.

3. Altered VLDL metabolism in sepsis

The assembly of VLDL particles is a complex and highly regulated process that occurs in the secretory pathway of hepatocytes. It represents an active export process of fuel carbons, mainly in the form of TG, and is an important route for cholesteryl ester and phospholipid secretion to the circulation. The biogenesis of VLDL has been mostly described as a two step process depending on the cellular availability of lipids, such as triglycerides, phospholipids, cholesterol, and cholesteryl esters, and it is absolutely dependent on the provision of functional apoB, which, in rodents, may be either the full length apoB-100 or the truncated form of apoB-48 (Davidson & Shelness, 2000). Firstly, during translocation to the lumen across the endoplasmic reticulum (ER) membrane, nascent apoB is lipidated by the essential chaperone microsomal triglyceride transfer protein (MTP) (Gordon & Jamil, 2000; Hussain et al., 2003; Liang & Ginsberg, 2001), originating a relatively small, dense, TG-poor lipoprotein particle. In the second stage, bulk of lipidation and final maturation of lipoprotein precursor occur in the ER and post-ER compartments to form mature VLDL (Gusarova et al., 2003; Kulinski et al., 2002). It is known that when MTP activity is low, or when lipid availability or synthesis is reduced, apoB is cotranslationally targeted for ER-associated degradation by both proteasome-dependent and non-dependent pathways (Fisher et al., 2001; Fisher & Ginsberg, 2002; Ginsberg & Fisher, 2009).

The apoB gene has been considered to be constitutively expressed (Pullinger et al., 1989) and VLDL assembly regulation as a post-transcriptional event. However, increasing evidence from in vivo and in vitro studies over the last years has shown changes in hepatic steady-state mRNA levels for apoB in several pathophysiological conditions, particularly under a variety of inflammatory conditions (Jura et al., 2004; Yokoyama et al., 1998).

VLDL secretion rate and composition can be modulated by a variety of factors, such as nutritional state (Gibbons & Burnham, 1991), endotoxin and proinflammatory cytokines (Aspichueta et al., 2006; Bartolome et al., 2007; Perez et al., 2006). Different mechanisms may be involved in the sepsis enhanced VLDL secretion (Fig. 2).

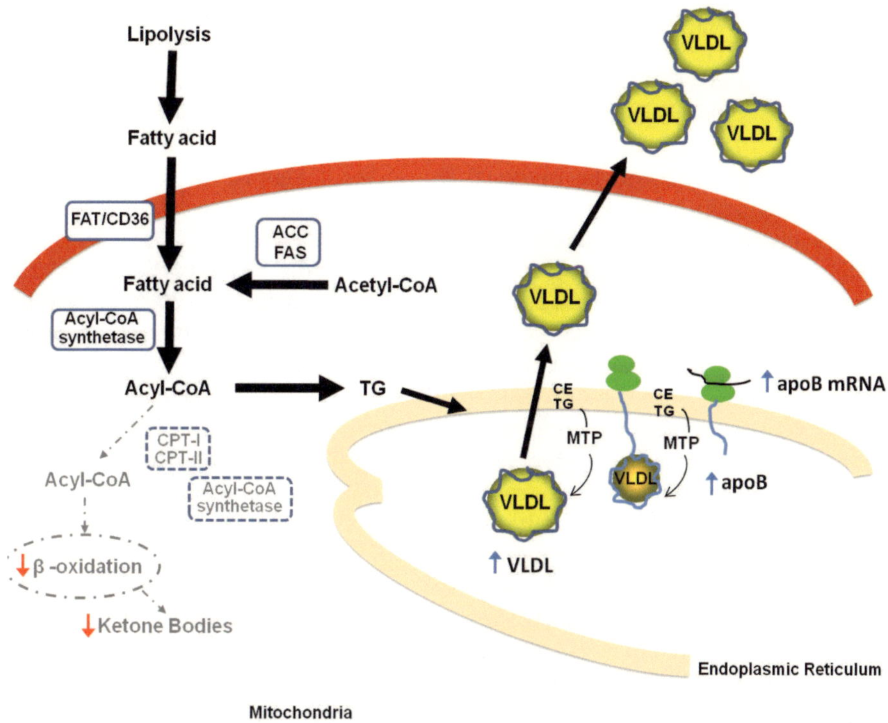

Fig. 2. Model of VLDL assembly and secretion during sepsis. FAT, fatty acid translocase; FAS, fatty acid synthase; ACC, Acetyl-CoA carboxylase; CPT, carnitine acyltransferase. Solid and blue arrows indicate increases, discontinuous and red arrows indicate decreases.

Our results suggest that specific mechanisms are involved in the temporal response to sepsis. In LPS treated rats we found that both fatty acids and hypertriglyceridemia, associated with VLDL-TG, peaked after 8 hours of endotoxin contact. During inflammation adipose tissue lipolysis is activated by pro-inflammatory mediators (Khovidhunkit et al., 2004; Zu et al., 2009) providing fatty acids for hepatic triglyceride synthesis, thus promoting VLDL secretion (Lanza-Jacoby et al., 1998). It has been reported that LPS enhance the expression of fatty acid translocase FAT/CD36, involved in fatty acid uptake (Memon et al., 1998a) and that endotoxin and cytokines suppressed mitochondrial acyl-CoA synthetase expression and activity (Memon et al., 1998b) but enhanced microsomal acyl-CoA synthetase. In addition, LPS administration to rats led to reduced carnitine acyltransferase I, lower ketogenic capacity (Takeyama et al., 1990) and decreased levels of serum ketone bodies (Bartolome et al., 2010). Evidences also established a relationship between increased de novo fatty acid synthesis and enhanced secretion of VLDL-TG in rodents treated with LPS or cytokines (Feingold et al., 1992; Lanza-Jacoby & Tabares, 1990). Taken all together, high amounts of fatty acids are directed away from mitochondrial oxidation and are available for their esterification into TG and secreted within VLDL. However, previous works done in our laboratory did not support the proposed hypothesis since levels of fatty acid synthase mRNA or rate of TG synthesis measured as the incorporation of [^{3}H]acetate or [^{3}H]oleate did not change after 18 h of LPS treatment (Aspichueta et al., 2006).

The high availability of lipids in the septic hepatocyte would protect apoB from degradation leading to an increased number of secreted VLDL particles (Phetteplace et al., 2000). In fact, we detected an elevation of 5 fold in the number of circulating VLDL particles, measured as apoB quantities, at 8 h from LPS administration, without any modification in apoB transcript level. The increment in VLDL-TG is of greater magnitude (8 fold), indicating that during the first phase of the septic response TG-rich VLDL particles accumulate in the circulation (Bartolome et al., 2010).

Different mechanisms seem to be involved in the second phase of septic response. The serum fatty levels drop below controls, which would suggest a lower availability of fatty acids of extrahepatic origin for hepatic VLDL-TG secretion.

Endotoxic rats showed a higher number (10 fold) of circulating VLDL particles in rats at 18 h, but the content of the lipid in each VLDL is reduced (Aspichueta et al., 2006; Bartolome et al., 2010). This was accompanied by high levels of *apob* gene transcript, which could provide for high apoB availability increasing the secretion of lipid poor VLDL particles. Using intact rats in the fasted state, injected with the LPL inhibitor Triton WR-1339, we have shown that the TG and cholesterol secreted into VLDL released by the liver to the blood in 2 h was not enhanced by LPS administration to the same extent as the VLDL-apoB production was (Aspichueta et al., 2005). In this way, hepatocytes isolated from 18 hour LPS-treated rats secreted TG-poor VLDL, and although secretion was highly stimulated, global triglyceride secretion in VLDL remained unchanged. This was related to unchanged rates of fatty acid esterification, measured as [^{3}H]oleate incorporation into TG (Aspichueta et al., 2005; Aspichueta et al., 2006).

In septic hypertriglyceridemic rats, 24 h after sepsis induction, the increase in plasma TG was associated to a decrease in VLDL-TG clearance rate, due to suppressed mRNA levels, protein mass and activity of LPL in peripheral tissues (Lanza-Jacoby et al., 1997; Lanza-Jacoby & Tabares, 1990). Thus, in the early phase of the septic reaction hypertriglyceridemia is mostly due to high VLDL secretion driven by availability of lipids in the hepatocyte; and during the second phase, hypertriglyceridemia would be the result of LPL inhibition, and the increase in apoB transcription would be responsible for the increased secretion of VLDL particles (Fig.3).

4. Zonation of VLDL secretion during sepsis

It has been suggested that parenchymal capacity for VLDL secretion is zonated. Zonation refers to a phenotypic heterogeneity that is well established in many essential liver functions (Jungermann & Katz, 1989). While some authors suggested that VLDL secretion might be higher in perivenous (PV) hepatocytes because of their higher capacity for fatty acid synthesis (Guzman & Castro, 1989), others proposed that it could be concentrated in the periportal (PP) area (Kang & Davis, 2000) since higher expression of the cholesterol synthesis rate-limiting enzyme 3-hydroxy-3-methylglutaryl-CoA reductase was found (Singer et al., 1984).

Zonation has also been evidenced in non parenchymal liver cells. Kupffer cells are more abundant and larger in the PP than in the PV zone (Bouwens et al., 1992), and expression of IL-6, a key cytokine acting on hepatocytes in response to endotoxin, occur preferentially in the PP region (Fang et al., 1998).

After 18 h of endotoxin treatment, highly pure rat PP and PV hepatocyte subpopulations, assessed by cytometry, were maintained in suspension for 2 h. Endotoxin treatment provoked zonation of VLDL secretion. The induction in VLDL-apoB secretion was markedly higher in PP hepatocytes (~90%) than in PV cells (~38%). In addition, the increase in the VLDL associated lipid, particularly in triglycerides, was lower than the enhance in apoB output, consequently producing changes in VLDL features which were triglyceride poor (Aspichueta et al., 2005). Endotoxin doubled apoB mRNA and increased by 50% MTP mRNA in PP hepatocytes when compared to their fasted controls, the increase in apoB genetic expression was of a lesser extend in PV cells. Regarding to de novo synthesis of lipids for VLDL assembly, the incorporation of [^{3}H]acetate into TG and cholesterol did not change by endotoxin challenge.

We concluded that periportal and perivenous hepatocytes exhibited similar capabilities for VLDL assembly and secretion in normal conditions; and, only the endotoxic condition led PP hepatocytes to a marked increase in TG-poor VLDL secretion (Fig 4).

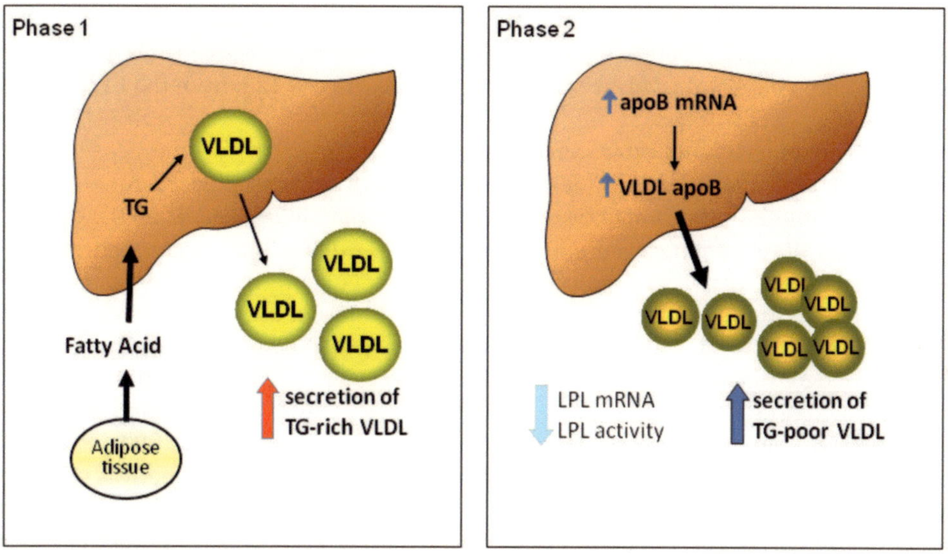

Fig. 3. Proposed model for the biphasic response to endotoxin in VLDL metabolism. In the first phase the stimulation of lipolysis provides fatty acids that are taken by the liver and esterified to be secreted into TG-rich VLDL. In the second phase apoB mRNA levels are increased providing the apolipoprotein for secretion of TG-poor VLDL.

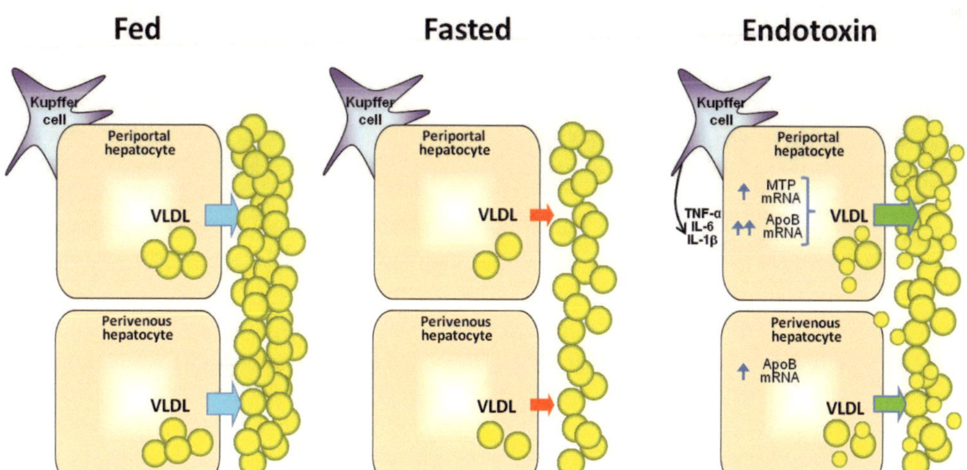

Fig. 4. Model of VLDL secretion by periportal and perivenous hepatocytes in fed state and 18 h after fasting or endotoxin treatment. Endotoxin effect when compared with the fasted state is marked with ⇨

5. Kupffer cell mediators and VLDL secretion

During the acute phase of the septic response, Kupffer cells, the resident macrophages in the liver, release a plethora of soluble bioactive molecules, among them soluble pro-inflammatory mediators as cytokines, particularly TNF-α, IL-6 and IL-1β. These cytokines would act locally on nearby hepatocytes as paracrine factors promoting VLDL secretion and many other metabolic changes that accompany the inflammatory reaction.

We confirmed a rapid release of TNF-α and IL-6 into the bloodstream in rats after 2 h of LPS injection (1 mg/Kg bw), whereas the IL-1β maximum level was observed at 6 h and the rise was less accentuated. Basal levels were recovered in all cases at 12 h from the LPS treatment (Bartolome et al., 2008).

Administration of cytokines to animals has been shown to mimic the sepsis induced alterations in lipid metabolism. TNF-α, IL-6 and IL-1β administered to rodents induce triglyceride synthesis and promote rises in VLDL-TG (Khovidhunkit et al., 2004). In the case of TNF-α and IL-6 administration, the hypertriglyceridemia has been reported to be secondary to higher lipolysis in peripheral tissues; consequently more fatty acids in blood are available and can be recruited by liver. In some studies, the three cytokines have been shown to stimulate hepatic de novo fatty acid synthesis (Feingold et al., 1989) and TG secretion (Feingold et al., 1991; Nonogaki et al., 1995), and decrease adipose tissue LPL activity (Feingold et al., 1994; Popa et al., 2007). Nevertheless, the reduction in LPL was delayed several hours with respect to hypertriglyceridemia (Esteve et al., 2005; Popa et al., 2007) and blockade of TNF-α or IL-6 function in septic mice inhibited hypertriglyceridemia without affecting LPL activity (Feingold et al., 1994).

In order to address the role of Kupffer cells in VLDL oversecretion during endotoxemia, we analyzed the response of rat primary hepatocytes to the direct effect of LPS-stimulated KC or unstimulated products. Hepatocytes were cultured for 8 h with the conditioned medium containing the mediators generated in 16 h by Kupffer cells after a previous 4 h culture with or without LPS. The exposure of hepatocytes to unstimulated KC conditioned medium resulted in doubled the secretion VLDL particles of normal composition. Cells cultured in LPS stimulated KC medium secreted further more VLDL particles that were enriched in PL (Bartolome et al., 2008). Regarding to apoB expression, KC products multiplied by two the abundance of apoB mRNA and no further increment was caused by specific LPS-triggered products. In any case was MTP mRNA modified. The high PL available would protect apoB from degradation, explaining the increase in apoB secretion in cells challenged by LPS-KC medium.

There are few studies investigating the direct effect of cytokines on VLDL secretion, and contradictory results have been reported using different cell types. In HepG2 cells IL-6 and IL-1β were found to reduce apoB secretion although apoB mRNA levels were increased (Yokoyama et al., 1998). However, in IL-6 treated murine hepatocytes, enhanced apoB synthesis, which corresponded with high apoB mRNA levels, was found to be the primary mechanism for increased lipoprotein secretion (Sparks et al., 2010). They also found that IL-6 did not alter the decay rate of apoB mRNA transcripts, concluding that it favours secretion of apoB-containing lipoproteins by increasing availability of apoB through changes in *apob* gene transcription (Sparks et al., 2010).

Our studies in rat hepatocyte cultures, have demonstrated that the inflammatory cytokines TNF-α, IL-6 and IL-1β, over a wide range of concentrations, enhanced VLDL-apoB secretion linked to upregulation of apoB mRNA expression (Bartolome et al., 2007; Bartolome et al.,

2008; Perez et al., 2006). IL-1β was the most potent and was the only one presenting a dose-response effect. The effect of the three cytokines was redundant, as the increase was not additive when they were combined. However, none of the treatments with cytokines modified the amount of TG and total lipids secreted as components of VLDL, suggesting that these particles are lipid poor.

We conclude that Kupffer cells play a role in the rise of VLDL secretion detected during the inflammatory processes and that the three cytokines TNF-α, IL-6 and IL-1β may be involved, nevertheless other Kupffer cells mediators are necessary to accomplish increased lipid association.

6. Higher apoB availability within the hepatocytes

As stated before, the assembly of VLDL is a complex process that depends on the availability of lipids and apoB (Davidson & Shelness, 2000).

Since we have found that under LPS treatment VLDL-apoB secretion was always increased, and given that not always enhanced apoB secretion is linked to high levels of apoB transcript, we hypothesized that during the acute phase response, transcriptional or post-transcriptional regulation affecting apoB mRNA levels might occur supplying more apoB for VLDL assembly.

During the first phase of the septic response we detected elevated circulating VLDL-apoB and -TG after 8 h of LPS treatment without altered apoB transcript levels. Taking into account that at this time point of the septic response, circulating fatty acid levels were elevated, we propose that fatty acid uptake by the liver is increased and large amounts of TG are synthesized. Since the N-terminus of apoB acquires neutral lipids in the endoplasmic reticulum membrane (Hussain et al., 2008), more nucleation sites are expected to be generated in apoB leading to increased apoB secretion. This could result in an increased hepatic secretion of triglycerides in VLDL particles, which would accumulate in the circulation, even in the absence of augmented levels of hepatic apoB mRNA (Bartolome et al., 2010).

In the second phase of the septic response, after 18 h of LPS challenge, enhanced VLDL-apoB secretion is accompanied by increased apoB mRNA levels (Bartolome et al., 2010). In addition, hepatocytes isolated 18 h after LPS administration presented higher levels of apoB transcript and secreted more VLDL particles, been this effect more marked in PP cells. At this time point of the septic response, lipid poor VLDL particles are secreted (Aspichueta et al., 2005) and lipid synthesis is not modified (Aspichueta et al., 2006). Therefore, the increase in *apob* gene transcript would provide the additional apoB necessary to enhance VLDL-apoB secretion. Similarly, the inflammatory cytokines TNF-α (Bartolome et al., 2007), IL1-β (Bartolome et al., 2010) and IL-6 (Perez et al., 2006) augmented the levels of apoB mRNA and secretion of VLDL particles without changing the amounts of lipid secreted in the VLDL.

Our hypothesis was that endotoxin-enhanced VLDL-apoB secretion was driven by higher transcription rates. However, we did not find a rise in transcription rate of *apob* gene when we measured the incorporation of 5′-[α-^{32}P]-UTP into newly synthesized RNA in liver nuclei from 16 h LPS-treated rats (Bartolome et al., 2010). We reported that global transcription rate in endotoxic liver was nearly two times higher than in control rats as expected in the acute phase response for up-regulating the positive proteins. However, the transcription rate of apoB gene was unaffected after 16 h of LPS challenge in the treated animals. It cannot be discarded that transcriptional activation may occur transiently during other stages of the APR.

Another aspect involved in regulating mRNA level is the modulation of mRNA stability through regulatory elements residing in the 3'- and 5'-untranslated region (UTR) and adequate RNA binding proteins. HuR is an important protein in stabilizing inflammatory AU-rich elements (ARE)-bearing RNAs. Human apoB mRNA has been reported to contain ARE sequences at 3'-UTRs and bioinformatic analysis of rat apoB transcript revealed the presence of AU-rich regions. Our results demonstrated the specific binding of stabilizing HuR protein to the rat apoB mRNA, although there were no superior binding in livers from LPS treated rats. Consequently, in our conditions it is not likely that apoB mRNA half-life was extended by HuR binding, but we can not discard a role for other stabilizing proteins or changes in the mRNA degradation pathway, but further analysis is need (Fig 5).

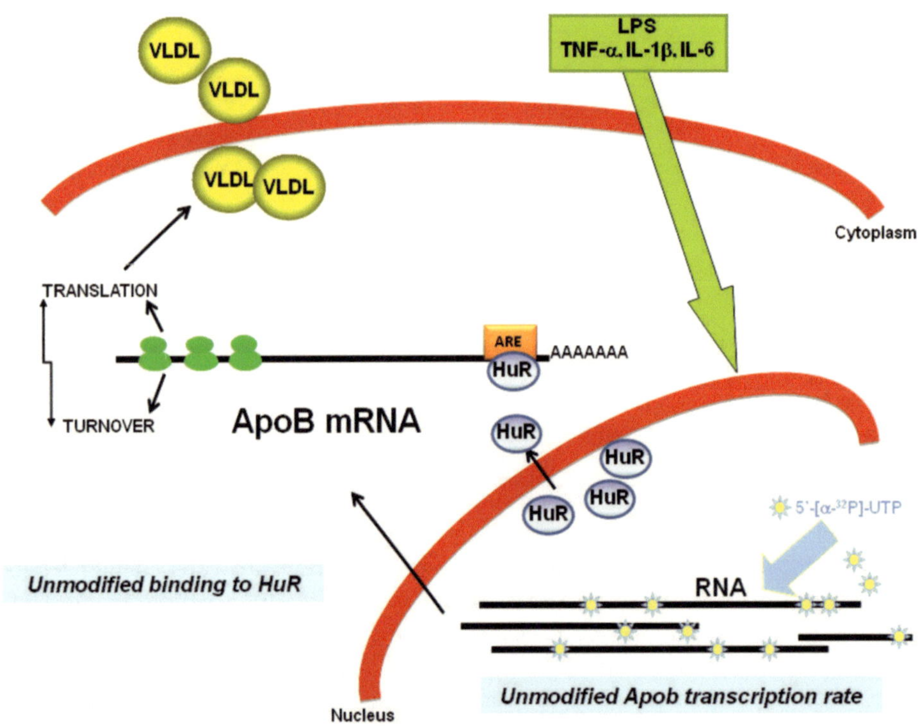

Fig. 5. Endotoxin induce increase in apoB mRNA without altering transcription rate or HuR protein binding.

7. Conclusion

During the septic response, altered VLDL metabolism is responsible for the lipemia of sepsis. Entotoxin promoted changes are biphasic. In the early stage hypertriglyceridemia is accompanied by increased circulating fatty acids levels and a rise in large TG-rich VLDL, whereas the later stage is characterized by high levels of hepatic apoB transcript and TG-poor VLDL accumulation. In the later stage, the endotoxin induced VLDL secretion is more accentuated in periportal cells. Kupffer cells released products directly promote VLDL assembly and secretion and increase apoB mRNA levels, among these products the cytokines TNF–α, IL-6 and IL-1β and other mediator/s could play a role in the enhancement of VLD secretion.

8. Acknowledgments

This work was supported by the Basque Government (IT336-10).

9. References

Adeli, K., Taghibiglou, C., Van Iderstine, SC., & Lewis, GF. (2001). Mechanisms of hepatic very low-density lipoprotein overproduction in insulin resistance. *Trends Cardiovasc. Med.*, Vol.11, No.5, pp. 170-176, ISSN 1050-1738

Andersen, SK., Gjedsted, J., Christiansen, C., & Tonnesen, E. (2004). The roles of insulin and hyperglycemia in sepsis pathogenesis. *J. Leukoc. Biol.*, Vol.75, No.3, pp. 413-421, ISSN 0741-5400

Aspichueta, P., Perez, S., Ochoa, B., & Fresnedo, O. (2005). Endotoxin promotes preferential periportal upregulation of VLDL secretion in the rat liver. *J. Lipid Res*, Vol.46, No.5, pp. 1017-1026, ISSN 0022-2275

Aspichueta, P., Perez-Agote, B., Perez, S., Ochoa, B., & Fresnedo, O. (2006). Impaired response of VLDL lipid and apoB secretion to endotoxin in the fasted rat liver. *J. Endotoxin. Res*, Vol.12, No.3, pp. 181-192, ISSN 0968-0519

Barcia, AM&Harris, HW. (2005). Triglyceride-rich lipoproteins as agents of innate immunity. *Clin. Infect. Dis.*, Vol.41 Suppl 7pp. S498-S503, ISSN 1058-4838

Bartolome, N., Arteta, B., Martinez, MJ., Chico, Y., & Ochoa, B. (2008). Kupffer cell products and interleukin 1beta directly promote VLDL secretion and apoB mRNA up-regulation in rodent hepatocytes. *Innate Immun.*, Vol.14, No.4, pp. 255-266, ISSN 1753-4259

Bartolome, N., Aspichueta, P., Martinez, MJ., Vazquez-Chantada, M., Martinez-Chantar, ML., Ochoa, B., & Chico, Y. (2010). Biphasic adaptative responses in VLDL metabolism and lipoprotein homeostasis during Gram-negative endotoxemia. *Innate. Immun.*, ISSN 1753-4259 Epub ahead of print

Bartolome, N., Rodriguez, L., Martinez, MJ., Ochoa, B., & Chico, Y. (2007). Upregulation of apolipoprotein B secretion, but not lipid, by tumor necrosis factor-alpha in rat hepatocyte cultures in the absence of extracellular fatty acids. *Ann. N. Y Acad. Sci.*, Vol.1096, pp. 55-69, ISSN 0077-8923

Bouwens, L., De, BP., Vanderkerken, K., Geerts, B., & Wisse, E. (1992). Liver cell heterogeneity: functions of non-parenchymal cells. *Enzyme*, Vol.46, No.1-3, pp. 155-168, ISSN 0013-9432

Davidson, NO&Shelness, GS. (2000). APOLIPOPROTEIN B: mRNA editing, lipoprotein assembly, and presecretory degradation. *Annu. Rev. Nutr.*, Vol.20pp. 169-193, ISSN 0199-9885

Esteve, E., Ricart, W., & Fernandez-Real, JM. (2005). Dyslipidemia and inflammation: an evolutionary conserved mechanism. *Clin. Nutr.*, Vol.24, No.1, pp. 16-31, ISSN 0261-5614

Fang, C., Lindros, KO., Badger, TM., Ronis, MJ., & Ingelman-Sundberg, M. (1998). Zonated expression of cytokines in rat liver: effect of chronic ethanol and the cytochrome P450 2E1 inhibitor, chlormethiazole. *Hepatology*, Vol.27, No.5, pp. 1304-1310, ISSN 0270-9139

Feingold, KR., Hardardottir, I., Memon, R., Krul, EJ., Moser, AH., Taylor, JM., & Grunfeld, C. (1993). Effect of endotoxin on cholesterol biosynthesis and distribution in serum lipoproteins in Syrian hamsters. *J. Lipid Res.*, Vol.34, No.12, pp. 2147-2158, ISSN 0022-2275

Feingold, KR., Marshall, M., Gulli, R., Moser, AH., & Grunfeld, C. (1994). Effect of endotoxin and cytokines on lipoprotein lipase activity in mice. *Arterioscler. Thromb.*, Vol.14, No.11, pp. 1866-1872, ISSN 1049-8834

Feingold, KR., Soued, M., Adi, S., Staprans, I., Neese, R., Shigenaga, J., Doerrler, W., Moser, A., Dinarello, CA., & Grunfeld, C. (1991). Effect of interleukin-1 on lipid metabolism in the rat. Similarities to and differences from tumor necrosis factor. *Arterioscler. Thromb.*, Vol.11, No.3, pp. 495-500, ISSN 1049-8834

Feingold, KR., Soued, M., Serio, MK., Moser, AH., Dinarello, CA., & Grunfeld, C. (1989). Multiple cytokines stimulate hepatic lipid synthesis in vivo. *Endocrinology*, Vol.125, No.1, pp. 267-274, ISSN 0013-7227

Feingold, KR., Staprans, I., Memon, RA., Moser, AH., Shigenaga, JK., Doerrler, W., Dinarello, CA., & Grunfeld, C. (1992). Endotoxin rapidly induces changes in lipid metabolism that produce hypertriglyceridemia: low doses stimulate hepatic triglyceride production while high doses inhibit clearance. *J. Lipid Res*, Vol.33, No.12, pp. 1765-1776, ISSN 0022-2275

Fisher, EA&Ginsberg, HN. (2002). Complexity in the secretory pathway: the assembly and secretion of apolipoprotein B-containing lipoproteins. *J Biol Chem.*, Vol.277, No.20, pp. 17377-17380, ISSN 0021-9258

Fisher, EA., Pan, M., Chen, X., Wu, X., Wang, H., Jamil, H., Sparks, JD., & Williams, KJ. (2001). The triple threat to nascent apolipoprotein B. Evidence for multiple, distinct degradative pathways. *J. Biol. Chem.*, Vol.276, No.30, pp. 27855-27863, ISSN 0021-9258

Gianturco, SH., Ramprasad, MP., Song, R., Li, R., Brown, ML., & Bradley, WA. (1998). Apolipoprotein B-48 or its apolipoprotein B-100 equivalent mediates the binding of triglyceride-rich lipoproteins to their unique human monocyte-macrophage receptor. *Arterioscler. Thromb. Vasc. Biol.*, Vol.18, No.6, pp. 968-976, ISSN 1079-5642

Gibbons, GF&Burnham, FJ. (1991). Effect of nutritional state on the utilization of fatty acids for hepatitic triacylglycerol synthesis and secretion as very-low-density lipoprotein. *Biochem. J.*, Vol.275 (Pt 1)pp. 87-92, ISSN 0264-6021

Ginsberg, HN (2002). New perspectives on atherogenesis: role of abnormal triglyceride-rich lipoprotein metabolism. *Circulation*, Vol.106, No.16, pp. 2137-2142, ISSN 0009-7322

Ginsberg, HN&Fisher, EA. (2009). The ever-expanding role of degradation in the regulation of apolipoprotein B metabolism. *J. Lipid Res.*, Vol.50 Supplpp. S162-S166, ISSN 0022-2275

Gordon, DA&Jamil, H. (2000). Progress towards understanding the role of microsomal triglyceride transfer protein in apolipoprotein-B lipoprotein assembly. *Biochim. Biophys. Acta*, Vol.1486, No.1, pp. 72-83, ISSN 0006-3002

Grunfeld, C., Zhao, C., Fuller, J., Pollack, A., Moser, A., Friedman, J., & Feingold, KR. (1996). Endotoxin and cytokines induce expression of leptin, the ob gene product, in hamsters. *J. Clin. Invest.*, Vol.97, No.9, pp. 2152-2157, ISSN 0021-9738

Gusarova, V., Brodsky, JL., & Fisher, EA. (2003). Apolipoprotein B100 exit from the endoplasmic reticulum (ER) is COPII-dependent, and its lipidation to very low density lipoprotein occurs post-ER. *J. Biol. Chem.*, Vol.278, No.48, pp. 48051-48058, ISSN 0021-9258

Guzman, M&Castro, J. (1989). Zonation of fatty acid metabolism in rat liver. *Biochem. J.*, Vol.264, No.1, pp. 107-113, ISSN 0264-6021

Hardardottir, I., Grunfeld, C., & Feingold, KR. (1994). Effects of endotoxin and cytokines on lipid metabolism. *Curr. Opin. Lipidol.*, Vol.5, No.3, pp. 207-215, ISSN 0957-9672

Harris, HW., Gosnell, JE., & Kumwenda, ZL. (2000). The lipemia of sepsis: triglyceride-rich lipoproteins as agents of innate immunity. *J Endotoxin. Res.*, Vol.6, No.6, pp. 421-430, ISSN 0968-0519

Harris, HW., Johnson, JA., & Wigmore, SJ. (2002). Endogenous lipoproteins impact the response to endotoxin in humans. *Crit Care Med.*, Vol.30, No.1, pp. 23-31, ISSN 0090-3493

Hussain, MM., Rava, P., Pan, X., Dai, K., Dougan, SK., Iqbal, J., Lazare, F., & Khatun, I. (2008). Microsomal triglyceride transfer protein in plasma and cellular lipid metabolism. *Curr. Opin. Lipidol.*, Vol.19, No.3, pp. 277-284, ISSN 0957-9672

Hussain, MM., Shi, J., & Dreizen, P. (2003). Microsomal triglyceride transfer protein and its role in apoB-lipoprotein assembly. *J Lipid. Res.*, Vol.44, No.1, pp. 22-32, ISSN 0957-9672

Jungermann, K&Katz, N. (1989). Functional specialization of different hepatocyte populations. *Physiol. Rev.*, Vol.69, No.3, pp. 708-764, ISSN 0031-9333

Jura, J., Wegrzyn, P., Zarebski, A., Wladyka, B., & Koj, A. (2004). Identification of changes in the transcriptome profile of human hepatoma HepG2 cells stimulated with interleukin-1 beta. *Biochim. Biophys. Acta*, Vol.1689, No.2, pp. 120-133, ISSN 0006-3002

Kang, S&Davis, RA. (2000). Cholesterol and hepatic lipoprotein assembly and secretion. *Biochim. Biophys. Acta*, Vol.1529, No.1-3, pp. 223-230, ISSN 0006-3002

Khovidhunkit, W., Kim, MS., Memon, RA., Shigenaga, JK., Moser, AH., Feingold, KR., & Grunfeld, C. (2004). Effects of infection and inflammation on lipid and lipoprotein metabolism: mechanisms and consequences to the host. *J. Lipid Res*, Vol.45, No.7, pp. 1169-1196, ISSN 0022-2275

Kitchens, RL&Thompson, PA. (2003). Impact of sepsis-induced changes in plasma on LPS interactions with monocytes and plasma lipoproteins: roles of soluble CD14, LBP, and acute phase lipoproteins. *J. Endotoxin. Res*, Vol.9, No.2, pp. 113-118, ISSN 0968-0519

Kitchens, RL., Thompson, PA., Munford, RS., & O'Keefe, GE. (2003). Acute inflammation and infection maintain circulating phospholipid levels and enhance lipopolysaccharide binding to plasma lipoproteins. *J. Lipid Res*, Vol.44, No.12, pp. 2339-2348, ISSN 0022-2275

Kulinski, A., Rustaeus, S., & Vance, JE. (2002). Microsomal triacylglycerol transfer protein is required for lumenal accretion of triacylglycerol not associated with ApoB, as well as for ApoB lipidation. *J Biol Chem.*, Vol.277, No.35, pp. 31516-31525, ISSN 0021-9258

Lanza-Jacoby, S., Phetteplace, H., Sedkova, N., & Knee, G. (1998). Sequential alterations in tissue lipoprotein lipase, triglyceride secretion rates, and serum tumor necrosis factor alpha during Escherichia coli bacteremic sepsis in relation to the development of hypertriglyceridemia. *Shock*, Vol.9, No.1, pp. 46-51, ISSN 1073-2322

Lanza-Jacoby, S., Sedkova, N., Phetteplace, H., & Perrotti, D. (1997). Sepsis-induced regulation of lipoprotein lipase expression in rat adipose tissue and soleus muscle. *J. Lipid Res.*, Vol.38, No.4, pp. 701-710, ISSN 0022-2275

Lanza-Jacoby, S&Tabares, A. (1990). Triglyceride kinetics, tissue lipoprotein lipase, and liver lipogenesis in septic rats. *Am. J. Physiol.*, Vol.258, No.4 Pt 1, pp. E678-E685, ISSN 0002-9513

Levels, JH., Abraham, PR., van den, EA., & van Deventer, SJ. (2001). Distribution and kinetics of lipoprotein-bound endotoxin. *Infect. Immun.*, Vol.69, No.5, pp. 2821-2828, ISSN 1098-5522

Liang, J&Ginsberg, HN. (2001). Microsomal triglyceride transfer protein binding and lipid transfer activities are independent of each other, but both are required for secretion of apolipoprotein B lipoproteins from liver cells. *J. Biol. Chem.*, Vol.276, No.30, pp. 28606-28612, ISSN 0021-9258

McGuinness, OP (2005). Defective glucose homeostasis during infection. *Annu. Rev. Nutr.*, Vol.25pp. 9-35, ISSN 0199-9885

Memon, RA., Feingold, KR., Moser, AH., Fuller, J., & Grunfeld, C. (1998a). Regulation of fatty acid transport protein and fatty acid translocase mRNA levels by endotoxin and cytokines. *Am. J. Physiol*, Vol.274, No.2 Pt 1, pp. E210-E217, ISSN 0002-9513

Memon, RA., Fuller, J., Moser, AH., Smith, PJ., Feingold, KR., & Grunfeld, C. (1998b). In vivo regulation of acyl-CoA synthetase mRNA and activity by endotoxin and cytokines. *Am. J. Physiol*, Vol.275, No.1 Pt 1, pp. E64-E72, ISSN 0002-9513

Memon, RA., Staprans, I., Noor, M., Holleran, WM., Uchida, Y., Moser, AH., Feingold, KR., & Grunfeld, C. (2000). Infection and inflammation induce LDL oxidation in vivo. *Arterioscler. Thromb. Vasc. Biol.*, Vol.20, No.6, pp. 1536-1542, ISSN 1079-5642

Nonogaki, K., Fuller, GM., Fuentes, NL., Moser, AH., Staprans, I., Grunfeld, C., & Feingold, KR. (1995). Interleukin-6 stimulates hepatic triglyceride secretion in rats. *Endocrinology*, Vol.136, No.5, pp. 2143-2149, ISSN 0013-7227

Perez, S., Aspichueta, P., Ochoa, B., & Chico, Y. (2006). The 2-series prostaglandins suppress VLDL secretion in an inflammatory condition-dependent manner in primary rat hepatocytes. *Biochim. Biophys. Acta*, Vol.1761, No.2, pp. 160-171, ISSN 0006-3002

Phetteplace, HW., Sedkova, N., Hirano, KI., Davidson, NO., & Lanza-Jacoby, SP. (2000). Escherichia coli sepsis increases hepatic apolipoprotein B secretion by inhibiting degradation. *Lipids*, Vol.35, No.10, pp. 1079-1085, ISSN 0024-4201

Popa, C., Netea, MG., van Riel, PL., van der Meer, JW., & Stalenhoef, AF. (2007). The role of TNF-alpha in chronic inflammatory conditions, intermediary metabolism, and cardiovascular risk. J. Lipid Res., Vol.48, No.4, pp. 751-762, ISSN 0022-2275

Pullinger, CR., North, JD., Teng, BB., Rifici, VA., Ronhild de Brito, AE., & Scott, J. (1989). The apolipoprotein B gene is constitutively expressed in HepG2 cells: regulation of secretion by oleic acid, albumin, and insulin, and measurement of the mRNA half-life. *J Lipid Res*, Vol.30, No.7, pp. 1065-1077, ISSN 0022-2275

Singer, II., Kawka, DW., Kazazis, DM., Alberts, AW., Chen, JS., Huff, JW., & Ness, GC. (1984). Hydroxymethylglutaryl-coenzyme A reductase-containing hepatocytes are distributed periportally in normal and mevinolin-treated rat livers. *Proc. Natl. Acad. Sci. U S. A.*, Vol.81, No.17, pp. 5556-5560, ISSN 0027-8424

Sparks, JD., Cianci, J., Jokinen, J., Chen, LS., & Sparks, CE. (2010). Interleukin-6 mediates hepatic hypersecretion of apolipoprotein B. *Am. J. Physiol Gastrointest. Liver Physiol*, Vol.299, No.4, pp. G980-G989, ISSN 0193-1857

Takeyama, N., Itoh, Y., Kitazawa, Y., & Tanaka, T. (1990). Altered hepatic mitochondrial fatty acid oxidation and ketogenesis in endotoxic rats. *Am. J. Physiol*, Vol.259, No.4 Pt 1, pp. E498-E505, ISSN 0002-9513

Taskinen, MR (2003). Diabetic dyslipidaemia: from basic research to clinical practice. *Diabetologia*, Vol.46, No.6, pp. 733-749, ISSN 0012-186X

Triantafilou, M&Triantafilou, K. (2005). The dynamics of LPS recognition: complex orchestration of multiple receptors. *J Endotoxin. Res.*, Vol.11, No.1, pp. 5-11, ISSN 0968-0519

Van Lenten, BJ., Fogelman, AM., Haberland, ME., & Edwards, PA. (1986). The role of lipoproteins and receptor-mediated endocytosis in the transport of bacterial lipopolysaccharide. *Proc. Natl. Acad. Sci. U. S. A*, Vol.83, No.8, pp. 2704-2708, ISSN 0027-8424

Vreugdenhil, AC., Snoek, AM., van, ', V., Greve, JW., & Buurman, WA. (2001). LPS-binding protein circulates in association with apoB-containing lipoproteins and enhances endotoxin-LDL/VLDL interaction. *J. Clin. Invest*, Vol.107, No.2, pp. 225-234, ISSN 0021-9738

Yokoyama, K., Ishibashi, T., Yi-qiang, L., Nagayoshi, A., Teramoto, T., & Maruyama, Y. (1998). Interleukin-1beta and interleukin-6 increase levels of apolipoprotein B mRNA and decrease accumulation of its protein in culture medium of HepG2 cells. *J. Lipid Res*, Vol.39, No.1, pp. 103-113, ISSN 0022-2275

Zu, L., He, J., Jiang, H., Xu, C., Pu, S., & Xu, G. (2009). Bacterial endotoxin stimulates adipose lipolysis via toll-like receptor 4 and extracellular signal-regulated kinase pathway. *J Biol. Chem.*, Vol.284, No.9, pp. 5915-5926, ISSN 0021-9285

11

Peroxisome Proliferator-Activated Receptor β/δ (PPAR β/δ) as a Potential Therapeutic Target for Dyslipidemia

Emma Barroso, Lucía Serrano-Marco, Laia Salvadó,
Xavier Palomer and Manuel Vázquez-Carrera
*Department of Pharmacology and Therapeutic Chemistry,
Spanish Biomedical Research Centre in Diabetes and Associated Metabolic Disorders(CIBERDEM)-Instituto de SaludCarlos III and IBUB,
(Biomedicine Institute of the University of Barcelona),
Faculty of Pharmacy, University of Barcelona, Barcelona,
Spain*

1. Introduction

Dyslipidemia is a powerful predictor of cardiovascular disease in patients at high risk (Turner et al., 1998), such as type 2 diabetic patients. Lowering of LDL-C is the prime target for treatment (2002), but even with intensification of statin therapy, a substantial residual cardiovascular risk remains (Barter et al., 2007; Miller et al., 2008; Fruchart et al., 2008; Shepherd et al., 2006). This may partly be due to atherogenic dyslipidemia. This term is commonly used to describe a condition of abnormally elevated plasma triglycerides and low high-density lipoprotein cholesterol (HDL-C), irrespective of the levels of LDL-C (Grundy, 1995). In addition to these key components, increased levels of small, dense LDL-C particles are also present, which in conjunction with the former components conform the also called "lipid triad" (Shepherd et al., 2005). Other abnormalities include accumulation in plasma of triglyceride-rich lipoproteins (TLRs), including chylomicron and very-low-density lipoprotein (VLDL) remnants. This is reflected by elevated plasma concentrations of non-HDL-C and apolipoprotein B-100 (apoB). Postprandially, there is also accumulation in plasma of TLRs and their remnants, as well as qualitative alterations in LDL and HDL particles. Thus, hypertriglyceridemia is associated with a wide spectrum of atherogenic lipoproteins not measured routinely (Taskinen, 2003). The presence of this lipid plasma profile with high triglyceride and low HDL-C levels have been shown to increase the risk of cardiovascular events independent of conventional risk factors (Bansal et al., 2007; Barter et al., 2007; deGoma et al., 2008). In fact, guidelines recommend modifying high triglyceride and low HDL-C as secondary therapeutic targets to provide additional vascular protection (2002). The presence of atherogenic dyslipidemia is seen in almost all patients with triglycerides > 2.2 mmol/l and HDL-C < 1.0 mmol/l, virtually all of whom have type 2 diabetes or abdominal obesity and insulin resistance (Taskinen, 2003). Most of these alterations are also characteristic of metabolic syndrome, which is defined as the clustering of multiple metabolic abnormalities, including abdominal obesity, dyslipidemia (high serum triglycerides and low serum HDL-C levels), glucose intolerance and hypertension (Eckel et al., 2005; Grundy et al., 2005).

2. Hypertriglyceridemia is crucial in the pathogenesis of atherogenic dyslipidemia

It is now recognized that the atherogenic dyslipidemia is mainly initiated by the hepatic overproduction of the plasma lipoproteins carrying triglycerides, the VLDL, which induce a sequence of lipoprotein changes leading to atherogenic lipid abnormalities in type 2 diabetes mellitus and metabolic syndrome (Adiels et al., 2008). Under these pathological conditions, the presence of insulin resistance at the level of adipose tissue leads to enhanced lypolisis and reduced free fatty acid (FFA) uptake and esterification which results in increased flux into the liver of FFA, which are either oxidized or esterified for triglyceride production, leading to hepatic steatosis and oversecretion into plasma of larger triglyceride-rich VLDL particles (Chan & Watts, 2011). These particles compete with chylomicrons and its remnants for clearance pathways regulated by lipoprotein lipase, an endothelial-bound enzyme, and by hepatic receptors, thereby exacerbating postprandial dyslipidemia. In addition, insulin resistance increases hepatic secretion of apoC-III, which is attached to VLDL delaying the catabolism of TRLs by inhibiting lipoprotein lipase and binding of remnant TRLs to hepatic clearance receptors (Chan & Watts, 2011). Finally, expansion of the VLDL triglyceride pool leads to cholesterol depletion and triglyceride enrichment of LDL and HDL through cholesteryl ester transfer protein, which facilitates the movement of cholesterol esters to VLDL, intermediate-density lipoprotein (IDL) and LDL from cholesterol ester rich HDL, leading to the accumulation in plasma of small, dense LDLs and a reduction in HDLs (Taskinen, 2003).

Since residual risk remains even after achieving an optimal LDL-C concentration with statins (Barter et al., 2007), probably due to other risk factors, such as high triglycerides, low HDL-C levels, defective glucose metabolism and other non-lipid-related risk factors (Kannel, 1983; Castelli, 1992; Lorenzo et al., 2010; Cederberg et al., 2010), the development of new drugs aimed at improving risk reduction is necessary. Among the new drugs for the treatment of the risk factors leading to the residual risk, PPARβ/δ activators might have a promising future. Interestingly, PPARβ/δ agonists have been demonstrated to be effective raising HDL-C and lowering triglyceride concentrations (Kersten, 2008). In addition to their lipid-modifying properties, PPARβ/δ agonists improve insulin resistance, which may also confer protection against the development of dyslipidemia (Coll et al., 2010a). This review summarizes the effects of PPARβ/δ on dyslipidemia identified during the last few years.

3. The PPAR family

PPARs are members of the nuclear receptor superfamily of ligand-activated transcription factors that regulate the expression of genes involved in fatty acid uptake and oxidation, lipid metabolism and inflammation (Kersten et al., 2000). To be transcriptionally active, PPARs need to heterodimerize with the 9-*cis* retinoic acid receptor (RXR) (NR2B) (Figure 1). PPAR-RXR heterodimers bind to DNA-specific sequences called peroxisome proliferator-response elements (PPREs), consisting of an imperfect direct repeat of the consensus binding site for nuclear hormone receptors (AGGTCA) separated by one nucleotide (DR-1). These sequences have been characterized within the promoter regions of PPAR target genes. The binding occurs in such a way that PPAR is always oriented to the DNA's 5'-end, while RXR is to the 3'-end. In the absence of ligand, high-affinity complexes are formed between PPAR-RXR heterodimers and nuclear receptor co-repressor proteins, which block transcriptional activation by sequestering the heterodimer from the promoter. Binding of the ligand to PPAR induces a conformational change resulting in dissociation of co-repressor proteins, so that the PPAR-RXR heterodimer can then bind to PPREs. Moreover, once activated by the ligand, the heterodimer recruits co-activator proteins that promote the initiation of transcription (Feige et al., 2006). As a consequence of these changes in transcriptional activity, binding of ligands to the receptor results in changes in the expression level of mRNAs encoded by PPAR target genes. In a specific cellular context, the activity of PPARs regulating the transcription of their target genes depends on many factors (relative expression of the PPARs, the promoter context of the target gene, the presence of co-activator and co-repressor proteins, etc.).

Thus, the transcriptional activity of PPARs is modulated by co-activators and co-repressors (Feige et al., 2006). One of the best described PPAR co-activators is PPARγ coactivator 1 α (PGC-1α). Silencing mediator for retinoic and thyroid hormone receptor (SMRT) and the nuclear receptor co-repressor (NCoR) are co-repressors that interact with the PPARs in the absence of ligands (Zamir et al., 1997). Receptor-interacting protein 140 (RIP140), an important metabolic regulator, is another ligand-dependent co-repressor which interacts with PPARs.

Finally, PPAR activity is also regulated at the post-transcriptional level by phosphorylation, ubiquitinylation, and sumoylation (for a detailed review see (Feige et al., 2006)).

However, the regulation of gene transcription by PPARs extends beyond their ability to trans-activate specific target genes in an agonist-dependent manner. PPARs also regulate gene expression independently of binding to PPREs. They cross-talk with other types of transcription factors and influence their function without binding to DNA, through a mechanism termed receptor-dependent trans-repression (Daynes & Jones, 2002). Most of the anti-inflammatory effects of PPARs are probably explained by this mechanism (Kamei et al., 1996; Li et al., 2000). Thus, through this DNA-binding independent mechanism, PPARs suppress the activities of several transcription factors, including nuclear factor κB (NF-κB), activator protein 1 (AP-1), signal transducers and activators of transcription (STATs) and nuclear factor of activated T cells (NFAT). There are three main trans-repression mechanisms by which ligand-activated PPAR-RXR complexes negatively regulate the activities of other transcription factors. First, trans-repression may result from competition for limiting amounts of shared co-activators. Under conditions in which the levels of specific co-activators are rate-limiting, activation of PPAR may suppress the activity of other transcription factors that use the same co-activators (Delerive et al., 1999; Delerive et al., 2002). In the second mechanism, activated PPAR-RXR heterodimers are believed to act through physical interaction with other transcription factors (for example AP-1, NF-κB, NFAT or STATs). This association prevents the transcription factor from binding to its response element and thereby inhibits its ability to induce gene transcription (Desreumaux et al., 2001). The third trans-repression mechanism relies on the ability of activated PPAR-RXR heterodimers to inhibit the phosphorylation and activation of certain members of the mitogen-activated protein kinase (MAPK) cascade (Johnson et al., 1997), preventing activation of downstream transcription factors.

The PPAR family consists of three members, PPARα (NR1C1 according to the unified nomenclature system for the nuclear receptor superfamily), PPARβ/δ (NR1C2) and PPARγ (NR1C3) (Auwerx et al., 1999). PPARα was the first PPAR to be identified and is the molecular target of the fibrate hypolipidemic class of drugs. This PPAR isotype is expressed primarily in tissues with a high level of fatty acid catabolism such as liver, brown fat, kidney, heart and skeletal muscle (Braissant et al., 1996). PPARγ has a restricted pattern of expression, mainly in white and brown adipose tissues and macrophages, whereas other tissues such as skeletal muscle and heart contain limited amounts. The γ isotype is the molecular target for the anti-diabetic drugs, thiazolidinediones. PPARβ/δ is ubiquitously expressed and, for this reason, was initially thought to be a "housekeeping gene" (Kliewer et al., 1994). However, studies with knockout mice (Barak et al., 2002; Peters et al., 2000; Tan et al., 2001) and the development of specific and high-affinity ligands for this receptor have shown that PPARβ/δ is a potential molecular target for prevention or treatment of several disorders. In this review we will highlight the role of PPARβ/δ in those metabolic processes with potential for treating dyslipidemia.

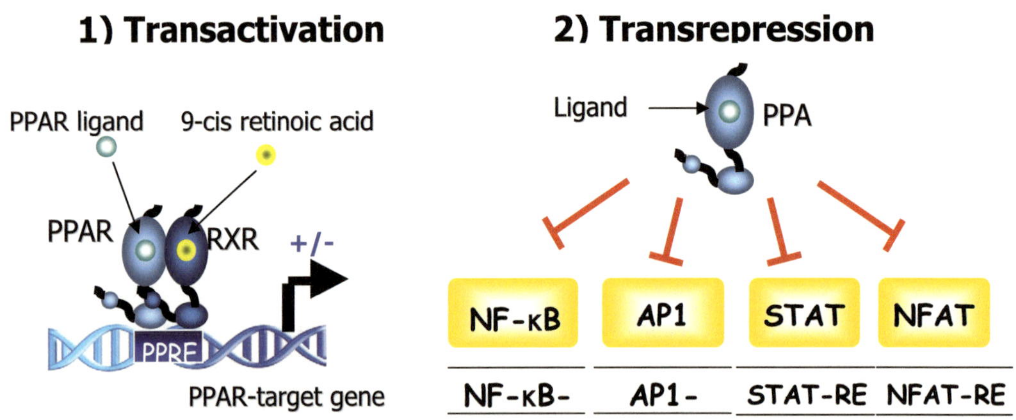

Fig. 1. Molecular mechanisms of Peroxisome Proliferator-Activated Receptors (PPARs). PPARs are ligand-activated transcription factors that regulate gene expression through two mechanisms: transactivation and transrepression. In transactivation PPAR-RXR heterodimers bind to DNA-specific sequences called peroxisome proliferator-response elements (PPREs), which are located in the promoter regions of genes involved in glucose and fatty acid metabolism. PPARs may also regulate gene expression through a DNA-independent mechanism called transrepression. Through this mechanism, PPARs inhibit the activity of several transcription factors such as NF-κB, which leads to anti-inflammatory effects. STAT denotes signal transducers and activators of transcription.

4. PPARβ/δ-specific features and ligands

The crystal structure of the ligand-binding domain of the PPARβ/δ isotype, which was first cloned in *Xenopus laevis* (Dreyer et al., 1992), revealed an exceptionally large pocket of approximately 1300 Å^3. This pocket is similar to that of PPARγ, but much larger than the pockets of other nuclear receptors (Takada et al., 2000; Xu et al., 1999), which may explain, at least in part, the great variety of natural and synthetic ligands that bind to and activate this nuclear receptor. Saturated (14 to 18 carbons) and polyunsaturated (20 carbons in length) fatty acids have affinities for PPARβ/δ in the low micromolar range (Xu et al., 1999; Forman et al., 1997; Yu et al., 1995; Krey et al., 1997). In addition, all-trans-retinoic acid (vitamin A) (Shaw et al., 2003) and fatty acids derived from VLDL (Chawla et al., 2003) can activate PPARβ/δFinally, the availability of three synthetic ligands (GW501516, GW0742 and L-165041) that activate PPARβ/δ at very low concentrations both in vivo and in vitro with high selectivity over other PPAR isotypes (Sznaidman et al., 2003) led to a huge increase in experimental studies on the role of PPARβ/δ in cellular processes. The EC_{50} for these compounds assessed with recombinant human PPARβ/δ were 1.0 nM for GW0742, 1.1 nM for GW501516 and 50 nM for L-165041 (Berger et al., 1999; Sznaidman et al., 2003).

5. Role of PPARβ/δ in lipoprotein metabolism

Treatment of the atherogenic dyslipidemia associated with type 2 diabetes mellitus and metabolic syndrome requires lowering triglycerides, increasing HDL-C and increasing the size of the LDL-C particle. Studies using the PPARβ/δ agonist GW501516 have demonstrated that this drug increased HDL-C (79%), and decreased triglycerides (56%), LDL-C (29%) and fasting insulin levels (48%) in obese rhesus monkeys, a model for human obesity and its associated metabolic disorders (Oliver, Jr. et al., 2001). A decrease in small dense LDL was also observed in treated animals (Oliver, Jr. et al., 2001). It has been suggested that the increase in HDL-C levels after PPARβ/δ treatment is caused by enhanced cholesterol efflux stimulated by a higher expression of the reverse cholesterol transporter ATP-binding cassette A1 (ABCA1) in several tissues, including human and mouse macrophages and intestinal cells and fibroblasts (Leibowitz et al., 2000; van, V et al., 2005). Apart from these beneficial effects of PPARβ/δ activation on HDL levels, treatment with this compound also increased HDL particle size in primates (Wallace et al., 2005), an effect which is thought to be protective against the progression of coronary artery disease in humans (Rosenson et al., 2002). In addition, PPARβ/δ activation reduces cholesterol absorption through a mechanism that may involve, at least in part, reduced intestinal expression of Niemann-Pick C1-like 1 (Npc1l1), the proposed target for the inhibitor of cholesterol absorption ezetimibe (van, V et al., 2005). However, additional studies are necessary to clearly demonstrate that the effects of these drugs are mediated through PPARβ/δ activation.

In obese and diabetic db/db mice, administration of a PPARβ/δ agonist modestly increased HDL particles, without affecting triglyceride levels (Leibowitz et al., 2000), whereas in a shorter treatment with GW501516 a reduction in plasma free fatty acids and triglyceride levels was observed in db/db mice, but not in mice exposed to a high fat diet (Tanaka et al., 2003).

In mice, deletion of PPARβ/δ led to enhanced LDL and triglyceride levels (Akiyama et al., 2004). It has been proposed that the increase in triglycerides observed in these PPARβ/δ-null mice is caused by a combination of increased VLDL production and decreased plasma triglyceride clearance, as demonstrated by a decrease in postheparin LPL activity and increased hepatic expression of the LPL inhibitors Angptl3 and 4 (Akiyama et al., 2004). Recent findings obtained by our laboratory indicate that additional mechanisms can also contribute to the hypotriglyceridemic effect of PPARβ/δ (Barroso et al., 2011). Interestingly, the main factor influencing hepatic triglyceride secretion is fatty acid availability (Lewis, 1997). In liver, fatty acids are either incorporated into triglycerides or oxidized by mitochondrial β-oxidation. An increase in fatty acid oxidation in liver would thus reduce the availability of fatty acids and subsequent hepatic triglyceride secretion. However, it was unknown whether the hypotriglyceridemic effect observed following PPARβ/δ activation involved increased hepatic fatty acid oxidation and the mechanisms implicated. The rate-limiting step for mitochondrial β-oxidation is the transport of fatty acid into mitochondria by liver carnitine palmitoyltransferase-1 (CPT1a). This fatty acid transporter is under the control of both PPARs and AMP-activated protein kinase (AMPK), which detects low ATP levels and in turn increases oxidative metabolism (Zhang et al., 2009) by reducing the levels of malonyl-CoA. Interestingly, PPARβ/δ activation can increase the activity of AMPK and the increase in fatty acid oxidation in human skeletal muscle cells following GW501516 treatment is dependent on both PPARβ/δ and AMPK (Kramer et al., 2007). It is worth noting that a recent discovered protein, lipin 1, plays an important role in hepatic fatty acid oxidation since it determines whether fatty acids are incorporated into triglycerides or undergo mitochondrial β-oxidation. In addition, the expression and compartmentalization of lipin 1 controls the secretion of hepatic triglycerides (Bou et al., 2009). Thus, in the cytoplasm, lipin 1 promotes triglyceride accumulation and phospholipid synthesis by functioning as an Mg^{2+}-dependent phosphatidate phosphatase (phosphatidic acid phosphatase-1, PAP-1). In contrast, in the nucleus lipin 1 acts as a transcriptional co-activator linked to fatty acid oxidation by regulating the induction of PGC-1α-PPARα-target genes (Finck et al., 2006). Lipin 1 induces PPARα gene expression and forms a complex with PPARα and PGC-1α leading to the induction of genes involved in fatty acid oxidation, including *Cpt1a* and *Mcad* (medium chain acyl-CoA dehydrogenase) (Finck et al., 2006).

When we examined the effects a high-fat diet (HFD) on hypertriglyceridemia and on the hepatic fatty acid oxidation pathway, we observed that exposure to HFD caused hypertriglyceridemia that was accompanied by reduced hepatic mRNA levels of PGC-1α and lipin 1, reduced hepatic phospho-AMPK levels and increased activity of extracellular-signal-regulated kinase 1/2 (ERK1/2) (Figure 2). Interestingly, drug treatment reduced hypertriglyceridemia, and restored hepatic phosphorylated levels of AMPK and ERK1/2. GW501516 treatment increased nuclear lipin 1 protein levels, leading to amplification of the PGC-1α-PPARα signaling system, as demonstrated by the increase in PPARα levels and PPARα-DNA binding activity and the increased expression of PPARα-target genes involved in fatty acid oxidation. These effects of GW501516 were accompanied by an increase in plasma β-hydroxybutyrate levels, demonstrating enhanced hepatic fatty acid oxidation.

The maintenance of AMPK phosphorylation following GW501516 treatment was accompanied by the recovery in the expression levels of *Lipin 1* and *Pgc-1α* and the increase in the mRNA levels of the *Vldl receptor* (Figure 2). Although we cannot rule out direct transcriptional activation of these genes by PPARβ/δ since it has been suggested that *Lipin 1*, the *Vldl receptor* (Sanderson et al., 2010) and *Pgc-1α* (Hondares et al., 2007) might be PPARβ/δ-target genes, most effects of GW501516 might be the result of the increase in AMPK phosphorylation (Kramer et al., 2007). In fact, it has been reported that this kinase upregulates the expression of *Lipin 1* (Higashida et al., 2008), the *Vldl receptor* (Zenimaru et al., 2008) and *Pgc-1α* (Lee et al., 2006b). The increase in AMPK phosphorylation following GW501516 treatment might involve several mechanisms. Since inhibitory crosstalk between ERK1/2 and AMPK has been reported (Du et al., 2008), the increase in phospho-AMPK levels could be the result of the inhibition by GW501516 of the phosphorylation of ERK1/2 induced by the HFD, which is in agreement with our previous study reporting that

GW501516 prevents LPS-induced ERK1/2 phosphorylation in adipocytes (Rodriguez-Calvo et al., 2008). It is important to note that a previous study found that obesity leads to increased hepatic ERK1/2 activity and that caloric restriction blunts this increase and improves insulin sensitivity (Zheng et al., 2009). In our study, the improvement in glucose tolerance caused by GW501516 was also accompanied by the reduction in phospho-ERK1/2 levels. An additional mechanism could involve SIRT1, since it has recently been reported that pharmacological PPARβ/δ activation increases the expression of SIRT1 (Okazaki et al., 2010), a deacetylase which regulates AMPK activity (Ruderman et al., 2010) through LKB1 acetylation (Lan et al., 2008), and might be essential to the regulatory loop involving PPARα, PGC-1α and Lipin 1 (Sugden et al., 2010). However, our findings made this possibility unlikely given that the increase in SIRT1 levels induced by GW501516 did not modify the acetylation status of LKB1. Interestingly, we showed that GW501516 increased the AMP/ATP ratio in liver, indicating that, in line with a previous study in skeletal muscle cells (Kramer et al., 2007), the underlying mechanism responsible for the increase in AMPK phosphorylation induced by this drug could be a modification of the cellular energy status. Previous studies have suggested that the reduction in ATP levels caused by GW501516 can be the result of a specific inhibition of one or more complexes of the respiratory chain, an effect on the ATP synthase system, or to mitochondrial uncoupling (Kramer et al., 2007). These potential changes would reduce the yield of ATP synthesis by the mitochondria, leading to AMPK activation.

In agreement with the reported regulation of PGC-1α (Canto et al., 2009; Jeninga et al., 2010; Lee et al., 2006a) and Lipin 1 (Higashida et al., 2008) by AMPK, exposure to the HFD reduced both *Pgc-1α* and *Lipin 1* expression. The reduction in Lipin 1 was likely to be the result of the decrease of PGC-1α, since it has been reported that genetic reduction of hepatic PGC-1α decreases the expression of *Lipin 1* (Estall et al., 2009). In addition, it has been shown that physiological stimuli that increase mitochondrial fatty acid oxidation induce *Pgc-1α* gene expression, which in turn activates the expression of *Lipin 1* (Finck et al., 2006). Interestingly, it has been reported that upregulation of *Lipin 1* in liver increases PPARα activity by two mechanisms: transcriptional activation of the *Ppara* gene and direct coactivation of PPARα in cooperation with PGC-1α (Finck et al., 2006). Thus, Lipin 1 is considered to be an inducible "booster" that amplifies pathways downstream PGC-1α-PPARα, mainly mitochondrial fatty acid oxidation (Finck et al., 2006). In agreement with this, GW501516 treatment prevented the reduction in PGC-1α, increased the nuclear protein levels of Lipin 1 and amplified the PGC-1αPPARα pathway, as demonstrated by the increase in the transcriptional activation of *Pparα* and the increase in PPARα transcriptional activity. These effects subsequently enhanced hepatic fatty acid oxidation, as shown by the increase in β-hydroxybutyrate levels. The reduction in PGC-1α and Lipin 1 levels caused by the HFD and their restoration after GW501516 treatment observed in our study might also contribute to the changes of plasma triglyceride levels, since both proteins are involved in the control of hepatic triglyceride secretion and fatty acid oxidation (Zhang et al., 2004; Chen et al., 2008; Estall et al., 2009). Overall, these data implicated PGC-1α and Lipin 1 in the hypotriglyceridemic effect of PPARβ/δ and complemented the findings of a previous study reporting that elevated plasma triglyceride levels in PPARβ/δ-null mouse were related to a combination of increased VLDL production and decreased plasma triglyceride clearance (Akiyama et al., 2004).

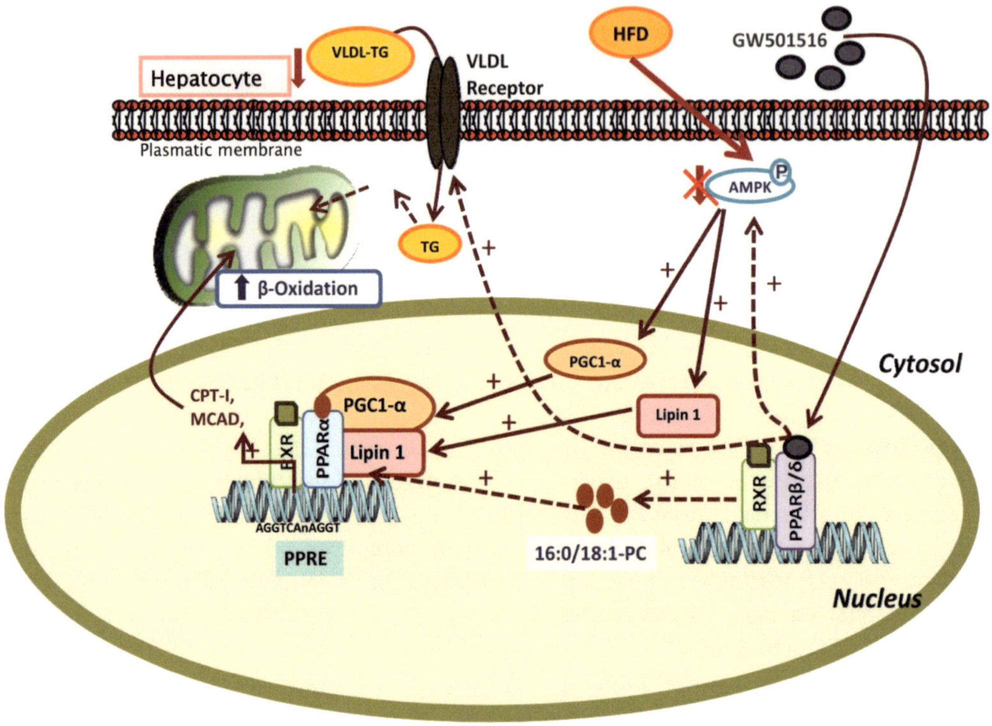

Fig. 2. A schematic of the potential effects of GW501516 (dashed lines) on liver metabolism is shown. Drug treatment with the PPARβ/δ agonist GW501516 prevents the reduction in phospho-AMPK levels and the subsequent increase in phospho-ERK1/2 levels caused by the HFD. In addition, GW501516 prevents the reduction in PGC-1α and increases Lipin 1 protein levels in the nucleus leading to amplification of the PPARα-PGC-1α pathway, which subsequently induces hepatic fatty acid oxidation. This pathway is additionally increased by GW501516 through the enhanced synthesis of the hepatic PPARα endogenous ligand 16:0/18:1-PC. As a result of the increase in this pathway the availability of fatty acids to be secreted as triglycerides might be compromised. The increase in the hepatic levels of the Vldl receptor can also contribute to reduce plasma triglyceride levels.

The data reported in our study also demonstrated that PPARβ/δ activation by GW501516 can amplify the PPARα pathway by an additional mechanism. Previous studies had demonstrated that hepatic fatty acid synthase (FAS) was necessary for the normal activation of PPARα target genes but did not identify the ligand involved in this process (Chakravarthy et al., 2005). Recently, this endogenous PPARα ligand was identified as 16:0/18:1-phosphatidilcholine (PC) (Chakravarthy et al., 2009). The synthesis of this ligand requires FAS activity, which yields palmitate (16:0), whereas 16:0/18:1-PC is generated through the enzymatic activity of CEPT1 (Chakravarthy et al., 2009). Subsequent binding of 16:0/18:1-PC to PPARα in the nucleus turns on PPARα-dependent genes and affects hepatic lipid metabolism. Interestingly, activation of PPARβ/δ by GW501516 induces FAS expression in liver as a result of increased glycolysis and the pentose phosphate shunt (Lee et al., 2006a). Our findings confirmed that GW501516 also increased *Cept1* expression and the levels of 16:0/18:1-PC, contributing to further amplification of the PPARα pathway.

The increase in fatty acid oxidation caused by GW501516 was apparently inconsistent with its lack of effects on hepatic triglyceride levels observed in our study. Several reasons may account for this. First, similar to the effects of GW501516, which restores Lipin 1 levels, hepatic *Lipin 1* overexpression leads to increased liver triglyceride content (Finck et al., 2006). This apparently conflicts with the effects of Lipin 1 on fatty acid oxidation, but it has been explained by hepatic triglyceride sequestration secondary to diminished triglyceride secretion, increased fatty acid uptake, or the PAP activity of Lipin 1 (Finck et al., 2006). Second, in our study we reported an additional possibility, the increase caused by GW501516 in the expression of the *Vldl receptor* in liver. The huge increase of this receptor observed in liver after GW501516 treatment might also reduce plasma triglyceride levels by increasing VLDL uptake by the liver. However, this can also lead to an increase in hepatic triglyceride content. Third, it has been reported that GW501516 improves hyperglycemia by increasing glucose flux through the pentose phosphate pathway and enhancing fatty acid synthesis in liver (Lee et al., 2006a). In that study, GW501516 increased liver triglyceride content but the authors reported that although this might raise concerns that long-term drug treatment might cause hepatic steatosis, they did not observe signs of fatty liver with treatment up to 6 months. In addition, long-term GW501516 treatment has been shown to reduce body weight and levels of circulating and liver triglycerides (Wang et al., 2004; Tanaka et al., 2003). In summary, our findings indicated that PPARβ/δ activation by GW501516 amplified the PPARα-PGC1-α pathway through the restoration of AMPK activity, contributing to the hypotriglyceridemic effect of this drug.
In humans, there are conflicting reports as to whether PPARβ/δ polymorphisms are associated with changes in plasma lipoproteins. Thus, while some studies found an association between a PPARβ/δ polymorphism and plasma lipids (Skogsberg et al., 2003), this was not confirmed in other studies (Gouni-Berthold et al., 2005). These discrepancies could be caused by differences in gender or the influence of gene-environment interactions, since a recent study reported that the association between the PPARβ/δ -87T>C polymorphism and plasma HDL-cholesterol might be sex-specific, women showing a stronger association, and that this association was only observed in subjects consuming a low-fat diet (Robitaille et al., 2007). The authors of this study concluded that the presence of the PPARβ/δ -87T>C polymorphism, which may result in enhanced PPARβ/δ activity, is associated with lower risk of suffering metabolic syndrome and that this association depends on the amount of fat consumed. In summary, the findings available at present on the effects of PPARβ/δ activation on lipoprotein metabolism are so promising that PPARβ/δ drugs are now in clinical trials for the treatment of human dyslipidemia.

6. Role of PPARβ/δ in insulin resistance

As stated above insulin resistance plays a crucial role in the development of hypertrigliceridemia, resulting in a sequence of lipoprotein changes leading to atherogenic dyslipidemia. Thus, those drugs, such as the PPARβ/δ ligands, which improve insulin resistance may also contribute to ameliorate the atherogenic dyslipidemia.

6.1 PPARβ/δ, inflammation and insulin resistance in adipose tissue

The expansion of adipose tissue, mainly in the form of visceral obesity, may contribute to enhanced inflammation in this tissue and insulin resistance through several processes. First, macrophages can infiltrate in adipose tissue, which contributes to the overproduction of inflammatory cytokines, such as tumor necrosis factor α (TNF-α and interleukin 6 (IL-6) (Gustafson et al., 2009). Indeed, the infiltration of macrophages into adipose tissue correlates with the degree of insulin resistance (Mathieu et al., 2010). Second, as visceral fat (which is very sensitive to lipolytic stimuli) increases, so does the rate of lipolysis. This leads to increased free fatty acid (FFA) mobilization and elevated levels of circulating FFA. Several studies have consistently demonstrated that elevations of plasma FFA produce insulin resistance in diabetic patients and in nondiabetic subjects (Boden et al., 1991; Boden, 1997). Saturated FFA are potent activators of the Toll-like receptor-4 (TLR4) (Mathieu et al., 2006) and recent evidence suggests that inflammatory processes induced by obesity and a high-fat diet cause systemic insulin resistance via a mechanism involving this receptor (Shi et al., 2006). TLR-4 is expressed in virtually all human cells and binds a wide spectrum of exogenous and endogenous ligands, including bacterial lipopolysaccharide (LPS) (Akira et al., 2006). In the presence of LPS, the TLR4 complex (including CD-14 and an accessory protein, MD-2), recruits the adaptor protein, myeloid differentiation factor-88 (MyD88), which in turn recruits interleukin-1 receptor-associated kinase (IRAK). This leads to the activation of the pro-inflammatory transcription factor NF-κB (Shoelson et al., 2006) and the subsequent enhanced expression of several inflammatory mediators (including IL-6 and monocyte chemoattractant protein-1 [MCP-1]). These observations indicate that saturated FFA derived from adipocytes and from high-fat diets activate TLR and the inflammatory pathway in adipocytes and macrophages, which contribute to the synthesis and production of cytokines such as TNF-α (Nguyen et al., 2007). In addition, high-fat diets raise plasma LPS to a concentration that is high enough to increase body weight, fasting glycemia and inflammation (Cani et al., 2007). Furthermore, LPS receptor-deleted mice (CD14 mutants) are hypersensitive to insulin, and the development of insulin resistance, obesity and diabetes in this animal model is delayed in response to a high-fat diet (Cani et al., 2007). Experiments performed in our laboratory have demonstrated that the PPARβ/δ agonist GW501516 inhibits LPS-induced cytokine expression and secretion by preventing NF-κB activation in adipocytes (Rodriguez-Calvo et al., 2008). Of note, NF-κB activation by LPS requires mitogen-activated protein kinase (MAPK)–extracellular signal–related kinase (ERK)1/2 (MEK1/2) activation, since inhibition of this pathway reduces LPS-induced cytokine production in adipocytes (Chung et al., 2006). In agreement with this role of ERK1/2 in inflammation in adipocytes, the expression of pro-inflammatory cytokines in these cells drops when they are exposed to LPS in the presence of the MAPK pathway inhibitor U0126. Interestingly, in white adipose tissue from PPARβ/δ-null mice we observed increased ERK1/2 phosphorylation and NF-κB activity and higher expression of IL-6 compared with wild-type mice (Rodriguez-Calvo et al., 2008). Moreover, in the white adipose tissue of a genetic model of obesity and diabetes, the Zucker diabetic fatty (ZDF) rat, the reduction in the expression of PPARβ/δ correlated with an increase in ERK1/2 phosphorylation and NF-κB activity. These findings suggest that PPARβ/δ activation prevents LPS-induced NF-κB activation via ERK1/2, thereby reducing the production of pro-inflammatory cytokines involved in the development of insulin resistance.

In addition, it has been suggested that IL-6 is another of the mediators linking obesity-derived chronic inflammation with insulin resistance through activation of signal transducer and activator of transcription 3 (STAT3), with subsequent up-regulation of suppressor of cytokine signaling 3 (SOCS3). Recently we have demonstrated that the PPARβ/δ agonist GW501516 prevents both IL-6-dependent reduction in insulin-stimulated Akt phosphorylation and glucose uptake in adipocytes (Serrano-Marco et al., 2011). In addition, this drug treatment abolished IL-6-induced SOCS3 expression in differentiated 3T3-L1 adipocytes. This effect was associated with the capacity of the drug to prevent IL-6-induced STAT3 phosphorylation on Tyr^{705} and Ser^{727} residues in vitro and in vivo. Moreover, GW501516 prevented IL-6-dependent induction of ERK1/2, a serine-threonine-protein kinase involved in serine STAT3 phosphorylation. Furthermore, in white adipose tissue from PPARβ/δ-null mice, STAT3 phosphorylation (Tyr^{705} and Ser^{727}), STAT3 DNA-binding activity and SOCS3 protein levels were higher than in wild-type mice. Several steps in STAT3 activation require its association with heat shock protein 90 (Hsp90), which was prevented by GW501516 as revealed in immunoprecipitation studies. Consistent with this finding, the STAT3-Hsp90 association was enhanced in white adipose tissue from PPARβ/δ-null mice compared to wild-type mice. Collectively, our findings indicate that PPARβ/δ activation prevents IL-6-induced STAT3 activation by inhibiting ERK1/2 and preventing the STAT3-Hsp90 association, an effect that may contribute to the prevention of cytokine-induced insulin resistance in adipocytes.

6.2 PPARβ/δ, inflammation and insulin resistance in skeletal muscle cells

FFAs may cause insulin resistance in skeletal muscle through several mechanisms, including effects on metabolism (Roden et al., 1996; Haber et al., 2003), signaling (Hirabara et al., 2007; Silveira et al., 2008) and mitochondrial function (Schrauwen et al., 2010; Hirabara et al., 2010). In addition, FFAs activate pro-inflammatory pathways, linking the development of this pathology to a chronic low-grade systemic inflammatory response (Wellen & Hotamisligil, 2005). In addition to FFA-induced inflammation through TLR, an additional pathway leads to FFA-mediated inflammation. This pathway involves intracellular accumulation of fatty acid derivatives. Once fatty acids are taken up by skeletal muscle cells they are either stored as fatty acid derivatives or undergo β-oxidation in the mitochondria. In the presence of high plasma FFA, fatty acid flux in skeletal muscle cells exceeds its oxidation, which leads to the accumulation of fatty acid derivatives, such as diacylglycerol (DAG), which can then activate a number of different serine kinases that negatively regulate insulin action. Thus, DAG is a potent allosteric activator of protein kinase Cθ (PKCθ), which is the most abundant PKC isoform in skeletal muscle (Griffin et al., 1999; Cortright et al., 2000; Itani et al., 2000). This PKC isoform inhibits the action of insulin by phosphorylating certain serine residues on insulin receptor substrate 1 (IRS1), including Ser^{307} in the rodent IRS-1 protein (reviewed in ref. (Gual et al., 2005)). This phosphorylation impairs insulin-receptor signaling through several distinct mechanisms (Hotamisligil et al., 1996). PKCθ also impairs insulin sensitivity by activating another serine kinase, IκB kinase β (IKKβ) (Perseghin et al., 2003). In addition to phosphorylating IRS-1 in Ser^{307}, IKKβ phosphorylates IκB. Thus, it activates the pro-inflammatory transcription factor NF-κB, which has been linked to fatty acid-induced impairment of insulin action in skeletal muscle in rodents (Kim et al., 2001; Yuan et al., 2001). Once activated, NF-κB regulates the expression of multiple inflammatory mediators, including IL-6. This cytokine correlates strongly with insulin resistance and type 2 diabetes (Pickup et al., 1997; Kern et al., 2001; Pradhan et al., 2001) and its plasma levels are 2-3 times higher in patients with obesity and type 2 diabetes than in lean control subjects (Kern et al., 2001).

Accumulation of fatty acid derivatives can be attenuated by mitochondrial β-oxidation. The rate-limiting step for β-oxidation of long-chain fatty acids is their transport into mitochondria via CPT-1. The activity of this enzyme is inhibited by malonyl-CoA, the product of acetyl-CoA carboxylase, which, in turn, is inhibited by AMPK. This kinase is a metabolic sensor that detects low ATP levels and increases oxidative metabolism (Reznick & Shulman, 2006), by reducing the levels of malonyl-CoA. Interestingly, activation of fatty acid oxidation by overexpressing CPT-1 in cultured skeletal muscle cells (Sebastian et al., 2007) and in mouse skeletal muscle (Bruce et al., 2009) improves lipid-induced insulin resistance. Hence, this approach may provide a valid therapeutic strategy to prevent this pathology. Activation of PPARβ/δ by its ligands (including GW501516) enhances fatty acid catabolism in adipose tissue and skeletal muscle, thereby delaying weight gain (for a review see (Barish et al., 2006)). This increase in fatty acid oxidation in human skeletal muscle cells following PPARβ/δ activation by GW501516 is dependent on both PPARβ/δ and AMPK (Kramer et al., 2007). AMPK is activated by GW501516 by modulating the ATP:AMP ratio (Kramer et al., 2007). Despite these data, little information was available on whether the increase in fatty acid oxidation attained after PPARβ/δ activation prevented fatty acid-induced inflammation and insulin resistance in skeletal muscle cells. However, we have recently reported that the PPARβ/δ ligand GW501516 prevented palmitate-induced inflammation and insulin resistance in skeletal muscle cells (Coll et al., 2010b). Treatment with GW501516 enhanced the expression of two-well known PPARβ/δ-target genes involved in fatty acid oxidation, CPT-1 and pyruvate dehydrogenase kinase 4 (PDK-4), and increased the phosphorylation of AMPK. This prevented the reduction in fatty acid oxidation caused by palmitate exposure. In agreement with these changes, GW501516 treatment reversed the increase in DAG and PKCθ activation caused by palmitate. These effects were abolished in the presence of the CPT-1 inhibitor etomoxir, thereby implicating increased fatty acid oxidation in the changes. Consistent with these findings, PPARβ/δ activation by GW501516 blocked palmitate-induced NF-κB DNA-binding activity. Likewise, drug treatment inhibited the increase in IL-6 expression caused by palmitate in C2C12 myotubes and human skeletal muscle cells, as well as the protein secretion of this cytokine. Overall, these findings indicate that PPARβ/δ attenuates fatty acid-induced NF-κB activation and the subsequent development of insulin resistance in skeletal muscle cells by reducing DAG accumulation. Interestingly, it has been suggested that the hypotrigliceridemic effect of GW501516 in humans is dependent of the increase in CPT-1 expression observed in skeletal muscle (Riserus et al., 2008).

7. Conclusion

Reduction of LDL-C, the main target of hypolipidemic therapy, has been proved effective reducing morbidity and mortality associated to CVD. However, a high proportion of patients receiving statins, the most lipid-lowering family of drugs used, do not reach optimal LDL-C levels. In addition, even in those patients reaching the optimal LDL-C levels following statin treatment, a residual risk remains, probably due to the presence of other risk factors, including the presence of atherogic dyslipidemia (described by the presence of high triglycerides, low HDL-C levels, and the presence of small dense LDL particles), glucose metabolism alterations and additional non-lipid-related risk factors. Several studies have confirmed that PPARβ/δ plays an important role in the regulation of lipoprotein metabolism, leading to reductions in the levels of plasma triglycerides and LDL-C and increases in HDL-C in different animal models. Taken together, these effects attained following PPARβ/δ activation on lipoprotein metabolism are so promising that this nuclear receptor has been considered a therapeutic target to prevent and treat dyslipidemia. However, as with any drug designed for human therapy, a great deal of research will be needed on the efficacy and safety of PPARβ/δ activators before they reach clinical use.

8. Acknowledgments

The author's work that is summarized in this review was supported by grants from the Ministerio de Ciencia e Innovación of Spain (SAF2009-06939). CIBER de Diabetes y Enfermedades Metabólicas Asociadas (CIBERDEM) is an Instituto de Salud Carlos III project. L.S-M. and L.S. were supported by FPI grants from the Spanish Ministerio de Ciencia e Innovación. We would like to thank the University of Barcelona's Language Advisory Service for its help.

9. References

Third Report of the National Cholesterol Education Program (NCEP) Expert Panel on Detection, Evaluation, and Treatment of High Blood Cholesterol in Adults (Adult Treatment Panel III) final report. *Circulation* 2002;106:3143-421.

Adiels M, Olofsson SO, Taskinen MR, Boren J. Overproduction of very low-density lipoproteins is the hallmark of the dyslipidemia in the metabolic syndrome. *Arterioscler Thromb Vasc Biol* 2008;28:1225-36.

Akira S, Uematsu S, Takeuchi O. Pathogen recognition and innate immunity. *Cell* 2006;124:783-801.

Akiyama TE, Lambert G, Nicol CJ et al. Peroxisome proliferator-activated receptor beta/delta regulates very low density lipoprotein production and catabolism in mice on a Western diet. *J Biol Chem* 2004;279:20874-81.

Auwerx J, Baulieu E, Beato M et al. A unified nomenclature system for the nuclear receptor superfamily. *Cell* 1999;97:161-63.

Bansal S, Buring JE, Rifai N, Mora S, Sacks FM, Ridker PM. Fasting compared with nonfasting triglycerides and risk of cardiovascular events in women. *JAMA* 2007;298:309-16.

Barak Y, Liao D, He W et al. Effects of peroxisome proliferator-activated receptor delta on placentation, adiposity, and colorectal cancer. *Proc Natl Acad Sci U S A* 2002;99:303-8.

Barish GD, Narkar VA, Evans RM. PPAR delta: a dagger in the heart of the metabolic syndrome. *J Clin Invest* 2006;116:590-597.

Barroso E, Rodriguez-Calvo R, Serrano-Marco L et al. The PPAR{beta}/{delta} Activator GW501516 Prevents the Down-Regulation of AMPK Caused by a High-Fat Diet in Liver and Amplifies the PGC-1{alpha}-Lipin 1-PPAR{alpha} Pathway Leading to Increased Fatty Acid Oxidation. *Endocrinology* 2011;152:1848-59.

Barter P, Gotto AM, LaRosa JC et al. HDL cholesterol, very low levels of LDL cholesterol, and cardiovascular events. *N Engl J Med* 2007;357:1301-10.

Berger J, Leibowitz MD, Doebber TW et al. Novel peroxisome proliferator-activated receptor (PPAR) gamma and PPARdelta ligands produce distinct biological effects. *J Biol Chem* 1999;274:6718-25.

Boden G. Role of fatty acids in the pathogenesis of insulin resistance and NIDDM. *Diabetes* 1997;46:3-10.

Boden G, Jadali F, White J et al. Effects of fat on insulin-stimulated carbohydrate metabolism in normal men. *J Clin Invest* 1991;88:960-966.

Bou KM, Sundaram M, Zhang HY et al. The level and compartmentalization of phosphatidate phosphatase-1 (lipin-1) control the assembly and secretion of hepatic VLDL. *J Lipid Res* 2009;50:47-58.

Braissant O, Foufelle F, Scotto C, Dauca M, Wahli W. Differential expression of peroxisome proliferator-activated receptors (PPARs): tissue distribution of PPAR-alpha, -beta, and -gamma in the adult rat. *Endocrinology* 1996;137:354-66.

Bruce CR, Hoy AJ, Turner N et al. Overexpression of carnitine palmitoyltransferase-1 in skeletal muscle is sufficient to enhance fatty acid oxidation and improve high-fat diet-induced insulin resistance. *Diabetes* 2009;58:550-558.

Cani PD, Amar J, Iglesias MA et al. Metabolic endotoxemia initiates obesity and insulin resistance. *Diabetes* 2007;56:1761-72.

Canto C, Gerhart-Hines Z, Feige JN et al. AMPK regulates energy expenditure by modulating NAD+ metabolism and SIRT1 activity. *Nature* 2009;458:1056-60.

Castelli WP. Epidemiology of triglycerides: a view from Framingham. *Am J Cardiol* 1992;70:3H-9H.

Cederberg H, Saukkonen T, Laakso M et al. Postchallenge glucose, A1C, and fasting glucose as predictors of type 2 diabetes and cardiovascular disease: a 10-year prospective cohort study. *Diabetes Care* 2010;33:2077-83.

Chakravarthy MV, Lodhi IJ, Yin L et al. Identification of a physiologically relevant endogenous ligand for PPARalpha in liver. *Cell* 2009;138:476-88.

Chakravarthy MV, Pan Z, Zhu Y et al. "New" hepatic fat activates PPARalpha to maintain glucose, lipid, and cholesterol homeostasis. *Cell Metab* 2005;1:309-22.

Chan DC, Watts GF. Dyslipidaemia in the metabolic syndrome and type 2 diabetes: pathogenesis, priorities, pharmacotherapies. *Expert Opin Pharmacother* 2011;12:13-30.

Chawla A, Lee CH, Barak Y et al. PPARdelta is a very low-density lipoprotein sensor in macrophages. *Proc Natl Acad Sci U S A* 2003;100:1268-73.

Chen Z, Gropler MC, Norris J, Lawrence JC, Jr., Harris TE, Finck BN. Alterations in hepatic metabolism in fld mice reveal a role for lipin 1 in regulating VLDL-triacylglyceride secretion. *Arterioscler Thromb Vasc Biol* 2008;28:1738-44.

Chung S, Lapoint K, Martinez K, Kennedy A, Boysen SM, McIntosh MK. Preadipocytes mediate lipopolysaccharide-induced inflammation and insulin resistance in primary cultures of newly differentiated human adipocytes. *Endocrinology* 2006;147:5340-5351.

Coll T, Barroso E, Alvarez-Guardia D et al. The Role of Peroxisome Proliferator-Activated Receptor beta/delta on the Inflammatory Basis of Metabolic Disease. *PPAR Res* 2010a;2010.

Coll T, Alvarez-Guardia D, Barroso E et al. Activation of peroxisome proliferator-activated receptor-{delta} by GW501516 prevents fatty acid-induced nuclear factor-{kappa}B activation and insulin resistance in skeletal muscle cells. *Endocrinology* 2010b;151:1560-1569.

Cortright RN, Azevedo JL, Zhou Q et al. Protein kinase C modulates insulin action in human skeletal muscle. *American Journal of Physiology-Endocrinology and Metabolism* 2000;278:E553-E562.

Daynes RA, Jones DC. Emerging roles of PPARs in inflammation and immunity. *Nat Rev Immunol* 2002;2:748-59.

deGoma EM, Leeper NJ, Heidenreich PA. Clinical significance of high-density lipoprotein cholesterol in patients with low low-density lipoprotein cholesterol. *J Am Coll Cardiol* 2008;51:49-55.

Delerive P, De Bosscher K, Vanden Berghe W, Fruchart JC, Haegeman G, Staels B. DNA binding-independent induction of I kappa B alpha gene transcription by PPAR alpha. *Molecular Endocrinology* 2002;16:1029-39.

Delerive P, De BK, Besnard S et al. Peroxisome proliferator-activated receptor alpha negatively regulates the vascular inflammatory gene response by negative cross-talk with transcription factors NF-kappaB and AP-1. *J Biol Chem* 1999;274:32048-54.

Desreumaux P, Dubuquoy L, Nutten S et al. Attenuation of colon inflammation through activators of the retinoid X receptor (RXR)/peroxisome proliferator-activated receptor gamma (PPARgamma) heterodimer. A basis for new therapeutic strategies. *J Exp Med* 2001;193:827-38.

Dreyer C, Krey G, Keller H, Givel F, Helftenbein G, Wahli W. Control of the peroxisomal beta-oxidation pathway by a novel family of nuclear hormone receptors. *Cell* 1992;68:879-87.

Du J, Guan T, Zhang H, Xia Y, Liu F, Zhang Y. Inhibitory crosstalk between ERK and AMPK in the growth and proliferation of cardiac fibroblasts. *Biochem Biophys Res Commun* 2008;368:402-7.

Eckel RH, Grundy SM, Zimmet PZ. The metabolic syndrome. *Lancet* 2005;365:1415-28.

Estall JL, Kahn M, Cooper MP et al. Sensitivity of lipid metabolism and insulin signaling to genetic alterations in hepatic peroxisome proliferator-activated receptor-gamma coactivator-1alpha expression. *Diabetes* 2009;58:1499-508.

Feige JN, Gelman L, Michalik L, Desvergne B, Wahli W. From molecular action to physiological outputs: peroxisome proliferator-activated receptors are nuclear receptors at the crossroads of key cellular functions. *Prog Lipid Res* 2006;45:120-159.

Finck BN, Gropler MC, Chen Z et al. Lipin 1 is an inducible amplifier of the hepatic PGC-1alpha/PPARalpha regulatory pathway. *Cell Metab* 2006;4:199-210.

Forman BM, Chen J, Evans RM. Hypolipidemic drugs, polyunsaturated fatty acids, and eicosanoids are ligands for peroxisome proliferator-activated receptors alpha and delta. *Proc Natl Acad Sci U S A* 1997;94:4312-17.

Fruchart JC, Sacks FM, Hermans MP et al. The Residual Risk Reduction Initiative: a call to action to reduce residual vascular risk in dyslipidaemic patient. *Diab Vasc Dis Res* 2008;5:319-35.

Gouni-Berthold I, Giannakidou E, Faust M, Berthold HK, Krone W. The peroxisome proliferator-activated receptor delta +294T/C polymorphism in relation to lipoprotein metabolism in patients with diabetes mellitus type 2 and in non-diabetic controls. *Atherosclerosis* 2005;183:336-41.

Griffin ME, Marcucci MJ, Cline GW et al. Free fatty acid-induced insulin resistance is associated with activation of protein kinase C theta and alterations in the insulin signaling cascade. *Diabetes* 1999;48:1270-1274.

Grundy SM. Atherogenic dyslipidemia: lipoprotein abnormalities and implications for therapy. *Am J Cardiol* 1995;75:45B-52B.

Grundy SM, Cleeman JI, Daniels SR et al. Diagnosis and management of the metabolic syndrome. An American Heart Association/National Heart, Lung, and Blood Institute Scientific Statement. Executive summary. *Cardiol Rev* 2005;13:322-27.

Gual P, Le Marchand-Brustel Y, Tanti JF. Positive and negative regulation of insulin signaling through IRS-1 phosphorylation. *Biochimie* 2005;87:99-109.

Gustafson B, Gogg S, Hedjazifar S, Jenndahl L, Hammarstedt A, Smith U. Inflammation and impaired adipogenesis in hypertrophic obesity in man. *Am J Physiol Endocrinol Metab* 2009.

Haber EP, Hirabara SM, Gomes AD, Curi R, Carpinelli AR, Carvalho CR. Palmitate modulates the early steps of insulin signalling pathway in pancreatic islets. *FEBS Lett* 2003;544:185-88.

Higashida K, Higuchi M, Terada S. Potential role of lipin-1 in exercise-induced mitochondrial biogenesis. *Biochem Biophys Res Commun* 2008;374:587-91.

Hirabara SM, Curi R, Maechler P. Saturated fatty acid-induced insulin resistance is associated with mitochondrial dysfunction in skeletal muscle cells. *J Cell Physiol* 2010;222:187-94.

Hirabara SM, Silveira LR, Abdulkader F, Carvalho CR, Procopio J, Curi R. Time-dependent effects of fatty acids on skeletal muscle metabolism. *J Cell Physiol* 2007;210:7-15.

Hondares E, Pineda-Torra I, Iglesias R, Staels B, Villarroya F, Giralt M. PPARdelta, but not PPARalpha, activates PGC-1alpha gene transcription in muscle. *Biochem Biophys Res Commun* 2007;354:1021-27.

Hotamisligil GS, Peraldi P, Budavari A, Ellis R, White MF, Spiegelman BM. IRS-1-mediated inhibition of insulin receptor tyrosine kinase activity in TNF-alpha- and obesity-induced insulin resistance. *Science* 1996;271:665-68.

Itani SI, Zhou Q, Pories WJ, MacDonald KG, Dohm GL. Involvement of protein kinase C in human skeletal muscle insulin resistance and obesity. *Diabetes* 2000;49:1353-58.

Jeninga EH, Schoonjans K, Auwerx J. Reversible acetylation of PGC-1: connecting energy sensors and effectors to guarantee metabolic flexibility. *Oncogene* 2010;29:4617-24.

Johnson TE, Holloway MK, Vogel R et al. Structural requirements and cell-type specificity for ligand activation of peroxisome proliferator-activated receptors. *J Steroid Biochem Mol Biol* 1997;63:1-8.

Kamei Y, Xu L, Heinzel T et al. A CBP integrator complex mediates transcriptional activation and AP-1 inhibition by nuclear receptors. *Cell* 1996;85:403-14.

Kannel WB. High-density lipoproteins: epidemiologic profile and risks of coronary artery disease. *Am J Cardiol* 1983;52:9B-12B.

Kern PA, Ranganathan S, Li C, Wood L, Ranganathan G. Adipose tissue tumor necrosis factor and interleukin-6 expression in human obesity and insulin resistance. *Am J Physiol Endocrinol Metab* 2001;280:E745-E751.

Kersten S. Peroxisome proliferator activated receptors and lipoprotein metabolism. *PPAR Res* 2008;2008:132960.

Kersten S, Desvergne B, Wahli W. Roles of PPARs in health and disease. *Nature* 2000;405:421-24.

Kim JK, Kim YJ, Fillmore JJ et al. Prevention of fat-induced insulin resistance by salicylate. *Journal of Clinical Investigation* 2001;108:437-46.

Kliewer SA, Forman BM, Blumberg B et al. Differential expression and activation of a family of murine peroxisome proliferator-activated receptors. *Proc Natl Acad Sci U S A* 1994;91:7355-59.

Kramer DK, Al-Khalili L, Guigas B, Leng Y, Garcia-Roves PM, Krook A. Role of AMP kinase and PPARdelta in the regulation of lipid and glucose metabolism in human skeletal muscle. *J Biol Chem* 2007;282:19313-20.

Krey G, Braissant O, L'Horset F et al. Fatty acids, eicosanoids, and hypolipidemic agents identified as ligands of peroxisome proliferator-activated receptors by coactivator-dependent receptor ligand assay. *Mol Endocrinol* 1997;11:779-91.

Lan F, Cacicedo JM, Ruderman N, Ido Y. SIRT1 modulation of the acetylation status, cytosolic localization, and activity of LKB1. Possible role in AMP-activated protein kinase activation. *J Biol Chem* 2008;283:27628-35.

Lee CH, Olson P, Hevener A et al. PPARdelta regulates glucose metabolism and insulin sensitivity. *Proc Natl Acad Sci U S A* 2006a;103:3444-49.

Lee WJ, Kim M, Park HS et al. AMPK activation increases fatty acid oxidation in skeletal muscle by activating PPARalpha and PGC-1. *Biochem Biophys Res Commun* 2006b;340:291-95.

Leibowitz MD, Fievet C, Hennuyer N et al. Activation of PPARdelta alters lipid metabolism in db/db mice. *FEBS Lett* 2000;473:333-36.

Lewis GF. Fatty acid regulation of very low density lipoprotein production. *Curr Opin Lipidol* 1997;8:146-53.

Li M, Pascual G, Glass CK. Peroxisome proliferator-activated receptor gamma-dependent repression of the inducible nitric oxide synthase gene. *Mol Cell Biol* 2000;20:4699-707.

Lorenzo C, Wagenknecht LE, Hanley AJ, Rewers MJ, Karter AJ, Haffner SM. A1C between 5.7 and 6.4% as a marker for identifying pre-diabetes, insulin sensitivity and secretion, and cardiovascular risk factors: the Insulin Resistance Atherosclerosis Study (IRAS). *Diabetes Care* 2010;33:2104-9.

Mathieu P, Lemieux I, Despres JP. Obesity, inflammation, and cardiovascular risk. *Clin Pharmacol Ther* 2010;87:407-16.

Mathieu P, Pibarot P, Despres JP. Metabolic syndrome: the danger signal in atherosclerosis. *Vasc Health Risk Manag* 2006;2:285-302.

Miller M, Cannon CP, Murphy SA, Qin J, Ray KK, Braunwald E. Impact of triglyceride levels beyond low-density lipoprotein cholesterol after acute coronary syndrome in the PROVE IT-TIMI 22 trial. *J Am Coll Cardiol* 2008;51:724-30.

Nguyen MT, Favelyukis S, Nguyen AK et al. A subpopulation of macrophages infiltrates hypertrophic adipose tissue and is activated by free fatty acids via Toll-like receptors 2 and 4 and JNK-dependent pathways. *J Biol Chem* 2007;282:35279-92.

Okazaki M, Iwasaki Y, Nishiyama M et al. PPARbeta/delta regulates the human SIRT1 gene transcription via Sp1. *Endocr J* 2010;57:403-13.

Oliver WR, Jr., Shenk JL, Snaith MR et al. A selective peroxisome proliferator-activated receptor delta agonist promotes reverse cholesterol transport. *Proc Natl Acad Sci U S A* 2001;98:5306-11.

Perseghin G, Petersen K, Shulman GI. Cellular mechanism of insulin resistance: potential links with inflammation. *Int J Obes Relat Metab Disord* 2003;27 Suppl 3:S6-11.

Peters JM, Lee SS, Li W et al. Growth, adipose, brain, and skin alterations resulting from targeted disruption of the mouse peroxisome proliferator-activated receptor beta(delta). *Mol Cell Biol* 2000;20:5119-28.

Pickup JC, Mattock MB, Chusney GD, Burt D. NIDDM as a disease of the innate immune system: association of acute-phase reactants and interleukin-6 with metabolic syndrome X. *Diabetologia* 1997;40:1286-92.

Pradhan AD, Manson JE, Rifai N, Buring JE, Ridker PM. C-reactive protein, interleukin 6, and risk of developing type 2 diabetes mellitus. *JAMA* 2001;286:327-34.

Reznick RM, Shulman GI. The role of AMP-activated protein kinase in mitochondrial biogenesis. *J Physiol* 2006;574:33-39.

Riserus U, Sprecher D, Johnson T et al. Activation of peroxisome proliferator-activated receptor (PPAR)delta promotes reversal of multiple metabolic abnormalities, reduces oxidative stress, and increases fatty acid oxidation in moderately obese men. *Diabetes* 2008;57:332-39.

Robitaille J, Gaudet D, Perusse L, Vohl MC. Features of the metabolic syndrome are modulated by an interaction between the peroxisome proliferator-activated receptor-delta -87T>C polymorphism and dietary fat in French-Canadians. *Int J Obes (Lond)* 2007;31:411-17.

Roden M, Perseghin G, Petersen KF et al. The roles of insulin and glucagon in the regulation of hepatic glycogen synthesis and turnover in humans. *J Clin Invest* 1996;97:642-48.

Rodriguez-Calvo R, Serrano L, Coll T et al. Activation of peroxisome proliferator-activated receptor beta/delta inhibits lipopolysaccharide-induced cytokine production in adipocytes by lowering nuclear factor-kappaB activity via extracellular signal-related kinase 1/2. *Diabetes* 2008;57:2149-57.

Rosenson RS, Otvos JD, Freedman DS. Relations of lipoprotein subclass levels and low-density lipoprotein size to progression of coronary artery disease in the Pravastatin Limitation of Atherosclerosis in the Coronary Arteries (PLAC-I) trial. *Am J Cardiol* 2002;90:89-94.

Ruderman NB, Xu XJ, Nelson L et al. AMPK and SIRT1: a long-standing partnership? *Am J Physiol Endocrinol Metab* 2010;298:E751-E760.

Sanderson LM, Boekschoten MV, Desvergne B, Muller M, Kersten S. Transcriptional profiling reveals divergent roles of PPARalpha and PPARbeta/delta in regulation of gene expression in mouse liver. *Physiol Genomics* 2010;41:42-52.

Schrauwen P, Schrauwen-Hinderling V, Hoeks J, Hesselink MK. Mitochondrial dysfunction and lipotoxicity. *Biochim Biophys Acta* 2010;1801:266-71.

Sebastian D, Herrero L, Serra D, Asins G, Hegardt FG. CPT I overexpression protects L6E9 muscle cells from fatty acid-induced insulin resistance. *Am J Physiol Endocrinol Metab* 2007;292:E677-E686.

Serrano-Marco L, Rodriguez-Calvo R, El K, I et al. Activation of Peroxisome Proliferator-Activated Receptor-{beta}/-{delta} (PPAR-{beta}/-{delta}) Ameliorates Insulin Signaling and Reduces SOCS3 Levels by Inhibiting STAT3 in Interleukin-6-Stimulated Adipocytes. *Diabetes* 2011;60:1990-1999.

Shaw N, Elholm M, Noy N. Retinoic acid is a high affinity selective ligand for the peroxisome proliferator-activated receptor beta/delta. *J Biol Chem* 2003;278:41589-92.

Shepherd J, Barter P, Carmena R et al. Effect of lowering LDL cholesterol substantially below currently recommended levels in patients with coronary heart disease and diabetes: the Treating to New Targets (TNT) study. *Diabetes Care* 2006;29:1220-1226.

Shepherd J, Betteridge J, Van GL. Nicotinic acid in the management of dyslipidaemia associated with diabetes and metabolic syndrome: a position paper developed by a European Consensus Panel. *Curr Med Res Opin* 2005;21:665-82.

Shi H, Kokoeva MV, Inouye K, Tzameli I, Yin H, Flier JS. TLR4 links innate immunity and fatty acid-induced insulin resistance. *J Clin Invest* 2006;116:3015-25.

Shoelson SE, Lee J, Goldfine AB. Inflammation and insulin resistance. *J Clin Invest* 2006;116:1793-801.

Silveira LR, Fiamoncini J, Hirabara SM et al. Updating the effects of fatty acids on skeletal muscle. *J Cell Physiol* 2008;217:1-12.

Skogsberg J, Kannisto K, Cassel TN, Hamsten A, Eriksson P, Ehrenborg E. Evidence that peroxisome proliferator-activated receptor delta influences cholesterol metabolism in men. *Arterioscler Thromb Vasc Biol* 2003;23:637-43.

Sugden MC, Caton PW, Holness MJ. PPAR control: it's SIRTainly as easy as PGC. *J Endocrinol* 2010;204:93-104.

Sznaidman ML, Haffner CD, Maloney PR et al. Novel selective small molecule agonists for peroxisome proliferator-activated receptor delta (PPARdelta)--synthesis and biological activity. *Bioorg Med Chem Lett* 2003;13:1517-21.

Takada I, Yu RT, Xu HE et al. Alteration of a single amino acid in peroxisome proliferator-activated receptor-alpha (PPAR alpha) generates a PPAR delta phenotype. *Mol Endocrinol* 2000;14:733-40.

Tan NS, Michalik L, Noy N et al. Critical roles of PPAR beta/delta in keratinocyte response to inflammation. *Genes Dev* 2001;15:3263-77.

Tanaka T, Yamamoto J, Iwasaki S et al. Activation of peroxisome proliferator-activated receptor delta induces fatty acid beta-oxidation in skeletal muscle and attenuates metabolic syndrome. *Proc Natl Acad Sci U S A* 2003;100:15924-29.

Taskinen MR. Diabetic dyslipidaemia: from basic research to clinical practice. *Diabetologia* 2003;46:733-49.

Turner RC, Millns H, Neil HA et al. Risk factors for coronary artery disease in non-insulin dependent diabetes mellitus: United Kingdom Prospective Diabetes Study (UKPDS: 23). *BMJ* 1998;316:823-28.

van d, V, Kruit JK, Havinga R et al. Reduced cholesterol absorption upon PPARdelta activation coincides with decreased intestinal expression of NPC1L1. *J Lipid Res* 2005;46:526-34.

Wallace JM, Schwarz M, Coward P et al. Effects of peroxisome proliferator-activated receptor alpha/delta agonists on HDL-cholesterol in vervet monkeys. *J Lipid Res* 2005;46:1009-16.

Wang YX, Zhang CL, Yu RT et al. Regulation of muscle fiber type and running endurance by PPARdelta. *PLoS Biol* 2004;2:e294.

Wellen KE, Hotamisligil GS. Inflammation, stress, and diabetes. *J Clin Invest* 2005;115:1111-19.

Xu HE, Lambert MH, Montana VG et al. Molecular recognition of fatty acids by peroxisome proliferator-activated receptors. *Mol Cell* 1999;3:397-403.

Yu K, Bayona W, Kallen CB et al. Differential activation of peroxisome proliferator-activated receptors by eicosanoids. *J Biol Chem* 1995;270:23975-83.

Yuan MS, Konstantopoulos N, Lee JS et al. Reversal of obesity- and diet-induced insulin resistance with salicylates or targeted disruption of IKK beta. *Science* 2001;293:1673-77.

Zamir I, Zhang J, Lazar MA. Stoichiometric and steric principles governing repression by nuclear hormone receptors. *Genes Dev* 1997;11:835-46.

Zenimaru Y, Takahashi S, Takahashi M et al. Glucose deprivation accelerates VLDL receptor-mediated TG-rich lipoprotein uptake by AMPK activation in skeletal muscle cells. *Biochem Biophys Res Commun* 2008;368:716-22.

Zhang BB, Zhou G, Li C. AMPK: an emerging drug target for diabetes and the metabolic syndrome. *Cell Metab* 2009;9:407-16.

Zhang Y, Castellani LW, Sinal CJ, Gonzalez FJ, Edwards PA. Peroxisome proliferator-activated receptor-gamma coactivator 1alpha (PGC-1alpha) regulates triglyceride metabolism by activation of the nuclear receptor FXR. *Genes Dev* 2004;18:157-69.

Zheng Y, Zhang W, Pendleton E et al. Improved insulin sensitivity by calorie restriction is associated with reduction of ERK and p70S6K activities in the liver of obese Zucker rats. *J Endocrinol* 2009;203:337-47.

12

Liver Glucokinase and Lipid Metabolism

Anna Vidal-Alabró, Andrés Méndez-Lucas, Jana Semakova, Alícia G. Gómez-Valadés and Jose C. Perales
Department of Physiological Sciences II, University of Barcelona, Barcelona, Spain

1. Introduction

Control of energy metabolism is crucial for optimal functioning of organs and tissues. Amongst all nutrients, glucose is the principal energy source for most cells and, therefore, minimum blood glucose levels must be guaranteed. Alterations in glycaemia can lead to hyperglycaemic states (producing protein glycosylation and toxicity in glucose-sensitive cells) or hypoglycaemic states (that can affect brain function), both harmful. Therefore, mechanisms must exist to keep glycaemia in a narrow physiological range (4-8 mM) independently of the nutritional state. To achieve control of blood glucose levels, our body has a complex, interorgan signaling system using nutrients (glucose, lipids, amino acids), hormones (insulin, glucagon, ghrelin, etc.) and the autonomic nervous system. In response to these signals, organs and tissues (mainly intestine, endocrine pancreas, liver, skeletal muscle, adipose tissue, brain and adrenal glands) adapt their function to energetic requirements.

The liver plays a pivotal role in the maintenance of glucose homeostasis by continuously adapting its metabolism to energetic needs. In the fed state, when blood glucose levels are high and there is insulin, liver takes-up part glucose to replenish glycogen stores. Besides, when glucose stores are full, the liver has the capacity to synthesize lipids *de novo* from glucose for-long term energy storage. Lipids are packaged in very low-density lipoprotein (VLDL) particles and then transported to the adipose tissue. Conversely during starvation, when glycaemia falls and glucagon increases, the liver produces glucose to maintain circulating glucose levels by breaking down glycogen stores or by synthesizing glucose de novo through gluconeogenesis. Gluconeogenesis, as an energy-consuming pathway, is linked to β-oxidation of fatty acids (fuel supplier pathway).

From this introduction on the regulation of glucose homeostasis, one can appreciate the close relation that exists between carbohydrate metabolism and lipid metabolism in the liver. Therefore, alterations in hepatic carbohydrate metabolic pathways may directly affect hepatic and/or blood lipid levels. Particularly, this chapter will focus on evaluating the incidence of glucokinase (GK) –the first enzyme of the glycolytic pathway in the liver- on lipidemia and on hepatic lipid content. But first, an introductory overview of the physiology behind the first-pass metabolism of dietary glucose in the liver will be presented.

2. Liver glucose metabolism

After a meal rich in carbohydrates, high levels of glucose reach the liver via portal vein. Glucose enters passively the hepatocyte through GLUT-2, a facilitated glucose transporter, and then is rapidly phosphorylated by GK at the sixth carbon to obtain glucose-6-phosphate which cannot escape the cell. From a functional perspective, it is important to recognize that both GLUT2 and glucokinase are expressed in cell types in which glucose metabolism has to vary accordingly to extracellular glucose concentration (glucose sensors). The high Km for glucose of both proteins, and the absence of product inhibition by glucose-6-phosphate, ensure that glucose uptake and phosphorylation in these cells are proportional to extracellular glucose concentration throughout the physiological range of glycaemia
The product of GK reaction, glucose-6-phosphate, is the gateway to the major pathways of glucose utilization: glycogen synthesis, glycolysis, oxidation of glucose and pentose phosphate pathway. It should be noted that hepatic glycolysis provides pyruvate principally for lipid synthesis rather than for oxidation. As glucose is the main substrate for fatty acid synthesis, hepatic glycolytic enzymes can be considered an extension of the lipogenic pathway. Glucose, insulin and parasympathetic nervous system orchestrate these glucose metabolic pathways in the fed state, with the aim of maintaining normal levels of blood sugar.

2.1 Glycogen synthesis

Two enzymes, glycogen synthase and glycogen phosphorylase, control glycogen levels. Both enzymes are regulated by phosphorylation and allosteric modulators. Specifically in the fed state, insulin activates glycogen synthase (limiting enzyme for glycogen synthesis) by promoting its dephosphorylation and, at the same time inhibits glycogen phosphorylase (important for glycogen breakdown). Meanwhile, glucose-6-phosphate binding to glycogen synthase favours its dephosphorylation, promoting glycogen synthase activity (Bollen, 1998; Agius, 2008). As a result, glucose coming from bloodstream fills hepatic glycogen stores.

2.2 Lipogenesis *de novo*

Hepatic lipogenesis is induced upon ingestion of excess carbohydrates to convert extra carbohydrates to triglyceride for long-time energy storage. Once inside the hepatocyte, glucose enters glycolytic pathway and provides pyruvate, which enters mitochondrion where it is converted into acetyl-CoA by pyruvate dehydrogenase. On the other side, in the cytoplasm glucose is also oxidized through the pentose phosphate pathway and NADPH is obtained. Acetyl-CoA will serve for fatty acid and also cholesterol synthesis. The initial steps for fatty acid synthesis are the transfer of acetyl-CoA from mitochondria to the cytoplasm and its conversion into malonyl-CoA under the action of the enzyme acetyl-CoA carboxylase. Importantly, malonyl-CoA is a regulatory molecule because it inhibits carnitine palmitoyltransferase-1, a rate limiting enzyme in β-oxidation of fatty acids. Therefore, increasing malonyl-CoA favours lipogenesis. Malonyl-CoA is elongated using NADPH under the action of the enzyme fatty acid synthase. Once obtained, fatty acids can be esterified with glycerol to form diglyceride and triglyceride. Most of the triglyceride is produced for export to the adipose tissue, but in order to be secreted, it must be packaged in very low-density lipoprotein (VLDL) particles together with cholesterol, phospholipids and apolipoprotein B (Figure 1).

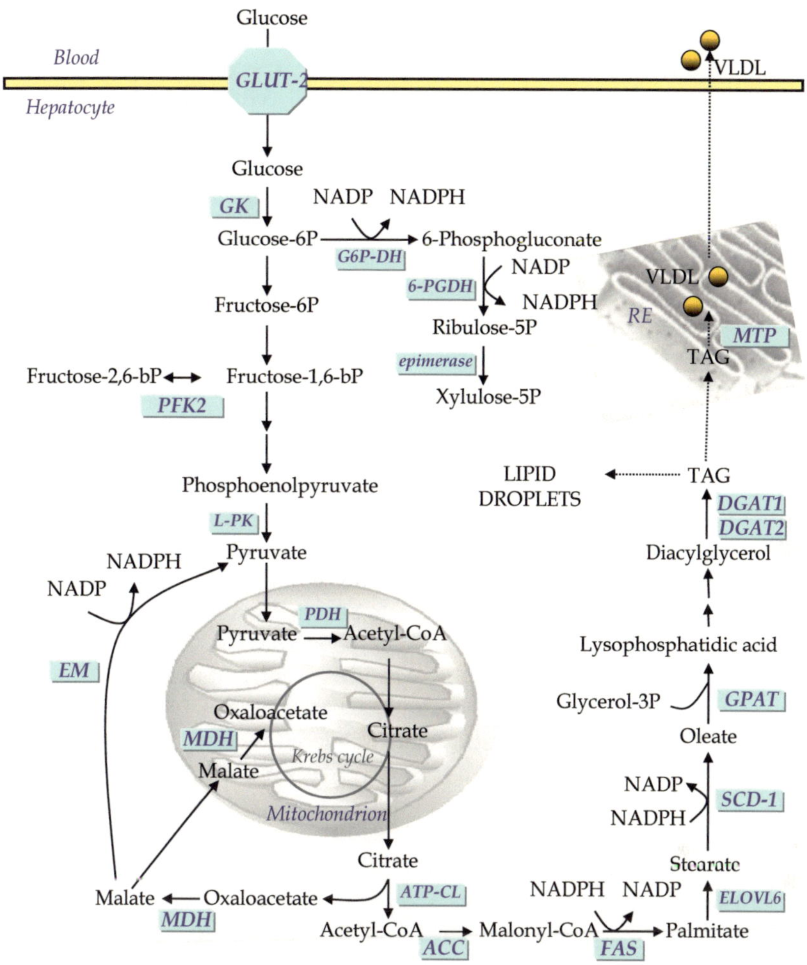

Fig. 1. Scheme of de novo lipogenesis from glucose. Once inside the hepatocyte, glucose is metabolized on one hand through glycolysis to pyruvate (GK means glucokinase; PFK-2, 6, phosphofructo-2-kinase/ fructose-2,6-bisphosphatase; L-PK, liver-pyruvate kinase). On the other hand, glucose is oxidized through pentose phosphate pathway to obtain NADPH (G6P-DH means glucose-6-phosphate dehydrogenase; 6-PGDH, 6-phosphogluconate dehydrogenase). Pyruvate enters the mitochondrion to obtain citrate (PDH means, pyruvate dehydrogenase; MDH, malate dehydrogenase and EM, malic enzyme). De novo synthesis of fatty acids starts with citrate (ATP-CL means ATP citrate lyase; ACC, acetyl-CoA carboxylase) and after suffering elongation and desaturation reactions (ELOVL6 means elongase that catalyzes the conversion of palmitate to stearate; SCD-1, stearoyl-coenzyme A desaturase), fatty acids are converted to triglyceride (TAG) (GPAT means glycerol-3-phosphate acyltransferase; DGAT, diacylglycerol acyltransferase). Triglyceride can be stored in the liver but are mostly packaged into VLDL (very low-density lipoprotein) and secreted to bloodstream (MTP means microsomal triglyceride transfer protein). Original artwork.

In mammals, hepatic lipogenesis is controlled by several transcription factors, mainly SREBP-1c (sterol regulatory element binding protein 1c) and ChREBP (carbohydrate-responsive element-binding protein), but also by PPAR-γ (peroxisome proliferator-activated receptor gamma), LXR-α (liver X receptor alpha) and XBP1, all of them regulated by nutritional and hormonal conditions.

SREBP-1c plays a major role in the induction of lipogenic genes by insulin. SREBP-1c is a member of the bZIP transcription factor family that was originally identified as a mediator of sterol signaling (Wang, 1994), and is produced as a precursor form that reside in the endoplasmic reticulum in an inactive state. On one hand insulin stimulates SREBP-1c gene transcription, and on the other hand, induces the maturation of SREBP-1c precursor (Shimomura, 1998). Mature SREBP-1c moves to nucleus and activates transcription of several lipogenic genes with SRE (sterol regulatory elements) sequences in their promoters, for instance fatty acid synthase (FAS), stearoyl-Coenzyme A desaturase 1 (SCD-1), etc. (Figure 2) (Foretz, 1999; Ferre, 2010).

Glucose regulates genes of glycolytic and lipogenic pathways by activating ChREBP (Iizuka, 2008). ChREBP is a transcription factor that binds to ChoRE sequences present in the promoter of ACC (acetyl Coenzyme-A carboxylase), fatty acid synthase (FAS), stearoyl-Coenzyme A desaturase 1 (SCD-1), L-pyruvate kinase (L-PK), etc. (Uyeda, 2006). Under basal conditions, ChREBP is phosphorylated at Ser196 and remains in the cytosol. When glycaemia increase, glucose enters the hepatocyte and is metabolized. Therefore there is an increase in some glucose metabolites such as xylulose-5P, which promotes ChREBP dephosphorylation (Kabashima, 2003). Then, ChREBP rapidly moves to the nucleus and will activate transcription of its target genes (Figure 2).

SREBP-1c and ChREBP are also transcriptionally activated by liver X receptor apha (LXR-α), which could be a glucose sensor although it is controversial (Mitro, 2007; Denechaud, 2008). LXR-α is classically activated by oxysterols and it is important for the transcription of some lipogenic genes, a part form SREBP-1c and ChREBP, since their promoters contain LXRE (LXR response element) sequences (Chen, 2004; Cha, 2007).

XBP1, a transcription factor best known as a key regulator of the unfolded protein response (UPR), has been surprisingly associated with *de novo* fatty acid synthesis in the liver. It seems to be induced by diet carbohydrates and its deletion in mice causes hypocholesterolemia and hypotriglyceridemia, attributed to diminished hepatic lipid production (Lee, 2008). But, there are still some questions about its function to answer: what is its binding site in the promoter regions of these genes? Does it act alone or in partnership with other known transcription factors such as SREBP, ChREBP and LXR?

In summary, hepatic lipogenesis is regulated by several transcription factors that may probably work synergistically (Figure 2). With this complex system, carbons from glucose can be directed to fatty acid synthesis only when there is substrate availability and glycogen depots have been replenished. Altered fatty acid synthesis in the liver can lead to changes in lipid secretion, and consequently to dyslipidemia (Ginsberg, 2006).

2.3 Inhibition of hepatic glucose production

During fasting, liver produces glucose that enters bloodstream in order to maintain glycaemia, ensuring fuel supply for brain and red blood cells. But after a meal, when diet glucose arrives, hepatocytes must switch glucose production to glucose uptake. Insulin and high glucose levels coordinate the inhibition of glycogenolysis and gluconeogenesis (glucose producing pathways).

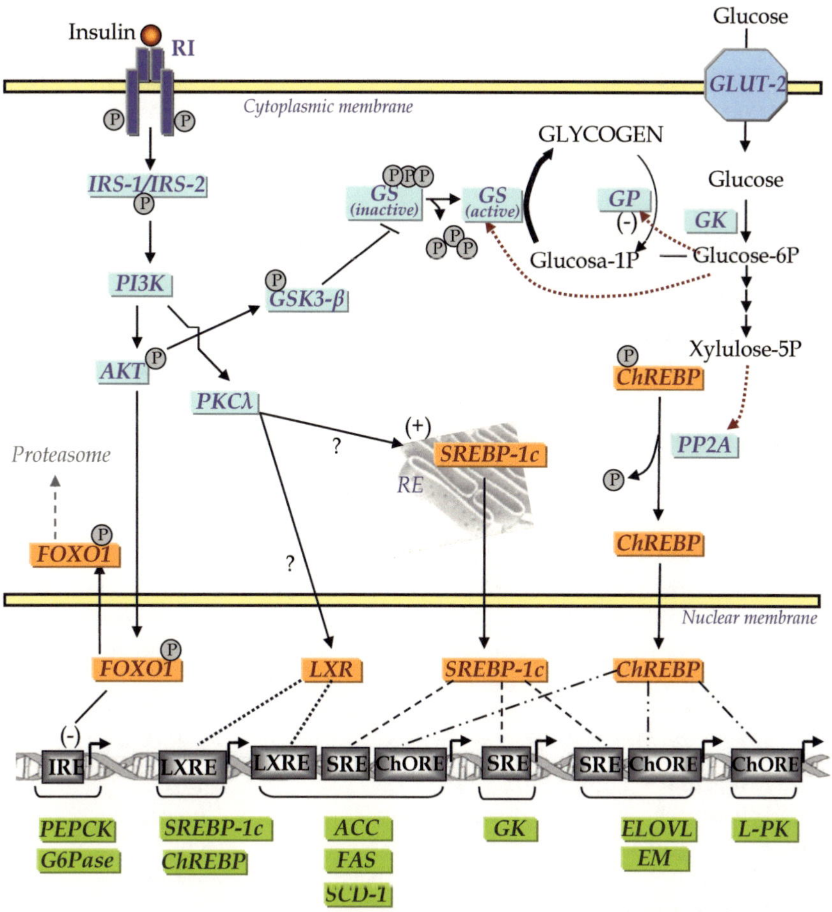

Fig. 2. Main regulatory mechanisms of hepatic metabolism in fed state. Insulin and glucose direct gene transcription to switch from glucose producing pathways to glucose uptake and storage. Briefly, insulin signaling promotes the phosphorylation of FOXO1 that results in its nuclear exclusion and proteasome degradation; consequently, transcription of gluconeogenic genes is inhibited. Besides, insulin stimulates transcription of lipogenic genes through SREBP-1c activation and probably through LXR-α, as well. Finally, insulin signaling causes activation of glycogen synthase function. Glucose also controls allostericaly glycogen synthesis and promote transcription of lipogenic genes via activation of ChREBP. IR means insulin receptor, IRS, insulin receptor substrate; PI3K, phosphoinositide 3-kinse; AKT, Ser/Thr protein kinase; GSK3-β, glycogen synthase kinase 3.beta; FOXO1, forkhead box O1; PCK, protein kinase C; LXR, liver X receptor; SREBP-1c, sterol regulatory element binding protein 1c; ChREBP, carbohydrate response element binding protein; GS, glycogen synthase; GP, glycogen phosphorylase; GK, glucokinase; PP2A, protein phosphatase 2A); IRE, insulin response element; LXRE liver X receptor response element; SRE, sterol regulatory elements; ChORE, carbohydrate-response elements; PEPCK-C, cytosolic phosphoenolpyruvate carboxykinase; G6Pase, glucose-6-phosphatase; ACC, Acyl-CoA carboxylase; FAS, fatty acid synthase; SCD-1, stearoyl-CoA desaturase 1; ELOVL , EM, malic enzyme and L-PK, liver-pyruvate kinase. Original artwork.

Insulin directly inhibits the transcription of gluconeogenic genes by promoting the phosphorylation of FOXO1 (forkhead box O), a transcription factor necessary for the induction of gluconeogenesis in conjunction with PGC-1α (PPAR-gamma coactivator 1-alpha) (Puigserver, 2003). In addition, SREBP-1c promotes the inhibition of some gluconeogenic genes. Insulin also represses glycogenolysis by phosphorylating glycogen synthase (Bollen, 1998). On the other hand, insulin regulates hepatic glucose production indirectly: a) it suppresses lipolysis in adipose tissue causing a reduction in glycerol (gluconeogenic substrate) availability; b) it inhibits glucagon secretion in the pancreas; and c) it activates hypothalamic pathways important for glucose homeostasis.

Synergistically with insulin, glucose inhibits glycogenolysis allosterically (Bollen, 1998). Glucose inhibition on gluconeogenesis is mediated by glucose metabolites, specifically fructose-2,6-bisphosphate (Wu, 2001) and xylulose-5-phosphate (Massillon, 1998).

3. Glucokinase regulates the fate of glucose carbons in the liver

In order to enter the lipogenic pathway, glucose must be metabolized. The first and rate-limiting step is the phosphorylation of glucose at the 6th carbon to obtain glucose-6-phosphate. This reaction is catalyzed by glucokinase (GK; EC 2.7.1.1), a member of the hexokinase family. However, GK differs from other hexokinases in its particular kinetic properties: affinity for glucose that is within the physiological plasma concentration range ($S_{0.5}$ for glucose of 8 mM), positive cooperativity for glucose although it is a monomeric enzyme, and lack of inhibition by glucose-6-phosphate (Table 1).

	HEXOKINASES 1-3	GLUCOKINASE
Molecular weight	100 KDa	50 KDa
Substrates	Hexoses	Glucose
$S_{0.5}$ for glucose	< 0.5 mM	8 mM
Kinetic	Hyperbolic	Sigmoidal
Product inhibition	Yes	No

Table 1. Hexokinase family kinetic properties

As a result of its kinetic characteristics, intracellular glucose phosphorylation rate inside the hepatocyte correlates with glycaemia. Hence, GK can be considered an intracellular glucose sensor. Consequently, apart from hepatocytes, GK is expressed in glucosensitive cells of the pancreas, hypothalamus, anterior pituitary gland, and entero-endocrine K and L cells of the gut (Schuit, 2001; Zelent, 2006; Vieira, 2007; Iynedjian, 2009), all of them crucial in the control of the whole-body glucose homeostasis.

Liver contains 99.9% of the body GK. Therefore, is not surprising that this enzyme influences intermediary metabolism and energy storage. GK reaction controls the flux of glucose through several metabolic pathways: glycolysis, glucose oxidization, glycogenesis, triglyceride synthesis, phospholipids and cholesterol synthesis, glycogenolysis and gluconeogenesis. For that reason, GK is an enzyme highly regulated in the liver, both at the transcriptional and the post-transcriptional level.

3.1 Regulation of GK activity in the liver

Gck gene has two distinct promoters and one of them directs gene transcription specifically in the liver (Postic, 1995). Hepatic GK expression responds to nutritional changes; it is activated by insulin and inhibited by glucagon. Insulin induction of Gck gene expression is through the PI_3-kinase/Akt signaling. However, no IRE (insulin response element) has been described in Gck promoter, and it is not clear which transcription factor mediates insulin-directed Gck expression. SREBP-1c is a candidate to mediate insulin-directed expression of Gck, although controversial results exist (Foretz, 1999; Gregory, 2006). Probably, SREBP-1c is not essential for rapid induction of GK transcription, but it can have a role for long-term expression. Other candidates to mediate insulin-dependent expression of Gck gene are the complex HIF-α/HNF-4/p300 (Roth, 2004), and ERR-α -estrogen-related receptor alpha- (Zhu, 2010).

GK can be modulated by covalent modifications such as nitrosylation and phosphorylation. However, the physiological importance of these modifications is still not determined. More importantly, protein interaction affects GK activity and even intracellular distribution. It has been described that GK in the liver can interact with GKRP (glucokinase regulatory protein), BAD (Bcl-xL/Bcl-2-Associated Death Promoter), PFK-2 (6-phosphofructo-2-kinase/fructose-2,6-bisphosphatase), GKAP (glucokinase-associated protein), etc. (Massa, 2010). From all GK protein partners, GKRP is the best studied and has high physiological relevance in the liver.

3.1.1 Post-transcriptional regulation by GKRP

GKRP regulation of GK affects both the activity and subcellular localization of the enzyme. GKRP is a competitive inhibitor with respect to glucose. Van Shaftingen *et al* proposed a mechanistic model (Van Shaftingen, 2004); GKRP exists in two conformations, one with low affinity for GK and the other with high affinity. Fructose-1-phosphate and fructose-6-phosphate bind to the same binding site in the GKRP protein. When fructose-1-phosphate is bound to GKRP, GKRP adopts a conformation with low affinity for GK, and on the contrary, when the binding of fructose-6-phosphate to GKRP favours its interaction with GK.

But, Kamata *et al* also described that GK can exist in different conformations with different affinity for glucose (Kamata, 2004); in the absence of glucose, the enzyme exists in a super-open conformation thermodynamically stable and with low affinity for substrate. When glucose binds to it, there is a conformational change to an open form and next to a closed conformation that binds ATP. Then the catalytic cycle completes, after reaction products are released, GK can relax to an open or to a super-open conformation, depending on glucose concentrations (considering that the open conformation has higher affinity for glucose). GK conformation is important for GKRP protein interaction, as it can only take place when GK is in the super-open conformation (Anderka, 2008). From these conformational models of GKRP and GK, one can extrapolate the exquisite influence of carbohydrate concentration in regulating GKRP/GK binding and, consequently, GK phosphorylating activity.

GKRP also plays a fundamental role in importing GK to the nucleus, as it can be deduced from animals null for GKRP that present GK permanently in the cytosol (Farrelly, 1999). At low glucose concentrations, GKRP binds to GK and the formation of GKRP/GK complex results in entry and sequestration of both proteins in the nucleus of hepatocytes. However, it is still not resolved how GK is translocated to the nucleus. On the other hand, in metabolic states with high glucose concentrations, accompanied or not by high fructose levels, and sufficient ATP, there is the dissociation of the GKRP/GK complex. GK has a nuclear export signal sequence. Therefore, once dissociated from the complex, GK can be exported to the cytoplasm (Shiota, 1999). Insulin also favours the dissociation of the complex.

The physiological function of GKRP consists of inhibiting GK activity by sequestering it to the nucleus. GKRP binding also serves to stabilize GK protein and protect it from degradation. Thus, thanks to GKRP a big reservoir of GK exists in the nucleus of the hepatocyte at low glucose concentration. After a meal, this reservoir of GK can be rapidly mobilized (translocation is complete within 30 minutes) to the cytosol in order to promote glucose uptake and storage in the liver. This regulation process is much more fast and efficient than the synthesis de novo of GK promoted by insulin. Conversely, when glucose uptake has finished, GK returns to the nucleus in order to save energy because, on one hand, this translocation avoids the futile cycle between glucose and glucose-6-phosphate, and on the other hand, it ends the glucose signal generated by GK activity that activate transcription of glycolytic and lipogenic genes (Figure 3). The consequence of GK translocation to the nucleus in the post-absorptive state is the induction of glycogenolysis and gluconeogenesis.

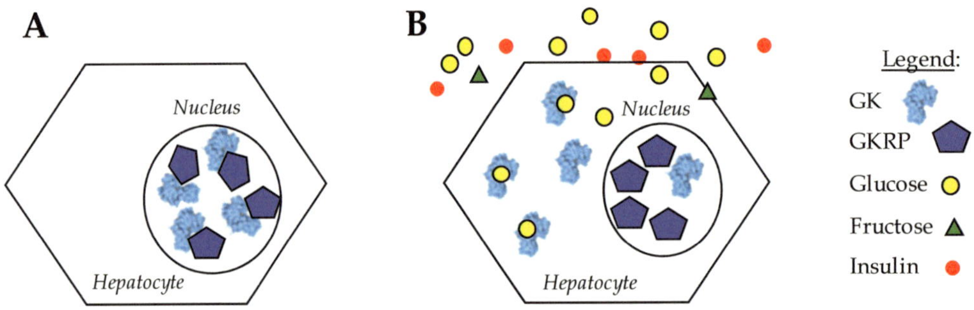

Fig. 3. Subcellular localization of GK regulated by GKRP. (A) During fasting, GK is sequestered in the nucleus where it remains bound to GKRP and inactive. After a meal, nutritional signals (i.e. insulin, glucose and fructose) induce the dissociation of the GK/GKRP complex and free GK translocates to the cytosol. Original artwork.

To summarize, thanks to its kinetic properties and its subtle regulation, GK enables the liver to adapt its metabolism for glucose uptake or glucose production as required, and consequently to regulate energy homeostasis.

3.2 GK modulation in the liver: impact on carbohydrate and lipid metabolism

Numerous natural mutations in GK gene have been associated to disease (Gloyn, 2003 & Osbak, 2009), reinforcing the concept that it is a crucial enzyme in the control of whole-body glucose homeostasis. Mutations that cause decrease or loss of GK activity are associated to maturity onset diabetes of the young-2 (MODY-2) or to permanent neonatal diabetes mellitus (PNDM). In diabetes, as a result of impairment in insulin secretion, the capacity of the liver to uptake glucose is diminished. On the other hand, activating mutations of GK cause persistent hyperinsulinemic hypoglycemia in infancy (PHHI). The phenotype of all these pathologies is mainly dominated by GK function in the pancreatic β-cell, where it regulates glucose-dependent insulin secretion. As insulin controls hepatic GK transcription and influences GKRP regulation, it is difficult to elucidate which are the specific consequences of these mutations on hepatic GK independently of insulin.

Some animal models have been developed to study the specific role of liver GK on metabolism.

3.2.1 Genetic suppression of hepatic GK

A liver specific GK knock-out was obtained using the LoxP-Cre system (Postic, 1999). Transgenic mice showed mild hyperglycemia and hyperinsulinemia in basal conditions, without changes in hepatic glycogen, plasma non-esterified fatty acids, triglycerides or β-hydroxybutyrate. In hyperglycaemic clamp studies, reduced hepatic glucose uptake and glycogen levels were observed in KO animals; however, results on lipid profile were not provided.

3.2.2 Genetic overexpression of GK in the liver

Several liver GK gain-of-function studies, both using transgenic animals and by means of adenovirus gene transfer, have been performed in healthy animals and models of diabetes such as streptozotocin induced type I and type II induced by ingestion of high fat/high carbohydrate diet. Due to heterogeneity, these studies will be examined according to the animal model and analysis conditions.

a. Overexpression of GK in the liver of fed, healthy animals is summarized in Table 2 (Ferre, 1996a, 1996b, 2003; O'Doherty, 1999; Scott, 2003).

Study variables	Ferre 1996a, 1996b Ferre 2003		O'Doherty 1999; Scott 2003	
Animal model	*Mus musculus*		*Rattus norvegicus*	
	Transgenic		Adenoviral gene transfer	
	PEPCK-C promoter		CMV promoter	
GK activity over control	x 2		x 3	x 6.4
Age at analysis	2 months	12 months	5 days post-injection (Rats 200-250 g)	
Glycaemia	decrease	-	no change	Decrease
Blood lactate	-		increase	Increase
Blood triglycerides	~ increase	-	~ increase	Increase
NEFA	~ increase	-	no change	increase
Insulin	decrease	increase	no change	decrease
Hepatic glucose-6-P	increase	~ increase	-	-
Hepatic glycogen	increase	decrease	no change	no change
Hepatic triglycerides	no change	increase	-	-
Modulation of enzymes and transcription factors	↑ L-PK ↓PEPCK-C, GLUT-2, TAT	-	↑ L-PK, ACC1, FAS, G6Pase. No change in PEPCK-K	-

Table 2. Hepatic GK overexpression studies in healthy fed animals. Comments: decrease, increase and no change are referred to control group. "~" means no statistically significant; "-", no determined; "CMV", cytomegalovirus; "PEPCK-C", cytosolic phosphoenolpyruvate carboxykinase; "L-PK", liver pyruvate kinase; "TAT", tyrosine aminotransferase; "ACC1", Acetyl-Coenzyme A carboxylase 1; "FAS", fatty acid synthase; and "G6Pase", glucose-6 phosphatase.

In these models, enhancing hepatic glucose uptake by GK overexpression results in a direct reduction of glycaemia. As a consequence of lower blood glucose levels, pancreatic β-cell secretes less insulin. Therefore, a decrease in insulinemia is a secondary effect of increasing hepatic GK activity. But, O'Doherty et al demonstrate that the influence of GK activity on blood glucose and insulin levels could be dose-dependent, as it occurs only with high doses of their transgene. In the hepatocyte, glucose-6-phosphate derived from GK activity is directed to glycogen synthesis and, consequently, hepatic glycogen levels are increased in the study by Ferre et al. However, glycogen content is not modified by GK overexpression in the study of O'Doherty et al, maybe for intrinsic limitations. In both animal models, increasing GK activity results in glucose signaling that activates transcription of glycolytic and lipogenic genes. Lipogenic proteins together with high availability of citrate and ATP (derived from augmented glucose metabolism) lead to enhanced *de novo* lipogenesis in the liver, and consequently, higher secretion of VLDL to bloodstream that could explain the observed increase in blood triglycerides. Augmented blood fatty acids might be explained by insulin levels; low levels of this hormone result in low inhibition of lipolysis in the adipose tissue, and consequently fatty acids raise in the bloodstream. Importantly, Ferre et al show that long-term GK overexpression drives to hyperinsulinemia and hepatic steatosis.

b. Studies of GK overexpression in the liver of fasted, healthy mice are listed in Table 3 (Hariharan, 1997; O'Doherty, 1999; Desai, 2001; Ferre, 2003 & Scott, 2003)

Study variables	Hariharan 1997	Desai 2001	Ferre 2003	O'Doherty 1999 Scott 2003
Animal model	*M. musculus* Transgenic	*M. musculus* Adenovirus	*M. musculus* Transgenic	*R. norvegicus* Adenovirus
Promoter	apoA1-SV40	RSV	PEPCK-C	CMV
GK activity over control	x5	x1.5	x2	x2.1 or x3
Age at analysis	5 weeks	3 weeks post-injection	12 months	4-5 days post-injection
Glycaemia	Decrease	no change	-	no change
Blood lactate	Decrease	no change	-	~ decrease
Blood triglycerides	no change	no change	increase	increase
NEFA	~ increase	no change	-	no change
Insulin	Decrease	decrease	increase	no change
Hepatic glucose-6-P	-	-	~ increase	-
Hepatic glycogen	-	-	no change	increase
Hepatic triglycerides	-	-	increase	-
Modulation of enzymes and transcription factors	-	-	-	↑ L-PK, ACC1 No change: PEPCK-C, PFK-2

Table 3. Hepatic GK overexpression studies in healthy fasted animals. Comments: decrease, increase and no change are referred to control group. "~" means no statistically significant; "-", no determined; "CMV", cytomegalovirus; "RSV", rose sarcoma virus; "apoA1-SV40", apolipoprotein A1 enhancer and simian vacuolating virus 40 promoter; "PEPCK-C", cytosolic phosphoenolpyruvate carboxykinase; "L-PK", liver pyruvate kinase; "ACC1", Acetyl-Coenzyme A carboxylase 1; "PFK-2", 6-phosphofructo-2-kinase/fructose-2,6-bisphosphatase.

In fast state, the influence of hepatic GK overexpression on glycaemia is not clear. Hariharan et al showed a decrease in glycaemia, accompanied by a decrease in insulinemia that could explain a reduction of glycolysis in skeletal muscle, causing the observed decline in serum lactate. Low insulin levels can also explain the increment of blood fatty acids. Interestingly, 20-weeks old mice were smaller than controls and presented reduced body mass index. On the contrary, long-term analysis of transgenic mice developed by Ferre et al showed that increasing GK activity in the liver lead to hepatic steatosis, hyperglycemia, hyperinsulinemia, obesity and insulin resistance. On the other hand, adenoviral gene transfer models for hepatic GK overexpression in fasting revealed induction of lipogenesis and consequently a tendency to increase blood triglycerides, without affecting glycaemia.

c. Studies on hepatic GK overexpression in the context of type 1 diabetes mellitus: This is an autoimmune disease with specific destruction of insulin-producing β-cells in the pancreas, and results in loss of insulin production. As insulin stimulates the transcription of Gck gene in the liver, type 1 diabetic subjects do not have GK protein in their livers and consequently hepatic glucose metabolism is impaired. Gene therapy has been tested to restore liver glucose uptake capacity by increasing hepatic GK protein (Ferre, 1996a; Morral, 2002, 2007). In type 1 diabetic liver, all models present a similar phenotype. When restoring glucose signaling in diabetic hepatocytes via GK, glucose catabolic pathways are induced and, on the contrary, hepatic glucose production is inhibited. Consequently there is a reduction of diabetic hyperglycemia accompanied by incremented hepatic glycogen depots and de novo lipogenesis. Decreasing blood glucose levels forces muscle and adipose tissue to use fatty acids as energetic substrates, and in consequence, serum fatty acids are decreased in type 1 diabetic mice expressing GK in the liver. Lower blood fatty acids, together with increased glucose metabolism in the liver, inhibit hepatic β-oxidation of fatty acids. Therefore, these models suggest that hepatic overexpression of GK in type 1 diabetes leads to normoglycaemia thanks to increments in hepatic glucose uptake and fatty acid oxidation in peripheral tissues.
d. Finally, hepatic GK overexpression in the context of type 2 diabetes: type 2 diabetes is a complex metabolic disorder caused by two physiologic defects: insulin resistance in combination with insulin secretion deficiency. Type 2 diabetes is characterized by glucose metabolism alterations such as failure of insulin to inhibit hepatic gluconeogenesis and impaired skeletal muscle glucose uptake. However, lipid metabolism is also altered. This is often reflected by increased circulating free fatty acids and triglycerides together with increased fat accumulation in non-adipose tissues. Thus, changes in the equilibrium between glucose and fatty acid metabolism in liver and muscle could be responsible for glucose homeostasis alterations. Obesity, hyperinsulinemia, in combination with hyperglycemia, inhibits fatty acid oxidation in many tissues. As a result, lipogenesis is favored over fatty acid oxidation leading to an increase in fat accumulation and a decrease in energy expenditure. A hypothetical strategy for type 2 diabetes therapy is increasing glucokinase activity, with the aim of enhancing glucose uptake in the liver that could contribute to gluconeogenesis inhibition with consequent restoration of glycaemia. If glycaemia is restored, plasma insulin levels could be secondarily lowered and it could be able to elevate energy expenditure and reduce obesity.

However, liver GK activity is increased in mild type 2 diabetes, but diminished in morbid obese diabetic patients. Animal diabetic models linked to obesity, show that GK deficiency in the liver occurs only in the case of obesity, and in severe or long-term forms of the disease. Although hepatic GK expression is different depending on disease stage, some strategies based on increasing GK activity in the liver have been tested in some models of high fat diet induced type 2 diabetes (Desai, 2001 & Ferre, 2003) , in obesity models (Wu, 2005 & Torres, 2009) and in transgenic mice with hepatic insulin resistance (Okamoto, 2007). All these studies have in common that the increase in hepatic GK activity produces glycaemia normalization. Hepatic GK, through glycolysis and glycogenesis activation, increases blood glucose clearance while it inhibits hepatic glucose production. On the other hand, liver GK activity results in increased malonyl-CoA, a lipogenic substrate and inhibitor of β-oxidation. It is difficult to draw clear conclusions when evaluating consequences of liver GK overexpression on lipid metabolism in type 2 diabetic models. Wu et al report an expected increase in hepatic and serum triglycerides, together with higher serum fatty acids. However, Wu et al report that, although hepatic fatty acid β-oxidation was decreased, muscle increased fatty acid oxidation as a consequence of lower glycaemia and insulinemia. Conversely, Desai et al showed no changes in hepatic and serum lipid levels. Otherwise, Torres et al & Okamoto et al obtained an increase in serum triglycerides with no changes in fatty acid levels. The most striking model is presented by Ferre et al: under high fat diet, liver GK-transgenic mice became insulin resistant faster than controls and showed hepatic steatosis. It contrasts with results obtained in GK gene locus transgenic mice (Shiota, 2001). Besides exhibiting a reduction of the blood glucose concentration, mice with a greater than normal amount of GK also exhibited a dramatic resistance to the development of hyperglycemia and hyperinsulinemia normally brought on by consumption of a high fat diet.

Taken together, all these models have convincingly demonstrated that increasing GK protein in the liver leads to a direct reduction of glycaemia, but sometimes it can be accompanied with the risk of serious alterations in lipid metabolism deriving in hepatic steatosis and/or overt dyslipidemia. This aspect is essential when considering the possibility of using GK overexpression in the liver for diabetes therapy. At this point, it would be important to find out which are the causes of the different phenotypes observed in those animal models of hepatic GK overexpression previously described. There are several possible reasons:

a. Species-specific results: one possibility is that GK overexpression in mouse liver may be more effective stimulating glucose disposal than the same degree of expression in a larger animal such as rat.
b. Side-effects of gene transfer technology: when using adenoviral gene transfer, adenoviruses involve *per se* hepatic metabolic changes. When using transgenic, germ-line manipulated animals overexpress GK throughout life, including intrauterine life, possibly resulting in compensatory changes in insulin secretion, insulin action, or in other metabolic variables that do not occur with acute manipulation of GK via adenovirus technology.
c. Promoter that directs transgene expression can affect two important variables. On one hand, taking into account the metabolic hepatic zonation concept (Jungermann, 1995), the promoter determines which set of hepatocytes express the transgene. It is well known that physiological GK expression predominates in the perivenous area of the liver (Moorman, 1991; Jungerman, 1995 & Jungerman, 2000). However, most studies of hepatic GK gain of function did not use perivenous promoters. For instance, Ferre et al used a PEPCK promoter that directs the transgene to the periportal area of the liver, specialized in gluconeogenesis. In contrast, RSV or CMV promoters are ubiquitous promoters that transfect both perivenous and periportal hepatocytes. On the other hand, promoter directs the regulation of transgene expression by nutrients and hormones. For instance, GK under the PEPCK promoter is expressed under glucagon signaling and is inhibited by glucose

and insulin. Therefore, hepatic GK transgenic mice described by Ferre et al express GK at the periportal area of the liver during fasting, and not in fed state.

d. Transgene dose: Desai et al and O'Doherty et al described different metabolic impact of hepatic GK overexpression depending on the dose of transgene that they used.

In our laboratory we aimed to re-examine the conclusions of these studies and the differentiated effects that GK activity could have on the metabolism, clearly differentiated, of periportal and perivenous hepatocytes. To evaluate the issue, we have developed a hydrodynamic gene transfer technique that served us to pursuit GK overexpression studies exclusively in perivenous liver (Liu, 1999; Zhang, 1999; Gomez-Valades, 2006; Budker, 2006 & Suda, 2007). With the injection of a plasmid for green fluorescent protein (GFP) and immunohistochemistry for PEPCK (periportal marker), we could visualize that hydrodynamic injection generate two separate populations of hepatocytes: green hepatocytes that expressed GFP and red hepatocytes showing PEPCK-C staining (Figure 4). We could conclude that in our conditions the hydrodynamic gene transfer technique delivered the transgene only in the hepatocytes surrounding the central vein of the liver acinus.

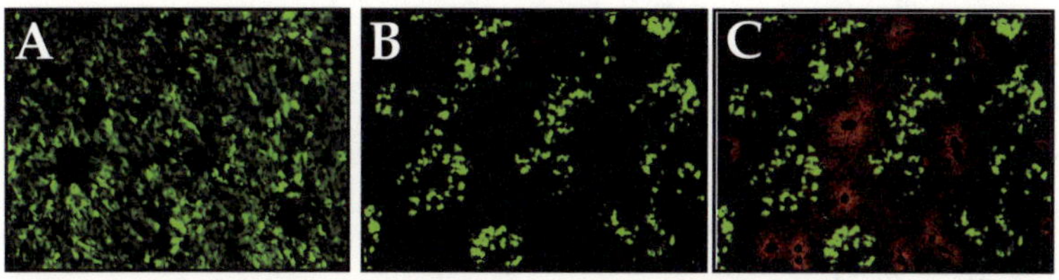

Fig. 4. Visualization of liver transfection achieved with adenoviral and hydrodynamic gene transfer techniques. (A) Healthy mice were injected with $5.5 \cdot 10^9$ IU of an adenovirus that codified for the green fluorescent protein (GFP). Green fluorescence was observed in liver sections (200X), demonstrating a homogeneous presence of the transgene all over the liver acinus. (B) A plasmid for GFP was hydrodynamically injected to healthy mice and, as it can see appreciated in liver sections, resulted in non-homogenous green fluorescence signal. (C) Slices from hydrodynamically-injected mice were immunostained for PEPCK-C (red signal), a periportal marker.

Our results represent the first attempt to overexpress pGK in perivenous hepatocytes. The first approach was the hydrodynamic injection of a plasmid with the Gck gene to healthy mice (Vidal-Alabró; publication pending). Forty-eight hours post-injection, increased GK in perivenous hepatocytes had clear effects on glucose homeostasis (Figure 5A). There was a reduction of glycaemia and insulinemia in the fed state, probably as a direct consequence of increased hepatic glucose uptake. Therefore perivenous GK gain of function reproduced results of periportal GK (Ferre, 1996), and liver-homogeneous GK overexpression (O'Doherty, 1999; Desai, 2001 & Scott, 2003). However, 16 hours-fasted mice did not show differences in blood glucose and insulin levels (data not shown), as Desai et al and O'Doherty et al had obtained with adenoviral GK transfer. Fifty days post-injection, perivenous GK overexpressing-mice presented blood glucose levels similar to control animals but accompanied by hyperinsulinism (Figure 5B). Long-term augmented GK activity in perivenous liver resulted in hepatic insulin resistance, since mice presented a phenotype very similar to liver-specific insulin receptor knock-out mice named LIRKO (Michael, 2000). Briefly, hyperinsulinism was probably due to reduced hepatic insulin clearance. Since peripheral tissues were still insulin-sensitive, hyperinsulinism inhibited lipolysis and induced lipogenesis in adipose tissue. Adipose tissue function together with reduced hepatic lipogenesis *de novo* could explain the observed decrease in circulating triglycerides and free fatty acids. Although having increased GK activity in the liver, neither glycogen synthesis nor glycolysis was stimulated in those mice. Besides, gluconeogenesis was not inhibited in fed state. Therefore, considering the bibliography, our perivenous model resembled transgenic mice that expressed GK transgene under PEPCK-C promoter at periportal hepatocytes (Ferre, 2003). However, periportal GK overexpressing model showed whole-body insulin resistance linked to obesity and hepatic steatosis. It must be considered that their analysis was in 12 months old mice. If the study was extended to 12 months, we would be able to tell if hepatic insulin resistance observed in our mice model leads to general insulin resistance or, on the contrary, confirm its resemblance to LIRKO animals.

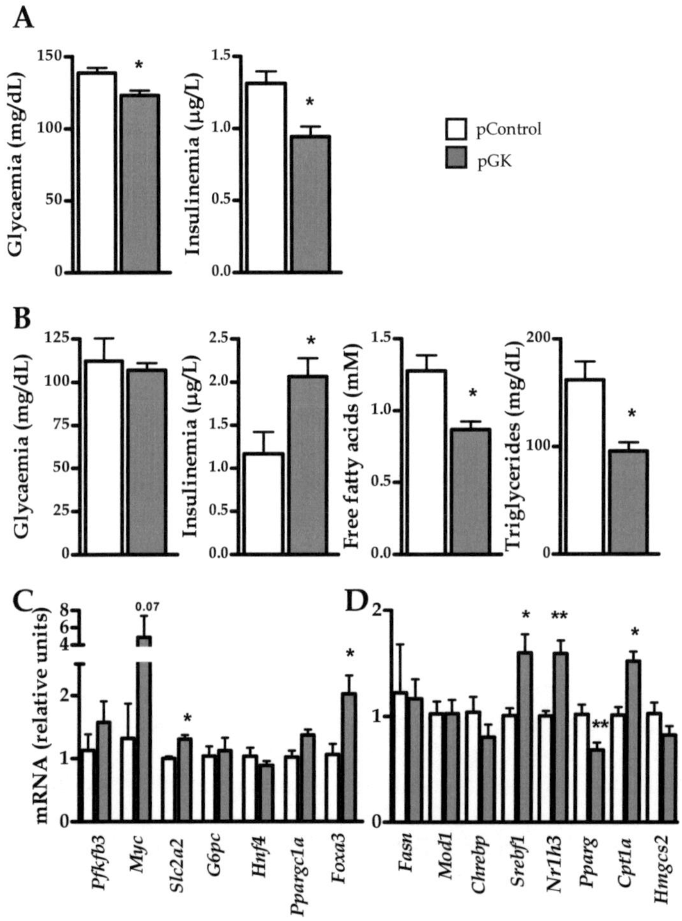

Fig. 5. Analysis of GK-overexpressing healthy mice. (A) Shows glycaemia and insulinemia, 48 hours post-injection of the plasmid that contained the GK gene. Columns represent media ± standard error. (B) 50 days post-injection results on serum nutrients (glucose, free fatty acids and triglycerides) together with insulin levels are represented. (C) After 50 days post-injection, expression of glycolytic and gluconeogenic genes from liver were analyzed by Real-Time PCR. Calculations were done following ΔΔCt algorithm (Applied Biosystems), using β-microglobulin gene expression as a housekeeping gene. (D) The same for lipogenic and lipolysis genes. * $p<0.05$ and ** $p<0.01$ vs control, determined by t-Student.

In the context of type 1 diabetes induced with streptozotocin, perivenous liver GK gain of function restored hepatic glucose uptake and reduced gluconeogenesis. Therefore, typical increases in hepatic glucose depots (glycogen, triglyceride) occurred and resulted in a reduction of diabetic glycaemia, albeit small. But, perivenous GK expressing mice showed a significant increase in triglyceride and free fatty acid serum concentration, and hepatic lipids (Figure 6) (Vidal-Alabró; publication pending). Therefore our work in type 1 diabetes model reproduces those of periportal GK overexpression (Ferre, 1996a) and those of liver homogeneous GK overexpression (Morral, 2002, 2007) in terms of glycaemia. However, our results on lipid metabolism are more deleterious, probably because perivenous hepatocytes have higher lipogenic potential than periportal hepatocytes (Jungermann, 1995).

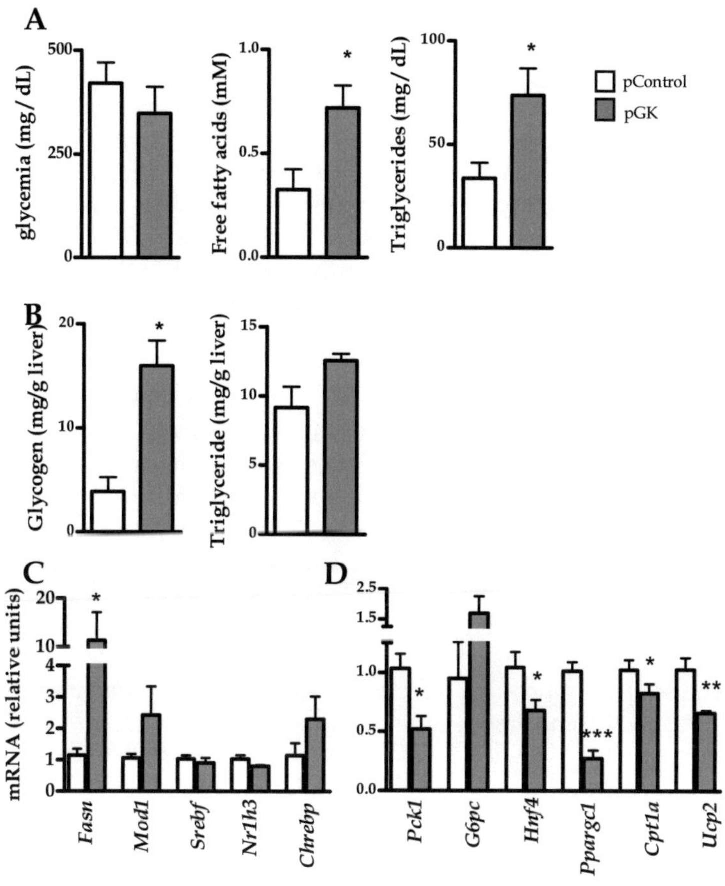

Fig. 6. Analysis of perivenous GK overexpression in type 1 diabetic mice. (A) Shows glycaemia, serum triglycerides and free fatty acids, 48 hours post-injection of the plasmid that contained the GK gene. Columns represent media ± standard error. (B) Hepatic glucose storage was evaluated by measuring glycogen and triglyceride levels. (C) Expression of lipogenic genes in the liver was analyzed by Real-Time PCR. Calculations were done following ΔΔCt algorithm (Applied Biosystems), using β-microglobulin gene expression as a housekeeping gene. (D) The same for gluconeogenic and lipolysis genes. * $p<0.05$, ** $p< 0.01$ and *** $p<0.001$ vs control, determined by t-Student.

All in all, our review of the literature together with our own results on the subject will convey that pGK-overexpression in the liver, independent of zonation, will result in changes in glycaemia but with the risk of non-desirable lipid alterations and insulin resistance. However, several undetermined factors influence the results obtained in GK overexpression studies, reinforcing the concept that hepatic GK is a key regulator of whole-body homeostasis, so that little changes in its activity and/or in its regulation affect glucose and lipid metabolism.

4. GKRP modulates the impact of GK activity on glucose and lipid homeostasis

GKRP is the best-known regulator of the hepatic GK at the post-transcriptional level. Therefore, impairments in GKRP should affect GK and consequently glucose metabolism, since GK plays a central role in glucose homeostasis. Nevertheless, mutations in the GKRP gene (Gckr) that caused disease or alterations in glucose metabolism have never been described until now. Recently, several whole-genome analysis have associated polymorphisms in the Gckr gene with fast hypoglycemia and increased serum triglyceride in humans, even though these subjects have reduced risk to type 2 diabetes (Køster, 2005; Sparsø, 2007; Vaxillaire, 2008; Orho-Melander, 2008 & Beer, 2009). The mechanism underlying this phenotype seems to be a reduction in GK inhibition by the variant regulatory protein (Beer, 2009). But, before exploring this issue it should be convenient to consider some aspects of GKRP biology.

Although GKRP research has been focused in the liver, there are evidences that the GKRP protein is also present in hypothalamic neurons (Schuit, 2001; Alvarez, 2002 & Roncero, 2009). GK/GKRP system in the hypothalamus could play a role in glucose-sensing important for the regulation of energy homeostasis by balancing energy intake, expenditure and storage. On the other hand, there is some controversy in the literature as to whether GKRP also regulates GK in pancreatic β-cells. The vast majority of studies state that GKRP is not expressed in rodent β-cells. However, it has been demonstrated that human islets express GKRP at very low levels (Beer, 2009). This issue should be revisited because of the recent publication of several genome-wide association studies that associate GK, GCKR, G6PC2, MTNR1B with type 2 diabetes risk linked to β-cell function (Reiling, 2009 & Bonetti, 2011). Whether, β-cell GK function is affected directly by a hypothetic pancreatic GKRP, or indirectly by liver GKRP impaired activity, still needs clarification. Another question that remains to be resolved is whether GKRP is also expressed and functional in other GK expressing cells, for instance, in the gut and in the pituitary gland.

Consequently, when considering studies of genome-wide association, mutant GKRP protein might affect GK activity in the brain, in the liver and perhaps in the β-cell. Therefore it is difficult to explain the phenotype only taking into account the hepatic GK/GKRP system. The same occurs with the characterization of GKRP-deficient mice (Farrelly, 2002 & Grimsby, 2000). GKRP knock-out mice models, whether heterozygous or homozygous, had normal weight. Interestingly focusing in liver analysis, those mice displayed reduced production of hepatic GK protein while having the same levels of GK mRNA than control animals, and GK protein was localized exclusively in the cytoplasm. That showed the importance of hepatic GKRP in stabilizing and protecting the intracellular GK pool. These animal models exhibited impaired postprandial glycemic control, with lower hepatic glycogen content and lack of inhibition of PEPCK-C gene expression, albeit with no noteworthy loss in insulin secretion or changes in fasting blood glucose concentrations. Moreover, when challenged with a high-sucrose/high-fat diet the knock-out and normal mice gained body weight at a similar rate but the knock-out mice were hyperglycaemic and hyperinsulinemic. Importantly, no changes in plasma triglycerides and non-esterified fatty acids were observed in basal conditions as well as with a high-sucrose/high-fat diet. In summary, absence of GKRP results in decreased hepatic GK protein content, affecting glucose metabolism without disturbing lipid parameters.

On the other hand, GKRP gain of function in the liver has also been assessed. In vitro studies with HepG2 cells simultaneously transduced with an adenoviral vector expressing GKRP and another adenoviral vector for GK had significantly elevated GK protein and activity levels compared with cells transduced with the GK adenovirus alone (Slosberg, 2001). These data suggest that GKRP serves to stabilize and protect a pool of GK protein (i.e., extend half-life), and is consistent with data obtained in GKRP knock-out studies. But in vivo studies revealed a more complicated situation. Adenoviral-mediated hepatic overproduction of GKRP in mice with high-fat diet-induced diabetes resulted in 23% decrease in GK enzymatic activity. Although reduction of GK activity is commonly associated to diabetes, hepatic GKRP-expressing mice had improved fasting and glucose-induced glycaemia with a concomitant increase in insulin sensitivity and TAG levels, and a decrease in leptin levels. A possible explanation for discrepancies between in vivo and in vitro results on GK levels when overexpressing GKRP is that GK expression in vivo is influenced by insulin and other physiological regulators. To understand how decreased GK activity improved type 2 diabetes phenotype in this model, a possibility is that GK activity may be applied in a more efficient manner toward metabolizing blood glucose. The subcellular compartmentalization by scaffolding proteins of enzymes or signaling proteins into clusters is often used as a means of increasing system efficiencies.

Coming back to genome-wide studies that associate Gckr with fast hypoglycemia and high triglycerides, Beer et al reported that P446L-GKRP has reduced regulation by physiological concentrations of fructose-6-phosphate, resulting indirectly in increased GK activity (Beer, 2009). They predicted that this increased GK activity in the liver enhanced glycolytic flux, promoting hepatic glucose metabolism and elevating concentrations of malonyl-CoA, a substrate for *de novo* lipogenesis, providing a mutational mechanism for the reported association of this variant with raised triglycerides and lower glucose levels. However, their predictions are conflictive with in vivo studies by Slosberg et al (Slosberg, 2001), since GKRP gain of function reduced hepatic GK activity and also resulted in a decrease of blood glucose levels accompanied by an increase of blood triglycerides. Therefore, any other undetermined factor/s must exist to really understand the complex physiology of the GK/GKRP system. Another possibility is that brain P446L-GKRP and β-cell P446L-GKRP (if existent) may exert determinant influences on phenotype.

Another study that may bring light to this issue, relates to defects in glucokinase translocation identified in Zucker diabetic fatty (ZDF) (Fujimoto, 2004 & Shin, 2007). Although having normal GK protein content, GK was predominantly localized in the nucleus regardless of plasma glucose and insulin levels. Nevertheless, sorbitol restored GK translocation. Clearly, there must be two distinct mechanisms bringing about the dissociation of GK from GKRP. How they are related and what differentiate them are questions currently under investigation. Since this defect was discovered in early stage of diabetes, it could cause of the progression to diabetes seen in the adult ZDF rat. Consistently, a MODY-2 mutation in the Gck gene has been reported to increase the physical interaction of GK and GKRP (García-Herrero, 2007). But, again these data are in conflict with other studies that reported some new GK mutations causing MODY-2 that reduced GK inhibition by GKRP (Veiga-da-Cunha, 1996; Gloyn, 2005 & Sagen, 2006). Once more, it is difficult to draw conclusions, but the importance of proper GK/GKRP function on metabolism and disease is reinforced, as subtle changes in its activity and/or regulation lead to contrary phenotypes.

Several naturally occurring activating mutations have been described that are localized at the same region where synthetic GK activators bind (Kamata, 2004; Heredia, 2006 & Matschinsky, 2009). Both activating mutations and synthetic activators stabilize the open conformation of the GK protein, resulting in higher affinity for glucose and a reduction of the interaction between GK and GKRP, since the super-open conformation of the enzyme (inactive) is not possible. In humans, activation of GK by naturally occurring mutations is associated to persistent hyperinsulinemic hypoglycemia of the infancy (PHHI), syndrome with a heterogeneous phenotype even in the same family but generally with a normal lipid profile. On the other hand, GK activation through administration of GK activation drugs has been tested for their potential in the therapy of type 2 diabetes, considering principally their capacity to increase glucose-stimulated insulin release at the β-cell (Grimsby, 2003; Brocklehurst, 2004; Efanov, 2005; Leighton, 2005; Coope, 2006 & Matschinsky, 2009). Whole-body effects of glucokinase activator drugs demonstrated a dose-dependent reduction of glycaemia, associated with increased insulin secretion in the pancreas and net glucose uptake in the liver. Besides, the administration of a GK activator prevented the development of diabetes in a diet-induced obesity animal model (Grimsby, 2003). Surprisingly, most in vivo studies with GK activators drugs do not show the lipid profile (Grimsby, 2003; Brocklehurst, 2004; Efanov, 2005; Leighton, 2005 & Coope, 2006), except one where treatment of ob/ob mice with GK activator PSN-GK1 did not produce any significant change blood lipids (Fyfe, 2007).

With all this puzzling background, we intended to study the expression of an activated mutant form of GK with the aim to decipher the metabolic consequences in the liver of having a GK not regulated by GKRP, with theoretical antidiabetic properties. Particularly we proposed the overexpression of glucokinase A456V (identified in patients of persistent hyperinsulinemic hypoglycemia of the infant), with a $S_{0.5}$ for glucose of 3 mM instead of 8 mM for the wild-type enzyme (Christesen, 2002), and without GKRP regulation (Heredia, 2006). We postulated that GK-A456V overexpression (also as a model for the liver-specific consequences of activating drugs on GK) could increase glucose uptake compared with the wild-type enzyme at equal levels of expression, whilst the metabolic fate of glucose might be different from that of wild-type GK due to its different capacity of interaction with other regulating proteins (GKRP and maybe PFK-2).

By means of hydrodynamic gene transfer of an expression plasmid for GK-A456V in healthy mice, we have been able to demonstrate that the perivenous overexpression of GK-A456V results in a sustained improvement in blood glucose, insulinemia and glucose tolerance, in the absence of dyslipidemia or hepatic lipidosis nor long-term insulin resistance (Vidal-Alabró; publication pending). Importantly, GK-A456V protein levels were similar to GK-control group, suggesting GK-A456V stability although not being directly regulated by GKRP. Its mechanism of action could be explained by its lower $S_{0.5}$ for glucose, so that glucose uptake is stimulated in later phases after ingestion (post absorptive phase) and during early fasting. It is tempting to speculate that glucose taken-up in perivenous liver, both in postprandial and post-absorptive periods, could be directed towards the glycolytic and oxidative metabolism and not through the pentose phosphate pathway that would favor lipid biosynthesis. This hypothesis is reinforced by results published by Wu et al (Wu, 2005) in which adenovirus expression of wild-type GK in the liver activate the pentose phosphate pathway, in marked contrast to the overexpression of the kinase domain from PFK-2 that stimulates flux through the glycolytic pathway. Surprisingly, GK-A456V transfected animals showed a marked increase in glucose-6-phosphatase. GK overexpression in perivenous hepatocytes does not significantly affect Glc6Pase expression, suggesting that zonation is an important experimental variable not sufficiently addressed to date in the field.

Transfecting GK-A456V in type 1 diabetic mice induced with streptozotocin, also caused an important reduction of diabetic hyperglycemia without dyslipidemia, in contrast with GK overexpression. Again, an induction of glucose-6-phosphatase transcription was observed in the liver GK-A456V -expressing animals (Figure 7) (Vidal-Alabró; publication pending).

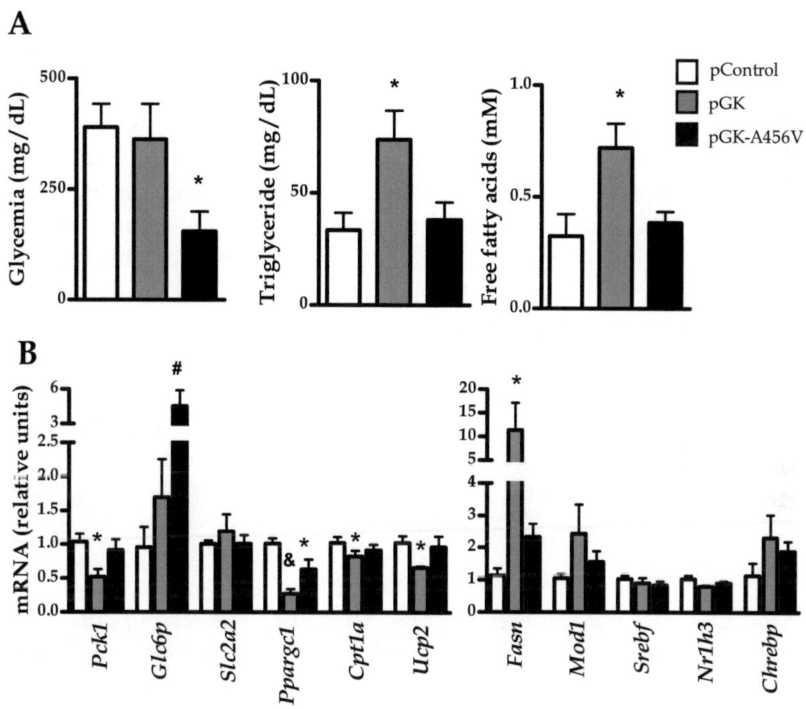

Fig. 7. Study of GK-A456V expression in the liver of type 1 diabetic mice. (A) Shows glycaemia, serum triglyceride and free fatty acid levels, 48 h post-injection of the plasmid for the GK-A456V gene. Columns represent media ± standard error. (B) Expression of gluconeogenic and lipolysis genes from liver was analyzed by Real-Time PCR. Calculations were done following ΔΔCt algorithm (Applied Biosystems), using β-microglobulin gene expression as a housekeeping gene. (C) The same for lipogenic genes. * $p<0.05$, # $p<0.05$ vs control and pGK, and & $p<0.001$ vs control and $p<0.05$ vs pGK-A456V, as determined by One-way ANOVA.

Our results lead us to consider the physiology of glucose-6-phosphatase in the context of glucose and lipid metabolism. Glucose-6-phosphatase dephosphorylates glucose-6-phosphate in the endoplasmic reticulum to obtain glucose, as the last step in the gluconeogenic pathway. Its transcription is regulated by insulin, so that it is repressed in fed state and induced during fasting. However, glucose induces transcription of this enzyme although the physiological significance of this induction is still not resolved (Nordlie, 2010). Finally glucose-6-phosphatase deficiency causes severe hyperlipidemia and hepatic steatosis (Bandsma, 2002, 2008), therefore giving rise that this enzyme may also participate or influence the GK/GKRP system in the regulation of hepatic glucose fate. To support this hypothesis, Reiling and colleagues described combined effects of single-nucleotide polymorphisms in GK, GKRP and glucose-6-phosphatase on fasting plasma glucose and type 2 diabetes (Reiling, 2009). Therefore, it is a field that needs further exploration.

5. Conclusion

Subtle changes in GK activity or in GKRP function have consequences in glucose and lipid metabolism. However, further studies must be done to completely understand the mechanism underlying GK/GKRP biology. Our results on increasing GK protein in the liver of both healthy and insulin-deficient mice (lacking endogenous GK) resulted in dyslipidemia. On the other hand, our analysis of the metabolic consequences of GK-GKRP deregulation by overexpressing a GK activating mutant (GKA456V) in the liver of both healthy and type 1 diabetic mice demonstrates an impact on glycaemia in the absence of dyslipidemia or hepatic lipid deposition. These data provide novel insights into the capacity of the complex GK-GKRP to influence the fate of metabolized glucose in the liver, providing a framework for further research on GK activating drugs in the liver.

We conclude that GKRP regulation impairment and GK-A456V altered kinetics greatly influence liver metabolism, in line with results in humans carrying a mutant GKRP (Køster, 2005; Sparsø, 2007; Vaxillaire, 2008 & Orho-Melander, 2008). Besides, it suggests that activating GK exclusively in the liver could be a feasible strategy to funnel excess glucose from the diet out of circulation, widening the scope for GK synthetic activators research.

6. Acknowledgments

We thank Sandra M. Ocampo, Francesc X. Blasco and the Research Support Services from the Biology Unit of Bellvitge (University of Barcelona) for their technical assistance, and Dr. Maria Molas for invaluable assistance in reviewing the manuscript. A.V.A received a fellowship from DURSI (Generalitat de Catalunya), A.M.L. received a fellowship from F.P.I. (Ministerio de Educación y Ciencia, Spain). This study was supported by a grant from the Ministerio de Educación y Ciencia (BFU2006-02802 and BFU2009-07506).

7. References

Agius, L. (2008). Glucokinase and molecular aspects of liver glycogen metabolism. *The Biochemical Journal,* Vol.414, No.1, (August 2008), pp. 1-18, ISSN 0264-6021

Alvarez, E., Roncero, I, Chowen, J.A., Vázquez, P. & Blázquez, E. (2002). Evidence that glucokinase regulatory protein is expressed and interacts with glucokinase in rat brain. *Journal of neurochemistry,* Vol. 80, No. 1, (January 2002), pp. 45-53, ISSN 0022-3042

Anderka, O., Boyken, J., Aschenbach, U., Batzer, A., Boscheinen, O. & Schmoll, D. (2008). Biophysical characterization of the interaction between hepatic glucokinase and its regulatory protein. *The Journal of Biological Chemistry,* Vol.283, No. 46, (November 2008), pp. 31333-31340, ISSN 0021-9258

Beer, N.L., Tribble, N.D., McCulloch, L.J., Roos, C., Johnson, P.R., Orho-Melander, M. & Gloyn, A.L. (2009). The P446L variant in GCKR associated with fasting plasma glucose and triglyceride levels exerts its effect through increased glucokinase activity in liver. *Human Molecular Genetics,* Vol 18, No. 21, (November 2009), pp. 4081-4088, ISSN 0964-6906

Bollen, J., Keppens, S. & Stalmans, W. (1998). Specific features of glycogen metabolism in the liver. *The Biochemical Journal,* Vol.336, No.1, (November 1998), pp. 19-31, ISSN 0264-6021

Bonetti, S., Trombetta, M., Boselli, M.L., Turrini, F., Malerba, G., Trabetti, E., Pignatti, P.F., Bonora, E. & Bonadonna, R.C. (2011). Variants of GCKR affect both β-cell and kidney function in patients with newly diagnosed type 2 diabetes: the Verona newly diagnosed type 2 diabetes study 2. *Diabetes care,* Vol. 34, No. 5, (May 2011), pp 1205-1210, ISSN 0149-5992

Brocklehurst, K. J., Payne, V.A., Davies, R.A., Carroll, D., Vertigan, H.L., Wightman, H.J., Aiston, S., Waddell, I.D., Leighton, B., Coghlan, M.P. & Agius, L. (2004). Stimulation of hepatocyte glycose metabolism by a novel small molecule glucokinase activators. *Diabetes,* Vol. 53, No. 3, (March 2004), pp. 535-541, ISSN 0012-1797

Budker, V.G., Subbotin, V.M., Budker, T., Sebestyén, M.G., Zhang, G. & Wolff, J.A. (2006). Mechanism of plasmid delivery by hydrodynamic tail vein injection. II. Morphological studies. *The journal of gene medicine,* Vol. 8, N. 7, (July 2006), pp. 874-888, ISSN 1099-498X

Cha, J.Y. & Repa, J.J. (2007). The liver X receptor (LXR) and hepatic lipogenesis. The carbohydrate-response element-binding protein is a target gene of LXR. *The Biochemical Journal,* Vol.282, No. 1, (January 2007), pp. 743-751, ISSN 0264-6021

Chen, G., Liang, G., Ou, J., Goldstein, J. L. & Brown, M.S. (2004). Central role for liver X receptor in insulin-mediated activation of Srebp-1c transcription and stimulation of fatty acid synthesis in liver. *Proceedings of the National Academy of Sciences,* Vol. 101, No. 31, (August 2004), pp. 11245-11250, ISSN 0027-8424

Christesen, H.B., Jacobsen, B.B., Odili, S., Buettger, C., Cuesta-Munoz, A., Hansen, T., Brusgaard, K., Massa, O., Magnuson, M.A., Shiota, C., Matschinsky, F.M & Barbetti, F. (2002). The second activating glucokinase mutation (A456V): implications for glucose homeostasis and diabetes therapy. *Diabetes,* Vol. 51, No. 4, (April 2002), pp. 1240-1246, ISSN 0012-1797

Coope, G.J., Atkinson, A.M., Allot, C., McKerrecher, D., Johnstone, C., Pike, K.G., Holme, P.C., Vertigan, H., Gill, D., Coghlan, M.P. & Leighton, B. (2006). Predictive blood glucose lowering efficacy by glucokinase activators in high fat fed female Zucher rats. *British Journal of pharmacology,* Vol. 149, No. 3, (October 2006), pp. 328-335, ISSN 0007-1188

Denechaud, P.D., Bossard, P., Lobaccaro, J.A., Millatt, L., Staels, B., Girard, J. & Postic, C. (2008). ChREBP, but not LXRs, is required for the induction of glucose-regulated genes in mouse liver. *The Journal of Clinical Investigation,* Vol. 118, No. 3, (March 2008), pp. 956-964, ISSN 0021-9738

Desai, U.J., Slosberg, E.D., Boettcher, B.R., Caplan, S.L., Fanelli, B., Stephan, Z., Gunther, V.J, Kaleko, M. & Connelly, S. (2001). Phenotypic correction of diabetic mice by adenovirus-mediated glucokinase expression. *Diabetes,* Vol. 50, No. 10, (October 2001), pp. 2287-2295, ISBN 0012-1797

Efanov, A.M., Barrett, D.G., Brenner, M.B., Briggs, S.L., Delaunois, A., Durbin, J.D., Giese, U., Guo, H., Radloff, M., Gil, G.S., Sewing, S., Wang, Y., Weixhert, A., Zaliani, A. & Gromada, J. (2005). A novel glucokinase activator modulates pancreatic islet and hepatocyte function. *Endocrinology,* Vol. 146, No. 9, (September 2005), pp. 3696-3701, ISSN 0013-7227

Farrely, D., (1999). Mice mutant for glucokinase regulatory protein exhibit decreased liver glucokinase: a sequestration mechanism in metabolic regulation. *Proceedings of the National Academy of Sciences,* Vol. 96, No. 25, (December 1999), pp. 14511-14516, ISSN 0027-8424

Ferre, P. & Foufelle, F. (2010). Hepatic steatosis: a role for *de novo* lipogenesis and the transcription factor SREBP-1c. *Diabetes, Obesity and Metabolism,* Vol.12, (October 2010), pp. 83-92, ISSN 1462-8902

Ferre, T., Pujol, A., Riu, E., Bosch, F. & Valera, A. (1996a). Correction of diabetic alterations by glucokinase. *Proceedings of the National Academy of Sciences,* Vol. 93, No. 14, (July 1996), pp. 7225-7230, ISSN 0027-8424

Ferre, T., Riu, E., Bosch, F.& Valera, A. (1996b). Evidence from transgenic mice that glucokinase is rate limiting for glucose utilization in the liver. *The FASEB Journal,* Vol. 10, No. 10, (August 1996), pp. 1213-1218, ISSN 0892-6638

Ferre, T., Riu, E., Franckhauser, S., Agudo, J & Bosch, F. (2003). Long-term overexpression of glucokinase in the liver of transgenic mice leads to insulin resistance. *Diabetologia,* Vol. 46, No. 12, (December, 2003), pp. 1662-1668, ISSN 0012-186X

Foretz, M., Guichard, C., Ferre, P. & Foufelle, F. (1999). Sterol regulatory element binding protein-1c is a major mediator of insulin action on the hepatic expression of glucokinase and lipogenesis-related genes. *Proceedings of the National Academy of Sciences,* Vol. 96, No. 22, (October 1999), pp. 12737-12742, ISSN 0027-8424

Fujimoto, Y., Donahue, E. D. & Shiota, M. (2004). Defect in glucokinase translocation in Zucher diabetic fatty rats. *American Journal of Physiology. Endocrinology and Metabolism,* Vol. 287, No. 3, (September 2004), pp. E414-E423, ISSN 0193-1849

Fyfe, M.C., White, J.R., Taylor, A., Chatfield, R., Wargent, E., Printz, R.L., Suplice, T., McCormack, J.G., Procter, M.J., Teynet, C., Widdowson, P.S. & Wong-Kai-In, P. (2007). Glucokinase activator PSN-GK1 displays enhanced antihyperglycaemic and insulinotropic actions. *Diabetologia,* Vol. 50, No. 6, (June 2007) pp. 1277-1287, ISSN 0012-186X

García-Herrero, C.M., Galán, M., Vincent, O., Flández, B., Gargallo, M., Delgado-Alvarez, E., Blázquez, E. & Navas, M.A. (2007). Functional analysis of human glucokinase gene mutations causing MODY2: exploring the regulatory mechanisms of glucokinase activity. *Diabetologia,* Vol. 50, No. 2, (February 2007), pp. 325-333, ISSN 0012-186X

Gavrilova, O., Haluzik, M., Matsuse, K., Custon, J.J., Johnson, L., Dietz, K.R., Nicol, C.J., Vinson, C., Gonzalez, F.J. & Reitman, M.L. (2003). Liver peroxisome proliferator-activated receptor gamma contributes to hepatic steatosis, triglyceride clearance, and regulation of body fat mass. *The Journal of Biological Chemistry,* Vol.278, No. 36, (September 2003), pp. 34268-34276, ISSN 0021-9258.

Ginsberg, H.N., Zhang,Y., Hernandez-Ono, A. (2006). Metabolic Syndrome: Focus on Dyslipidemia. *Obesity*, Vol.14, Suppl.1, (February 2006), pp. 41S-49S, ISSN 1930-7381.

Gloyn, A.L. (2003). Glucokinase (GCK) mutations in hyper- and hypoglycemia: maturity-onset diabetes of the young, permanent neonatal diabetes, and hyperinsulinemia of infancy. *Human mutation,* Vol. 22, No. 5, (November 2003), pp. 353-362, ISSN 1059-7794

Gloyn, A.L., Odili, S., Zelent, D., Buettger, C., Castleden, H.A., Steele, A. M., Stride, A., Shiota, C., Magnuson, M.A., Lorini, R., d'Annunzio, G., Stanley, C.A., Kwagh, J., van Schaftingen E., Veiga-da-Cunha, M., Barbetti, F., Dunten, P., Han, Y., Grimsby, J., Taub, R., Ellard, S., Hattersley, A. T.& Matschinsky, F.M. (2005). Insights into the structure and regulation of glucokinase from a novel mutation (V62M), which causes maturity-onset diabetes of the young. *The Journal of Biological Chemistry,* Vol. 280, No. 14, (April 2005), pp 14105-14113, ISSN 0021-9258

Gómez-Valadés, A. G., Vidal-Alabro, A., Molas, M., Boada, J., Bermúdez, J., Bartrons, R. & Perales, J.C. (2006). Overcoming diabetes-induced hyperglycemia through inhibition of hepatic phosphoenolpyruvate carboxykinase (GTP) with RNAi. *Molecular Therapy,* Vol. 13, No. 2; (February 2006), pp. 401-410, ISSN 1525-0016

Gregori, C., Guillet-Deniau, I., Girard, J., Decaux, J.F. & Pichard, A.L. (2006). Insulin regulation of glucokinase gene expression: evidence against a role for sterol regulatory element binding protein 1 in primary hepatocytes. *FEBS Letters,* Vol. 580, No. 2, (January 2006), pp. 410-414, ISSN 0014-5793

Grimsby, J., Coffey, J.W., Dvorozniak, M.T., Magram, J., Li, G., Matschinsky, F.M., Shiota, C., Kaur, S., Magnuson, M.A. & Grippo, J.F. (2000). Characterization of glucokinase regulatory protein-deficient mice. *The Journal of biological chemistry,* Vol. 275, No. 11, (March 2000), pp. 7826-7831, ISSN 0021-9258

Grimsby, J., Sarabu, R., Corbett, W.L., Haynes, N.E., Bizzarro, F.T., Coffey, J.W., Guertin, K.R., Hilliard, D.W., Kester, R.F., Mahaney, P.E., Marcus, L., Qi, L., Spence, C.L., Tengi, J., Magnuson, M.A., Chu, C.A., Dvorozniak, M.T., Matschinsky, F.M. & Grippo, J.F. (2003). Allosteric activators of glucokinase: potential role in diabetes therapy. *Science,* Vol. 301, No. 5631, (July 2003), pp. 370-373, ISSN 0036-8075

Hariharan, N., Farrelly, D., Hagan, D., Hillyer, D., Arbeeny, C., Sabrah, T., Treloar, A., Brown, K., Kalinowski, S. & Mookhtiar, K. (1997). Expression of human hepatic glucokinase in transgenic mice liver results in decreased glucose levels and reduced body weight. *Diabetes,* Vol. 46, No. 1, (January 1997), pp. 11-16, ISSN 0012-1797

Heredia, V.V., Carlson, T.J, Garcia, E. & Sun, S. (2006). Biochemical basis of glucokinase activation and the regulation by glucokinase regulatory protein in naturally occurring mutations. *The Journal of biolobical chemistry,* Vol. 281, No. 52, (December 2006), pp. 40201-40207, ISSN 0021-9258

Iizuka, K. & Horikawa, Y. (2008). ChREBP: A Glucose-activated Transcription Factor Involved in the Development of Metabolic Syndrome. *Endocrine Journal.* Vol. 55, No. 4, (August 2008), pp. 617-624, ISSN 0918-8959

Iynedjian, P.B., (2009). Molecular physiology of mammalian glucokinase. *Cellular and Molecular Life Sciences,* Vol. 66, No. 1, (January 2009), pp. 27-42, ISSN 1420-682X

Jungermann, K., (1995). Zonation of metabolism and gene expression in liver. *Histochemistry and cell biology,* Vol. 103, No. 2,(February 1995), pp. 81-91, ISSN 0948-6143

Jungermann, K. & Kietzmann, T. (2000). Oxygen: modulator of metabolic zonation and disease of the liver. *Hepatology,* Vol. 31, No. 2, (February 2000), pp. 255-260, ISSN 0270-9139

Kabashima, T., Kawaguchi, T., Wadzinski, B.E. & Uyeda, K. (2003). Xylulose-5-phosphate mediates glucose-induced lipogenesis by xylulose-5-phosphate-activated protein phosphatase in rat liver. *Proceedings of the National Academy of Sciences,* Vol. 100, No. 9, (April, 2003), pp. 5107-5112, ISSN 0027-8424

Kamata, K., Mitsuya, M., Nishimura, T., Eiki, J. & Nagata, Y. (2004). Structural basis for allosteric regulation of the monomeric allosteric enzyme human glucokinase. *Structure,* Vol. 12, No. 3, (March 2004), pp. 429-438, ISSN 0969-2126

Køster, B., Fenger, M., Poulsen, P., Vaag, A. & Bentzen, J. (2005). Novel polymorphisms in the GCKR gene and their influence on glucose and insulin levels in a Danish twin population. *Diabetic medicine: a journal of the British Diabetic Association*, Vol. 22; No. 12 (December 2005), ISSN 0742-3071

Lee, A., Scappa, E.F., Cohen, D.E. & Glimcher, L.H. (2008) Regulation of Hepatic Lipogenesis by the Transcription Factor XBP1. *Science,* Vol. 320, No. 5882, (June 2008), pp. 1492-1496, ISSN 0036-8075

Leighton, B., Atkinson, A. & Coghlan, M.P., (2005). Small molecule glucokinase activators as novel anti-diabetic agents. *Biochemical Society transactions,* Vol. 33, No. Pt 2, (April 2005), pp. 371-374, ISSN 0300-5127

Liu, F., Song, Y. & Liu, D. (1999). Hydrodynamics-based transfection in animals by systemic administration of plasmid DNA. *Gene Therapy,* Vol. 6, No. 7, (July 1999), pp. 1258-1266, ISSN 0969-7128

Massa, M.L., Gagliardino, J.J. & Francini, F. (2011). Liver glucokinase: an overview on the regulatory mechanisms of its activity. *IUBMB Life,* Vol. 63, No. 1, (January 2011), pp. 1-6, ISSN 1521-6543

Massillon, D., Chen, W., Barzilai, N., Prus-Wertheimer, D., Hawkins, M., Liu, R., Taub, R. & Rossetti, L. (1998). Carbon flux via the pentose phosphate pathway regulates the hepatic expression of the glucose-6-phosphatase and phosphoenolpyruvate carbokykinase genes in conscious rats. *The Journal of Biological Chemistry,* Vol.273, No. 1, (January 1998), pp. 228-234, ISSN 0021-9258.

Matschinsky, F.M. Assessing the potential of glucokinase activators in diabetes therapy. *Nature reviews. Drug discovery,* Vol 8, No. 5, (May 2009), pp. 399-416, ISSN 1474-1776

Michael, M.D., Kulkarni, R.N., Postic, C., Previs, S.F., Shulman, G.I., Magnuson, M.A. & Kahn, C.R. (2000). Loss of insulin signaling in hepatocytes leads to severe insulin resistance and progressive hepatic dysfunction. *Molecular Cell,* Vol. 6, No. 1, (July 2000), pp. 87-97, ISSN 1097-2765

Mitro, N., Mak, P.A., Vargas, L., Godio, C., Hampton, E., Molteni, V., Kreusch, A. & Saez, E. (2007). The nuclear receptor LXR is a glucose sensor. *Nature,* Vol. 445, (January 2007), pp. 219-223, ISSN 0028-0836

Moorman, A.F., de Boer, P.A., Charles, R. & Lamers, W.H. (1991). Pericentral expression pattern of glucokinase mRNA in the rat liver lobulus. *FEBS letters,* Vol. 287, No. 1-2, (August 1991), pp. 47-52, ISSN 0014-5793

Morral, N., McEvoy, R., Dong, H., Meseck, M., Altomonte, J., Thung, S. & Woo, S.L. (2002). Adenovirus-mediated expression of glucokinase in the liver as an adjuvant treatment for type 1 diabetes. *Human gene therapy,* Vol. 13; No. 13, (September 2002), pp. 1561-1570, ISSN 1043-0342

Morral, N., Edenberg, H.J., Witting, S.R., Altomonte, J., Chu, T. & Brown, M. (2007). Effects of glucose metabolism on the regulation of genes of fatty acid synthesis and triglyceride secretion in the liver. *Journal of lipid research,* Vol. 48, No. 7, (July 2007), pp. 1499-1510, ISSN 0022-2275

Nordlie, R.C. & Foster, J.D. (2010). A retrospective review of the roles of multifunctional glucose-6-phosphatase in blood glucose homeostasis: Genesis of the tuning/retuning hypothesis. *Life sciences,* Vol. 87, No. 11-12, (September 2010), pp. 339-349, ISSN 0024-3205

O'Doherty, R.M., Lehman, D.L., Télémaque-Potts, S. & Newgard, C.B. (1999). Metabolic impact of glucokinase overexpression in liver: lowering of blood glucose in fed rats is accompanied by hyperlipidemia. *Diabetes,* Vol. 48, No. 10, (October, 1999), pp. 2022-2027, ISSN 0012-1797

Okamoto, Y., Ogawa, W., Nishizawa, A., Inoue, H., Teshigawara, K., Kinoshita, S., Matsuki, Y., Watanabe, E., Hiramatsu, R., Sakaue, H., Noda, T. & Kasuga, M. (2007). Restoration of glucokinase expression in the liver normalizes postprandial glucose disposal in mice with hepatic deficiency of PDK1. *Diabetes,* Vol. 56, No. 4, (April 2007), pp. 1000-1009, ISSN 0012-1797

Orho-Melander, M., Melander, O., Guiducci, C., Perez-Martinez, P., Corella, D., Roos, C., Tewhey, R., Rieder, M.J., Hall, J., Abecasis, G., Tai, E.S., Welch, C., Arnett, D.K., Lyssenko, V., Lindholm, E., Saxena, R., de Bakker, P.I., Burtt, N., Voight, B.F., Hirschhorn, J.N., Tucker, K.L., Hedner, T., Tuomi, T., Isomaa, B., Eriksson, K.F., Taskinen, M.R., Wahlstrand, B., Hughes, T.E., Parnell, L.D., Lai, C.Q., Berglund, G., Peltonen, L., Vartiainen, E., Jousilahti, P., Havulinna, A.S., Salomaa, V., Nilsson, P., Groop, L., Altshuler, D., Ordovas, J.M. & Kathiresan, S. (2008). Common missense variant in the glucokinase regulatory protein gene is associated with increased plasma triglyceride and C-reactive protein but lower fasting glucose concentrations. *Diabetes,* Vol. 57, No. 11, (November 2008), pp. 3112-3121, ISSN 0012-1797

Osbak, K.K., Colclough, K., Saint-Martin, C., Beer, N.L., Bellanné-Chantelot, C., Ellard, S. & Gloyn, A.L. (2009). Update on mutations in glucokinase (GCK), which cause maturity-onset diabetes of the young, permanent neonatal diabetes, and hyperinsulinemic hypoglycemia. *Human mutation,* Vol. 30, No. 11, (November, 2009), pp. 1512-1526, ISSN 1059-7794

Postic, C., Niswender, K.D., Decaux, J.F., Parsa, R., Shelton, K.D., Gouhot, B., Pettepher, C.C., Granner, D.K., Girard, J. & Magnuson, M.A. (1995). *Genomics,* Vol. 29, No. 3, (October 1995), pp. 740-750, ISSN 0888-7543

Postic, C., Shiota, M., Niswender, K.D., Jetton, T.L., Chen, Y., Moates, J.M., Shelton, K.D., Lindner, J., Cherrington, A.D. & Magnuson, M.A. (1999) Dual roles for glucokinase in glucose homeostasis as determined by liver and pancreatic beta cell-specific gene knock-outs using Cre recombinase. *The Journal of Biological Chemistry,* Vol.274, No. 1, (January 1999), pp. 305-315, ISSN 0021-9258.

Puigserver, P., (2003). Insulin-regulated hepatic gluconeogenesis through FOXO1-PGC-1alpha interaction. *Nature,* Vol. 423, (May 2003), pp. 550-555, ISSN 0028-0836

Reiling, E., van't Riet, E., Groenewould, M.J., Welschen, L.M., van Hove, E.C., Nijpels, G., Maassen, J.A., Dekker, J.M. & 't Hart, L.M. (2009). Combined effects of single-nucleotide polymorphisms in GCK, GCKR, G6PC2 and MTNR1B on fasting plasma glucose and type 2 diabetes risk. *Diabetologia,* Vol. 52, No. 9, (September 2009) pp. 1866-1870, ISSN 0012-186X

Roncero, I., Sanz, C., Alvarez, E., Vázquez, P., Barrio, P.A. & Blázquez, E. (2009). Glucokinase and glucokinase regulatory proteins are functionally coexpressed before birth in the rat brain. *Journal of Neuroendocrinology,* Vol. 21; No. 12, (December 2009), pp. 973-981, ISSN 0953-8194

Roth, U., Curth, K., Unterman, T.G., & Kietzmann, T. (2004). The transcription factors HIF-1 and HNF-4 and the coactivator p300 are involved in insulin-regulated glucokinase gene expression via the phosphatidylinositol 3-kinase/ protein Kinase B pathway. *The Journal of Biological Chemistry,* Vol.279, No. 4, (January 2004), pp. 2623-2631, ISSN 0021-9258.

Sagen, J.V., Odili, S., Bjørkhaug, L., Zelent, D., Buettger, C., Kwagh, J., Stanley, C., Dahl-Jørgensen, K., de Beaufort, C., Bell, G.I., Han, Y., Grimsby, J., Taub, R., Molven, A., Søvik, O., Njølstad, P.R. & Matschinsky, F.M. (2006). From clinicogenetic studies of maturity-onset diabetes of the young to unravelling complex mechanisms of glucokinase regulation. *Diabetes,* Vol. 55, No. 6, (June 2006), pp. 1713-1722, ISSN 0012-1797

Schuit, F.S., Huypens, P., Heimberg, H. & Pipeleers, D.G. (2001). Glucose Sensing in Pancreatic β-Cells. A Model for the Study of Other Glucose-Regulated Cells in Gut, Pancreas, and Hypothalamus. *Diabetes,* Vol. 50, No. 1, (January 2001), pp. 1-11, ISSN 0012-1797

Scott, D.K., Collier, J.J., Doan, T.T., Bunnell, A.S., Daniels, M.C., Eckert, D.T. & O'Doherty, R.M. *Molecular and cellular biochemistry,*Vol. 254, No. 1-2, (December 2003), pp. 327-337, ISSN 0300-8177

Shimomura, I., Shimano, H., Korn, B.S., Bashmakow, Y., & Horton, J.D. (1998). Nuclear sterol regulatory element-binding proteins activate genes responsible for the entire program o unsaturated fatty acid biosynthesis in transgenic mouse liver. *The Journal of Biological Chemistry,* Vol.273, No. 52, (December 1998), pp. 35299-35306, ISSN 0021-9258.

Shin, J.S., Torres, T.P., Catlin, R.L., Donahue, E.P. & Shiota, M. (2007). A defect in glucose-induced dissociation of glucokinase from the regulatory protein in Zucker diabetic fatty rats in the early stage of diabetes. *American Journal of Phisiology. Regulatory, integrative and comparative physiology.* Vol. 292, No. 4, (April 2007), pp. R1381-R1390, ISSN 0363-6119

Shiota, C., Coffey, J., Grimbsy, J., Grippo, J.F. & Magnuson, M.A. (1999). Nuclear import of hepatic glucokinase depends upon glucokinase regulatory protein, whereas export is due to a nuclear export signal sequence in glucokinase. *The Journal of Biological Chemistry,* Vol. 274, No. 52, (December 1999), pp. 37125-37130, ISSN 0021-9258.

Shiota, M., Postic, C., Fujimoto, Y., Jetton, T.L., Dixon, K., Pan, D., Grimsby, J., Grippo, J.F., Magnuson, M.A. & Cherrington, A.D. (2001). Glucokinase gene locus transgenic mice are resistant to the development of obesity-induced type 2 diabetes. *Diabetes,* Vol. 50, No. 3, (March 2001), pp. 622-629, ISSN 0012-1797

Slosberg, E.D., Desai, U.J., Fanelli, B., St. Denny, I., Connelly, S., Kaleko, M., Boettcher, B.R. & Caplan, S.L. (2001). Treatment of type 2 diabetes by adenoviral-mediated overexpression of the glucokinase regulatory protein. *Diabetes,* Vol. 50, No. 8, (August 2001), pp. 1813-1820, ISSN 0012-1797

Sparsø, T., Andersen, G., Nielsen, T., Burgdorf, K.S., Gjesing, A.P., Nielsen, A.L., Albrechtsen, A., Rasmussen, S.S., Jørgensen, T., Borch-Johnsen, K., Sandbæk, A., Lauritzen, T., Madsbad, S., Hansen, T. & Pedersen, O. (2008). The GCKR rs780094 polymorphism is associated with elevated fasting serum triacylglycerol, reduced fasting and OGTT-related insulinaemia, and reduced risk of type 2 diabetes. *Diabetologia,* Vol. 51, No. 1, (January 2008), pp. 70-75, ISSN 0012-186X

Suda, T., Gao, X., Stolz, D.B. & Liu, D. (2007). Structural impact of hydrodynamic injection on mouse liver. *Gene Therapy,* Vol. 14, No. 2, (January 2007), pp. 129-137, ISSN 0969-7128

Torres, T.P., Catlin, R.L., Chan, R., Fujimoto, Y., Sasaki, N., Printz, R.L., Newgard, C.B. & Shiota, M. (2009). Restoration of hepatic glucokinase expression corrects hepatic glucose flux and normalizes plasma glucose in zucker diabetic fatty rats. *Diabetes,* Vol. 58, No. 1, (January 2009), pp. 78-86, ISSN 0012-1797

Uyeda, K. & Repa, J.J. (2006). Carbohydrate response element binding protein, ChREBP, a transcription factor coupling hepatic glucose utilization and lipid synthesis. *Cell Metabolism,* Vol. 4, No. 2, (August 2006), pp. 107-110, ISSN 1550-4131

Van Shaftingen, E. & Veiga da Cunha, M. (2004). Discovery and role of glucokinase regulatory protein, In: *Glucokinase and Glycemic Disease: From Basics to Novel Therapeutics,* Matschinsky, F.M., Magnuson, M.A. (eds), pp. 193-207, Karger, ISBN 3-8055-7744-3, Basel (Switzerland)

Vaxillaire, M., Cavalcanti-Proença, C., Dechaume, A., Tichet, J., Marre, M., Balkau, B. & Froguel, P., for the DESIR Study Group (2008). The common P446L polymorphism in GCKR inversely modulates fasting glucose and triglyceride levels and reduces type 2 diabetes risk in the DESIR prospective general French population. *Diabetes,* Vol. 57, No. 8, (August 2008), pp. 2253-2257, ISSN 0012-1797

Veiga-da-Cunha, M., Xu, L.Z., Lee, Y.H., Marotta, D., Pilkis, S.J. & Van Schaftingen, E. (1996). Effect of mutations on the sensitivity of human beta-cell glucokinase to liver regulatory protein. *Diabetologia,* Vol. 39, No. 10, (October 1996), pp. 1173-1179, ISSN 0012-186X

Vieira, E., Salehi, A & Gylfe, E. (2007). Glucose inhibits glucagon secretion by a direct effect on mouse pancreatic alpha cells. *Diabetologia,* Vol. 50. No. 2, (February 2007), pp. 370-379, ISSN 0012-186X

Wang, X., Sato, R., Brown, MS., Hua, X. & Goldstein, JL. (1994). SREBP-1, a membrane-bound transcription factor released by sterol-regulated proteolysis. *Cell,* Vol. 77, No.1, (April 1994), pp. 53-62, ISSN 0092-8674.

Wu, C., Okar, D.A., Newgard, C.B. & Lange, A.J. (2001) Overexpression of 6-phosphofructo-2-kinase/fructose-2,6-bisphosphatase in mouse liver lowers blood glucose by suppressing hepatic glucose production. *The Journal of Clinical Investigation,* Vol. 107, No. 1, (January 2001), pp. 91-98, ISSN 0021-9738

Wu, C., Kang, J.E., Peng, L.J., Li, H., Khan, S.A., Hillard, C.J., Okar, D.A. & Lange, A.J. (2005) Enhancing hepatic glycolysis reduces obesity: differential effects on lipogenesis depend on site of glycolytic modulation. *Cell Metabolism,* Vol. 2, No. 2, (August 2005), pp. 131-140, ISSN 1550-4131

Zelent, D., Golson, M.L., Koeberlein, B., Quintens, R., van Lommel, L., Buettger, C., Weik-Collins, H., Taub, R., Grimsby, J., Schuit, F., Kaestner, K.H. & Matschinsky, F.M. (2006). A Glucose Sensor Role for Glucokinase in Anterior Pituitary Cells. *Diabetes,* Vol. 55, (July 2006), pp. 1923-1929, ISSN 0012-1797

Zhang, G., Budker, V. & Wolff, J.A. (1999). High levels of foreign gene expression in hepatocytes after tail vein injections of naked plasmid DNA. *Human Gene Therapy,* Vol. 10, No. 10, (July 1999), pp. 1735-1737, ISSN 1043-0342

Zhu, L.L., Liu, Y., Cui, A.F., Shao, D., Liang, J.C., Liu, X.J., Chen, Y., Gupta, N., Fang, F.D., & Chang, Y.S. (2010). PGC-1alpha coactivates estrogen-related receptor-alpha to induce the expression of glucokinase. *American Journal of Physiology. Endocrinology and metabolism.* Vol 298. No. 6, (June 2010), pp.E1210-8, ISSN 0193-1849

13

Liver Sinusoidal Endothelial Cells and Regulation of Blood Lipoproteins

Dmitri Svistounov[1], Svetlana N. Zykova[1,2], Victoria C. Cogger[1], Alessandra Warren[1], Aisling C. McMahon[1], Robin Fraser[3] and David G. Le Couteur[1]

[1]*Centre for Education and Research on Ageing and ANZAC Research Institute, University of Sydney and Concord RG Hospital, Sydney,*
[2]*Department of Nephrology, University Hospital of Northern Norway, Tromsø,*
[3]*University of Otago, Christchurch,*
[1]*Australia*
[2]*Norway*
[3]*New Zealand*

1. Introduction

Dyslipidaemia is a well-described major independent risk factor for cardiovascular disease (Lin et al.). It is well established that the liver plays the central role in lipid metabolism and liver malfunction is one of the main sources of dyslipidemia (Watson et al., 2003). However, most of the studies so far have focused on the role of hepatocytes in lipid turnover. Indeed, hepatocytes do play a central role in liver lipid metabolism, but they are not alone. Hepatocytes do not have direct contact with the circulation. Any blood-borne lipoprotein particle must first pass through a filter comprised of a layer of endothelial cells, lining the walls of liver sinusoids, before it can contact the liver parenchyma. Likewise, lipoproteins remodelled or synthesized by the liver encounter the same barrier before they reach systemic circulation.

2. The structure of the hepatic sinusoid

The hepatic sinusoids are small blood vessels, comparable to capillaries in size, that perfuse the hepatocytes. However, unlike the capillaries in other tissues, sinusoids are formed by a discontinuous endothelium that lacks any significant underlying basement membrane. Walls of sinusoids are formed by the liver sinusoidal endothelial cells (LSECs). LSECs are separated from liver parenchyma by the perisinusoidal extravascular space, known as the space of Disse (Figure 1A). LSECs contribute only 15-20% of all liver cells but comprise 70% of the population of sinusoidal cells in the liver (Arias, 1990; Arii and Imamura, 2000; Blouin et al., 1977; Knook and Sleyster, 1976).

The LSECs are perforated by trans-cytoplasmic pores called fenestrae, which do not have any intervening diaphragmatic membrane, and thus are fully patent holes through the cell (Figure 1A-B). This specialized lace-like morphology of the LSECs minimizes any barrier to the bi-directional transfer of solutes and particulate substrates between the sinusoidal blood and hepatocytes, whilst retaining the capacity and substantial surface area to undergo interactions with circulating blood cells including immune cells (Cogger and Le Couteur, 2009; Fraser et al., 1995; Wisse et al., 1996). Fenestrae are not uniformly distributed over the LSEC surface but are aggregated into groups of tens to hundreds in gossamer thin areas of cytoplasm and towards the periphery of the cell. These areas of fenestral aggregations are termed sieve plates (Figure 1B). Between 60-75% of fenestrae are found within sieve plates in rats (Vidal-Vanaclocha and Barbera-Guillem, 1985) but isolated fenestrae are also frequently observed on the LSEC surface.

The LSEC becomes fenestrated at an early gestational stage (Enzan et al., 1997; Martinez-Hernandez and Amenta, 1993; Nonaka et al., 2007; Smedsrod et al., 2009). The porosity of the sinusoids depends on the number and especially the size or diameter of the fenestrae. The diameter of fenestrae has a normal distribution curve of about 50-200nm (Cogger and Le Couteur, 2009). Gaps larger than about 200nm are regarded as artifacts formed during specimen preparation for electron microscopy (Akinc et al., 2009; Fraser et al., 1978; Fraser et al., 1980; Hilmer et al., 2005a).

Fenestrae have been found in many species including such diverse species as man, rat, mouse, guinea pig, sheep, goat, rabbit, fowl, monkey, baboon, bat, kitten, dog, turtle and fish (Cogger and Le Couteur, 2009).

The fenestrated endothelium was first suggested as a filter of chylomicrons by Wisse in 1970 (Wisse, 1970) from their reported diameters (Fraser et al., 1968) and termed the "liver sieve" once sieving was confirmed (Fraser et al., 1978; Naito and Wisse, 1978). Fenestrae allow the transfer of a wide range of substrates including plasma and plasma molecules, such as plasma proteins, some lipoproteins and colloidal particles (Le Couteur et al., 2005). The latter also include artificial chylomicron-like nanospheres such as Intralipid, but also small viruses leading to hepatitis, viral vectors for DNA manipulation of hepatocytes.

The fenestrated LSEC can be defined as an ultrafiltration system because it is a low pressure system with pores approximately 100nm in diameter. Specifically, the liver sieve can be described as a Loeb–Sourirajan ultrafiltration system, with the LSECs providing the thin porous layer (Baker, 2004). The transfer of fluid across an ultrafiltration system can be calculated using the Hagen Poiseuille equation for ultrafiltration where the flux of fluid is proportional to the number of pores and the radius of the pores to the power of four (Baker, 2004; Le Couteur et al., 2006; Warren et al., 2005). Therefore small changes in the size of fenestrae has profound effects on the size and number of substrates and macromolecules that can gain passage into the space of Disse. Indeed, manipulation of fenestrae diameter might have a role in regulating the transfer of substrates in response to physiological changes, such as feeding and fasting (O'Reilly et al., 2010).

The space of Disse is the extravascular space lying between the hepatocytes and LSECs. It contains some components of extracellular matrix and most components of blood plasma filtered through LSEC's sieve plates. Extracellular matrix in the space of Disse contains fibronectin and collagen type I ,III, V, and VI. Collagen type IV is also present but unlike its sheet-like polymeric presentation in typical basement membranes, here it appears in the form of discontinuous aggregates (Martinez-Hernandez and Amenta, 1993). Of note, basement membrane has not been identified in liver sinusoids in any non-pathological state or developmental stage until old age (Enzan et al., 1997; Martinez-Hernandez and Amenta, 1993; Nonaka et al., 2007; Smedsrod et al., 2009), where its appearance is believed to be a sign of age-related degeneration and – possibly – a cause of pathology.

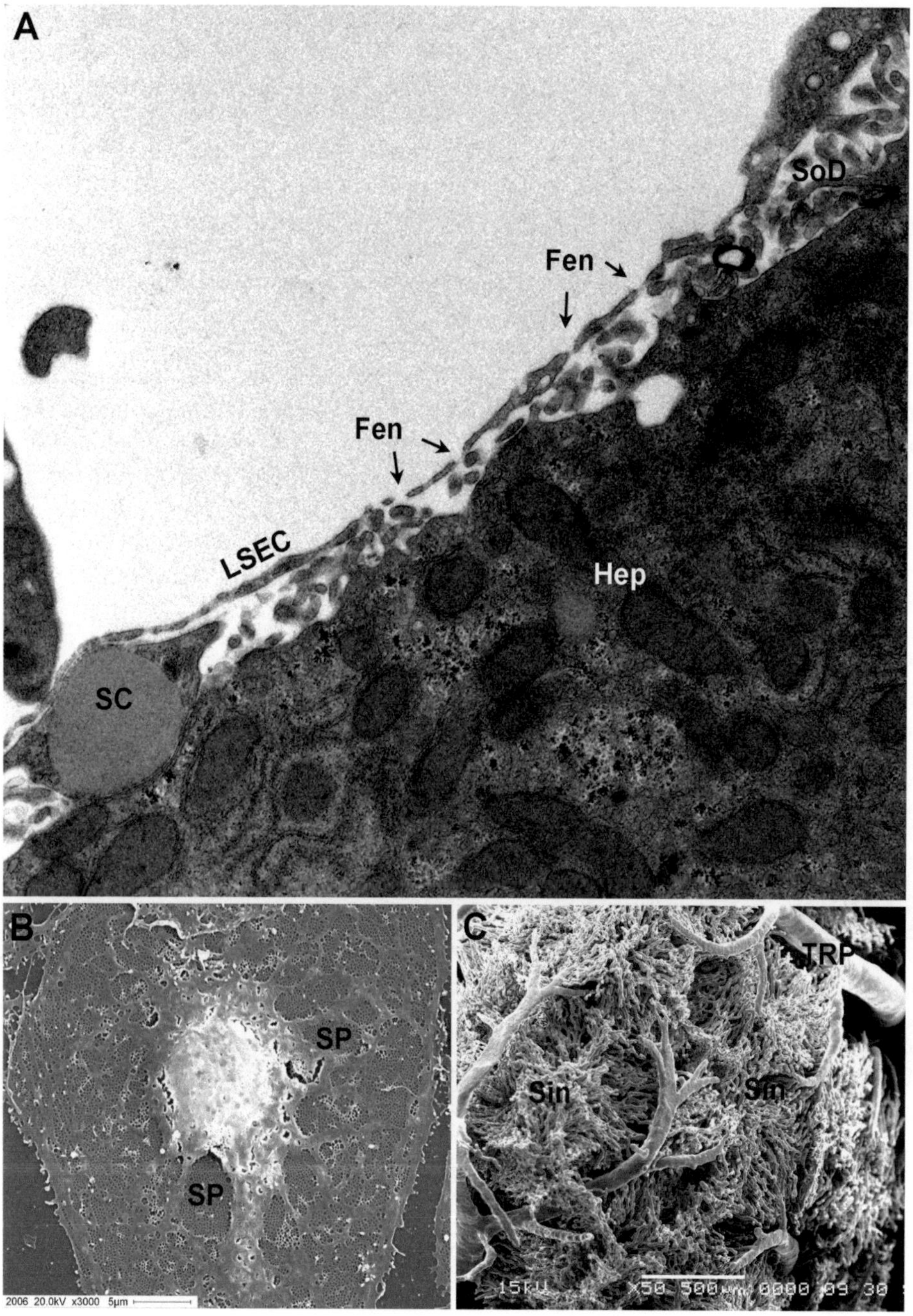

Fig. 1. A: Transmission electron micrograph showing liver sinusoidal endothelial cell (LSEC) perforated by fenestrae (Fen). (Hep) – hepatocyte, (SoD) - space of Disse, (SC) - stellate cells with lipid droplet in space of Disse. B: Scanning electron micrograph of an isolated liver sinusoidal endothelial cell showing fenestrae clustered into sieve plates (SP). C: Scanning electron micrograph of a vascular cast showing branches of the portal vein (TPV) with surrounding sinusoidal network (Sin). (Preparations performed by A Warren).

Multiple microvilli from the the sinusoidal surface of the hepatocytes protrude into the space of Disse and increase the available surface area for the recognition, transport and diffusion of substrates to and from the liver (Cogger and Le Couteur, 2009; Fraser et al., 1995; Wisse et al., 1996).

There are three other cell types residing in the liver sinusoids apart from the LSECs: Kupffer cells (resident liver macrophages), stellate cells and pit cells. Kupffer cells represent only 20% of all the population of liver sinusoidal cells but 80-90% of all tissue macrophages in the body (Knook and Sleyster, 1976). They generally reside within the lumen of the liver sinusoids and take up bacteria and other large particles, such as cell debris, from the circulation by phagocytosis. In response to bacterial infection, Kupffer cells produce cytokines and a number of soluble pro-inflammatory factors that promote influx and activation of neutrophils (Smedsrod et al., 1994; Smedsrod et al., 2009) and may alter the porosity of the sinusoids to promote cirrhosis (Dobbs et al., 1994). Together, LSECs (pinocytosis) and Kupffer cells (phagocytosis) constitute the hepatic reticuloendothelial system (RES), the most powerful scavenger system of mammals and other terrestrial vertebrates (Aschoff, 1924; Kawai et al., 1998).

3. The normal function of the LSEC in regulation of blood lipids

Because of the LSECs fenestrae, all lipoproteins except large chylomicrons have unimpeded access to the hepatocytes. After delivering triglycerides to peripheral tissues, chylomicrons become processed into so-called "chylomicron remnants" that carry significant amounts of cholesterol and are highly pro-atherogenic (Fujioka and Ishikawa, 2009; Karpe et al., 1994). At the same time they become small enough to pass through LSECs fenestrae (Fujioka and Ishikawa, 2009) and can be taken up by hepatocytes, which allows liver parenchyma to be the major site for removal of pro-atherogenic chylomicron remnants from the blood (Cooper, 1997; Dietschy et al., 1993) under normal circumstances. However, fast and efficient blood clearance of highly atherogenic chylomicron-remnants by hepatocytes requires well fenestrated LSECs.

4. Ageing of the LSEC and regulation of blood lipids

Many important diseases, particularly cardiovascular diseases, that result in disability and death, occur late in life, indicating that aging itself is a key risk factor. Old age is associated with significant changes in the cells of the hepatic sinusoid. Previously, it has been considered that the liver does not undergo significant aging changes because of its large functional reserve, regenerative capacity and dual blood supply (Popper, 1986). Only a few descriptions of the aging liver have been generally established, such as an increase in the number of polyploid and binucleate hepatocytes (Schmucker, 1998) and "brown atrophy", which is a reduction in liver mass accompanied by the deposition of the aging pigment, lipofuscin (Popper, 1986). Today it has become clear that age-related changes in hepatic structure and function are significant and influence systemic exposure to xenobiotics, endogenous substances associated with disease and medications (McLean and Le Couteur, 2004). Thus, such changes in the liver have implications for many diseases of aging and the aging process itself.

It has now been reported that old age is associated with substantial ultrastructural changes in the LSECs and space of Disse in intact livers of the rat (Jamieson et al., 2007; Le Couteur et al., 2001), human (McLean et al., 2003), the mouse (Ito et al., 2007; Warren et al., 2005) and the non-human primate, *Papio hamadryas* (Cogger et al., 2003). The findings have been replicated in at least three separate centres around the world (Furrer et al.; Ito et al., 2007; Le Couteur et al., 2001; Stacchiotti et al., 2008). These changes have been termed 'pseudocapillarization' because the aging sinusoids become similar to capillaries seen in other non-fenestrated vascular beds (Le Couteur et al., 2001). Unlike 'capillarization' seen in the hepatic sinusoid in cirrhosis of the liver, aging is not associated with any of the typical changes apparent on light microscopy, such as bridging fibrosis and nodular regeneration (Le Couteur et al., 2001; Le Couteur et al., 2008). In old age, LSEC thickness is increased by approximately 50% and there is a similar reduction of about 50% in the porosity and number of fenestrae (Figure 2). These changes are associated with perisinusoidal basal lamina deposition in many old livers and some scattered collagen in the space of Disse. The effect of aging on the diameter of fenestrae has been inconsistent between species, however there is a trend towards a reduction in diameter of around 5-10% (Le Couteur et al., 2008). Isolated LSECs typically retain some of these ultrastructural changes. Fenestrae diameter was reduced in old age from 194±1 nm to 185±1 nm in isolated rat LSECs (O'Reilly et al., 2009).

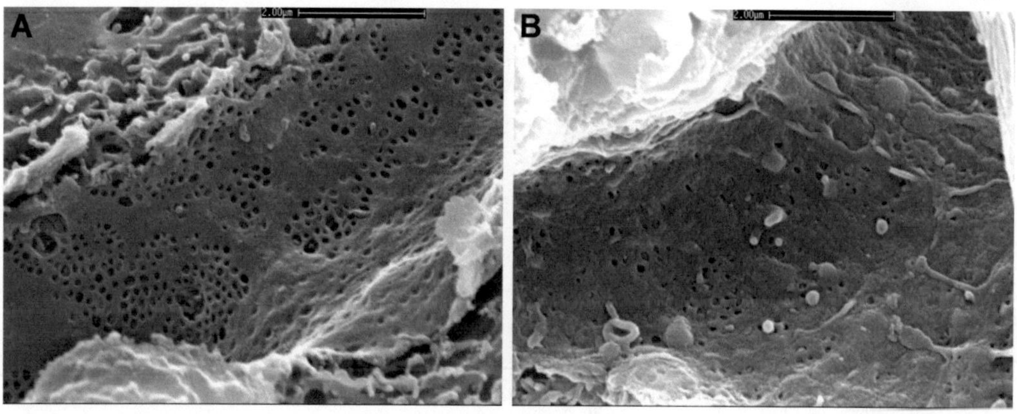

Fig. 2. Scanning electron micrographs of the liver sinusoid of a young (A) and old (B) rat. The loss of fenestrae perforating the endothelial cell surface in the old liver is apparent. (Preparations performed by A Warren).

Fenestrations have a role in the transfer of lipoproteins from blood to the hepatocyte, therefore it is likely that pseudocapillarization of sinusoids will impair lipoprotein clearance by the liver and contribute to dyslipidaemia in older people (Le Couteur et al., 2002). Atherosclerosis increases dramatically with old age and its complications affect most older people (Lakatta and Levy, 2003). The clearance of chylomicron remnants is significantly impaired in older people (Borel et al., 1998; Krasinski et al., 1990) and in those aged 65 years and older, remnant-like lipoprotein cholesterol is associated with the development of coronary artery disease (Simons et al., 2001). To determine whether age-related defenestration impairs the transfer of lipoproteins across the LSECs, the multiple indicator dilution method was used to study lipoprotein disposition in perfused rat livers (Hilmer et al., 2005b). In young livers, lipoproteins (approximately 50 nm diameter) entered the entire extracellular space whereas in old livers, the lipoproteins were confined to the vascular space. These results strongly suggest that age-related pseudocapillarization impairs the hepatic disposition of lipoproteins and thus plays a role in age-related dyslipidaemia.

Matrix heparan sulfate proteoglycans bind and sequester lipoprotein remnants (Williams, 2008). In old age, formation of basal lamina beneath LSECs leads to a change in the proportions of extracellular matrix components and may result in impaired passage of lipoproteins across the space of Disse. However, the importance of this pathway in lipoprotein turnover has not been studied sufficiently, especially in connection to aging.

A reduction in caloric intake by about 40% increases maximum life expectancy and is associated with a delay in the onset of most age-associated disorders and pathology (Everitt et al., 2005). It has also been demonstrated that caloric restriction delays the onset of pseudocapillarization in rats. In the old caloric restricted rats, endothelial thickness was significantly less and fenestrae porosity was significantly greater than in the old ad libitum fed rats. Moreover, caloric restriction prevented the age-related increase in perisinusoidal collagen IV staining (Jamieson et al., 2007). The finding that caloric restriction influences pseudocapillarization suggests that the latter is secondary to the aging process and thus potentially reversible. As a consequence, modulation of LSEC fenestrations might be a therapeutic target for the treatment of age-related dyslipidemia and prevention of vascular disease. On the other hand, early onset of pseudocapillarization and dyslipidemia occur in a transgenic mouse model of Werner syndrome, a rare premature aging syndrome in humans.

Another hallmark of old age - the reduction in liver size as a fraction of body weight - is usually in the order of 25-35% (Le Couteur and McLean, 1998) and is associated with a decrease in the number of hepatocytes. In addition, several studies have shown that the total hepatic blood flow is reduced by about 30-50% (Le Couteur and McLean, 1998). Liver perfusion, which is the blood flow per mass of liver, is also reduced in old age but to a lesser extent than total blood flow. Mechanisms for these changes remain unclear; however, a recent study using high resolution *in vivo* microscopy has shown how pseudocapillarization might contribute to these phenomena. There was a 14% reduction in the numbers of perfused sinusoids with old age and a 35% reduction in sinusoidal blood flow (Ito et al., 2007). Narrower sinusoids with thickened LSECs and swollen stellate cells with abundant lipid droplets were also observed. It was concluded that these changes caused age-related reduction in hepatic perfusion and hepatic blood flow by blocking the sinusoids (Ito et al., 2007). The clearance of highly extracted substrates from the circulation is dependent on blood flow, therefore the age-related reduction in hepatic blood flow has a dramatic effect on the liver's overall function (Le Couteur and McLean, 1998), including the clearance of lipoproteins.

It is reasonable to conclude that pseudocapillarization, in combination with a reduction in hepatic blood flow, are two major factors contributing to age-related dyslipidemia.

5. Scavenger function of LSEC in clearance of oxidized lipoproteins

Another unique feature of LSECs is extraordinary endocytic activity. LSECs are rich in coated pits and vesicles and other organelles associated with endocytosis. Although LSECs constitute only 2.8 % of the total liver volume, they contain about 15% of the total lysosomal volume and about 45% of the pinocytic vesicle volume of the liver (Blouin et al., 1977). Moreover, specific activities of several lysosomal enzymes are higher in LSECs than in other liver cells (Knook and Sleyster, 1980). LSECs express a set of high-affinity endocytic receptors for soluble macromolecular waste products, generated during normal tissue turnover, blood clotting, inflammatory processes and pathological conditions (McCourt et al., 1999; Skogh et al., 1985; Smedsrod, 2004; Smedsrod et al., 1994; Smedsrod et al., 2006; Smedsrod et al., 1997; Smedsrod et al., 1990). Connective tissue macromolecules including hyaluronan, chondroitin sulphate, collagen α-chain, Procollagen Propeptides (PICP, PINP and PIIINP), products released during cell death such as lysosomal enzymes and metabolic byproducts including oxidized low density lipoproteins (oxLDLs), advanced glycation end products, and immune complexes and microbial CpG motifs are exclusively cleared from the blood circulation by mannose receptor-mediated or scavenger receptor-mediated endocytosis in LSECs (Elvevold et al., 2008; Malovic et al., 2007; Martin-Armas et al., 2006; Skogh et al., 1985; Smedsrod, 2004; Smedsrod et al., 1997; Smedsrod et al., 1990).

LSECs express several different scavenger receptors including scavenger receptors -A, scavenger receptors-B, and scavenger receptors-H (Hughes et al., 1995; Malerod et al., 2002). However, stabilin-1 and stabilin-2 have been recognised as the main scavenger receptors on LSECs (Hansen et al., 2005; Hansen et al., 2002; McCourt et al., 1999; Politz et al., 2002; Zhou et al., 2000). Following receptor mediated endocytosis in LSECs most of the ligands are rapidly degraded intra-lysosomally. Thus, LSECs represent a major site of scavenging and degradation of harmful waste macromolecules from the circulation and have therefore been termed 'scavenger endothelial cells' (Seternes et al., 2002).

LSEC endocytosis of oxLDL may also be implicated in the development of atherosclerosis. Atherosclerosis begins as a progressive, chronic inflammatory condition characterized by thickening of the arterial intima through proliferation of intimal smooth muscle cells, which has been shown to be precipitated by cholesterol-rich LDL and triglycerides derived from chylomicron remnants (Fischer-Dzoga et al., 1976). This may then advance to a complex plaque, which can ultimately lead to serious cardiovascular complications, such as myocardial infarction and stroke from occluded arteries. The oxidative modification of LDL has been suggested to play an important role in the development of these events (Steinberg, 1997, 2009). LDL can undergo *in vivo* oxidation in the arterial walls (Yla-Herttuala et al., 1989) and in plasma (Avogaro et al., 1988; Holvoet et al., 1998b). The process starts within the LDL particle with oxidation of polyunsaturated fatty acids which generates a great number of various intermediate and end-products. Formation of free and organic radicals launches a chain reaction that causes fragmentation of both lipid and protein constituents of LDL. Formation of reactive aldehydes, such as malondialdehyde, 4-hydroxynonenal and glyoxal results in chemical modification of side chain amino groups of the lysine residues of apoB-100, which in turn leads to an increased net negative surface charge of the molecule (Baynes and Thorpe, 1999; Fu et al., 1996; Jialal and Devaraj, 1996; Oorni et al., 2000; Witztum and Steinberg, 1991; Young and McEneny, 2001). Therefore, the oxidative modification of LDL involves changes in both the protein and the lipid components of the LDL-particle. This in turn induces changes in surface charge and conformation, which renders LDL a ligand for scavenger receptors, and reduces or abolishes its affinity to the LDL receptor (Berliner and Heinecke, 1996; Li et al., 2011).

In arterial intima, oxLDLs are taken up by macrophages via scavenger receptors. This induces foam cell formation and subsequent atheroma development (Henriksen et al., 1981, 1983; Steinbrecher et al., 1984). Oxldls are commonly present in atherosclerotic lesions of experimental animals and humans (Palinski et al., 1989; Yla-Herttuala et al., 1989). OxLDL has also been identified in plasma of healthy individuals (Avogaro et al., 1988; Ehara et al., 2001; Itabe and Takano, 2000). In patients with cardiovascular disease, plasma levels of oxLDL have been reported to be approximately fourfold higher than in healthy subjects (Ehara et al., 2001; Holvoet et al., 1998b). In addition to cardiovascular disease, increased levels of oxLDL are associated with ageing (Brinkley et al., 2009) and certain age-related pathologies, such as Alzheimer's disease (Kankaanpaa et al., 2009), glomerulosclerosis (Lee, 1999), and diabetes mellitus (Lopes-Virella et al., 1999).

Therefore, timely clearance and maintenance of low circulatory levels of oxLDLs appear to be important for the prevention of atherosclerosis (Holvoet et al., 1998b; Itabe, 2003). Previously, it has been shown that intravenously injected radiolabeled oxLDLs are rapidly removed from blood by uptake in Kupffer cells and LSECs (Ling et al., 1997; Van Berkel et al., 1991). However, a recent study demonstrated that Kupffer cells are only active in uptake of heavily oxidized LDL (Li et al., 2011). which is mainly present in atherosclerotic plaques (Yla-Herttuala et al., 1989) or formed as an artifact during *in vitro* oxLDL preparation. At the same time, LSECs hold an exclusive role in the uptake of mildly oxidized LDL from the circulation (Li et al., 2011). Mildly oxidized LDL is the major form of oxLDL found in the blood (Chang et al., 1997; Holvoet et al., 1998a; Holvoet et al., 1998b), and has proatherogenic properties (Berliner et al., 1990; Watson et al., 1997; Witztum and Steinberg, 1991). Both stabilin-1 and stabilin-2 are involved in the endocytic uptake of oxLDL by LSECs. Stabilin-1, however, appears to be more important for the uptake of mildly oxidized LDL, which represents physiological blood-borne oxLDL, while stabilin-2 is important for uptake when there is greater LDL modification (Li et al., 2011).

The morphological changes in the LSEC in old age might also affect its role in endocytosis. Recently, *in vivo* microscopy was used to examine the real time uptake of scavenger receptor ligands by LSECs (Ito et al., 2007). Endocytosis was clearly diminished in old mice, particularly in the pericentral zone which may indicate hypoxic liver damage. The effect of old age on clearance of oxLDL by LSEC has not been examined yet. However, involvement of stabilin 1 and 2, the two major LSEC scavenger receptors, in the process of oxLDL uptake (Li et al., 2011) makes it likely that oxLDL clearance would be diminished in old age. This change would increase the level of oxLDL in the circulation, thereby promoting its extrahepatic concentration and increasing the risk of the development of atherosclerosis.

6. Conclusions

Age-related changes in morphology and function of LSECs apparently contribute to dyslipidemia and, as a consequence, to the development of cardiovascular disease. Old age is associated with reduced fenestrae in the LSEC which impedes the hepatic uptake of chylomicron remnants and possibly other lipoproteins. In addition, aging is associated with reduced LSEC endocytic capacity which will impact on circulating levels of oxLDL. Thus the LSEC is a novel therapeutic target for the treatment of age-related dyslipidemia and has great potential for the prevention of atherosclerosis and cardiovascular events.

7. References

Akinc, A., M. Goldberg, J. Qin, J. R. Dorkin, C. Gamba-Vitalo, M. Maier, K. N. Jayaprakash, M. Jayaraman, K. G. Rajeev, M. Manoharan, V. Koteliansky, I. Rohl, E. S. Leshchiner, R. Langer, and D. G. Anderson, 2009, Development of lipidoid-siRNA formulations for systemic delivery to the liver: Mol Ther, v. 17, p. 872-9.

Arias, I. M., 1990, The biology of hepatic endothelial cell fenestrae: Prog Liver Dis, v. 9, p. 11-26.

Arii, S., and M. Imamura, 2000, Physiological role of sinusoidal endothelial cells and Kupffer cells and their implication in the pathogenesis of liver injury: J Hepatobiliary Pancreat Surg, v. 7, p. 40-8.

Aschoff, L., 1924, Das reticulo-endotheliale System: Ergebnisse inn. Med Kinderheilk, v. 26, p. 1-118.

Avogaro, P., G. B. Bon, and G. Cazzolato, 1988, Presence of a modified low density lipoprotein in humans: Arteriosclerosis, v. 8, p. 79-87.

Baker, R. W., 2004, Membrane Technology and Applications: Hokoben NJ, John Wiley & Sons Ltd.

Baynes, J. W., and S. R. Thorpe, 1999, Role of oxidative stress in diabetic complications: a new perspective on an old paradigm: Diabetes, v. 48, p. 1-9.

Berliner, J. A., and J. W. Heinecke, 1996, The role of oxidized lipoproteins in atherogenesis: Free Radic Biol Med, v. 20, p. 707-27.

Berliner, J. A., M. C. Territo, A. Sevanian, S. Ramin, J. A. Kim, B. Bamshad, M. Esterson, and A. M. Fogelman, 1990, Minimally modified low density lipoprotein stimulates monocyte endothelial interactions: J Clin Invest, v. 85, p. 1260-6.

Blouin, A., R. P. Bolender, and E. R. Weibel, 1977, Distribution of organelles and membranes between hepatocytes and nonhepatocytes in the rat liver parenchyma. A stereological study: J Cell Biol, v. 72, p. 441-55.

Borel, P., N. Mekki, Y. Boirie, A. Partier, M. C. Alexandre-Gouabau, P. Grolier, and B. Beaufrere, 1998, Comparison of postprandial plasma vitamin A response in young and older adults: J Gerontol, v. 53, p. B133-140.

Brinkley, T. E., B. J. Nicklas, A. M. Kanaya, S. Satterfield, E. G. Lakatta, E. M. Simonsick, K. Sutton-Tyrrell, and S. B. Kritchevsky, 2009, Plasma oxidized low-density lipoprotein levels and arterial stiffness in older adults: the health, aging, and body composition study: Hypertension, v. 53, p. 846-52.

Chang, Y. H., D. S. Abdalla, and A. Sevanian, 1997, Characterization of cholesterol oxidation products formed by oxidative modification of low density lipoprotein: Free Radic Biol Med, v. 23, p. 202-14.

Cogger, V. C., and D. G. Le Couteur, 2009, Fenestrations in the liver sinusoidal endothelial cell, *in* I. Arias, A. Wolkoff, J. Boyer, D. Shafritz, N. Fausto, H. Alter, and A. Cohen, eds., The Liver: Biology and Pathobiology: Hokoben NJ, John Wiley & Sons, Ltd, p. 387-404.

Cogger, V. C., A. Warren, R. Fraser, M. Ngu, A. J. McLean, and D. G. Le Couteur, 2003, Hepatic sinusoidal pseudocapillarization with aging in the non-human primate: Exp Gerontol, v. 38, p. 1101-1107.

Cooper, A. D., 1997, Hepatic uptake of chylomicron remnants: J Lipid Res, v. 38, p. 2173-92.

Dietschy, J. M., S. D. Turley, and D. K. Spady, 1993, Role of liver in the maintenance of cholesterol and low density lipoprotein homeostasis in different animal species, including humans: J Lipid Res, v. 34, p. 1637-59.

Dobbs, B. R., G. W. Rogers, H. Y. Xing, and R. Fraser, 1994, Endotoxin-induced defenestration of the hepatic sinusoidal endothelium: a factor in the pathogenesis of cirrhosis?: Liver, v. 14, p. 230-3.

Ehara, S., M. Ueda, T. Naruko, K. Haze, A. Itoh, M. Otsuka, R. Komatsu, T. Matsuo, H. Itabe, T. Takano, Y. Tsukamoto, M. Yoshiyama, K. Takeuchi, J. Yoshikawa, and A. E. Becker, 2001, Elevated levels of oxidized low density lipoprotein show a positive relationship with the severity of acute coronary syndromes: Circulation, v. 103, p. 1955-60.

Elvevold, K., J. Simon-Santamaria, H. Hasvold, P. McCourt, B. Smedsrod, and K. K. Sorensen, 2008, Liver sinusoidal endothelial cells depend on mannose receptor-mediated recruitment of lysosomal enzymes for normal degradation capacity: Hepatology, v. 48, p. 2007-15.

Enzan, H., H. Himeno, M. Hiroi, H. Kiyoku, T. Saibara, and S. Onishi, 1997, Development of hepatic sinusoidal structure with special reference to the Ito cells: Microsc Res Tech, v. 39, p. 336-49.

Everitt, A., G. S. Roth, D. G. Le Couteur, and S. N. Hilmer, 2005, Calorie restriction versus drug therapy to delay the onset of aging diseases and extend life: Age, v. 27, p. 1-10.

Fischer-Dzoga, K., R. Fraser, and R. W. Wissler, 1976, Stimulation of proliferation in stationary primary cultures of monkey and rabbit aortic smooth muscle cells. I. Effects of lipoprotein fractions of hyperlipemic serum and lymph: Exp Mol Pathol, v. 24, p. 346-59.

Fraser, R., A. G. Bosanquet, and W. A. Day, 1978, Filtration of chylomicrons by the liver may influence cholesterol metabolism and atherosclerosis: Atherosclerosis, v. 29, p. 113-23.

Fraser, R., L. M. Bowler, W. A. Day, B. Dobbs, H. D. Johnson, and D. Lee, 1980, High perfusion pressure damages the sieving ability of sinusoidal endothelium in rat livers: Br J Exp Pathol, v. 61, p. 222-8.

Fraser, R., W. J. Cliff, and F. C. Courtice, 1968, The effect of dietary fat load on the size and composition of chylomicrons in thoracic duct lymph: Q J Exp Physiol Cogn Med Sci, v. 53, p. 390-8.

Fraser, R., B. R. Dobbs, and G. W. Rogers, 1995, Lipoproteins and the liver sieve: the role of fenestrated sinusoidal endothelium in lipoprotein metabolism, atherosclerosis, and cirrhosis: Hepatology, v. 21, p. 863-874.

Fu, M. X., J. R. Requena, A. J. Jenkins, T. J. Lyons, J. W. Baynes, and S. R. Thorpe, 1996, The advanced glycation end product, Nepsilon-(carboxymethyl)lysine, is a product of both lipid peroxidation and glycoxidation reactions: J Biol Chem, v. 271, p. 9982-6.

Fujioka, Y., and Y. Ishikawa, 2009, Remnant lipoproteins as strong key particles to atherogenesis: J Atheroscler Thromb, v. 16, p. 145-54.

Furrer, K., A. Rickenbacher, Y. Tian, W. Jochum, A. G. Bittermann, A. Kach, B. Humar, R. Graf, W. Moritz, and P. A. Clavien, Serotonin reverts age-related capillarization and failure of regeneration in the liver through a VEGF-dependent pathway: Proc Natl Acad Sci U S A, v. 108, p. 2945-50.

Hansen, B., P. Longati, K. Elvevold, G. I. Nedredal, K. Schledzewski, R. Olsen, M. Falkowski, J. Kzhyshkowska, F. Carlsson, S. Johansson, B. Smedsrod, S. Goerdt, and P. McCourt, 2005, Stabilin-1 and stabilin-2 are both directed into the early endocytic pathway in hepatic sinusoidal endothelium via interactions with clathrin/AP-2, independent of ligand binding: Exp Cell Res, v. 303, p. 160-73.

Hansen, B., D. Svistounov, R. Olsen, R. Nagai, S. Horiuchi, and B. Smedsrod, 2002, Advanced glycation end products impair the scavenger function of rat hepatic sinusoidal endothelial cells: Diabetologia, v. 45, p. 1379-88.

Henriksen, T., E. M. Mahoney, and D. Steinberg, 1981, Enhanced macrophage degradation of low density lipoprotein previously incubated with cultured endothelial cells: recognition by receptors for acetylated low density lipoproteins: Proc Natl Acad Sci U S A, v. 78, p. 6499-503.

Henriksen, T., E. M. Mahoney, and D. Steinberg, 1983, Enhanced macrophage degradation of biologically modified low density lipoprotein: Arteriosclerosis, v. 3, p. 149-59.

Hilmer, S. N., V. C. Cogger, R. Fraser, A. J. McLean, D. Sullivan, and D. G. Le Couteur, 2005a, Age-related changes in the hepatic sinusoidal endothelium impede lipoprotein transfer in the rat: Hepatology, v. 42, p. 1349-54.

Hilmer, S. N., V. C. Cogger, R. Fraser, A. J. McLean, D. Sullivan, and D. G. Le Couteur, 2005b, Age-related changes in the hepatic sinusoidal endothelium impede lipoprotein transfer in the rat: Hepatology, v. 42, p. 1349-1354.

Holvoet, P., J. M. Stassen, J. Van Cleemput, D. Collen, and J. Vanhaecke, 1998a, Oxidized low density lipoproteins in patients with transplant-associated coronary artery disease: Arterioscler Thromb Vasc Biol, v. 18, p. 100-7.

Holvoet, P., J. Vanhaecke, S. Janssens, F. Van de Werf, and D. Collen, 1998b, Oxidized LDL and malondialdehyde-modified LDL in patients with acute coronary syndromes and stable coronary artery disease: Circulation, v. 98, p. 1487-94.

Hughes, D. A., I. P. Fraser, and S. Gordon, 1995, Murine macrophage scavenger receptor: in vivo expression and function as receptor for macrophage adhesion in lymphoid and non-lymphoid organs: Eur J Immunol, v. 25, p. 466-73.

Itabe, H., 2003, Oxidized low-density lipoproteins: what is understood and what remains to be clarified: Biol Pharm Bull, v. 26, p. 1-9.

Itabe, H., and T. Takano, 2000, Oxidized low density lipoprotein: the occurrence and metabolism in circulation and in foam cells: J Atheroscler Thromb, v. 7, p. 123-31.

Ito, Y., K. K. Sorensen, N. W. Bethea, D. Svistounov, M. K. McCuskey, B. H. Smedsrod, and R. S. McCuskey, 2007, Age-related changes in the hepatic microcirculation of mice: Exp Gerontol, v. 48, p. 789-797.

Jamieson, H., S. N. Hilmer, V. C. Cogger, A. Warren, R. Cheluvappa, D. R. Abernethy, A. Everitt, R. Fraser, R. de Cabo, and D. G. Le Couteur, 2007, Caloric restriction reduces age-related pseudocapillarization of the hepatic sinusoid: Experimental Gerontology, v. 42, p. 374-8.

Jialal, I., and S. Devaraj, 1996, Low-density lipoprotein oxidation, antioxidants, and atherosclerosis: a clinical biochemistry perspective: Clin Chem, v. 42, p. 498-506.

Kankaanpaa, J., S. P. Turunen, V. Moilanen, S. Horkko, and A. M. Remes, 2009, Cerebrospinal fluid antibodies to oxidized LDL are increased in Alzheimer's disease: Neurobiol Dis, v. 33, p. 467-72.

Karpe, F., G. Steiner, K. Uffelman, T. Olivecrona, and A. Hamsten, 1994, Postprandial lipoproteins and progression of coronary atherosclerosis: Atherosclerosis, v. 106, p. 83-97.

Kawai, Y., B. Smedsrod, K. Elvevold, and K. Wake, 1998, Uptake of lithium carmine by sinusoidal endothelial and Kupffer cells of the rat liver: new insights into the classical vital staining and the reticulo-endothelial system: Cell Tissue Res, v. 292, p. 395-410.

Knook, D. L., and E. C. Sleyster, 1976, Separation of Kupffer and endothelial cells of the rat liver by centrifugal elutriation: Exp Cell Res, v. 99, p. 444-9.

Knook, D. L., and E. C. Sleyster, 1980, Isolated parenchymal, Kupffer and endothelial rat liver cells characterized by their lysosomal enzyme content: Biochem Biophys Res Commun, v. 96, p. 250-7.

Krasinski, S. D., J. S. Cohn, E. J. Schaefer, and R. M. Russell, 1990, Postprandial plasma retinyl ester response is greater in older subjects compared with younger subjects. Evidence for delayed plasma clearance of intestinal lipoproteins: J Clin Invest, v. 85, p. 883-892.

Lakatta, E. G., and D. Levy, 2003, Arterial and cardiac aging: major shareholders in cardiovascular disease enterprises: Part I: aging arteries: a "set up" for vascular disease: Circulation, v. 107, p. 139-146.

Le Couteur, D. G., V. C. Cogger, S. N. Hilmer, M. Muller, M. Harris, D. Sullivan, A. J. McLean, and R. Fraser, 2006, Aging, atherosclerosis and the liver sieve, *in* L. V. Clark, ed., New Research on Atherosclerosis: NY, Nova Science, p. 19-44.

Le Couteur, D. G., V. C. Cogger, A. M. A. Markus, P. J. Harvey, Z. L. Yin, A. D. Ansselin, and A. J. McLean, 2001, Pseudocapillarization and associated energy limitation in the aged rat liver: Hepatology, v. 33, p. 537-543.

Le Couteur, D. G., R. Fraser, V. C. Cogger, and A. J. McLean, 2002, Hepatic pseudocapillarisation and atherosclerosis in ageing: Lancet, v. 359, p. 1612-1615.

Le Couteur, D. G., R. Fraser, S. Hilmer, L. P. Rivory, and A. J. McLean, 2005, The hepatic sinusoid in aging and cirrhosis - Effects on hepatic substrate disposition and drug clearance: Clin Pharmacokinet, v. 44, p. 187-200.

Le Couteur, D. G., and A. J. McLean, 1998, The aging liver - Drug clearance and an oxygen diffusion barrier hypothesis: Clin Pharmacokinet, v. 34, p. 359-373.

Le Couteur, D. G., A. Warren, V. C. Cogger, B. Smedsrod, K. K. Sorensen, R. De Cabo, R. Fraser, and R. S. McCuskey, 2008, Old age and the hepatic sinusoid: Anat Rec (Hoboken), v. 291, p. 672-83.

Lee, H. S., 1999, Oxidized LDL, glomerular mesangial cells and collagen: Diabetes Res Clin Pract, v. 45, p. 117-22.

Li, R., A. Oteiza, K. K. Sorensen, P. McCourt, R. Olsen, B. Smedsrod, and D. Svistounov, 2011, Role of liver sinusoidal endothelial cells and stabilins in elimination of oxidized low-density lipoproteins: Am J Physiol Gastrointest Liver Physiol, v. 300, p. G71-81.

Lin, Y., S. S. Mousa, N. Elshourbagy, and S. A. Mousa, Current status and future directions in lipid management: emphasizing low-density lipoproteins, high-density lipoproteins, and triglycerides as targets for therapy: Vasc Health Risk Manag, v. 6, p. 73-85.

Ling, W., M. Lougheed, H. Suzuki, A. Buchan, T. Kodama, and U. P. Steinbrecher, 1997, Oxidized or acetylated low density lipoproteins are rapidly cleared by the liver in mice with disruption of the scavenger receptor class A type I/II gene: J Clin Invest, v. 100, p. 244-52.

Lopes-Virella, M. F., G. Virella, T. J. Orchard, S. Koskinen, R. W. Evans, D. J. Becker, and K. Y. Forrest, 1999, Antibodies to oxidized LDL and LDL-containing immune complexes as risk factors for coronary artery disease in diabetes mellitus: Clin Immunol, v. 90, p. 165-72.

Malerod, L., K. Juvet, T. Gjoen, and T. Berg, 2002, The expression of scavenger receptor class B, type I (SR-BI) and caveolin-1 in parenchymal and nonparenchymal liver cells: Cell Tissue Res, v. 307, p. 173-80.

Malovic, I., K. K. Sorensen, K. H. Elvevold, G. I. Nedredal, S. Paulsen, A. V. Erofeev, B. H. Smedsrod, and P. A. McCourt, 2007, The mannose receptor on murine liver sinusoidal endothelial cells is the main denatured collagen clearance receptor: Hepatology, v. 45, p. 1454-61.

Martin-Armas, M., J. Simon-Santamaria, I. Pettersen, U. Moens, B. Smedsrod, and B. Sveinbjornsson, 2006, Toll-like receptor 9 (TLR9) is present in murine liver sinusoidal endothelial cells (LSECs) and mediates the effect of CpG-oligonucleotides: J Hepatol, v. 44, p. 939-46.

Martinez-Hernandez, A., and P. S. Amenta, 1993, The hepatic extracellular matrix. I. Components and distribution in normal liver: Virchows Arch A Pathol Anat Histopathol, v. 423, p. 1 11.

McCourt, P. A., B. H. Smedsrod, J. Melkko, and S. Johansson, 1999, Characterization of a hyaluronan receptor on rat sinusoidal liver endothelial cells and its functional relationship to scavenger receptors: Hepatology, v. 30, p. 1276-86.

McLean, A. J., V. C. Cogger, G. C. Chong, A. Warren, A. M. Markus, J. E. Dahlstrom, and D. G. Le Couteur, 2003, Age-related pseudocapillarization of the human liver: J Pathol, v. 200, p. 112-117.

McLean, A. J., and D. G. Le Couteur, 2004, Aging biology and geriatric clinical pharmacology: Pharmacol Rev, v. 56, p. 163-184.

Naito, M., and E. Wisse, 1978, Filtration effect of endothelial fenestrations on chylomicron transport in neonatal rat liver sinusoids: Cell Tissue Res, v. 190, p. 371-82.

Nonaka, H., M. Tanaka, K. Suzuki, and A. Miyajima, 2007, Development of murine hepatic sinusoidal endothelial cells characterized by the expression of hyaluronan receptors: Dev Dyn, v. 236, p. 2258-67.

O'Reilly, J. N., V. C. Cogger, R. Fraser, and D. G. Le Couteur, 2010, The effect of feeding and fasting on fenestrations in the liver sinusoidal endothelial cell: Pathology, v. 42, p. 255-8.

O'Reilly, J. N., V. C. Cogger, and D. G. Le Couteur, 2009, Old age is associated with ultrastructural changes in isolated rat liver sinusoidal endothelial cells: J Electron Microsc (Tokyo).

Oorni, K., M. O. Pentikainen, M. Ala-Korpela, and P. T. Kovanen, 2000, Aggregation, fusion, and vesicle formation of modified low density lipoprotein particles: molecular mechanisms and effects on matrix interactions: J Lipid Res, v. 41, p. 1703-14.

Palinski, W., M. E. Rosenfeld, S. Yla-Herttuala, G. C. Gurtner, S. S. Socher, S. W. Butler, S. Parthasarathy, T. E. Carew, D. Steinberg, and J. L. Witztum, 1989, Low density lipoprotein undergoes oxidative modification in vivo: Proc Natl Acad Sci U S A, v. 86, p. 1372-6.

Politz, O., A. Gratchev, P. A. McCourt, K. Schledzewski, P. Guillot, S. Johansson, G. Svineng, P. Franke, C. Kannicht, J. Kzhyshkowska, P. Longati, F. W. Velten, and S. Goerdt, 2002, Stabilin-1 and -2 constitute a novel family of fasciclin-like hyaluronan receptor homologues: Biochem J, v. 362, p. 155-64.

Popper, H., 1986, Aging and the liver: Prog Liver Dis, v. VIII, p. 659-683.

Schmucker, D. L., 1998, Aging and the liver: an update: J Gerontol, v. 53A, p. B315-B320.

Seternes, T., K. Sorensen, and B. Smedsrod, 2002, Scavenger endothelial cells of vertebrates: a nonperipheral leukocyte system for high-capacity elimination of waste macromolecules: Proc Natl Acad Sci U S A, v. 99, p. 7594-7.

Simons, L. A., J. Simons, Y. Friedlander, and J. McCallum, 2001, Cholesterol and other lipids predict coronary heart disease and ischemic stroke in the elderly, but only in those below 70 years: Atherosclerosis, v. 159, p. 201-208.

Skogh, T., R. Blomhoff, W. Eskild, and T. Berg, 1985, Hepatic uptake of circulating IgG immune complexes: Immunology, v. 55, p. 585-94.

Smedsrod, B., 2004, Clearance function of scavenger endothelial cells: Comp Hepatol, v. 3 Suppl 1, p. S22.

Smedsrod, B., P. J. De Bleser, F. Braet, P. Lovisetti, K. Vanderkerken, E. Wisse, and A. Geerts, 1994, Cell biology of liver endothelial and Kupffer cells: Gut, v. 35, p. 1509-16.

Smedsrod, B., K. Elvevold, and I. Martinez, 2006, The liver sinusoidal endothelial cell: a cell type of controversial and confusing identity: 13th International Symposium on Cells of the Hepatic Sinusoid, v. 13th, p. 61-62.

Smedsrod, B., D. Le Couteur, K. Ikejima, H. Jaeschke, N. Kawada, M. Naito, P. Knolle, L. Nagy, H. Senoo, F. Vidal-Vanaclocha, and N. Yamaguchi, 2009, Hepatic sinusoidal cells in health and disease: Liver Int, v. 29, p. 490-501.

Smedsrod, B., J. Melkko, N. Araki, H. Sano, and S. Horiuchi, 1997, Advanced glycation end products are eliminated by scavenger-receptor-mediated endocytosis in hepatic sinusoidal Kupffer and endothelial cells: Biochem J, v. 322 (Pt 2), p. 567-73.

Smedsrod, B., H. Pertoft, S. Gustafson, and T. C. Laurent, 1990, Scavenger functions of the liver endothelial cell: Biochem J, v. 266, p. 313-27.

Stacchiotti, A., A. Lavazza, M. Ferroni, G. Sberveglieri, R. Bianchi, R. Rezzani, and L. F. Rodella, 2008, Effects of aluminium sulphate in the mouse liver: similarities to the aging process: Exp Gerontol, v. 43, p. 330-8.

Steinberg, D., 1997, Low density lipoprotein oxidation and its pathobiological significance: J Biol Chem, v. 272, p. 20963-6.

Steinberg, D., 2009, The LDL modification hypothesis of atherogenesis: an update: J Lipid Res, v. 50 Suppl, p. S376-81.

Steinbrecher, U. P., S. Parthasarathy, D. S. Leake, J. L. Witztum, and D. Steinberg, 1984, Modification of low density lipoprotein by endothelial cells involves lipid peroxidation and degradation of low density lipoprotein phospholipids: Proc Natl Acad Sci U S A, v. 81, p. 3883-7.

Van Berkel, T. J., Y. B. De Rijke, and J. K. Kruijt, 1991, Different fate in vivo of oxidatively modified low density lipoprotein and acetylated low density lipoprotein in rats. Recognition by various scavenger receptors on Kupffer and endothelial liver cells: J Biol Chem, v. 266, p. 2282-9.

Vidal-Vanaclocha, F., and E. Barbera-Guillem, 1985, Fenestration patterns in endothelial cells of rat liver sinusoids: J Ultrastruct Res, v. 90, p. 115-23.

Warren, A., P. Bertolino, V. C. Cogger, A. J. McLean, R. Fraser, and D. G. Le Couteur, 2005, Hepatic pseudocapillarization in aged mice: Exp Gerontol, v. 40, p. 807-12.

Watson, A. D., N. Leitinger, M. Navab, K. F. Faull, S. Horkko, J. L. Witztum, W. Palinski, D. Schwenke, R. G. Salomon, W. Sha, G. Subbanagounder, A. M. Fogelman, and J. A. Berliner, 1997, Structural identification by mass spectrometry of oxidized phospholipids in minimally oxidized low density lipoprotein that induce monocyte/endothelial interactions and evidence for their presence in vivo: J Biol Chem, v. 272, p. 13597-607.

Watson, K. E., B. N. Horowitz, and G. Matson, 2003, Lipid abnormalities in insulin resistant states: Rev Cardiovasc Med, v. 4, p. 228-36.

Williams, K. J., 2008, Molecular processes that handle -- and mishandle -- dietary lipids: J Clin Invest, v. 118, p. 3247-59.

Wisse, E., 1970, An electron microscopic study of the fenestrated endothelial lining of rat liver sinusoids: J Ultrastruct Res, v. 31, p. 125-50.

Wisse, E., F. Braet, D. Luo, R. De Zanger, D. Jans, E. Crabbe, and A. Vermoesen, 1996, Structure and function of sinusoidal lining cells in the liver: Toxicol Pathol, v. 24, p. 100-11.

Witztum, J. L., and D. Steinberg, 1991, Role of oxidized low density lipoprotein in atherogenesis: J Clin Invest, v. 88, p. 1785-92.

Yla-Herttuala, S., W. Palinski, M. E. Rosenfeld, S. Parthasarathy, T. E. Carew, S. Butler, J. L. Witztum, and D. Steinberg, 1989, Evidence for the presence of oxidatively modified low density lipoprotein in atherosclerotic lesions of rabbit and man: J Clin Invest, v. 84, p. 1086-95.

Young, I. S., and J. McEneny, 2001, Lipoprotein oxidation and atherosclerosis: Biochem Soc Trans, v. 29, p. 358-62.

Zhou, B., J. A. Weigel, L. Fauss, and P. H. Weigel, 2000, Identification of the hyaluronan receptor for endocytosis (HARE): J Biol Chem, v. 275, p. 37733-41.

14

Dyslipidemia and Cardiovascular Risk: Lipid Ratios as Risk Factors for Cardiovascular Disease

Telmo Pereira
College of Health Technologies, Polytechnic Institute of Coimbra
Portugal

1. Introduction

There are extensive epidemiological data demonstrating that high blood cholesterol levels increase cardiovascular risk, and that this risk is dependent on the levels of the different blood cholesterol fractions. Moreover, the reduction of total blood cholesterol has been clearly related to a reduction in the risk of stroke, coronary disease and overall cardiovascular death. However, the traditional cholesterol measurements tend to be most accurate at predicting risk for those at the lower and higher ends of the risk spectrum. Recent data has shown LDL-Cholesterol/HDL-Cholesterol ratio and even Total-Cholesterol/HDL-Cholesterol ratio, to be accurate predictors of cardiovascular risk. In fact, changes in ratios have been shown to be better indicators of successful CHD risk reduction than changes in absolute levels of lipids or lipoproteins. In the Helsinki Study, the LDL-C/HDL-C ratio had more prognostic value than LDL-C or HDL-C alone (Manninen, Tenkanen, Koskinen *et al*, 1992). The ratio was especially accurate at predicting risk among those who also had elevated triglyceride levels. The PROSPER trial, a retrospective analysis of 6,000 patients, found that the ratio of LDL-C/HDL-C was the most powerful measure of cardiovascular disease risk in elderly people (Packard, Ford, Robertson *et al*, 2005). The PROCAM Study, which included almost 11,000 men aged 36 to 65 who were studied for 4 to 14 years, found a continuous and graded relationship between the LDL-C/HDL-C ratio and CVD mortality (Cullen, Schulte, Assmann *et al*, 1997). In addition, comparison of individual LDL-C/HDL-C ratios from subjects in the Framingham Study clearly indicates that these ratios are significantly more robust predictors of CVD than the individual levels of LDL-C or HDL-C (Kannel, 2005).

2. Theoretical framework

2.1 Cardiovascular risk – Generalities

Cardiovascular diseases are an unavoidable topic when discussing health related issues, particularly in developed societies. Cardiovascular disease is the leading cause of mortality in these countries (World Health Organization, 2002), assuming a progressively more important role in developing countries and even in less developed countries. In the latter, we may consider the presence of a *double-frontier* of health risk. These countries show coexistence of important mortality indexes related to diseases whose prevalence is a demonstration to their stage of development (perinatal, nutritional and infectious health problems), with a more consistent presence of coronary disease, with increased percentage reaching 137% for males and 120% for females by the year 2010 (Yusuf, Reddy, Ounpuu *et al*, 2001).

In epidemiological terms, coronary heart disease and cerebrovascular disease represent the most significant expressions of cardiovascular disease, and were the main causes of mortality and morbidity worldwide, accounting for one third of total mortality in the year 2001 (American Heart Association, 2003). According to the World Health Organization, every year 16 million deaths occur from cardiovascular disease, and this number is expected to rise to 20 million in the first decade of the XXI century (World Health Organization, 2002). The singular importance of coronary heart disease is extraordinarily important and it is estimated that mortality by this disease had risen to 7.2 million individuals by the year 2001 (World Health Organization, 2002). However, in recent years, there has been a trend towards a decline in this disease in Western countries, with a concomitant increase in other lands, notably in Russia and Eastern European countries. In fact, in Western countries, the number of deaths from coronary per 100,000 inhabitants was 151 in 1972, dropping to 44 in 2004, in men aged 64 or less. Similar reductions were also observed in females (36 to 11 women per 100,000). Paradoxically, in Russia, there was a marked increase of this rate, from 169/100.000, in the year 1980, to 242/100.000 deaths, in the year 2005 (Allender, Scarborough, Black *et al*, 2008).

The onset of cardiovascular disease is consistently related to the presence of a group of cardiovascular risk factors, whose manipulation can be crucial to its prevention (see Table 1).

Reversible
Smoking
Arterial hypertension
Hyperlipidemia
Obesity
Sedentarism
Alcohol
Stress
Irreversible
Family history
Male gender
Age
Partially Reversible
Diabetes
Menopause

Table 1. Conventional cardiovascular risk factors.

Concerning reversible risk factors in which intervention could be decisive, we should highlight the relative importance of smoking, arterial hypertension and hypercholesterolaemia. Although the global fight against all reversible risk factors constitute a therapeutic imperative, the elimination of hypercholesterolemia would result in the single most important benefit against the incidence of coronary heart disease as well as other atherosclerotic vascular problems (Wilson, D'Augustine, Levy *et al*, 1998).

Regarding arterial hypertension, it always presents itself as a major risk factor, given its very high incidence and prevalence. Despite all the research carried out and considering all the remarkable therapeutic advances, the control of blood pressure levels only provides a reduction of about 40% in mortality from cerebrovascular disease and a more modest 20% reduction in mortality from coronary heart disease (Kaplan, 2002).

Diabetes is another important risk factor, with the particularity of becaming the major epidemy of this century given its substantial and consistent epidemiological growth. The high cardiovascular risk that diabetes provides is well illustrated by the prognostic similarity between a diabetic patient without clinical manifestations of coronary heart disease and a patient with a history of acute coronary events (Hafnner, Lethe, Ronnema *et al*, 1988).

Obesity is undoubtedly a major risk factor for cardiovascular disease (Higgins, Kannel, Garrison *et al*, 1988), now becoming a public health problem, given the alarming increase of its prevalence in industrialized countries. The pathogenic mechanisms involved in this situation are complex and not just related to the metabolic overload involved, but also determined by its close associations with arterial hypertension, type 2 diabetes, dyslipidemia, and inflammation (Higgins, Kannel, Garrison *et al*, 1988).

Smoking is consensually assumed as a relevant contributer to cardiovascular disease, both in the active as well as the passive form. Some studies indicate that smokers have a reduced life expectancy of about ten years (although this number is dose-dependent) and that this habit cancells the natural cardioprotection in women (Silva, 2000). In fact, the differences in cardiovascular risk amongst men and women are well known, largely documented by the classic time lag between genders, with a higher risk in males until the fifth decade of life, with a progressive increase in women of cardiovascular risk until the eighth decade of life, when the risk is similar in men and women. The explanation for this is closely linked to the production and subsequent estrogen deficiency (as a consequence of menopause) seen in different phases of a woman's life. But other factors must not be overlooked. For instance, If we consider only the lipid profile changes induced by menopause, on average a 10% increase in LDL-cholesterol, an 8% reduction in HDL-cholesterol and an elevation in triglycerides are expected. Nonetheless, these changes can be normalized by hormonal replacement therapy (Stampfer, Colditz, Willet *et al*, 1991). Oral contraception, by contrast, tends to cause an adverse impact on lipid profile. At present, the worrying rate of young women with acute coronary events, a situation rarely seen before, has directed special attention to factors that could be blamed for this surprising finding. The association of hormonal contraception with smoking has emerged as very common in this population, likely to concur not only for atherogenic metabolic features but also for potentially thrombotic coagulation disorders (Mosca, Grundy, Judelson *et al*, 1999).

The cardiovascular impact of alcohollic intake must also be considered. The cardiovascular impact of this behaviour is closely related to the amount of alcohol consumed. A moderate intake may confer some cardiovascular protection, particularly by raising HDL-cholesterol and reducing platelet aggregation, yet it may lead to a higher incidence of arterial hypertension and cerebrovascular disease. Patterns of high alcoholic consumption are an unusually hazardous behaviour, particularly for the heart, greatly increasing the risk of sudden death (Silva, 2000).

2.2 Cardiovascular risk – Dislipidemia

Lipids are a very heterogeneous group of compounds, and their influence on metabolism goes far beyond the misdeeds attributed to him. Lipids constitute an important source of energy storage, represented by triglycerides, and assume a great importance in the constitution of the brain (17% of its dry weight), the formation of hormones, lipoproteins, bile acids, vitamins, and in the structure of cell membranes. Cholesterol and Triglycerides are transported between various components of the organism by specific proteins called apoproteins. These constitute the protein fraction of lipoproteins whose lipid component includes phospholipids, cholesterol and Triglycerides. Lipoproteins are usually divided into six classes according to their composition, size, density and function: Quilomicra, VLDL (very low density lipoproteins), IDL (intermediate density lipoprotein), LDL (low density lipoprotein), HDL (high density lipoprotein) and Lipoprotein (a). The interaction of lipoproteins with a high number of enzymes, transport proteins and receptors, constitutes a complex metabolism where equilibrium is determined by intrinsic and extrinsic factors, and its unbalance leads to the pathophysiological cascade of atherosclerosis, with its well known clinical consequences (Silva, 2000). In very one-dimensional terms, fat from the diet is transported to the intestinal wall and integrated into large lipoprotein particles rich in triglycerides - the Quilomicra - which, when secreted by the lymphatic system eventually reach the bloodstream. The liver, in its turn, synthesizes other lipoproteins with high content of triglycerides, the VLDL. The extracellular lipoprotein-lipase degrades triglycerides of Quilomicra and VLDL into free fatty acids, which are deposited in tissues. Lipoproteins, by reducing their concentration in triglycerides, are converted into IDL, which are usually hydrolyzed by the hepatic lipase, and are than converted into LDL, which bind to specific liver or peripheral receptors. Meanwhile, in another cycle - the reverse transport of cholesterol - HDL particles pick up cholesterol deposited in the arterial wall and provide transportation to the liver, where it is subsequently excreted in the bile (Eckardstein, Hersberger & Roher, 2005).

The disorder of lipid metabolism is a key player for the occurrence of cardiovascular disease and particularly heart disease. For many years, cholesterol has been directly related to cardiovascular prognosis. This relationship is very consistent, as an increase of 2 to 3% in the incidence of coronary heart disease is expected for every 1% increase in total cholesterol (Carlson, Bottiger & Ahfeldt, 1979). A review of internationally published studies showed, however, that this association may be even stronger. Thus, a 10% increase in total cholesterol relates to a 38% increase in the risk of coronary-related mortality (Law, Wald & Thompson, 1994). More recently, several clinical studies on the primary and secondary prevention of coronary heart disease emphasized the importance of the LDL fraction (ILIB International Lipid Information Bureau, 2003) allowing the potential for the discrimination of cardiovascular risk. In fact, the risk of each patient may best be defined by the magnitude of the LDL-cholesterol rather than its total cholesterol, which is why international standards for the treatment of dyslipidemia have been oriented to listing the risk thresholds and treatment goals depending on the plasma levels of this lipoprotein. In practical terms, the determination of LDL-cholesterol may be derived by the Friedewald formula, where LDL Cholesterol = Total Cholesterol - HDL Cholesterol - VLDL cholesterol, VLDL cholesterol are derived from triglycerides/5.

For many years it was difficult to classify unequivocally Triglycerides as an independent risk factor for the occurrence of coronary heart disease, a situation presumably related to the wide fluctuations observed in their concentrations throughout the day, with the

heterogeneity of triglyceride-rich lipoproteins (Quilomicra and VLDL) and its inseparable association with other risk factors. However, several studies have demonstrated a clear correlation between their levels and the occurrence of coronary heart disease, indicating that the presence of high levels of Triglycerides leads to a 13% increase in the risk of cardiovascular disease in men and 37% in women (Castelli, 1986; Criqui, Heiss, Cohn *et al*, 1993; Hokanson & Austin, 1996; Assman, Schulte & von Eckardstein, 1996). With regard to HDL-cholesterol, its inverse relationship with the risk of coronary heart disease is well accepted. In fact, this risk is 2 to 3% lower for each 1mg/dl elevation of HDL-Cholesterol (Gordon, Probstfiel, Garrison *et al*, 1989). The protective properties of this fraction derive not only from its involvement in reverse cholesterol transport, but are also a consequence of its anti-inflammatory capacity and protection against LDL-cholesterol oxidation (Ansell, Navab, Watson *et al*, 2004). On the other hand, it is recognized that individuals with very low levels of HDL-cholesterol have a higher cardiovascular risk. This population is often characterized for having concomitant hypertriglyceridemia, obesity, a sedentary lifestyle, active tobacco intoxication and decreased glucose tolerance (World Health Organization, 1999). In fact, an increased occurrence of cardiovascular events is expected for levels of HDL-cholesterol below 40 mg/dl (1.0 mmol/L) in men and less than 46 mg/dl (1.2 mmol/L) in women (UK HDL-C Consensus Group, 2004).
Recent evidence further stresses the importance of determining the non-HDL-cholesterol, defined by the concentration of LDL-cholesterol + VLDL-cholesterol. This parameter can better translate the risk of cardiovascular mortality than LDL-cholesterol, as it expresses more accurately the lipoprotein atherogenicity (Cui, Blumenthal, Flaws *et al*, 2001).
In recent years, a large number of risk factors for vascular disease have emerged from the international literature (see Table 2), demonstrating the relevance of more complex lipid disorders for the pathophysiology of atherosclerosis. Other emerging risk factors are related to inflammatory markers, as well as by the presence of metabolic changes, subtle changes in coagulation, hormonal disturbances and psychological or behavioral disorders (ILIB International Lipid Information Bureau, 2003).

Lipidic	**Coagulation**
Lipoproteic remnants	Fibrinogen
Lipoprotein (a)	Von Willebrand Factor
Small and dense LDL	Factor VII
HDL subspecies	Plasminogen activator inhibitor (PAI-1)
apolipoprotein B	
Apolipoprotein A-1	**Psychological / Behavioral**
Inflammatory	Alcoholism
High-sensitivity CRP	Depression
Homocysteine	Social Isolation
Interleukin-6	Loss and social support
Cell adhesion molecule-1	Low socioeconomic status
Selectin-CD40	**Hormonal**
Metabolic	Loss of estrogen production (menopause)
Postprandial hyperinsulinemia (insulin resistance)	

Table 2. Emerging cardiovascular risk factors.

As we have seen, each stated factor conveys a certain risk to the affected population. However, in everyday clinical practice a large majority of patients have associations of these factors and, as such, have cardiovascular risks that express the magnitude of individual risk factors present in an exponential, rather than additive, trend (Yusuf, Giles, Croft *et al*, 1998; American Heart Association, 2002).

An alternative option, with very promising results in the context of cardiovascular risk stratification and assessment of the effectiveness of lipid-lowering interventions, is the use of lipid ratios, just as the LDL-Cholesterol/HDL-Cholesterol ratio and the Total-Cholesterol/HDL-Cholesterol ratio, which have the added advantage of being easy to use in clinical practice (Gotto, Whitney & Stein, 2000). Changes in these relations have in fact been shown to better indicate the reduction in cardiovascular risk compared with the absolute levels of conventionally used lipid measures (Natarajan, Glick, Criqui *et al*, 2003; Kannel, 2005). On the other hand, the estimated LDL-Cholesterol/HDL-Cholesterol ratio translates, albeit imperfectly, an approach to the relationship of plasma apolipoproteins (apo) A-1 and apo B (Walldius & Jungner, 2005), thus enriching the lipid characterization of each patient, with the possibility of a better discrimination of cardiovascular risk, particularly among groups at intermediate cardiovascular risk (Gotto, Whitney, Stein *et al*, 2000).

Several large studies have demonstrated that the LDL-Cholesterol/HDL-Cholesterol ratio is an excellent predictor of risk of coronary disease and an excellent way to monitor the impact of lipid-lowering therapies (Manninen, Tenkanen, Koskinen *et al*, 1992; Kannel, 2005; Cullen, Schulte, Assmann *et al*, 1997; Stampfer, Sacks, Salvini *et al*, 1991; Gaziano, Hennekens, O'Donnell *et al*, 1997). In the Helsinki Study, a clinical trial with a 5-year follow-up, involving more than 4000 middle-aged men with hyperlipidemia, the LDL-Cholesterol/HDL-Cholesterol ratio had a superior prognostic value compared with isolated values of LDL-Cholesterol and HDL-Cholesterol. The predictive ability of this ratio was particularly strong in patients with concomitant elevation of triglycerides. It was further shown that the LDL-Cholesterol/HDL-Cholesterol ratio together with the fasting triglyceride concentration, allowed the identification of a particular subgroup of patients that had a remarkable 70% reduction in the risk of coronary heart disease with gemfibrozil (lipid-lowering agent) therapy. In the PROSPER trial, a retrospective analysis of 6,000 patients, the LDL-Cholesterol/HDL-Cholesterol ratio was the stronger predictor of cardiovascular events in elderly patients (Packard, Ford, Robertson *et al*, 2005). From this study has emerged the recommendation of pharmacological intervention whenever the LDL-Cholesterol/HDL-Cholesterol ratio values exceed 3.3 units. Another study (PROCAM study) involving about 11,000 men aged between 36 and 65, followed over 4 to 14 years, has documented an extremely important and linear relationship between the LDL-Cholesterol/HDL-Cholesterol ratio and cardiovascular mortality (Cullen, Schulte, Assmann *et al*, 1997). In this study, cardiovascular mortality peaked for LDL-Cholesterol/HDL-Cholesterol values between 3.7 and 4.3 units. In line with these results is the Physician's Health Study, involving 15,000 men (40 to 84 years), where there was a 53% increase in the risk of an acute coronary event for each one-unit increase in the LDL-Cholesterol/HDL-Cholesterol ratio (Stampfer, Sacks, Salvini *et al*, 1991). In another mixed study, involving men and women under the age of 76, the LDL-Cholesterol/HDL-Cholesterol ratio showed a strong relationship with the risk of coronary events (Gaziano, Hennekens, O'Donnell *et al*, 1997), aspect reinforced in an analysis of patients from the Framingham Heart Study, where a clear superiority of LDL-Cholesterol/HDL-Cholesterol ratio in predicting cardiovascular events compared to the levels of isolated LDL-cholesterol and HDL-cholesterol was depicted (Kannel, 2005).

Another point that reinforces the superiority of the lipid ratios in the stratification of cardiovascular risk arises from the effect of dietary cholesterol on plasma lipid levels. Several studies have demonstrated that these ratios are not affected by dietary cholesterol (Greene, Zerner, Wood *et al*, 2005; Herron, Vega-Lopez, Earl *et al*, 2002). On the contrary, some studies have shown that dietary cholesterol interferes with LDL-cholesterol and HDL-cholesterol, with little variation in the ratio (McNamara, 2000). On average, the predicted change in the LDL-Cholesterol/HDL-Cholesterol ratio per 100 milligrams/day increase in dietary cholesterol is quite small, around 0.01 (McNamara, 2000).

2.3 Cardiovascular risk – Atherogenesis

To understand the sequence of events that occur at the vascular level, resulting in devastating clinical manifestations that are all too familiar, we must look a little closer at the physiology of this system.

One of the most important organs we have without doubt is the vascular endothelium. The endothelium is the inner portion of our vessels, which can be compared to a thin membrane that carpets the blood vessels, and its integrity is fundamental for the maintenance of several potentially unstable equilibria. In this sense, a huge amount of vascular wall or circulating factors are present in close relation to the endothelium, endlessly alternating between defense and aggression, aggression, with Nitric Oxide as the key protector. As the most egregious examples of interaction near the endothelium vicinity, we have the following associations: vasodilation/vasoconstriction; anti-trombotic/pro-trombotic; anti-inflamatory/pro-inflamatory, among others. The relative hegemony of each of these interacting factors will determine the final maintenance of endothelial integrity or, conversely, its dysfunction and destruction (Houston, 2002). Endothelial dysfunction is thus the initial phase of a cascade of events that flow until the onset of clinically overt disease. In a very simplified overview, once the endothelial barrier is compromised, an association of events takes place, mainly with a lipid flooding process of the vascular wall, with the mobilization of inflammatory cells, the expression of chemotactic factors, growth and proliferation of smooth muscle and connective tissue, among others. The histologic consequence of these processes ranges from an initial lipid streak that evolves for an atherosclerotic plaque that may progress to calcification, progressively reducing the vascular lumen (Silva, 2000).

Curiously, most clinical cases are not determined directly by the extreme portion of the atherosclerotic continuum. In other words, cardiovascular events do not usually stem from progressive and insidious arterial occlusion, with consequent ischemia of downstream areas. Of course, cardiovascular events tend to be characterized by their acute nature, that is, by their sudden and unpredictable occurrence. As such, the implicit pathophysiology should express facts that support real-life events. In fact, one of the most important factors in the emergence of cardiovascular events is related to the so-called "atherosclerotic plaque stability". Thus, plaques with a small lipid core, with small inflammation infiltrate, and fitted with a thick, tough outer layer will be less susceptible to disruption by various harmful factors, such as blood pressure, sympathetic activity and other vasoconstrictor stimuli. In contrast, plaques with a rich lipid core, inflammatory activity and a significant weak fibrous cap will present a higher risk of fracture and exposure of their internal contents (Ridolfi & Hutchins, 1977). This in turn will lead to the activation of several factors that promote clotting and platelet aggregation *in-sito* (Falk, 1991), which may also lead to a sudden reduction of the vascular lumen, or even its complete occlusion by thrombosis.

Thus, the atherosclerotic process brings with it a wide array of metabolic, inflammatory and coagulation phenomena, decisively contributing to its clinical expression. Herein lies the justification of the diverse therapeutic targets that aimed for in these patients.
The importance of hypercholesterolemia as a key-player in this cascade of events is unquestioned and widely demonstrated in the published literature. A perfect expression of the interaction between research and practice is surely the publication of recommendations and guidelines that assist clinicians in the rationalization of therapeutic means available. These emerge as regular updates of successive collections of published scientific data, outlined in an admirably succinct way so they can be strategically combined and applied to the most varied health systems worldwide. Regarding the core topic of this paper, we have to address the most relevant recommendations published by the European Society of Cardiology and the National Cholesterol Education Program (NCEP). These recomendations were prepared according to an individual-risk perspective, and the therapeutic goals are defined according to the expected individual risk at long-term. Table 3 sumarizes the NCEP guidelines, revealing a clear therapeutic aggressiveness increase based on individual risk, as well as the adoption of progressively reduced target LDL-cholesterol values.

	Target	**Therapeutic options**	
High risk 10-year risk> 20% Established cardiovascular disease Equivalents of Cardiovascular Disease	LDL<100 mg/dl	LDL<100 mg/dl-129 mg/dl Dietary intervention Drug treatment?	LDL≥130 mg/dl Dietary intervention Drug treatment
Intermediate risk ≥ 2 Risk Factors 10-year risk ≤ 20%	LDL<130 mg/dl	LDL≥130 mg/dl Dietary intervention Drug treatment	
10-year risk ≤ 10%	LDL<130 mg/dl	LDL 130-160 mg/dl Dietary intervention	LDL≥160 mg/dl Dietary intervention Drug treatment
Low risk 10-year risk ≤ 10% ≤ 1 risk factor	LDL<160 mg/dl	LDL 160-190 mg/dl Dietary intervention Drug treatment?	LDL≥190 mg/dl Dietary intervention Drug treatment

Table 3. Hypercholesterolemia treatment algorithm of the second Report of the Third National Cholesterol Education Program – NCEP (2001).

These recommendations also included some secondary therapeutic goals, including the attempt to reduce non-HDL cholesterol in patients with triglycerides above 200 mg/dl for values 30 mg/dL higher than the individual target for LDL-cholesterol. Another objective lies in promoting an increase in HDL-cholesterol. Although these objectives are based on a very interventionist philosophy, recent studies may impose additional requirements on these recommendations. In fact, the Heart Protection Study (Heart Protection Study

Collaborative Group, 2002) showed that a reduction of 30% compared to the more restrictive goal (LDL cholesterol <100 mg/dl) was related to an additional 30% reduction in the relative risk of coronary heart disease. The PROVE IT study (Cannon, Braunwald, McCabe *et al*, 2004), enrolled patients who had had acute coronary events and showed that larger reductions of LDL-cholesterol, to levels lower than 100 mg/dl, could significantly provide aditional benefit in terms of future cardiovascular mortality and morbidity.

According to these results one has to consider more challenging treatment goals. The aim is to reach values of LDL-cholesterol <70mg/dl in patients with very high cardiovascular risk, such as those combining several primary risk factors (with primary relevance for diabetics), in patients with primary risk factors that are poorly controlled (with special care to the ones that maintain smoking habits), in patients with multiple risk factors of the so-called metabolic syndrome (triglycerides ≥ 200 mg/dl, non-HDL-cholesterol> 130 mg/dl, HDL-cholesterol<40 mg/dl) and in patients with history of acute coronary events.

The establishment of a therapeutic basis grounded in the control of cardiovascular risk factors has demonstrated its strong validity, and is further reinforced for its effectiveness in terms of cost-benefit. Improved control of risk factors almost certainly contributed to the 50% reduction in cardiovascular mortality observed in the United States of America between 1980 and 1990, with 43% attributable to the verified pharmacological advances (Hunink, Glodman, Tosteson *et al*, 1997). In the Netherlands, similar results were observed, and primary prevention was responsible for a 40% decline in mortality from coronary heart disease between 1978 and 1985 (Grobee & Bots, 1996). The adoption of dietary measures in Finland, relying on an increase in the consumption of fruits and vegetables and a reduction of saturated fats intake, has resulted in a 65% reduction in mortality from coronary heart disease in a time horizon of 20 years (Pekka, Pirjo & Ulla, 2002).

Despite the promising results indicated by these data, only 35% of Americans with a formal indication for dietary or pharmacological therapy, according to the recommendations of the NCEP (2001), are complying with it (Hoerger, Bala, Bray *et al*, 1988). In Canada, a study carried out between 1988 and 1993, including patients at high cardiovascular risk admitted to hospitals, showed very low percentages in relation to lipid dosing prescription (28%) and early dietary (22%) or pharmacological (8%) therapy (The Clinical Quality Improvement Network (CQIN) Investigators, 1995).

In Europe, results have fallen below expectations. An important follow-up study - EUROASPIRE - between 1995 and 1996, envolving nine European countries, showed that 86% of the enrolled patients had hypercholesterolaemia. Nevertheless, only 32% were on medication, and among those treated only 21% had achieved the target lipid levels (EUROASPIRE Study Group, 1997; EUROASPIRE I and II Group, 2001).

In Asia and the Pacific, the outlook is not encouraging either. In patients hospitalized for acute coronary events, quite small rates of lipid profile dosing (1 to 58%) were observed, as well as for the prescription of diet (1 to 32%) or pharmacological (6 to 60%) therapy to patients with high Cholesterol levels (Asian-Pacific CHD Risk Factor Collaborative Group, 1998).

The control of risk factors in clinical practice is thus a vaguely realized desideratum. The EUROASPIRE study has clarified some trends from 1995 to 2000. If the positive results have raised expectations, with an improvement seen in the control of hypercholesterolemia and hypertension, they are still accompanied by other rather disappointing indicators, such as those of smoking habits, obesity and diabetes, whose prevalence has been steadily increasing (EUROASPIRE Study Group, 1997; EUROASPIRE I and Group II, 2001). In the

United States of America the results are also somewhat disappointing. In survivors of acute myocardial infarction or stroke, the control percentages for some primary risk factors are below expectations, particularly for smoking habits (18%), control of hypercholesterolemia (46%), diabetes (48%) and hypertension (53%) (Qureshi et al, 2001).
As in almost all chronic conditions, the real picture lags far behind the expectations and available resources. Regarding hypercholesterolemia, the current situation is even less understandable, given its clear and strong association with the prevailing causes of death and incapacity, and the public awareness of the problem and in consideration of the demonstrated effectiveness of the available lipid-lowering drugs, that may have a quite favorable impact upon the prognosis of patients.

3. Original research data

3.1 Aim

Given the demonstrated role-playing of blood cholesterol in the atherosclerotic continuum, we designed two studies to ascertain the usefulness of the LDL-cholesterol/HDL-cholesterol, Triglycerides/HDL-cholesterol and Total-cholesterol/HDL-cholesterol ratios in predicting cardiovascular risk, through its relation to cardiovascular events and peripheral arterial disease (PAD) in two different clinical and experimental settings.

3.2 Study 1 – Usefulness of the lipidic ratios predicting peripheral artery disease in hypertensive patients: A retrospective analysis

The importance of the lipidic profile is well established in atherosclerotic processes related to coronary artery disease. Its relation with atherosclerosis in other vascular territories, particularly the inferior limbs has also received strong support from several experimental settings and in different clinical contexts. In order to address wether the lipid ratios can predict the occurrence of obstructive peripheral artery disease (PAD) we conducted a cross-sectional study in a sample of hypertensive patients. The study population consisted of 920 Portuguese nationals, aged between 20 and 91 years (mean 64.23 + 12.30 years).

3.2.1 Methods

A total of 920 hypertensive patients (51.3% female, age 64.22 ± 12.01 years) were consecutively included in the study. None of the patients were taking drugs or were in situations known to affect lipoprotein metabolism. Total cholesterol, triglycerides and HDL cholesterol were measured. LDL cholesterol was obtained by Friedewald's formula (if triglycerides <3.39 mmol/l) or by ultracentrifugation. The LDL-Cholesterol/HDL-Cholesterol, Total Cholesterol/HDL-Cholesterol and Triglycerides/HDL-Cholesterol ratios were calculated in all patients. Blood pressure and heart rate were measured in standard conditions. Ankle-Brachial index (ABI) was estimated bilaterally as the ratio of ankle (left and right) systolic blood pressure and brachial (highest upper limb) systolic blood pressure. The normal range for ABI was 0.9-1.3 mmHg, and individuals with ABI<0.9 were classified as having peripheral arterial disease.
All data was processed using STATA for Windows, version 11.1. The distribution of the variables was tested for normality using the Kolmogorov-Smirnov test, and for homogeneity of variance by Levene's test. Simple descriptive statistics were used to characterize the sample and the distribution of variables. Logistic regression analysis was used to determine the influence of the lipidic parameters on the occurrence of PAD.

Groups were compared using the $\chi2$ test for categorical variables and the Student's t test (2 groups) or ANOVA with the post-hoc Tukey test (3 groups) for quantitative variables. A value of P≤0.05 was taken as the criterion of statistical significance for a 95% confidence interval.

3.2.2 Results

The general characteristics of the studied population are summarized in Table 4. Mean age was 64.23±12.30, with a similar proportion of men versus women (49% and 51%, respectively).

	Total (n=920)	**No PAD Patients** (n=803)	**PAD Patients** (n=117)	***p-value*** **(PAD versus No PAD)**
Age, years	64.23±12.30	63.23±12.30	69.88±8.15	<0.01
Sex, men:women	49:51	48:52	52:48	0.462
Body Mass Index, Kg/m²	28.79±11.85	28.92±12.53	27.94±5.31	0.416
CV events history, no:yes	88:12	90:10	75:25	<0.01
Tobacco Consumption, no:yes	89:11	89:11	88:12	0.856
Dyslipidemia, no:yes	40:60	42:58	26:74	<0.01
Diabetes, no:yes	66:34	68:32	54:46	<0.01
SBP, mmHg	150.14±20.69	148.97±19.60	157.81±25.59	<0.01
DBP, mmHg	86.28±10.91	86.59±10.63	84.20±12.43	0.025
Heart Rate, bpm	70.52±10.48	69.12±9.42	71.22±9.21	0.791
Plasma Glucose, mg/dl	112.42±39.65	111.35±39.10	119.61±42.60	0.035
Plasma Creatinine, mg/dl	0.88±0.22	0.87±0.21	0.96±0.26	<0.01
eGFR, ml/min/1.73m²	84.73±23.28	85.86±23.40	76.94±20.88	<0.01
ABI	1.09±0.14	1.12±0.12	0.8±0.10	<0.01

PAD – peripheral artery disease; CV – cardiovascular events; SBP – systolic blood pressure; DBP – diastolic blood pressure; eGFR – estimated Glomerular Filtration Rate; ABI – Ankle-Brachial Index

Table 4. Characteristics of the study population, in general and stratified for the presence or absence of peripheral artery disease.

Mean body mass index was 28.79±11.85, indicating an overwheighted population. With regard to cardiovascular risk factors, all patients were hypertensive, 60% had dyslipidemia and 34% were diabetic; 11% were smokers and 12% had a personal history of cardiovascular events (mainly Stroke). About 37% were medicated for cardiovascular pathologies, with 13.6% of the patients undertaking statins. This factor was controlled in all the multivariable analysis. Peripheral artery disease (PAD) was encountered in 117 patients (12.7%). Patients with PAD were older, and had a worst metabolic and hemodynamic profile. The proportion of patients with a personal history of cardiovascular events was also greater in patients with PAD (25% versus 10%, p<0.01). The Ankle-Brachial Index (ABI) was also significantly lower in patients with PAD, as expected. Interestingly, patients with PAD also had a significantly lower estimated glomerular filtration rate (76.94±20.88 ml/min/1.73m^2 versus 85.86±23.40 ml/min/1.73m^2 in patients without PAD).

Regarding the overall and the comparative lipidic profile (depicted in table 5), significant differences amongst patients with and without PAD were only observed for the three considered lipidic ratios, expressing higher values when PAD was present, and for the HDL-cholesterol, with the PAD patients reaching lower HDL levels (although tendencially, *p-value*=0.073).

	Total (n=920)	**No PAD Patients** (n=803)	**PAD Patients** (n=117)	***p-value*** **(PAD versus No PAD)**
Plasma Total Cholesterol, mg/dl	196.61±41.15	197.06±41.18	193.68±40.98	0.400
Plasma LDL-Cholesterol, mg/dl	116.31±37.62	116.17±41.18	193.68±40.98	0.763
Plasma HDL-Cholesterol, mg/dl	54.46±21.47	54.96±21.56	51.14±20.65	0.073
Plasma Triglicerides, mg/dl	134.84±67.88	134.20±41.18	139.09±66.02	0.460
LDL-Colesterol/HDL-Colesterol Racio	2.55±2.45	2.48±2.11	3.04±2.03	<0.01
Total Cholesterol/HDL-Colesterol Racio	4.15±2.95	4.06±2.48	4.80±2.05	<0.01
Triglicerídeos/HDL-Colesterol Racio	2.97±2.98	2.88±2.44	3.59±2.33	<0.01

Table 5. Lipid profile of the study population.

Figure 1 further ilustrates the differences in the lipidic ratios among patients with and without PAD, with all three considered ratios presenting significant differences between the considered groups.

A multivariable logistic regression analysis was also performed considering PAD as the dependent variable (dichotomized in normal/abnormal), and forcing each lipidic parameter (either individual lipis or lipid ratios) in a model adjusted for the conventional Framingham cardiovascular risk factors (age, sex, diabetes, blood pressure, smoking status and body mass index). The observed Odds Ratios (OR) with 95% confidence intervals is depicted in figure 2. Although there's an appreciable tendency of association with PAD in all lipid variables, it reaches statistical significancy only for the lipidic ratios. In fact, the OR for LDL-cholesterol, Total-cholesterol, HDL-cholesterol and Triglycerides were respectively 1.004 (IC: 0.999-1.010, p=0.1), 1.001 (IC: 0.996-1.007, p=0.4), 0.993 (IC: 0.980-1.004, p=0.2) and 1.001 (IC: 0.998-1.004, p=0.2). For the LDL-cholesterol/HDL-cholesterol ratio, the multiadjusted OR was 1.06 (IC: 0.999-1.120, p=0.052), with a marginally significant association with PAD. For the Total-cholesterol/HDL-cholesterol and the Triglycerides/HDL-cholesterol ratios, the adjusted OR were respectively 1.051 (IC: 1.011-1.200, p=0.01) and 1.050 (IC: 1.002-1.110, p=0.04). A further analysis showed that the association of the lipid ratios with PAD was tendencially linear, particularly for the Total-cholesterol/HDL-cholesterol ratio.

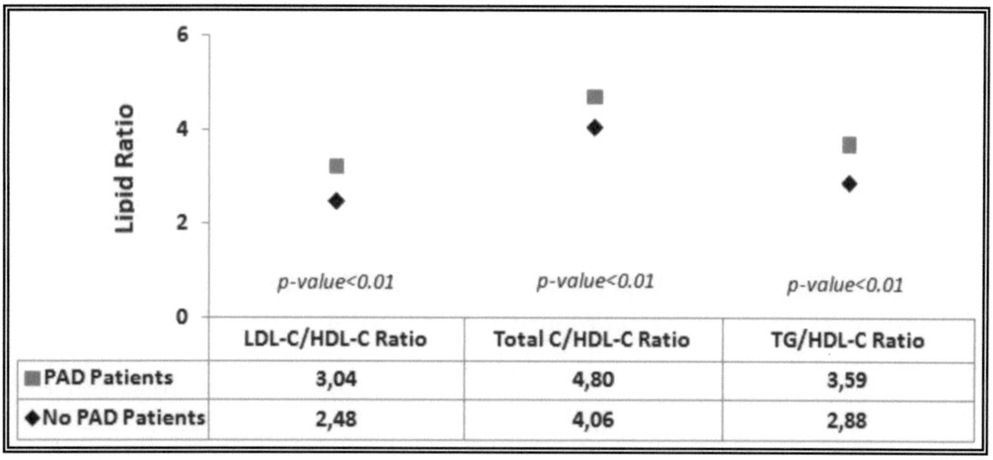

PAD - peripheral artery disease

Fig. 1. Representation of the comparative lipid ratios in patients with and without peripheral arterial disease.

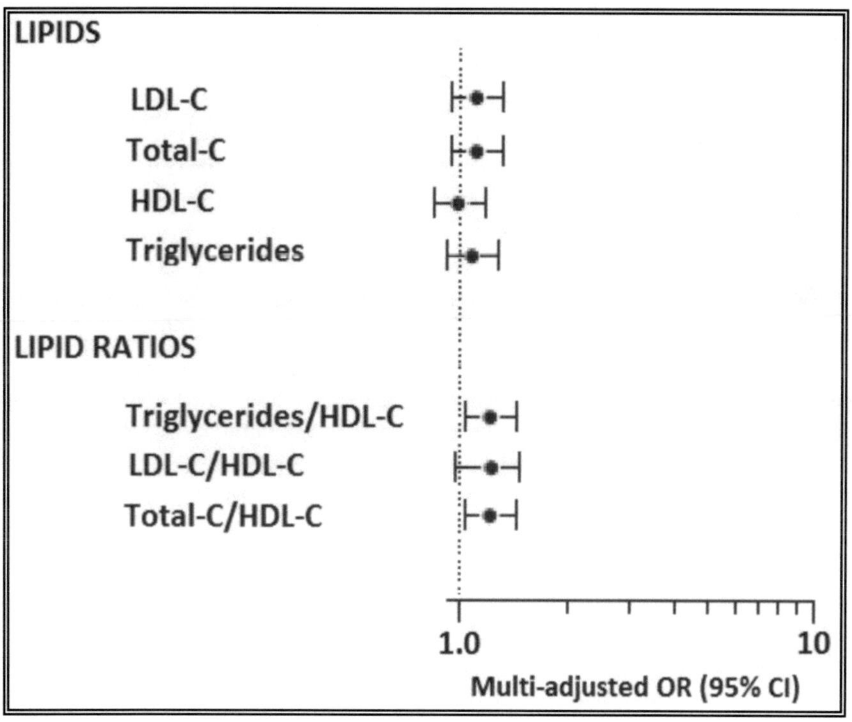

OR - Odds Ratio

Fig. 2. Adjusted Odds Ratios for Peripheral Artery Disease for the individual lipidic variables and for the lipidic ratios. The Odds Ratios are multi-adjusted to conventional Framingham cardiovascular risk factors.

3.3 Study 2 – Usefulness of the lipidic ratios in a low-to-moderate cardiovascular risk population: A sub-analysis of the EDIVA (Estudo de Distensibilidade Vascular) project

The EDIVA project was an epidemiological study assessing cardiovascular risk through sequential Pulse Wave Velocity measurement (Maldonado, Pereira, Polónia *et al*, 2011), but since serum lipids were available for all the included patients, we re-analyzed the EDIVA database aiming to address the delineated objective: to ascertain the usefulness of The LDL-Cholesterol/HDL-Cholesterol, Total Cholesterol/HDL-Cholesterol and Triglycerides/HDL-Cholesterol ratios in the general population. The study population consisted of 2200 Portuguese nationals (1290 men and 910 women), aged between 18 and 91 years (mean 46.33±13.76 years). Of these, 668 had low cardiovascular risk, and 1532 were patients with hypertension, diabetes and/or dyslipidemia. Individuals defined as having low cardiovascular risk were those who had had no chronic disease, had never been prescribed chronic pharmacological therapy, and had a normal physical exam, electrocardiogram, blood and urine tests, these characteristics having remained unchanged for at least two annual assessments. The patient group was under pharmacological therapy for at least one of the above pathologies.

3.3.1 Methods

The study's aims were explained to all participants and their informed consent was obtained. The methodology used to collect the data was approved by the Portuguese Data Protection Commission and the study was approved by the Ethics Committees of the hospitals involved. Mean follow-up was 2 years.

This was a prospective, multicenter, observational study monitoring the occurrence of major adverse cardiovascular events (MACE) - death, stroke, transient ischemic attack, myocardial infarction, unstable angina, peripheral arterial disease, revascularization or renal failure. Follow-up of the patients consisted of annual assessments including, blood pressure (BP) measurement, laboratory tests, including serum lipids, and clinical observation. Total cholesterol, triglycerides and HDL cholesterol were measured. LDL cholesterol was obtained by Friedewald's formula (if triglycerides <3.39 mmol/l) or by ultracentrifugation. The LDL-Cholesterol/HDL-Cholesterol, Total Cholesterol/HDL-Cholesterol and Triglycerides/HDL-Cholesterol ratios were calculated in all patients. At each consultation, the subjects' weight and height were measured and body mass index (BMI) was calculated in kg/m2. Blood pressure and heart rate were measured in standard conditions, in a supine position and after a 10-minute resting period, by an experienced operator and using a clinically validated (class A) sphygmomanometer (Colson MAM BP 3AA1-2®; Colson, Paris) (Pereira & Maldonado, 2005).Three measurements were taken and the arithmetic mean was used in the analysis. All participants underwent routine fasting laboratory tests. At the first consultation they filled out a questionnaire concerning relevant personal and family history, smoking habits, alcohol consumption and medication.

Data from the sample subjects were processed using STATA for Windows, version 11.1. The distribution of the variables was tested for normality using the Kolmogorov-Smirnov test, and for homogeneity of variance by Levene's test. Simple descriptive statistics were used to characterize the sample and the distribution of variables. Cox proportional hazards analysis was used to determine the influence of the lipidic parameters on the occurrence of the specified cardiovascular events. C-Statistics was calculated to address the reliability of the lipidic parameters as prognostic variables.

Groups were compared using the $\chi 2$ test for categorical variables and the Student's t test (2 groups) or ANOVA with the post-hoc Tukey test (3 groups) for quantitative variables. A value of $P \leq 0.05$ was taken as the criterion of statistical significance for a 95% confidence interval.

3.3.2 Results

The general characteristics of the study population are summarized in Table 6. Mean age was 46.33±13.77, indicating a relatively young sample, with similar proportions of men and women (59% and 41%, respectively). With regard to cardiovascular risk factors, 52% of the patients were hypertensive, 33% had dyslipidemia and 11% were diabetic; 17% were smokers and 15% had a family history of cardiovascular events. About 37% were medicated for cardiovascular pathologies, with 13.6% of the patients undertaking statins. This factor was controlled in all the multivariable analysis. Mean follow-up is currently 21.42±10.76 months. A total of 50 non-fatal MACE (2.2% of the sample) were recorded, including 27 cases of stroke, 19 of coronary events, 2 of renal failure and 2 of occlusive peripheral arterial disease.

		No MACE		MACE	
	Total	**Low Risk Patients**	**Patients**	**Patients**	***p-value*** **(MACE vs No MACE)**
N,%	2200	32%	66%	2%	
Age, years	46.33±13.77	40.00±13.42	49.03±13,14	50.00±10,21	0.360
Sex, men:women*	59:41	60:40	58:42	46:54	0.104
Body Mass Index, Kg/m²	27.18±5.50	25.90±4.21	27.71±4.45	28.59±5.75	0.348
Waist, cm	89.82±11,05	86.83±10,30	90.63±11,00	90.00±13,06	0.917
Family History, no:yes*	85:15	92:8	83:17	60:40	0.020
Tobacco Consumption, no:yes*	83:17	78:22	85:15	78:22	0.243
Hypertension, no:yes*	48:52	100:0	26:74	14:86	0.109
Dyslipidemia, no:yes*	67:33	100:0	53:47	60:40	0.311
Diabetes, no:yes*	89:11	100:0	85:15	86:14	0.941
SBP, mmHg	142.51±21.05	129.17±14.33	147.83±14.33	161.08±17.34	<0.001
DBP, mmHg	84.52±12.29	77.43±10.11	87.32±11.87	92.08±10.07	<0.001
PP, mmHg	57.99±15.29	51.74±11.90	60.05±15.86	66.20±12.93	<0.001
MAP, mmHg	103.85±14.02	94.68±1.26	107.48±13.52	117.14±11.43	<0.001
Heart Rate, bpm	70.56±12.24	68.21±12.58	71.49±11.87	78.20±13.01	0.001
Plasma Glucose, mg/dl	100.44±31.54	90.86±9.16	103.70±3.75	110.32±39.64	0.406
Plasma Creatinine, mg/dl	1.31±5.08	0.90±1.77	1.43±5.99	1.53±2.92	0.996

MACE – major acute cardiovascular events; SBP – systolic blood pressure; DBP – diastolic blood pressure; PP – pulse pressure; MAP – mean blood pressure

Table 6. General characteristics of the study cohort, depending on the presence of MACE and conventional cardiovascular risk factors.

Regarding the lipidic profile, patients with MACE presented higher levels of the different lipidic parameters, as illustrated in table 7, in particular the lipidic ratios were significantly higher in patients with MACE (5.76±1.74 versus 6.75±1.98 for Total Cholesterol/HDL-Cholesterol ratio, 3.24±1.32 versus 4.51±1.49 for LDL-Cholesterol/HDL-Cholesterol ratio, 3.17±1.34 versus 4.35±1.67 for Triglycerides/HDL-Cholesterol ratio, *p-value*<0.01). So, overall, the patients with MACE were characterized by an unfavorable metabolic profile compared to the asymptomatic patients.

	No MACE (n=2150)	**MACE** (n=50)	***p-value***
Plasma Total Cholesterol, mg/dl	221.37±34.01	238.43±36.12	<0,01
Plasma LDL-Cholesterol, mg/dl	141.37±31.22	163.26±41.12	<0,01
Plasma HDL-Cholesterol, mg/dl	41.22±11.07	36.19±7.28	<0,01
Plasma Triglicerides, mg/dl	156.37±34.01	181.43±36.12	<0,01
LDL-Colesterol/HDL-Colesterol Ratio	2.98±2.32	4.51±1.49	<0,01
Total Cholesterol/HDL-Colesterol Ratio	4.76±2.11	6.75±1.98	<0,01
Triglicerídeos/HDL-Colesterol Ratio	3.17±2.32	4.35±1.67	<0,01

MACE – major acute cardiovascular events; SBP – systolic blood pressure; DBP – diastolic blood pressure; PP – pulse pressure; MAP – mean blood pressure

Table 7. Lipid profile of the study cohort, stratified for the presence or absence of of MACE.

In the multivariable model analysis, adjusting for all conventional Framingham cardiovascular risk factors (age, sex, diabetes, blood pressure, smoking status and body mass index), the lipids ratios were associated with MACE, with stronger associations than the ones observed for the individual lipidic variables. Overall, the Total-Cholesterol/HDL-Cholesterol was found to be the best single predictor of MACE. In figure 3 we plot the hazard ratios for quintiles of the lipid ratios. A linear increase of the hazard ratios across quintiles of the Total-Cholesterol/HDL-Cholesterol is clearly depicted, while for the other ratios only the upper-extreme quintiles showed an important association with cardiovascular events.

Comparative data of risk association for those in the extreme quintiles of each lipidic variable is presented in figure 4. Of note, one can see that the combination of two individual lipidic components into a single variable provides stronger association with cardiovascular risk, as expressed by the depicted hazard ratios for the lipid ratios. On the other hand, the lipid ratio with the strongest association was the Total-Cholesterol/HDL-Cholesterol ratio, in line with the data depicted in figure 3.

The ROC curve analysis provided the Areas-Under-the-Curve (AUC, equivalent to the C-statistics) for the different lipid parameter considered in the analysis. The parameters with the biggest AUC were the Total-cholesterol/HDL-cholesterol ratio (AUC=0.703, IC:0.65-0.77) and the LDL-cholesterol/HDL-cholesterol (AUC=0.701, IC:0.64-0.79).

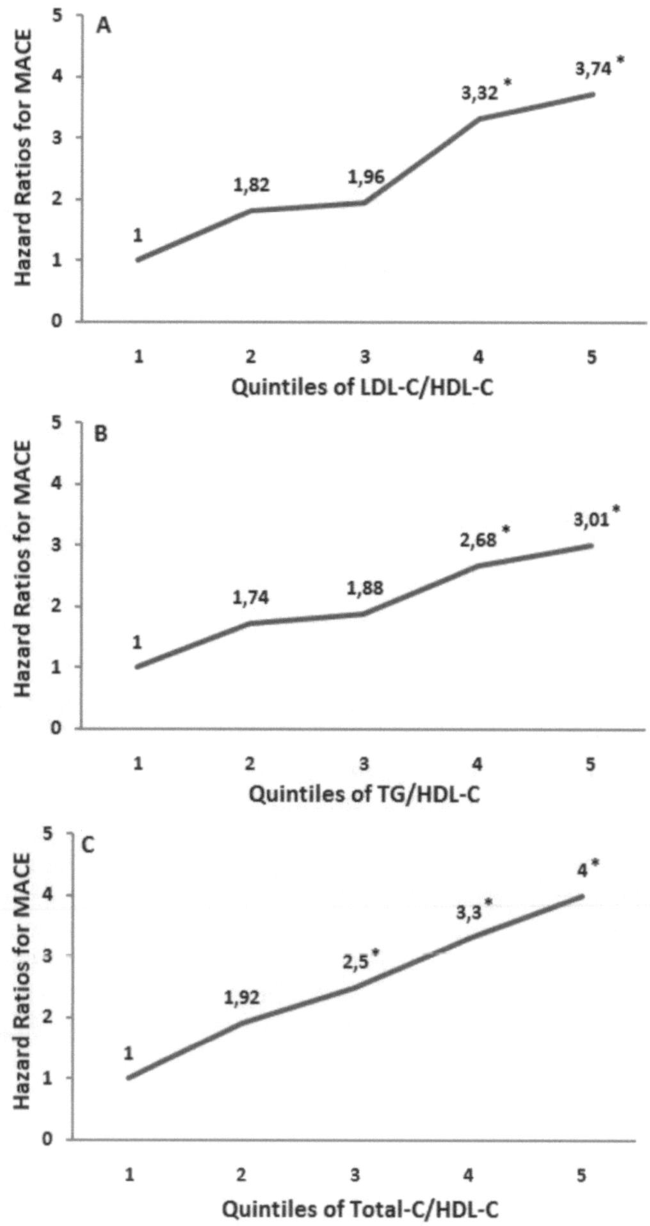

* *p-value<0.01.*

Fig. 3. Adjusted Hazard Ratios for major acute cardiovascular events distributed according to quintiles of the lipid ratios. A) Hazard ratios for quintiles of the LDL-Cholesterol/HDL-Cholesterol ratio; B) Hazard ratios for quintiles of the Triglycerides/HDL-Cholesterol ratio; C) Hazard ratios for quintiles of the Total-Cholesterol/HDL-Cholesterol ratio. The hazard ratios are multi-adjusted to conventional Framingham cardiovascular risk factors.

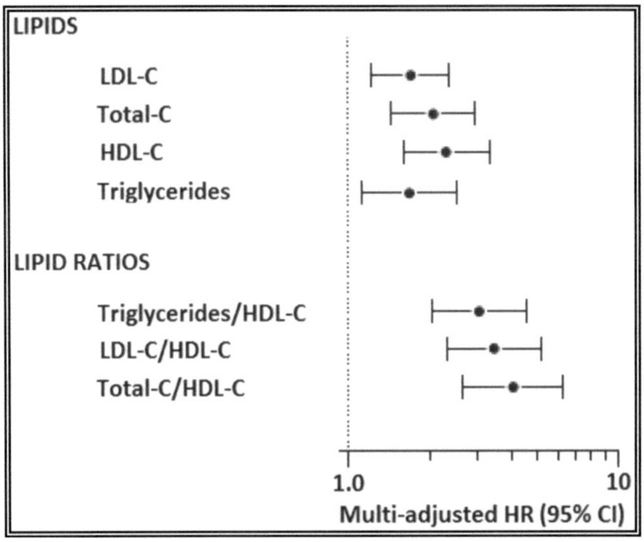

Fig. 4. Adjusted Hazard Ratios for major acute cardiovascular events amongst those in the extreme quintiles of each considered lipidic parameter. The hazard ratios are multi-adjusted to conventional Framingham cardiovascular risk factors.

4. Discussion and conclusions

As previously mentioned, cardiovascular disease, as an expression of atherosclerotic processes, is the leading cause of death in industrialized countries. The key role played by cholesterol in essential pathophysiologic processes that lead to the occurrence of clinically significant cardiovascular events is well recognized. In contemporary clinical practice, this notion is well entrenched, and the individual cardiovascular risk definition incorporates, among other factors, the lipid profile, including the Total Cholesterol, LDL Cholesterol, HDL Cholesterol and triglycerides. A practical evidence of the aforementioned is the fact that the major cardiovascular risk tables currently available (e.g. the Framingham score or the EuroSCORE), incorporate lipid parameters in the definition of thresholds of risk. On the other hand, therapeutic decisions and monitoring have been largely centered on the conventional lipid profile. Even the international recommendations (such as those issued by the National Cholesterol Education Program - NCEP, 2001) recommend target levels of LDL and HDL -cholesterol to determine cardiovascular risk and evaluate the effectiveness of lipid-lowering therapies. However, some studies have indicated important limitations of these parameters in the prediction of cardiovascular risk, particularly in patients with intermediate cardiovascular risk (Gotto, Whitney, Stein *et al*, 2000).
However, more recent evidence has suggested other lipidic components to optimize the definition of cardiovascular risk in clinical practice. In fact, several studies have expressed the superiority of the levels of apolipoprotein (apo) B, apo A-1 and its ratio, both in predicting cardiovascular events and in the evaluation of treatment efficacy (Packard & Marcovina, 2006; Yusuf , Hawken, Ounpuu, *et al*, 2004; Meisinger, Loewel, Mraz *et al*, 2005; Barter, Ballantyne, Carmena *et al*, 2006; Kim, Chang, Choi *et al*, 2005). In fact, considering that each lipidic particle contains one molecule of the atherogenic apo B, then its levels are a direct measure of the number of potentially atherogenic particles in the different

conventional lipid components (Walldius & Junger, 2006). In contrast, the concentration of apo A-1 translates the number of anti-atherogenic particles contained in the HDL-cholesterol, thus enclosing the conceptual framework of apoB/apoA-1 ratio as a measure of the ratio of atherogenic particles versus anti-atherogenic particles transported in the blood. Despite the growing enthusiasm about the potential of these emerging parameters for their best performance in the definition of cardiovascular risk, there still remain some questions that limit their dissemination in clinical practice. The central question is very practical, and focuses on the cost-benefit relation associated with a change in the traditional clinical approach. In fact, it is not yet clear whether the superiority of these new lipid parameters over the more conventional ones for risk stratification is enough to justify the additional cost inherent to their laboratory determination (Pischon, Girman, Sacks *et al*, 2005). Furthermore, despite the current literature supporting apolipoproteins as better predictors of cardiovascular events, its use may not be the most practical operational perspective. Moreover, it is not yet clear whether the replacement of conventional parameters for emerging ones will translate into clear clinical benefit, or if, conversely, it will confuse the various protagonists over the clinical decision frame.

In contrast to this line of argument, several studies have also emerged affirming quite clearly the advantages of using lipid ratios, based on conventional parameters, such as those studied in this work. This is based on the fact that, on the one hand, they add cardiovascular risk discriminative capacity to the individual lipid parameters, and on the other, they are more favorable than the apolipoproteins considering cost and immediate operationalization (Gotto, Whitney & Stein, 2000). As mentioned earlier, several studies have shown fairly consistently that changes in these ratios are favorable indicators of cardiovascular disease risk, above the absolute levels of individual lipids (Natarajan, Glick, Criqui *et al*, 2003; Kannel, 2005). Accumulating evidence in this regard is quite broad, spreading over several clinical frameworks (Manninen, Tenkanen, Koskinen *et al*, 1992; Kannel, 2005; Cullen, Schulte, Assmann *et al*, 1997; Stampfer, Sacks, Salvini *et al*, 1991; Gaziano, Hennekens, O'Donnell *et al*, 1997; Packard, Ford, Robertson *et al*, 2005). The results presented here clearly fall into this line, reinforcing the belief in the superiority of the lipid ratios, particularly the Total-Cholesterol/HDL-Cholesterol and the LDL-Cholesterol/HDL-Cholesterol ratios, over the classic lipid parameters, predicting peripheral arterial disease in hypertensive patients (in a high cardiovascular risk) and predicting future major cardiovascular events (including stroke and myocardial infarction) in a low-to-intermediate cardiovascular risk population.

One of the curious aspects extracted from the second presented study was the existence of a linear relationship for the Total-Cholesterol/HDL-Cholesterol ratio with the risk of MACE, something not apparent in the LDL-Cholesterol/HDL-Cholesterol ratio. This same result was reproduced in the Quebec Cardiovascular Study, in which more than 2.000 middle-aged men were followed for 5 years, monitoring the occurrence of major cardiovascular events (Lemieux, Lamarche, Couillard *et al*, 2001). The lipid parameters with better performance in predicting risk in this study were the Total-Cholesterol/HDL-Cholesterol ratio and the LDL-Cholesterol/HDL-Cholesterol ratio, although only the first stated ratio expressed a linear relationship with risk. One possible explenation for this result is metabolic in nature. In fact, it is well documented that patients with dyslipidemia showing high triglycerides and low HDL-cholesterol (generally patients with abdominal obesity and insulin resistance), often have marginal or even normal levels of LDL-Cholesterol (Lamarche, Després, Moorjani *et al*, 1996). Moreover, LDL-Cholesterol concentrations are often estimated indirectly from 3 measurements (Total-Cholesterol, Triglycerides and HDL-

Cholesterol), which may include a variation that can reach 25% (Schectman & Sasse, 1993), with a potential and quite significant impact in the LDL-Cholesterol/HDL-Cholesterol ratio, eventually under-estimated. By contrast, the two components included in the Total-Cholesterol/HDL-Cholesterol ratio are measured directly. Supporting the superiority of these ratios over the isolated lipid parameters, is their unique ability to reflect the bidirectional cholesterol traffic (in and outward) through the arterial intima in a way that the individual LDL and HDL-Cholesterol levels cannot reach (Kannel, 2005). Consistent with this assumption, another recent cohort prospective study, involving over 15.000 women followed over a period of 10 years, demonstrated that the Total-Cholesterol/HDL-Cholesterol ratio alongside the non-HDL Cholesterol were predictors of future cardiovascular events, as good or better than apolipoprotein fractions (Ridker, Rifai, Cook *et al*, 2005).

Of course, there are still unresolved issues, such as the definition of a cut-off in these ratios from which lipid-lowering therapy should be considered. The current guidelines of the NCEP (2001) recommend a cut-off of 2.5 for the ratio LDL-cholesterol/HDL-cholesterol. However, recent studies suggest that the risk of cardiovascular events begins to have significant expression for values between 3.3-3.7 (Cullen, Assmann & Schulte, 1997), in line with the results we reported here.

Given all the data currently available, as long as the fundamental reservations to the routine use of apolipoproteins are not exceeded, the use of lipid ratios in clinical practice is strongly advised, both in risk stratification and therapeutic decision and in monitoring its effectiveness.

5. Acknowledgments

The author sincerely thanks Dr Markus Carpenter for the linguistic assistance.

6. References

Allender, S.; Scarborough, P.; Preto, V., et al. (2008). *European cardiovascular disease statistics*. European Heart Network, Belgium.

American Heart Association. (2002). *Heart disease and stroke statistics – 2003 update*. Dallas, Tex: American Heart Association.

American Heart Association. (2003). Statistical facts sheet-populations. *International Disease Statistics*. Dallas, Tex: American Heart Association.

Ansell, B.J.; Navab, M.; Watson, K.E.; *et al.* (2004). Anti-inflamatory properties of HDL. *Rev Endocr Metab Disord*, 5:351-358.

Asian-Pacific CHD Risk Factor Collaborative Group. (1998). Risk factor management in CHD patients in Asia: current status. Atherosclerosis, 136:S31.

Assman, G.; Schulte, H.; von Eckardstein, A. (1996). Hypertriglyceridemia and elevated lipoprotein (a) are risk factors for major coronary events in middle-aged men. Am J Cardiol, 77: 1179-1184.

Barter, P.J.; Ballantyne, C.M.; Carmena, R.; *et al.* (2006). Apo B versus cholesterol in estimating cardiovascular risk and in guiding therapy: report of the thirty-person/ten-country panel. *J Intern Med*, 259:247–258.

Bots, M.L.; Grobee, D.E. (1996). Decline of coronary heart disease mortality in The Netherlands from 1987 to 1985: contributions of medical care and changes over time in presence of major cardiovascular risk factors. *J Cardiovasc Risk*, 3:271-276.

Cannon, C.P.; Braunwald, E.; McCabe, C.H.; *et al.* (2004). Pravastatin or Atorvastatin evaluation and infection therapy: thrombolisis in myocardial infarction 22 investigators. Intensive versus moderate lipi lowering with statins after acute coronary syndromes. *N Eng J Med*, 350:1495-1504.

Carlson, L.A.; Bottiger, L.E.; Ahfeldt, P.E. (1979). Risk factors for myocardial infarction in the Stockholm Prospective Study . A 14-year follow-up focusing on the role of plasma triglycerides and cholesterol. *Acta Med Scand*, 206:351-360.

Castelli, W.P. (1986). The triglyceride issue: a view from the Framingham. *Am Heart J*, 112:432-437.

Criqui, M.H.; Heiss, G.; Cohn, R. *et al.* (1993). Plasma triglyceride level and mortality from coronary heart disease. *N Eng J Med*, 328:1120-1125.

Cui, Y.; Blumenthal, R.S.; Flaws, J.A.; *et al.* (2001). Non-high-density lipoprotein cholesterol level as a predictor of cardiovascular disease mortality. *Arch Intern Med*, 161:1413-1419.

Cullen, P.; Schulte, H.; Assmann, G. (1997). The Munster Heart Study (PROCAM) Total Mortality in Middle-Aged Men is increased at low total and LDL cholesterol concentrations in smokers but not in nonsmokers. *Circulation*, 96:2128 - 2136.

Eckardstein, A.; Hersberger, M.; Roher, L. (2005). Current understanding of the metabolism and biological actions of HDL. Curr Opin Clin Nutr Metab Care, 8:147-152.

EUROASPIRE I and II Group. (2001). Clinical reality of coronary prevention guidelines: a comparison of EUROASPIRE I and II in nine countries. *Lancet*, 357:995-1001.

EUROASPIRE Study Group. (1997). EUROASPIRE: A European Society of Cardiology survey of secondary prevention of coronary heart disease: principal results. *Eur Heart J*, 18:1569-1582.

European guidelins on cardiovascular disease prevention in clinical practice. (2003). Third joint task force of european and other societies on cardiovascular disease prevention in clinical practice. *European J Card Prev and Rehab*, 10:S1-S10.

Falk, E. (1991). Coronary thrombosis: pathogenesis and clinical manifestations. *Am J Cardiol*, 68:28B-35B.

Gaziano, J.M.; Hennekens, C.H.; O'Donnell, C.J.; *et al.* (1997). Fasting triglycerides, high-density lipoprotein, and risk of myocardial infarction. *Circulation*, 96:2520 - 2525.

Gordon, D.J.; Probstfield, J.L.; Garrison, R.J.; *et al.* (1989). High-density lipoprotein cholesterol and cardiovascular disease: four prospective american studies. *Circulation*, 79:8-15.

Gotto, A.M.; Whitney, E.; Stein, E.A.; *et al.* (2000). Relation between baseline and on-treatment lipid parameters and first acute major coronary events in the Air Force/Texas Coronary Atherosclerosis Prevention Study (AFCAPS/Tex CAPS). *Circulation*, 101:477 - 484.

Gotto, A.M.; Whitney, E.; Stein, E.A.; *et al.* (2000). Relation between baseline and on-treatment lipid parameters and first acute major coronary events in the Air Force/Texas Coronary Atherosclerosis Prevention Study (AFCAPS/Tex CAPS). *Circulation*, 101:477–484.

Greene, C.M.; Zern, T.L.; Wood, R.J.; *et al.* (2005). Maintenance of the LDL cholesterol: HDL cholesterol ratio in an elderly population given a dietary cholesterol challenge. *J Nutr*, 135:2793 - 2798.

Haffner, S.M.; Letho, S.; Ronnema, T.; *et al.* (1988). Mortality from coronary heart disease in subjects with typo 2 diabetes and in non diabetic subjects with and without prior myocardial infarction. *N Eng J Med*, 339:229-234.

Heart Protection Study collaborative group.(2002). MRC/BHF Heart Protection Study of cholesterol lowering with sinvastatin in 20.536 high-risk individuals: a randomised placebo-controlled trial. Lancet, 360(9326):7-22.

Herron, K.J.; Vega-Lopez, S.; Conde, K.; et al. (2002). Pre-menopausal women classified as hypo-or hyper-responders, do not alter their LDL/HDL ratio following a high dietary cholesterol challenge. *J Am Coll Nutr*, 21:250 - 258.

Higgins, M.; Kannel, W.; Garrison, R.; *et al.* (1988). Hazards of obesity: the Framingham experience. *Acta Med Scand*, Suppl 723:23-36.

Hoerger, T.J.; Bala, M.V.; Bray, J.W.; *et al.* (1988). Treatment patterns and distribution of low-density lipoprotein cholesterol levels in treatment-eligible United States adults. *Am J Cardiol*, 82:61-65.

Hokanson, J.E.; Austin, M.A. (1996). Plasma triglyceride level is a risk factor for cardiovascular disease independent of high-density lipoprotein choloesterol level: a meta-analysis of population-based prospective studies. *J Cardiovasc Risk*, 3:213-219.

Houston, M. (2002). *Vascular Biology and Clinical Practice.* Hanley & Belfus Inc. Philadelphia.

Hunink, M.L.; Glodman, L.; Tosteson, A.N.A.; *et al.* (1997). The recent decline in mortality from coronary heart disease, 1980-1990: the effect of secular trends in risk factors and treatment. *JAMA*, 277:535-542.

ILIB International Lipid Information Bureau. (2003). *Dyslipidemia and coronary heart disease.* 3th Edition. 2003 International Lipid Information Bureau. New York.

Implications of recent clinical trials for the National Cholesterol Education Program Adult Treatment Panel III Guidelines. (2004). *Circulation*, 110:227-239.

Kannel, W.B. (2005). Risk stratification of dyslipidemia: Insights from the Framingham Study. *Curr Med Chem Cardiovasc Hematol Agents*, 3:187 - 193.

Kaplan's Clinical Hypertension. (2002). Lippincot Williams & Wilkins.

Kim, H.K.; Chang, S.A.; Choi, E.K.; *et al.* (2005). Association between plasma lipids, and apoliproteins and coronary artery disease: a cross-sectional study in a low-risk Korean population. *Int J Cardiol*, 101:435–440.

Lamarche, B.; Després, J.P.; Moorjani, S.; *et al.* (1996). Triglycerides and HDL.cholesterol as risk factors for ischemic heart disease: results from the Quèbec Cardiovascular Study. *Atherosclerosis*, 119:235-245.

Law, M.R.; Wald, N.J.; Thompson, S.G. (1994). By how much and how quickly does reduction in serum cholesterol concentratio lower risk of ischemic heart disease ? *BMJ*, 308:367-372.

Lemieux, I.; Lamarche, B.; Couillard, C ; *et al.* (2001). Total cholesterol/HDL cholesterol ratio vs LDL cholesterol/HDL cholesterol ratio as indices of ischemic heart disease risk in men. Arch Intern Med, 161:2685-2692.

Maldonado, J.; Pereira, T.; Polónia, J.; *et al.* (2011). Arterial stiffness predicts cardiovascular outcome in a low-to-moderate cardiovascular risk population: the EDIVA (Estudo de DIstensibilidade VAscular) project. *J Hypertens*, 29(4):669-75.

Manninen, V.; Tenkanen, L.; Koskinen, P.; *et al.* (1992). Joint effects of serum triglyceride and LDL cholesterol and HDL cholesterol concentrations on coronary heart disease risk in the Helsinki Heart Study. Implications for treatment. *Circulation*, 85:37 - 45.

Marcovina, S.; Packard, C.J. (2006). Measurement and meaning of apolipoprotein AI and apolipoprotein B plasma levels. *J Intern Med*, 259:437–446.

McNamara, D.J. (2000). The impact of egg limitations on coronary heart disease risk: Do the numbers add up? *J Am Coll Nutr*, 19:540S - 548S.

Meisinger, C.; Loewel, H.; Mraz, W.; *et al.* (2005). Prognostic value of apolipoprotein B and A-I in the prediction of myocardial infarction in middle-aged men and women: results from the MONICA/KORA Augsburg cohort study. *Eur Heart J*, 26:271–278.

Mosca, J.; Grundy, S.M.; Judelson, D.; *et al.* (1999). Guide to preventive cardiology in women. AHA/ACC scientific statement: consensus panel statement. *Circulation*, 99:2480-2484.

Natarajan, S.; Glick, H.; Criqui, M.; *et al.* (2003). Cholesterol measures to identify and treat individuals at risk for coronary heart disease. *Am J Prev Med*, 25:50 - 57.

Packard, C.J.; Ford, I.; Robertson, M.; *et al.* (2005). The PROSPER Study Group: Plasma lipoproteins and apolipoproteins as predictors of cardiovascular risk and treatment benefit in the PROspective Study of Pravastatin in the Elderly at Risk (PROSPER). *Circulation*, 112:3058 - 3065.

Pekka, P.; Pirjo, P.; Ulla, U. (2002). Influencing public nutrition for non-communicable disease prevention: from community intervention to national programme - experiences from Finland. *Public Health Nutr*, 5:245-251.

Pereira, T.; Maldonado, J. (2005). Performance of the Colson MAM BP 3AA1-2 automatic blood pressure monitor according to the European Society of Hypertension validation protocol. *Rev Port Cardiol*, 24:1341–1351.

Pischon, T.; Girman, C.J.; Sacks, F.M.; *et al.* (2005). Non-high-density lipoprotein cholesterol and apolipoprotein B in the prediction of coronary heart disease in men. *Circulation*, 112:3375–3383.

Qureshi, A.I.; Suri, M.F.K.; Guterman, L.R.; et al. (2001). Ineffective Secondary Prevention in Survivors of Cardiovascular Events in the US Population: Report From the Third National Health and Nutrition Examination Survey. Arch Intern Med, 161:1621-1628.

Ridker, P.M.; Rifai, N.; Cook, N.R.; *et al.* (2005). Non-HDL cholesterol, apolipoproteins A-1 and B100, standard lipid measures, lipid ratios, and CRP as risk factors for cardiovascular disease in women. JAMA, 294 (3):326-333.

Ridolfi, R.L.; Hutchins, G.M. (1977). Relationship between coronary artery lesions and myocardial infarcts: ulceration of atherosclerotic plaques precipitating coronary thrombosis. *Am Heart J*, 93:468.

Schectman, G.; Sasse, E. (1993). Variability of lipid measurements: relevance for the clinician. *Clin Chem*, 39:1495-1503.

Silva, J. (2000). *Colesterol, lípidos e doença vascular*. Lidel, Edições Técnicas Lda.

Stampfer, M.J.; Colditz, G.A.; Willet, W.C.; *et al.* (1991). Postmenopausal estrogen therapy and cardiovascular disease:ten-year follow-up from the Nurses Health Study. *N Eng J Med*, 325:756-762.

Stampfer, M.J.; Sacks, F.M.; Salvini, S.; *et al.* (1991). A prospective study of cholesterol apolipoproteins and the risk of myocardial infarction. *N Engl J Med*, 325:373 - 381.

The Clinical Quality Improvement Network (CQIN) Investigators. (1995). Low incidence of assessment and modification of risk factors in acue care patients at high risk for cardiovascular events, particularly among females and the elderly. *Am J Cardiol*, 76:570-573.

UK HDL-Consensus Group. (2004). Role of fibrates in reducing coronary risk: a UK consensus. *Curr Med Res Opin*, 20:241-247.

Walldius, G.; Junger, N. (2006). The apo B/apoA-I ratio: a strong, new risk factor for cardiovascular disease and a target for lipid-lowering therapy - a review of evidence. J Int Med, 259:493–519.

Walldius, G.; Jungner, I. (2005). Rationale for using apoliprotein B and apolipoprotein A-1 as indicators of cardiac risk and as targets for lipid-lowering therapy. *Eur Heart J*, 26:210 - 212.

Wilson, p.; D'Agostinho, R.B.; Levy, D.; *et al.* (1998). Prediction of coronary heart disease using risk factor categories. *Circulation*, 97:1837-1847.

World Health Organization. (1999). *Definition, diagnosis and classification of diabetes mellitus and its complications: report of a WHO consultation.* Part 1: Diagnosis and classification of diabetes mellitus. Geneva: World Health Organization.

World Health Organization. (2002). *The world health report 2002: reducing risks, promoting life.* Geneva: Worlf Health Organization.

Yusuf, H.R.; Giles, W.H.; Croft, J.B.; et al. (1998). Impact of multiple risk factor profiles on determining cardiovascular disease risk. Prev Med, 27:1-9.

Yusuf, S.; Hawken, S.; Ounpuu, S ; *et al.* (2004). Effect of potentially modifiable risk factors associated with myocardial infarctin in 52 countries (the INTERHEART study): case-control study. *Lancet*, 364:937–952.

Yusuf, S.; Reddy, S.; Ounpuu, S.; et al. (2001). Global burden of cardiovascular diseases part I: general considerations. *Circulation*, 104:2746-2753.

15

Dyslipidemia and Cardiovascular Disease

Hossein Fakhrzadeh and Ozra Tabatabaei-Malazy
Endocrinology & Metabolism Research Center,
Tehran University of Medical Sciences,Tehran,
Islamic Republic of Iran

1. Introduction

Four non-communicable diseases (NCDs) including cardiovascular disease (CVD), cancer, chronic respiratory disease, and diabetes were announced by World Health Organization (WHO) as the major causes of mortality in the world in 2008(Alwan, 2008). According to WHO prediction, in the next 10 years, mortality rate caused by NCDs will increase by 17 percent with the highest mortality rate in the regions of Africa (27 percent) and Eastern Mediterranean (EMRO, 25 percent) (Alwan, 2008). Fortunately more than 80 percent of heart disease, stroke, and type 2 diabetes mellitus incidence and almost one third of cancers could be prevented with appropriate interventions to reduce the effect of risk factors (Alwan, 2008).

Dyslipidemia, as a risk factor of CVD, is manifested by elevation or attenuation of plasma concentration of lipoproteins. Several methods have been used to classify the lipoproteins in respect to their density, physical, and chemical properties. Based on these classifications, different types of lipoproteins, including chylomicrones, IDL[1], VLDL[2], LDL[3], and HDL[4], and apolipoproteins (Apo), including Apo A, Apo B, Apo C, and Apo E, have been introduced. Generally, dyslipidemia is defined as the total cholesterol, LDL, triglycerides, apo B or Lp (a) levels above the 90th percentile or HDL and apo A levels below the 10th percentile of the general population (Dobsn et al., 1996).

CVD is the most common health problem worldwide. This disease is often manifested as coronary heart disease (CHD). According to the international reports, mortality of CHD in the developed countries is expected to reach almost 29 percent in women and 48 percent in men in years 1990-2020. These figures have been estimated to increase by 120 percent in women and 137 percent in men (Thom et al., 1998) in the developing countries.

Atherosclerosis is the most common cause of CHD. According to recent epidemiological studies, hypercholesterolemia and possibly coronary atherosclerosis are suggested as the sole risk factors of ischemic stroke. The results of a meta-analysis of 10 large cohort studies (Law et al., 1994) showed that for each 0.6 mmol/l reduction in serum cholesterol levels in

---

[1] Intermediate Density Lipoprotein
[2] Very Low Density Lipoprotein
[3] Low Density Lipoprotein
[4] High Density lipoprotein

those aged 60 years, the risk of CHD decreased by 27 percent, which manifested a calculated relative risk of 0.73. With three times reduction in serum cholesterol (1.80 mmol/l or 70mg/dl), the relative risk of CHD was 0.39 $(0.73)^3$ and risk reduction reached to 61 percent. The expected benefits of total cholesterol and LDL reduction seem to be in both primary and secondary prevention of CHD. Protective effects of HDL against initial coronary events in secondary prevention (Barter et al., 2007; Rosenson, 2007) was even observed in levels of higher than 75 mg/dl with long lifetime protection (Longevity Syndrome) and emancipation of the relative risk of coronary disease. Based on these observations, current attempt for stroke prevention is mostly focused on intensive treatment with lipid-lowering drugs (Gorelick et al., 1997).

In spite of a decline in cardiac events and coronary mortality rates, many people who are under appropriate treatment are still exposed to these events. In a population-based study regarding hypercholesterolemia awareness (Nieto et al., 1995), only 42% of population were informed of their hypercholesterolemia and only 4% were under lipid-lowering drug treatment. Need assessment to better understand the role of lipids and its subgroups including; VLDL, Small dense LDL, lipoprotein (a), and subgroups of HDL in pathogenesis of CVD calls for a general awareness regarding these topics. In this context, the major challenges would be: 1 - to identify those who need treatment (with or without past history of coronary artery disease), 2 - to develop more effective treatment strategies for patients with coronary artery disease (whether individuals were treated with lipid-lowering drugs or people who have not received adequate treatment), 3 - to adequately treat other high risk individuals such as diabetic, hypertensive, and old subjects.

1.1 Objective

Main objective of this chapter is to express the relationship between lipid disorders and CVD according to the top epidemiological studies in the world. Other minor objectives include; evaluation of role of dyslipidaemia in the incidence of CVD, and also assessment of the role of different types of lipoproteins in this area.

1.2 Expected outcomes

- To increase general awareness regarding the relationship between lipid disorders and CVD
- To reduce the morbidity and mortality of CVD (by primary or secondary prevention)

2. World epidemiological evidences of association between dyslipidemia and CVD

CVD is widespread among general population. Reports received from late 1990s indicate that the ultimate cause of death in adults is CVD (Murray & Lopez, 1997). It has been predicted that CVD will become the ultimate cause of disability in the world between years 2000-2025 (Murray & Lopez, 1997). Common lifestyle determinants such as western diet, physical inactivity, tobacco consumption and also increase in life expectancy are linked to elevation of CVD prevalence (Critchley et al., 1999).

According to data published from the autopsy studies in 1960s, the origin of early lesions of atherosclerosis in adults is mostly caused by consumption of Western diet. The prevalence and severity of fibroid plaques and calcified lesions as signs of CVD were significantly lower in Asia, underdeveloped countries and consumers of Mediterranean diet (Eggen et al., 1964).

2.1 Total and LDL cholesterol

Two decades after World War II, large population studies had been performed in different countries in order to determine risk factors of heart disease. The most famous studies include the Framingham Study, Chicago and Tecumseh in USA (Butler et al., 1985; Dawber et al., 1951; Dyer et al., 1981; Keys, 1970) and Seven Country Studies including studies in England, Sweden and Norway (Fager et al., 1981; Keys et al., 1984; Miller et al., 1977) in European countries. The major finding of these cohort studies was that in addition to serum cholesterol levels, other factors also are involved in development of coronary heart disease. Among the main risk factors, dyslipidemia, especially increase in LDL levels and decrease in HDL concentrations were considered as the important factors. Table-1 demonstrates the Population Attributable Factors (PARs) with its 99 percent confidence interval (CI) associated with lipids by sex and geographic region (Labarthe, 2011; Yusuf et al., 2004). In some countries, PAR estimation in women is based on small numbers which makes them less reliable.

Region	Lipids in men % (CI 99%)	Lipids in women % (CI 99%)	Lipids in both sexes % (CI 99%)
West Europe	36.7 (10.7-73.8)	47.9 (20.3-76.8)	44.6 (23.5-67.8)
Central & eastern Europe	38.7 (20.0-61.4)	26.8 (5.9-68.2)	35.0 (19.2-54.9)
Middle East	72.7 (58.8-83.2)	63.3 (32.0-86.3)	70.5 (57.8-80.7)
Africa	73.7 (55.2-86.4)	74.6 (49.1-90.0)	74.1 (59.7-84.6)
South Asia	60.2 (42.5-75.6)	52.1 (19.0-83.5)	58.7 (42.7-73.1)
China	41.3 (32.4-50.7)	48.3 (36.9-59.9)	43.8 (36.7-51.2)
Southeast Asia and Japan	68.7 (51.2-82.1)	64.5 (29.5-88.7)	67.7 (52.0-80.2)
Australia & New Zealand	48.7 (17.5-80.9)	14.9 (0.0-99.6)	43.4 (16.0-75.6)
South America	41.6 (20.2-66.6)	59.3 (30.5-82.9)	47.6 (29.6-66.2)
North America	60.0 (22.2-88.8)	32.2 (1.1-95.1)	50.5 (18.2-82.4)
Overall adjusted for age, sex & smoking	53.8 (48.3-59.2)	52.1 (44.0-60.2)	54.1 (49.6-58.6)
Overall adjusted for risk factors	49.5 (43.0-55.9)	47.1 (37.4-57.0)	49.2 (43.8-54.5)

Legend: CI: Confidence Interval.

Table 1. Population Attributable Factors (PARs) associated with lipids in men & women by geographic region.

In parallel to these large population studies, a series of case studies were also performed. In one study, serum lipid levels were evaluated in 500 men with a prior history of myocardial infarction. Overall 30 percent of study population had abnormal blood lipid levels (Goldstein et al., 1973). High levels of cholesterol in 8 percent, triglycerides in7 percent and concomitant high cholesterol and triglycerides in15 percent were reported by this study.
In normal individuals from different communities, plasma levels of lipids vary due to differences in genetic background and diet. For example, the average cholesterol levels, according to age, in western and Chinese men are 202 mg/dl and165 mg/dl, respectively (Caroll et al., 2005; Wu et al., 2004). Based on results of the National Health and Nutrition Examination Surveys (NHANES) from 1999 to 2004, the percentage of adults with triglyceride levels above 150 and 200 mg/dl in the United States, were 33 and 18 percent, respectively (Ford et al., 2009). In the United States, the NHANES from 2005 to 2008 found that 98.8 million adults have total cholesterol levels ≥ 200 mg/dl, 33.6% of them having a total cholesterol level ≥ 240 mg/dl (American Heart Association [AHA], 2011).
Table-2 shows the prevalence of high levels of total cholesterol (cholesterol ≥ 200 mg/dl), LDL (LDL cholesterol ≥130 mg/dl), and HDL (HDL cholesterol≤ 40 mg/dl) in adults aged ≥20 years, according to NHANES (American Heart Association [AHA], 2011).

	Non-Hispanic White		**Non-Hispanic Black**		**Mexican-American**	
	M	**F**	**M**	**F**	**M**	**F**
Total cholesterol						
200-239 mg/dl	41.2	47.0	37.0	41.2	50.1	46.5
≥ 240 mg/dl	13.7	16.9	9.7	13.3	16.9	14.0
LDL cholesterol						
≥130 mg/dl	30.5	32.0	34.4	27.7	41.9	31.6
HDL cholesterol						
≤ 40 mg/dl	29.5	10.1	16.6	6.6	31.7	12.2

Legend: M: Male; F: Female; LDL: Low Density Lipoprotein; HDL: High Density Lipoprotein.

Table 2. Proportion of USA adults aged ≥ 20 years with dyslipidemia by ethnicity and gender

In MONICA[5] project designed for more than 30 countries in different regions of WHO coverage except the US, the percentage of hypercholesterolemia for individuals aged between 35-64 years and total cholesterol levels between 5.2-7.8 mmol/l (approximately 200-300 mg/dl) was found to be lowest (20%) among the men in China-Beijing and highest (76%) in France-Strasbourg. The lowest percent of women with hypercholesterolemia (5%) was in Australia-Perth population and the highest percent (76%) was observed in Germany-Bremen (WHO MONICA project, 2008). However, these figures were different when the total cholesterol level >7.8 mmol/l was considered as hypercholesterolemia. None of the China-Beijing's men had the serum cholesterol levels >7.8 mmol/l (0%) while 15% of Switzerland-Ticino men had hypercholesterolemia (highest percent). for women these figures were 0% in China-Beijing and 14% in Lithuania-Kaunas (WHO MONICA project, 2008).

[5] Multinational MONItoring of trends and determinants in CArdiovascular disease

The WHO MONICA project showed (WHO MONICA project, 1989) that the average of total cholesterol in 30 studied areas varied from 158 mg/dl (in the Beijing, China) to 246 mg/dl (Loczamburk, Germany) for men and from 162 mg/dl (Beijing, China) to 246 mg/dl (Glasgow, UK) in women. In addition, there was a difference in prevalence of hypercholesterolemia in different regions, from 2 percent in Beijing, China to nearly 50 percent in Lille, France (WHO MONICA project, 1989). An intermediate reduction in cholesterol level of MONICA project study populations during 5-6 year follow-up was observed. The mean annual decrease in total serum cholesterol was 0.4-3 mg/dl (Dobsn et al., 1996).

The highest incidence of hyperlipidemia is shown in patients with premature coronary artery disease, which occurs before age 55 years in men and 65 years in women. Prevalence of dyslipidemia in these patients is equal to 80-88 percent, compared to 40-48 percent in age-matched controls without CHD (Genest et al., 1992; Roncaglioni et al., 1992). In these conditions, 12.5 percent of patients with a prior history of premature coronary disease and 58.5 percent of age-matched controls without prior history of coronary disease have normal lipid profiles.

MRFIT[6] study performed in more than 350,000 middle-aged men demonstrated (Stamler et al., 1986) that a sigmoid relationship (curvilinear) between total serum cholesterol level and prevalence of coronary artery disease especially in total cholesterol more than 240 mg/dl is presented (Figure-1).

The strongest association was found in population from United States and Finland, the intermediate association was observed in European population, and the least correlation was related to Japanese men and rural area of Greece. The relationship between serum cholesterol and incidence of CVD become stronger when the number of risk factors was increased (Kannel, 1983).

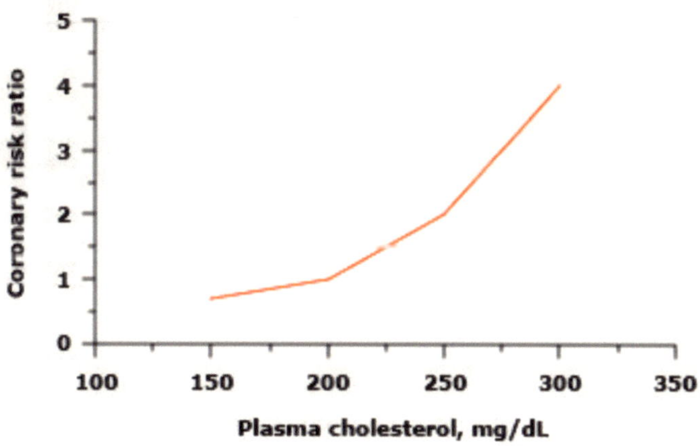

Fig. 1. Association between plasma cholesterol and coronary risk among MRFIT study

[6] Multiple Risk Factor Intervention Trial

Similar results were obtained from Framingham and Migration studies (Kannel et al., 1971, 1979). The Migration study is one of the strong studies evaluating the relationship between increased serum cholesterol and risk of CVD. This study was done in 1960 and compared Japanese men residing in Japan with immigrated Japanese to Honolulu and San Francisco. In Japanese men living in their native country, the mean total cholesterol levels and CHD rate were lower compared to immigrated population. In immigrated Japanese, those who live in Hawaii had lower lipid levels than those in San Francisco. Considering race similarity in this study, the reason for observed differences in rate of CHD and cholesterol levels can be related to differences in dietary cholesterol and fat consumption (Kagen et al., 1974).

However the results of other studies on immigrants were not always similar to the Migration study. In one study (Kushi et al., 1985), diet produced no effect on cholesterol levels or heart disease mortality. In General, the importance of age, sex and race on levels of cholesterol has been shown in population-based studies.

Invention of ultracentrifuge has facilitated measurement of the various lipid parameters. LRCP (Lipid Research Clinics Program) was one of the first surveys during 1970 that was conducted to determine the total cholesterol, HDL cholesterol, LDL cholesterol and triglyceride levels in American adults (Heiss et al., 1980). In another study, difference in distribution of cholesterol and its components in the blood in accordance to age were described (Glueek & Stein, 1979). In both sexes, the slope of total cholesterol curve is increased by increase in age until the end of middle-age. After that, by increasing the age, slope of the curve is downward until reaching the old age. Mean total cholesterol in men and women aged between 20 -50 years is similar, however, the levels of HDL cholesterol in women after puberty is higher than men (Rifkind & Segal, 1983).

Among patients with a prior history of myocardial infarction, an elevated total cholesterol following recovery was a major independent risk factor for reinfarction, death from heart disease and total mortality. Cardiovascular mortality is varied in different populations. The highest and lowest mortality rate was found in Finland and Japan, respectively, with a direct relationship to serum cholesterol levels (Rosenson, 2011).

2.2 HDL cholesterol

The negative relationship between low HDL cholesterol and the risk of heart disease is well stablished in the general population (Abbott et al., 1988; Abbott et al., 1998; Castelli, 1983; Gordon et al, 1989; Harper & Jacobson, 1999; Rosenson, 2005) (figure-2). In the Framingham Heart study, the protective role of HDL has been well described (Kannel et al., 1971).

Based on results of this study, by each 5 mg /dl decrease in serum levels of HDL (compared to mean normal values for men and women), the risk of myocardial infarction was increased by 25 percent.

Predictive role of HDL against coronary events was also well documented in patients with known heart disease. The results of Lipid and Care clinical trial showed that low levels of HDL cholesterol is a stronger predictor of heart disease incidence in presence of serum LDL cholesterol < 125 mg/dl than LDL cholesterol ≥ 125 mg/dl (Sacks et al., 2002). They also found that in serum LDL<125 mg/dl, each 10 mg /dl increase in HDL level, will cause 29 percent reduction in the incidence of cardiovascular events , while with the serum LDL cholesterol ≥ 125 mg/dl, this attenuation will be lowered to 10 percent. This association was also seen in post hoc analysis of TNT[7] study, in which 10000 known cases of CVD were under-treatment with different doses of statins (Barter et al., 2007).

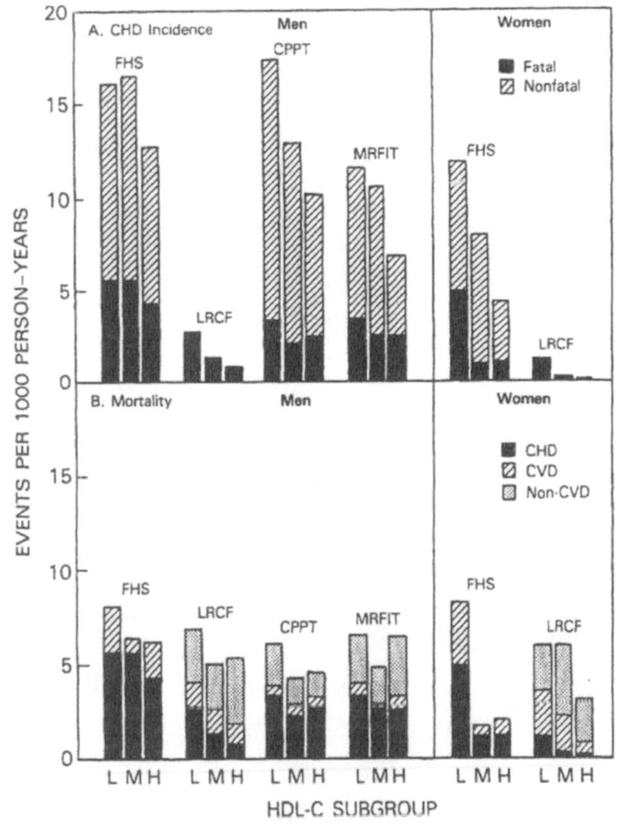

Legend: CHD: Coronary heart disease; L M H HDL: Low, middle, high, high density lipoprotein; CVD: Cardiovascular disease; FHS: Framingham Heart Study; LRCF: Lipid Research Clinics Prevalence Mortality Follow-up Study; CPPT: Lipid Research Clinics Coronary Primary Prevention Trial; MRFIT: Multiple Risk Factor Intervention Trial.

Fig. 2. Inverse association between HDL and CVD events.

As mentioned previously, the cardioprotective effect of HDL was shown to be present at serum levels higher than 60 mg/dl (Castelli et al., 1983). These effects are more prominent when the serum levels of HDL cholesterol reach 75 mg/dl and higher (Table-3).
In assessment of 18 relatives with familial hyperalfa–lipoproteinemia, the life long of these men and women were found to be 5 and 7 years, respectively, more than general population (Glueck et al., 1976).

---

[7] Treating to New Targets trial

In the Lipid Research Clinics study, the Framingham heart Study and the HHS[8] the ratio of LDL to HDL was shown to be the best predictor of cardiovascular events (Manninen et al., 1992; Kinosian et al., 1994). In HHS study, the risk of new coronary events such as myocardial infarction and sudden cardiac death in patients with LDL/HDL ≥ 5 and a concomitant serum triglycerides ≥ 200 mg /dl, was fourfold more than patients with lower LDL/HDL ratio and triglycerides levels. Overall, among men, an LDL/HDL ratio of ≥ 6.4 had 2–14 percent higher predictive value than serum total cholesterol or LDL levels. Among women the predictive value of LDL/HDL ≥ 5.6 was 25–45 percent greater than serum total cholesterol or LDL level (Kinosian et al., 1994).

HDL (mg/dl)	**Multiplier for cardiovascular risk**	
	men	**women**
30	1.82	----
35	1.49	----
40	1.22	1.94
45	1.00	1.55
50	0.82	1.25
55	0.67	1.00
60	0.55	0.80
65	0.45	0.64
70	----	0.52
75	Longevity syndrome	Longevity syndrome

Legend: HDL: High Density Lipoprotein.

Table 3. Inverse relation between plasma HDL-cholesterol levels and cardiovascular risk in men and women.

2.3 Triglycerides

The relationship between hypertriglyceridemia and CVD was determined in the population-based Stockholm prospective study (Carlson et al., 1979). In this study, 3,486 subjects were followed for 14.5 years. An independent relation between hypertriglyceridemia and CVD was observed in this study, which was stronger than the relationship between hypercholesterolemia and CVD. Meta-analysis of several large population-based prospective studies showed similar results (Hokanson & Austin, 1996). Based on this study, the univariate risk ratio (RR) of triglyceride, independent of HDL and other CVD risk factors, among men was 1.32 (95 percent CI, 1.26 to 1.39) and among women was 1.76 (95 percent CI, 1.50 to 2.07).

As mentioned previously in the HHS study, not only there is an interaction between triglycerides and total cholesterol/HDL ratio, but also an inverse association between triglycerides and HDL levels exists (Rosenson, 2011). Additionally, hypertriglyceridemia is associated with increased mortality in patients with known CHD and also reduces the

[8] Helsinki Heart Study

event–free survival after coronary artery bypass graft surgery (CABG) (Haim et al., 1999; Sprecher et al., 2000).

Nevertheless, because hypertriglyceridemia is an independent risk factor for CVD, measurement of triglycerides as a part of routine cholesterol screening is recommended by NECP ATPIII guidelines (Haim et al., 1999). Fasting triglyceride measurement is important for evaluating the risk of heart disease especially in cases who are suffering from diabetes, glucose intolerance, insulin resistance syndrome, obesity and low HDL. Although, triglyceride measurement is commonly done after 8–12 hours fasting, an association between nonfasting triglyceride levels and CVD is also present (Nordestgaard et al., 2007; Bansal et al., 2007).

2.4 Non-HDL cholesterol

Non–HDL cholesterol is defined as the difference between total and HDL cholesterols. Thus it includes LDL, Lp (a), IDL and VLDL (Ballantyne et al., 2000). In both LRCP study and the Women's Health Study non-HDL cholesterol has been suggested as a better tool for risk assessment of CVD than LDL levels (Cobbaert et al., 1997; Ridker et al., 2005). In the LRCP study in which the patients were followed for an average of 19 years, a 30 mg/dl difference in non–HDL and LDL concentrations, produced 19 and 15 percent, increase in mortality risk of CVD among men, respectively, and 11 and 8 percent, among women, respectively, (Cobbaert et al., 1997).

2.5 Lipoprotein (a)

Lipoprotein (a), also called Lp (a), is established as an independent risk factor for CVD. Lp (a) is a modified form of LDL with a structure similar to plasminogen (Steyrer et al., 1994) that could interfere with fibrinolysis by competing with plasminogen for binding to cells (Loscalzo et al., 1990; Palabrica et al., 1995). Lp (a) also binds to macrophages to promote foam cell formation and deposition of cholesterol in atherosclerotic plaques (Zioncheck et al., 1991). Thus, Lp (a) accelerates atherosclerosis process by impairing fibrinolysis and increasing LDL oxidation (Stein & Rosenson, 1997). Evidences of association between Lp (a) excess [Lp (a) levels above the 95th percentile] and CVD mostly come from 2 large meta-analyses that found positive continuous correlation between Lp (a) and risk of CVD events (Bennet et al., 2008; Emerging et al., 2009). The 24 cohort studies in the meta-analysis (Bennet et al., 2008) found a risk ratio of 1.13 (95 percent CI, 1.09 to 1.18) between the top and third bottom baseline Lp (a) levels after adjustment for multiple traditional cardiovascular risk factors. Lp (a) excess concentration is usually detected in patients with premature CHD. In one study 18.6 percent of patients with premature CHD had excess levels of Lp (a), while 12.7 percent of them had no dyslipidemia (Genest et al., 1992).

LP (a) increases the risk of cerebrovascular disease, peripheral vascular disease, myocardial infarction (MI), re–stenosis after angioplasty, and failure after CABG (Rosengren et al., 1990; Schaefer et al., 1994). 12 years and more follow–up of patients in the Framingham Heart study showed that Lp (a) can increase the risk of premature coronary heart disease by two-times (Bostom et al., 1996), and augment the risk of MI, intermittent claudication, cerebrovascular disease, and coronary artery stenosis. In the 4S[9] study an association between increased Lp (a) levels and overall mortality rate was also observed (Bostom et al., 1994).

---

[9] Scandinavian Simvastatin Survival Study

2.6 Apolipoproteins & atherogenic lipoprotein phenotype

There are limited prospective studies about the relationship between apolipoproteins (apo A-I and apo B) and the CVD risk. The QCS[10] was studied 2155 men aged between 45-76 years and reported a direct correlation between apo B levels and prevalence of ischemic heart disease over the future 5 years, [relative risk (RR) 1.4; 95 percent CI, 1.2 to 1.7] (Lamarche et al., 1996), independent of other risk factors of CVD. For apo A-I, a negative correlation (RR = 0.85; 95 percent CI, 0.7 to 1.0) was reported.

Since the measurement of apo B and apo A-I is an indicator of total atherogenic (IDL, VLDL, and LDL) and antiatherogenic particles (HDL), some studies (Lamarche et al., 1996; Meisinger et al., 2005; Yusuf et al., 2004; Walldius et al., 2001, 2005) proposed that measurements of apo B and apo A are more important predictors of the CVD than above measurements. The AMORIS[11] study evaluated this relationship in 175,553 subjects with 65 months follow up (Walldius et al., 2001). In the multivariate analysis the apo B concentration was significantly higher than LDL levels and served as a better predictor of CVD than LDL.

The results regarding the role of apolipoproteins in prediction of CVD risk are conflicting. Two studies; Women's Health Study and the Framingham Study obtained a similar predictive value for apo B/A-I ratio versus total cholesterol/ HDL ratio (Ridker et al., 2005; Ingelsson & Schaefer, 2007). However, in contrast to Health Professionals Follow-up Study (Pischon et al., 2005; Sniderman, 2005) and AMORIS study, apo A-I and apo B did not have any predictive value for CHD risk in ARIC[12] study (Sharrett et al., 2001). The explanation for these disparate results is not clear. However, it seems apolipoproteins have a potential role in CHD risk stratification. Standardization of laboratory methods and measurements to the same reference system, and establishing threshold and target values for diagnosis could help recognize the full potential of apolipoproteins (Srinivasan & Berenson, 2001; Denke, 2005).

Apo E is important in plasma lipid metabolism and Apo E gene affects plasma levels of LDL. Three major apo E isoforms are E2, E3, and E4, which are encoded by three common alleles at the APO E locus. The less common and the most common isoforms in society are E2 and E3, respectively. E4 allele is associated with higher plasma total cholesterol and LDL cholesterol levels and with risk of heart attack. In contrast, subjects with E2 allele have lower risk of heart attack compared to people with E4 isoform (Song et al., 2004).

Some clinical researches have focused on the relationship between small dense LDL particles and risk of CVD. This status, also called atherogenic lipoprotein phenotype, is usually associated with increased triglyceride, VLDL and LDL levels (Krauss, 1994). The Physician's Health Study showed that small dense LDL particles can increase three times the risk of CVD more than LDL cholesterol (Zambon et al., 1996). In QCS study, during 5 year follow up, 114 cases from a total of 2103 were diagnosed with heart disease. In this study, in multivariate analysis small dense LDL was more important predictor of CVD [odds ratio (OR) = 3.7; 95 percent CI, 1.4 to 9.7) than LDL (OR = 1.8; 95 percent CI, 1.2 to 2.9) (Lamarche et al., 1997). The Familial atherosclerosis Treatment Study (FATS) found that LDL subclasses were the most important predictor of coronary progression (Zambon et al., 1999). In the Pravastatin Limitation of Atherosclerosis in the Coronaries (PLAC-I) study showed that

---

[10] Quebec Cardiovascular Study

[11] Apolipoprotein-related MOrtality RISk

[12] Atherosclerosis risk in Communities

small LDL particle size (≤ 20.5 nm) could increase rate of coronary progression with OR= 5.0 and 95 percent CI, 1 to 9. High numbers of small LDL particles (>30 mg/dl) was the most important lipoprotein predictor in multivariate analysis (OR = 9.1; 95 percent CI, 2.1 to 39) (Otvos et al., 2002).

In the FATS[13] study 95 percent variance in regression of atherosclerosis in coronary arteries were related to changes in lipid profile. Adding the LDL density to the equation showed that almost 45 percent of the variance was related to changes in LDL density (Lamarche et al., 1997). In contrast, the CHS[14] reported that LDL particle concentration and not LDL size acted as a significant predictor of MI and angina in women, in which by every 100 nmol/l increase in LDL particle number, the OR of MI and angina increased by 11 percent (Kuller et al., 2002).

In Women's Health Study which assessed LDL particle size and concentration by NMR[15] , the LDL particle concentration was a strong predictor of CVD after adjustment for traditional risk factors (Blake et al., 2002).

EPIC[16]- Norfolk prospective Population Study examined NMR-measured LDL particle size and concentration (EI Harchaoui et al., 2007) and found that LDL particle concentration did not increase the prediction of CHD. After LDL particle concentration adjustment, LDL size was no longer associated with CHD.

Recently, some scientists from the University of Warwick in UK discovered a modified form of LDL, MGmin-LDL, also called super-sticky LDL, or very-bad LDL, that promotes CVD (Rabbani et al., 2011). High levels of this lipid are more common in diabetics and elderly patients. Diabetic subjects present almost four times more serum levels of MGmin-LDL than normal subjects. This may explain the high frequency of CVD in diabetics and elderly patients. Rabbani et al (Rabbani et al., 2011) found that secondary to hyperglycemia, LDL is glycated with methylglyoxal (MG) and makes a type of LDL with smaller, stickier and more atherogenic LDL than normal LDL. The MGmin-LDL can help to build fatty plaques. When these plaques grow, the wall of arteries become narrower and the blood flow reduces. Plaque rapture, an event that would eventually happen, triggers the blood clot cascades that could cause a heart attack or stroke. In elderly, the activity of the enzyme for detoxification of MGmin-LDL is reduced. They (Rabbani et al., 2011) also showed that metformin can block the glycation processes which might explain the cardioprotective effects of this drug. This discovery could lead to invention of new treatments for CVD prevention especially in type 2 diabetics and the elderly subjects.

3. Summary

The relationships described above can be summarized in the figure-3 (Ridker et al., 2005). This figure shows the adjusted Hazard ratios of future cardiovascular events among patients who are in the extreme quintiles of each measured marker. Black bars present 95 percent CI.

---

[13] Familial Atherosclerosis Regression Study

[14] Cardiovascular health Study

[15] Nuclear Magnetic Resonance

[16] European Prospective Investigation into Cancer and Nutrition

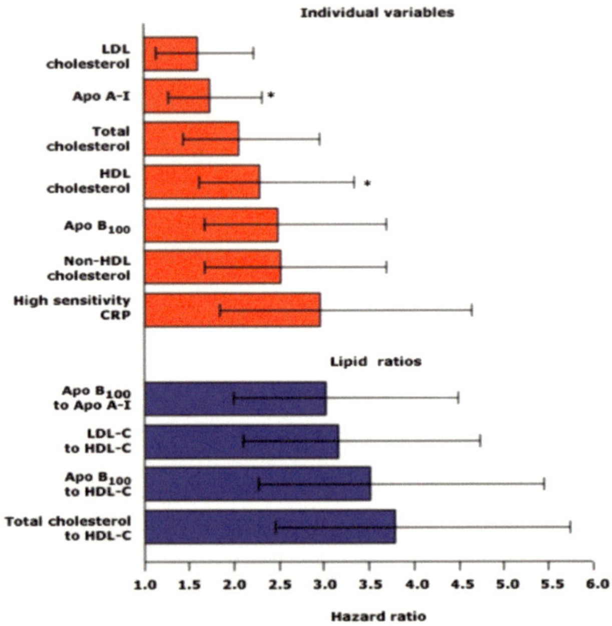

Legend: LDL: Low Density Lipoprotein; Apo A-I: Apolipoprotein A-I; HDL: High Density Lipoprotein; Apo B100: Apolipoprotein B100; CRP: C - reactive protein.

Fig. 3. Adjusted Hazard ratios for future cardiovascular events.

Today, interventional studies have investigated the effects of augmentation of HDL levels. The clinical trials which deal with this matter will be discussed in a separate part. In assessment of dyslipidemia two points should be stipulated:

1. Decline of coronary events could be possible by modifying the serum lipid levels in order to prevent or delay the reduction of vessel diameter, and also to stabilize atheroma plaques. Small plaques are mostly filled with lipid and are prone to disposable rupture, thrombosis, acute, serious and ultimately fatal atherosclerosis. Reduction of LDL leads to removal of fatty deposits from the inside of the atheroma plaque and makes them more stable. In addition, lowering the lipids levels can return the normal activity of vessel wall endothelium and its ability to produce nitric oxide, the main mediator of coronary vasodilation (Krauss, 1994).
2. During lipid-lowering drug therapy the cost-effectiveness of the treatment should be considered. This depends on the price of drugs as well as patient's risk. For example, at least cost-effectiveness includes patients with intermediate elevation of serum cholesterol, who, without any other risk factors, are under- lipid lowering agent therapy. In 4S study which was performed in patients with high risk of CVD, cost per year of life gain, was depended on age, sex and baseline levels of lipid. The range of this cost was varied from 3,800 $ U.S. for men aged 70 years and the mean serum cholesterol 309 mg/dl, to 27,400 $ U.S. for women aged 35 years and the average serum cholesterol 213 mg/dl (Johannessonet al., 1997). In other studies these figures were different from 19,000 $ U.S. to 56,000 $ U.S. which depends on drug dose and formulation used. Also, these costs were three folds, two folds and 1.3 folds more in women at age 40, 60 and 70 years, respectively, when compared with the men at age 40 years (Martens & Guibert, 1994; Thorvik et al., 1996).

4. References

Abbott RD, Wilson PWF, Kannel WB, Castelli WP (1988). High density lipoprotein cholesterol, total cholesterol screening, and myocardial infarction: the Framingham Study. *Arteriosclerosis*; 8: 207-11.

Abbott RD, Yano K, Hakim AA (1998). Changes in total and high - density lipoprotein holesterol over 10- and 20-year periods (the Honolulu Heart program). *Am J Cardiol*; 82: 172-8.

Alwan A (2008). 2008-2013 action plan for the global strategy for the prevention and control of noncommunicable diseases. *Report World Health Organization*.

Ballantyne CM, Grundy SM, Oberman A, et al (2000). Hyperlipidemia: diagnostic and therapeutic perspectives. *J Clin Endocrinol Metab*; 85:2089-112.

Bansal S, Buring JE, Rifai N, et al (2007). Fasting compared with nonfasting triglycerides and risk of cardiovascular events in women. *JAMA*; 298:309-16.

Barter P, Gotto AM, LaRosa JC, Maroni J, Szarek M, Grundy SM, et al (2007). HDL cholesterol, very low levels of LDL cholesterol, and cardiovascular events. *N Engl J Med*; 357: 1301-10.

Bennet A, Di Angelantonio E, Erqou S, et al (2008). Lipoprotein (a) levels and risk of future coronary heart disease: large-scale prospective data. *Arch Intern Med*; 168:598- 608.

Blake GJ, Otvos JD, Rifai N, Ridker PM (2002). Low-density lipoprotein particle concentration and size as determined by nuclear magnetic resonancespectroscopy as predictors of cardiovascular disease in women. *Circulation*; 106: 1930-7.

Blood cholesterol levels by sex, adults aged 35-64, latest available data MONICA project population, 4th August 2008, Available from: http://www.ktl.fi/publications/monica.

Bostom AG, Gagnon DR, Cupples LA, et al (1994). A prospective investigation of elevated LP (a) detected by electrophoresis and cardiovascular disease in women: the Framingham Heart Study. *Circulation*; 90: 1688-95.

Bostom AG, Cupples LA, Jenner JL, et al (1996). Elevated plasma lipoprotein (a) and coronary heart disease in men aged 55 years and younger: a prospective study. *JAMA*; 276: 544-48.

Butler WJ, Ostrander LDJ, Carman WJ (1985). Mortality from coronary heart disease in the Tecumseh Study: long-term effect of diabetes mellitus, glucose tolerance and other risk factors. *Am J Epidemiol*; 121: 541-7.

Carlson LA, Böttiger LE, Ahfeldt PE (1979). Risk factors for myocardial infarction in the Stockholm prospective study. A 14-year follow-up focussing on the role of plasma triglycerides and cholesterol. *Acta Med Scand*;206(5):351-60.

Caroll MD, Lacher DA, Sorlie PD, Cleeman JI, Gordon DJ, Wolz M, et al. (2005).Trends in serum lipids and lipoproteins of adults, 1960-2002. *JAMA*; 294:1773- 81.

Castelli WP (1983). Cardiovascular disease and multifactorial risk: Challenge of the 1980s. *Am Heart J*; 106: 1191-200.

Cobbaert C, Jukema JW, Zwinderman AH, et al (1997). Modulation of lipoprotein(a) atherogenicity by high density lipoprotein cholesterol levels in middle-aged men with symptomatic coronary artery disease and normal to moderately elevated serum cholesterol. Regression Growth Evaluation Statin Study (REGRESS) Study Group. *J Am Coll Cardiol*; 30:1491-9.

Critchley J, Liu J, Zhao D (2004). Explaining the increase in coronary heart disease mortality in Beijing between 1984 and 1999. *Circulation;* 110: 1236–44.

Dawber TR, Meadors GF, Moore FE Jr (1951). Epidemiological approaches to heart disease: the Framingham Study. *Am J Public Health;* 41: 279–86.

Denke MA (2005). Weighing in before the fight: low-density lipoprotein cholesterol and non-high-density lipoprotein cholesterol versus apolipoprotein B as the best predictor for coronary heart disease and the best measure of therapy. *Circulation;* 112: 3368–70.

Dobsn A, Filipiak B, Kuulasmaa K (1996). Relations of changes in coronary disease rates and changes in risk factor levels: methodological issues and a practical example. *Am J Epidemiol;* 143: 1025–34.

Dyer AR, Stamler J, Paul O (1981). Serum cholesterol and risk of death from cancer and other causes in three Chicago epidemiological studies. *J Chronic Dis;* 39: 249–60.

E'g'gen DA, Strong JP, McGill HCJ (1964). Calcification in the abdominal aorta: relationship to race, sex, and coronary atherosclerosis. *Arch Pathol;* 78: 575– 83.

El Harchaoui K, van der Steeg WA, Stroes ES, et al (2007). Value of low-density lipoprotein particle number and size as predictors of coronary artery disease in apparently healthy men and women: the EPIC-Norfolk Prospective Population Study. *J Am Coll Cardiol;* 49:547–53.

Emerging Risk Factors Collaboration, Erqou S, Kaptoge S, et al (2009). Lipoprotein(a) concentration and the risk of coronary heart disease, stroke, and nonvascular mortality. JAMA; 302:412– 23.

Fager G, Wiklund O, Olofsson SO, Wilhelmsen L, Bondjers G (1981). Multivariate analysis of apolipoproteins and risk factors in relation to acute myocardial infarction. *Arteriosclerosis;* 1: 273–7.

Ford ES, Li C, Zhao G, Pearson WS, Mokdad AH (2009). Hypertriglyceridemia and its pharmacologic treatment among US adults. *Arch Intern Med;* 169: 572–8.

Genest JJ Jr, Martin-Munley SS, McNamara JR, Ordovas JM, Jenner J, Myers RH, et al. (1992). Familial lipoprotein disorders in patients with premature coronary artery disease. *Circulation;* 85: 2025–33.

Glueck CJ, Gartside P, Fallat RW, et al (1976). Longevity syndromes: familial hypobeta and familial hyperalphalipoproteinemia. *J Lab Clin Med;* 88: 941–75.

Glueck CJ, Stein EA (1979). Treatment and management of hyperlipoproteinemia in childhood. In: Levy R, Rifkind B, Dennis B, Ernst N. Nutrition, Lipids, and Coronary Heart Disease, New York: Raven Press; pp. 285–307.

Goldstein JL, Hazzard WR, Schrott HG, Bierman EL, Motulsky AG (1973). Hyperlipidemia in coronary heart disease I. Lipid levels in 500 survivors of myocardial infarction. *J Clin Invest;* 52:1533–43.

Gordon DJ, Probstfield JL, Garrison RJ, Neaton JD, Castelli WP, Knoke JD, et al. (1989). High-density lipoprotein cholesterol and cardiovascular disease. Four prospective American studies. *Circulation;* 79: 8–15.

Gorelick PB, Schneck M, Berglund LF, Feinberg W, Goldstone J (1997). Status of lipids as a risk factor for stroke. *Neuroepidemiology;* 16: 107–15.

Haim M, Benderly M, Brunner D, et al (1999). Elevated serum triglyceride levels and long-term mortality in patients with coronary heart disease: the Bezafibrate Infarction Prevention (BIP) Registry. *Circulation;* 100: 475–82.

Harper CR, Jacobson TA (1999). New perspectives on the management of low levels of high-density lipoprotein cholesterol. *Arch Intern Med;* 159(10):1049-57.

Heiss G, Tamir I, Davis CEo (1980). Lipoprotein -Cholesterol distributions in selected North American populations: the Lipid Research Clinics Program Prevalence Study. *Circulation;* 61: 302-15.

High blood cholesterol and other lipids-statistics, 8 June 2011, Available from: www.americanheart.org

Hokanson IE, Austin MA (1996). Plasma triglyceride level is a risk factor in cardiovascular disease independent of high density lipoprotein cholesterol level: a meta - analysis of population - based prospective studies. *J Cardiovasc Risk;* 3: 213-9.

Ingelsson E, Schaefer EJ, Contois JH, et al (2007). Clinical utility of different lipid measures for prediction of coronary heart disease in men and women. *JAMA;* 298: 776-85.

Johannesson M, Jonsson B, Kjekshns J (1997). Cost-effectiveness of Simvastatin treatment to lower cholesterol levels in patients with coronary heart disease. *N Engl J Med;* 336: 332-6.

Kagan A, Harris BR, Winkelstein W Jr (1974). Epidemiologic studies of coronary disease and stroke in Japanese men living in Japan, Hawaii and California: demographic, physical, dietary and biochemical characteristics. *J Chronic Dis;* 27: 345-64.

Kannel WB, Castelli WP, Gordon T, McNamara PM (1971). Serum cholesterol, lipoproteins, and the risk of coronary heart disease: the Framingham Study. *Ann Intern Med;* 74: 1-12.

Kannel WB, Castelli WP, Gordon T (1979). Cholesterol in the prediction of atherosclerotic disease: new perspective based on the Framingham Heart Study. *Ann Intern Med;* 90: 85-91.

Kannel WB (1983). High-density lipoproteins: epidemiologic profile and risks of coronary artery disease. *Am J Cardiol;* 52:9B-12B.

Keys A (1970). Coronary heart disease in seven countries. *Circulation;* 41 (suppl 1): 1-199.

Keys A, Menotti A, Aravanis C, Blackburn H, Djordevic BS, Buzina R, et al. (1984). The seven countries study: 2289 deaths in 15 years. *Prev Med;* 13: 141-54.

Kinosian B, Glick H, Garland G (1994). Cholesterol and coronary heart disease: predicting risk s by levels and ratios. *Ann Intern Med;* 121: 641-7.

Krauss RM (1994). Heterogeneity of plasma low-density lipoproteins and atherosclerosis risk. *Curr Opin Lipidol;* 5: 339-49.

Kuller L, Arnold A, Tracy R, et al (2002). Nuclear magnetic resonance spectroscopy of lipoproteins and risk of coronary heart disease in the cardiovascular health study. *Arterioscler Thromb Vasc Biol;* 22:1175-80.

Kushi LH, Lew RA, Stare FJ (1985). Diet and 20-year mortality from coronary heart disease. The Ireland -Boston Diet-Heart Study. *N Engl J Med;* 312: 811-8.

Labarthe DR (2011). Coronary heart disease, In: *Epidemiology and prevention of cardiovascular disease: a global challenge,* Labarthe DR, pp. 59-87, Jones and Bartlett, ISBN-13: 978-0-7637-4689-6, Canada.

Lamarche B, Moorjani S, Lupien PJ, et al (1996). Apolipoprotein AI and B levels and the risk of ischemic heart disease during a five year follow up of men in the Quebec Cardiovascular Study. *Circulation;* 94: 273-278.

Lamarche B, Tchernof A, Mooljani S, et al (1997). Small, dense low-density lipoprotein particles as a predictor of the risk of ischemic heart disease in men: prospective results from the Quebec Study. *Circulation*; 95: 69–75.

Law MR, Wald NJ, Thompson SG (1994). By how much and how quickly does reduction in serum cholesterol concentration lower risk of ischemic heart disease? *BMJ*; 308: 367–72.

Loscalzo J, Weinfeld M, Fless GM, Scanu AM (1990). Lipoprotein(a), fibrin binding, and plasminogen activation. *Arteriosclerosis*; 10:240- 5.

Manninen V, Tenkanen L, Koskinen P, Huttunen JK, Manttar M, Heinonen OP, et al (1992). Joint effects of serum triglyceride and LDL–cholesterol and HDL- cholesterol concentrations on coronary heart disease risk in the Helsinki Heart Study: implications for treatment. *Circulation*: 85: 37–45.

Martens LL, Guibert R (1994). Cost–effectiveness analysis of Lipid - modifying therapy in Canada: comparison of HMG–COA reductase inhibitors in the primary prevention of coronary heart disease. *Clin Therapeut*; 16: 1052–62.

Meisinger C, Loewel H, Mraz W, Koenig W (2005). Prognostic value of apolipoprotein B and A–I in the prediction of myocardial infarction in middle-aged men and women: results from the MONICA/KORA Augsburg cohort study. *Eur Heart J*; 26:271–8.

Miller NE, Thelle DS, Forde OH, Mjos OD (1977). The TromsØ heart study. High-density Lipoprotein and coronary heart disease: a Prospective case–control study. *Lancet*; 1: 965–70.

Murray CJ, Lopez AD (1997). Mortality by cause for eight regions of the world: Global Burden of Disease Study. *Lancet*; 349: 1269–76.

Murray CJ, Lopez AD (1997). Alternative projections of mortality and disability by cause 1990–2020: Global Burden of Disease Study. *Lancet*; 349: 1498–504.

Nieto FJ, Alonso J, Chambliss LE (1995). Population awareness and control of hypertension and hypercholesterolemia: the atherosclerosis in communities study. *Arch Intern Med*; 155: 677–84.

Nordestgaard BG, Benn M, Schnohr P, Tybjaerg-Hansen A (2007). Nonfasting triglycerides and risk of myocardial infarction, ischemic heart disease, and death in men and women. *JAMA*; 298:299–308.

Otvos JD, Shalaurova I, Freedman DS, Rosenson RS (2002). Effects of pravastatin treatment on lipoprotein subclass profiles and particle size in the PLAC–I trial. *Atherosclerosis*; 160:41–8.

Palabrica TM, Liu AC, Aronovitz MJ, Furie B, Lawn RM, Furie BC (1995). Antifibrinolytic activity of apolipoprotein(a) in vivo: human apolipoprotein(a) transgenic mice are resistant to tissue plasminogen activator-mediated thrombolysis. *Nat Med*; 1:256- 9.

Pischon T, Girman CJ, Sacks FM, et al (2005). Non–high–density lipoprotein cholesterol and apolipoprotein B in the prediction of coronary heart disease in men. *Circulation*; 112: 3375–83.

Rabbani N, Godfrey L, Xue M, Shaheen F, Geoffrion M, Milne R, et al (2011). Glycation of LDL by methylglyoxal increases arterial atherogenicity. A possible contributor to increased risk of cardiovascular disease in diabetes. *Diabetes*; 60 (7): 1973–80.

Ridker PM, Rifai N, Cook NR, Bradwin G, Buring JE (2005). Non–HDL cholesterol, apolipoproteins A–I and B100, standard lipid measures, lipid ratios, and CRP as risk factors for cardiovascular disease in women. *JAMA*; 294:326- 33.

Rifkind BM, Segal P (1983). Lipid Research Clinics Program reference values for Hyperlipidemia and hypolipidemia. *JAMA*; 250: 1869-72.

Roncaglioni MC, Santoro L, D'Avanzo B, Negri E, Nobili A, Ledda A, et al. (1992). Role of family history in patients with myocardial infarction. An Italian case- control study. GISSI-EFRIM investigators. *Circulation*; 85: 2065-72.

Rosengren A, Wilhelmsen L, Eriksson E (1990). Lipoprotein (a) and coronary heart disease risk: a prospective case - control study in a general population sample of middle - aged men. *BMJ*; 301: 1248-51.

Rosenson RS (2005). Low HDL-C: a secondary target of dyslipidaemia therapy. *Am J Med*; 118: 1067-77.

Rosenson RS. Screening guidelines for dyslipidemia, May 2011, Available from: www.uptodate.com

Sacks FM, Tonkin AM, Craven T, Pfeffer MA, Shepherd J, Keech A, et al (2002). Coronary Heart disease in patients with low LDL-cholesterol: benefit of pravastatin in diabetics and enhanced role for HDL- cholesterol and triglycerides as risk factors. *Circulation*; 105: 1424-8.

Schaefer EI, Lamon - Fava S, Ianner I (1994). Lipoprotein (a) levels and risk of coronary heart disease in men: the Lipid Research Clinics Primary Prevention Trial. *JAMA*; 271: 999-1003.

Sharrett AR, Ballantyne CM, Coady SA, et al (2001). Coronary heart disease prediction from lipoprotein cholesterol levels, triglycerides, lipoprotein(a), apolipoproteins A-I and B, and HDL density subfractions: The Atherosclerosis Risk in Communities (ARIC) Study. *Circulation*; 104: 1108-13.

Sniderman AD (2005). Apolipoprotein B versus non-high-density lipoprotein cholesterol: and the winner is... *Circulation*; 112: 3366-7.

Song Y, Stampfer MJ, Liu S (2004). Meta-analysis: apolipoprotein E genotypes and the risk for coronary heart disease. *Ann Intern Med*; 141 (2): 137-47.

Sprecher DL, Pearce GL, Cosgrove DM, et al (2000). Relation of serum triglyceride levels to Relation of serum triglyceride levels to survival after coronary artery bypass grafting. *Am J Cardiol*; 86:285-8.

Srinivasan SR, Berenson GS (2001). Apolipoproteins B and A-I as predictors of risk of Coronary artery disease. *Lancet*; 358:2012-3.

Stamler, J, Wentworth, D, Neaton, JD (1986). Is relationship between serum cholesterol and risk of premature death from coronary heart disease continuous and graded? Findings in 356,222 primary screenees of the Multiple Risk Factor Intervention Trial (MRFIT). *JAMA*; 256:2823-8.

Stein IH, Rosenson RS (1997). Lipoprotein LP (a) excess and coronary heart disease. *Arch Intern Med*: 157: 1170-6.

Steyrer E, Durovic S, Frank S, et al (1994). The role of lecithin: cholesterol acyltransferase for lipoprotein (a) assembly. Structural integrity of low density lipoproteins is a prerequisite for Lp(a) formation in human plasma. *J Clin Invest*; 94: 2330- 40.

The WHO MONICA Project: Risk factors (1989). *Int J Epidemiol*; 339: 861-7.

Thom TJ, Kannel WB, Silbershats S (1998). Incidence, prevalence and mortality of cardiovascular diseases in the United States. In: Hurst's the Heart, 9th ed, Alexander R W, Schlant RC, Fuster V, Roberts R (Eds), McGraw Hill, New York, P.3.

Thorvik E, Aursnes I, Kristiansen IS, Waller HT (1996). Cost-effectiveness of cholesterol - lowering drugs :a review of the evidence. *Wiener Klin Wochensch*; 108: 234-43.

Walldius G, Jungner I, Holme I, et al (2001). High apolipoprotein B, low apolipoprotein A- I, and improvement in the prediction of fatal myocardial infarction (AMORIS study): a prospective study. *Lancet*; 358: 2026-33.

Walldius G, Jungner I (2005). Rationale for using apolipoprotein B and apolipoprotein A-I as indicators of cardiac risk and as targets for lipid-lowering therapy. *Eur Heart J*; 26: 210-2.

Wu Z, Yao C, Zhao D, Wu G, Wang W, Liu J, et al. (2004). Cardiovascular disease risk factor levels and their relations to CVD rates in China- results of Sino- MONICA project. *Eur J Cardiovasc Prev Rehabil*; 11: 275-83.

Yusuf S, Hawken S, Ôunpuu S, Dans T, Avezum A, Lanas F, et al. (2004). Effect of potentially modifiable risk factors associated with myocardial infarction in 52 countries (the INTERHEART study): case-control study. *Lancet*; 364: 937-52.

Zambon A, Brown BG, Hokansen LE, Brunzeel IL (1996). Hepatic lipase changes predict coronary artery disease regression in the Familial Atherosclerosis Treatment Study (Abstract). Circulation; 94: 1-539.

Zambon A, Hokanson JE, Brown BG, Brunzell JD (1999). Evidence for a new pathophysiological mechanism for coronary artery disease regression: hepatic lipase-mediated changes in LDL density. Circulation; 99: 1959- 64.

Zioncheck TF, Powell LM, Rice GC, et al (1991). Interaction of recombinant apolipoprotein(a) and lipoprotein(a) with macrophages. J Clin Invest; 87:767-71.

16

Cardiovascular Risk in Tunisian Patients with Bipolar I Disorder

Asma Ezzaher[1,2], Dhouha Haj Mouhamed[1,2], Anwar Mechri[2], Fadoua Neffati[1], Wahiba Douki[1,2], Lotfi Gaha[2] and Mohamed Fadhel Najjar[1]

[1]Laboratory of Biochemistry-Toxicology,
[2]Research Laboratory "Vulnerability to Psychotic Disorders LR 05 ES 10", Department of Psychiatry/Monastir University Hospital, Tunisia

1. Introduction

Bipolar disorder (previously also labeled manic-depressive illness) is typically referred to as an episodic, yet lifelong and clinically severe affective (or mood) disorder, affecting approximately 3.5% of the population (Marmol, 2008; Simon, 2003; Wittchen et al., 2003; Woods, 2000). The term bipolar disorder, however, encompasses several phenotypes of mood disorders, i.e. mania, hypomania or cyclothymia that may present with a puzzling variety of other symptoms and disorders. According to the Fourth Edition of the Diagnostic and Statistical Manual of Mental Disorders (DSM-IV) (American Psychiatric Association, 2004), the diagnostic classificatory system used in most epidemiological studies, bipolar disorder is defined by a set of specific symptom criteria. Bipolar type I requires the presence or the history of at least one manic or mixed episode. Although, typically, patients with a manic episode also experience major depressive episodes, bipolar disorder can be diagnosed even if only one manic episode and no past major depressive episodes are present. Bipolar disorder type II differs from type I only by presence of hypomanic but no manic episodes. Hypomanic episodes differ from mania by a shorter duration (at least 4 days instead of 1 week), and less severe impairment (not severe enough to cause marked impairment in social or occupational functioning, psychiatric hospitalization, or psychotic features). The DSM-IV also includes "cyclothymia" as a bipolar spectrum disorder with hypomanic as well as depressive episodes that do not meet criteria for major depression (American Psychiatric Association, 2004).

Bipolar disorder is a chronic disease that is associated with a potentially devastating impact on patients' wellbeing and social, occupational, and general functioning (Revicki et al., 2005). The disorder ranks as the sixth leading cause of disability in the world, with an economic burden that in the US alone that was estimated more than a decade ago at $7 billion in direct medical costs and $38 billion (1991 values) in indirect costs (Wyatt et al., 1991).

A number of reviews and studies have shown that people with severe mental illness, including bipolar disorder, have an excess mortality, being two or three times as high as that in the general population. This mortality gap, which translates to a 13-30 year shortened life expectancy in severe mental illness patients, has widened in recent decades, even in countries where the quality of the health care system is generally acknowledged to be good. About 60% of this excess mortality is due to physical illness especially cardiovascular disease. Additionally, several studies have found that after suicide and accidents, cardiovascular and all vascular diseases are the main leading causes of death in these patients (De Hert et al., 2011; Garcia-Portilla et al., 2009).

Patients with bipolar disorder, especially type I, are known to suffer a considerable number of associated pathologies that may manifest at earlier ages and with higher frequency than in the general population. The most recent studies have explored cardiovascular risk and the association with metabolic and endocrine disorders fundamentally, obesity and metabolic syndrome which are clearly associated with the development of cardiovascular disease (Angst et al., 2002; Sicras et al., 2008).

Cardiovascular disease, i.e. coronary heart disease, stroke, and peripheral vascular disease, are potentially preventable diseases. Thanks to epidemiological, experimental and clinical studies, the primary determinants of cardiovascular disease have been identified, as well as the efficacy of specific interventions. The prevalence of cardiovascular disease is increasing in less urbanized, developed populations across the world, as their lifestyles change to a so called "western style", with increasing consumption of dietary saturated fat, cholesterol and salt, cigarette smoking, decreased physical activity and the rise in cardiovascular risk factors including obesity and diabetes. Other known factors that contribute to cardiovascular disease risk are stress and high alcohol intake. Among all these factors, hypercholesterolemia is the leading cause of death from cardiovascular disease. As a result, public health agencies have attempted to reduce the prevalence of hypercholesterolemia through screening and by increasing public awareness and strategies for reducing it (Muntoni et al., 2009).

The exact mechanisms increasing the incidence of cardiovascular risk in bipolar patients remain to be clarified, but they possibly include industrialisation, stress, lack of exercise, dietary lipids (that is, omega-3 fatty acid deficiency) and increasing incidence of smoking and alcohol consumption and other factors (Ezzaher et al., 2010).

This study aims to investigate the principal factors predisposing to the cardiovascular risk in Tunisian bipolar I patients (cigarette smoking, hypertension, diabetes, obesity, lipid profile, hyperhomocysteinemia and metabolic syndrome) and to determine the association between these factors and the clinical and therapeutic characteristics of bipolar I disorder.

2. Patients and methods

2.1 Subjects

This study was approved by the local ethical committee and all subjects were of Tunisian origin. Our samples included 130 patients with bipolar I disorder (37.9 ± 12.1 years) from the psychiatry department of the University Hospital of Monastir, Tunisia, 45 women (37.5 ± 13.4 years) and 85 men (38.1 ± 11.4 years). Consensus on the diagnosis, according to the Diagnostic and Statistical Manual of Mental Disorders, fourth edition (DSM-IV) criteria (American Psychiatric Association, 2004), was made by psychiatrists. The exclusion criteria were age < 18 years, other psychiatric illnesses, epilepsy or mental retardation. The control group consisted of 175 volunteer subjects without psychiatric pathology. The mean age was 40.1 ± 14.0 years, and there were 73 women (42.0 ± 14.4 years) and 102 men (38.8 ± 13.6

years). All subjects were questioned about their age, gender, previous treatments and cigarette and alcohol consumption habits.
The clinical and socio-demographic characteristics are shown in table 1. Differences between patients and controls for body mass index (BMI) ($p < 0.001$) and smoking status ($p = 0.025$) were noted. Therefore, these variables were considered as potential confounder factors for this analysis.

	Patients (n = 130)		**Controls (n = 175)**		**p**
Gender: Men/Women (ratio)	85/45 (1.89)		102/73 (1.39)		0.143
Age (years) (mean ± SD)	37.9 ± 12.1		40.1 ± 14.0		0.840
BMI (kg/m²) (M ± ET)	27.1 ± 4.6		25.3 ± 4.1		**< 0.001**
	Nombre	**%**	**Nombre**	**%**	**p**
BMI (kg/m²)					
< 25	47	36.2	89	50.9	**< 0.001**
[25-30[	40	30.7	72	41.1	
≥ 30	43	33.1	14	8	
Cigarette smoking					
Yes	68	52.3	69	39.4	**0.025**
No	62	47.7	106	60.6	
Alcoholic beverages					
Yes	17	13.1	12	6.9	0.067
No	113	86,9	163	93.1	
Illness episode					
Depressive	21	16.2	-	-	-
Euthymic	73	56.1	-	-	-
Manic	36	27.7	-	-	-
Treatment					
Valproic acid	64	49.3	-	-	-
Lithium	12	9.2	-	-	-
Carbamazepine	10	7.7	-	-	-
Valproic acid and lithium	6	4.6	-	-	-
Antipsychotics	38	29.2	-	-	-

Antipsychotics: Haloperidol, Risperidone, Chlorpromazine, Olanzapine; BMI: body mass index

Table 1. Sociodemographic and therapeutic characteristics of studied population.

2.2 Samples

After a 12 h overnight fasting, venous blood for each patient was drawn in tubes containing lithium heparinate and immediately centrifuged. The plasma samples were stored at -20°C until the biochemical analysis.

2.3 Biochemical analysis

The methods of dosage and the normal values of the different biological parameters are shown in table 2.

Parameters	Assay	Automates	Normal values
Cholesterol	Enzymatic	Konelab 30 equipment (Thermo Electron Corporation, Ruukintie, Finland)	< 5.17 mmol/L
Triglycerides			< 1.7 mmol/L
c-HDL			Men: ≥ 1.1 mmol/L Women: ≥ 0.9 mmol/L
c-LDL			< 3.4 mmol/L
ApoA1	Immunoturbidimetry		1.2- 1.6 g/L
ApoB			0.7-1.3 g/L
Lp(a)			< 200 mg/L
Uric acid	Enzymatic		Men: 210-420 µmol/L Women: 150-360 µmol/L
Homocysteine	Fluorescence polarization (FPIA)	AxSYM® (Abbott Laboratories, Abbott Park, IL 60064, Barcelaneta, Puerto Rico)	< 15 µmol/L
Vitamin B12	Electrochemiluminescence	Elecsys 2010™ (Roche Diagnostics, Indianapolis, IN, USA)	≥ 187ng/L
Folate			≥ 3.7 µg/L
Insulin			< 17µU/mL

Table 2. Methods of dosage of the studied parameters.

2.4 Clinical evaluation

Body mass index (BMI) was calculated as weight (kg) divided by height (m^2). Obesity was defined when BMI ≥ 30 kg/m^2 and overweight when BMI ≥ 25 kg/m^2 (World Health Organization, 1997).

2.5 Criteria for metabolic syndrome

Metabolic syndrome (MS) was defined according to the National Cholesterol Education Program (NCEP) Adult Treatment Panel (ATP) III modified criteria and required fulfillment of at least three of the following five components: body mass index (BMI) ≥ 28.5 kg/m^2, triglycerides ≥ 1.7 mmol/L, high-density lipoprotein cholesterol (c-HDL) < 1.1 mmol/L (in men) and < 0.9 mmol/L (in women), blood pressure ≥ 130 /85 mmHg and fasting glucose (≥ 6.1 mmol/L) (National Cholesterol Education Program, 2002).

2.6 HOMA-IR determination

Insulin resistance (IR) was estimated using the Homeostasis Model of Assessment equation: HOMA-IR = [fasting insulin (mU/L) × fasting glucose (mmol/L)]/22.5. IR was defined as the upper quartile of HOMA-IR. Values above 2.5 were taken as abnormal and reflect insulin resistance (Ozdemir et al., 2007). Bipolar patients with diabetes (n = 21) were excluded in the HOMA-IR analysis.

2.7 Statistical analysis

Statistical analyses were performed using SPSS 17.0 (SPSS, Chicago, IL, USA). Quantitative variables were presented as mean ± SD and comparisons were performed using the Student's t test. Qualitative variable comparisons were performed using the Chi-squared test (χ^2) and Fisher's exact test (when n < 5). Comparisons between patients and controls in biological parameters were performed using analysis of variance (ANOVA) after adjustment for potential confounder factors. Odd ratios (ORs) and their 95% confidence interval (CI) were calculated and adjusted for potential confounder factors by binary logistic regression. The statistical significance level was set at $p < 0.05$. All variables with a p value < 0.25 between the two studied groups (patients and controls) were considered as potential confounder factors for this analysis.

3. Results

Table 3 shows the comparisons of biological variables between bipolar I patients and controls.

Biological variables	**Patients (n = 130)**	**Controls (n = 175)**	**p**	**p***
Triglycerides (mmol/L)	1.95 ± 1.55	1.23 ± 0.81	**< 0.001**	**< 0.001**
Cholesterol (mmol/L)	4.42 ± 0.99	4.37 ± 1.26	0.707	0.856
c-LDL (mmol/L)	2.14 ± 1.10	2.37 ± 1.38	0.118	0.047
c-HDL (mmol/L)				
Men (85/102)	1.04 ± 0.37	0.98 ± 0.29	0.192	0.017
Women (45/73)	1.17 ± 0.36	1.21 ± 0.48	0.542	0.702
ApoA1 (g/L)	1.20 ± 0.23	1.40 ± 0.67	**< 0.001**	**0.028**
ApoB (g/L)	0.82 ± 0.28	0.83 ± 0.24	0.784	0.777
ApoB/Apo A1	0.71 ± 0.26	0.65 ± 0.25	0.086	0.314
Lp(a) (mg/L)	243 ± 223	87 ± 129	**< 0.001**	**< 0.001**
Homocysteine (µmol/L)	15.8 ± 8.9	11.5 ± 5.0	**< 0.001**	**< 0.001**
Vitamin B12 (ng/L)	356 ± 198	360 ± 190	0.837	0.819
Folate (µg/L)	3.3 ± 0.9	5.1 ± 2.8	**< 0.001**	**<0.001**
Uric acid (µmol/L)				
Men (85/102)	311 ± 99	250 ± 107	**0.001**	**0.005**
Women (45/73)	246 ± 97	197 ± 73	**0.012**	0.408

* Lipid profile parameters, folatemia, vitamin B12 and uric acid were adjusted for gender, BMI, cigarette smoking, alcoholic beverages, diabetes and hypertension

*Hcys was adjusted for gender, BMI, cigarette smoking, alcoholic beverages, diabetes, hypertension, folatemia and vitamin B12

Table 3. Comparisons of biological variables between bipolar I patients and controls.

Compared with controls, patients had significantly higher triglycerides (1.95 ± 1.55 *Vs* 1.23 ± 0.81 mmol/L; p < 0.001), Lp(a) (243 ± 223 *Vs* 87 ± 129 mg/L; p < 0.001), homocysteine levels (15.8 ± 8.9 *Vs* 11.5 ± 5.0 µmol/L; p < 0.001) and uric acid (311 ± 99 *Vs* 250 ± 107 µmol/L; p = 0.001 in men; 246 ± 97 *Vs* 197 ± 73 µmol/L; p = 0.012 in women), and significantly lower ApoA1 (1.20 ± 0.23 *Vs* 1.40 ± 0.67 g/L; p < 0.001) and folate (3.3 ± 0.9 *Vs* 5.1 ± 2.8 µg/L; p < 0.001) levels. After adjustment for potential confounder factors, these differences remained significant for all of these parameters except for uric acid which is remained significantly higher only for men (table 3).

Table 4 reports the association between bipolar I disorder and cigarette smoking, alcoholic beverages, obesity, diabetes, hypertension, lipid profile parameters, hyperhomocysteinemia, hypofolatemia, hypovitamin B12 and, hyperuricemia.

Parameters	Patients (n = 130)	Controls (n = 175)	OR	IC 95%	p	OR*	p*
Cigarette smoking	52.3%	39.4%	1.68	1.06-2.66	**0.025**	-	-
Alcoholic beverages	13.1%	6.9%	2.04	0.94-4.44	0.067	-	-
Obesity (BMI ≥ 30 kg/m^2)	33.1%	8%	5.68	2.94-10.96	**< 0.001**	8.69	**< 0.001**
Diabetes ≥ *6.1 mmol/L*	16.1%	9.7%	1.79	0.90-3.55	0.092	1.60	0.325
Hypertension (≥ 130/85 mm Hg)	5.4%	16%	0.34	0.15-0.78	0.008	0.43	0.136
Hypercholesterolemia (≥ 5.17 mmol/L*)*	26.2%	26.9%	0.96	0.57-1.61	0.891	0.99	0.987
Hypertriglyceridemia (≥ 1.7 mmol/L*)*	53.1%	17.7%	4.10	2.44-6.90	**< 0.001**	3.71	**< 0.001**
HyperLDL (≥ 3.4 mmol/L)	13.1%	26.9%	0.39	0.22-0.73	0.002	0.48	< 0.001
¥*HypoHDL*	59.2%	58.3%	1.00	0.63-1.59	0.975	0.78	0.359
HyperLp(a) (≥ 200 mg/L)	47.7%	14.8%	5.25	3.04-9.07	**< 0.001**	4.48	**< 0.001**
Hyperhomocysteinemia (≥15 µmol/L)	39.2%	18%	2.80	1.66-4.72	**< 0.001**	1.95	**0.038**
Hypovitamin B12 (< 187 ng/L)	21.2%	14.9%	0.69	0.34-1.38	0.296	0.62	0.215
Hypofolatemia (< 3.7 µg/L)	66.2%	36.2%	3.44	2.13-5.54	**< 0.001**	3.69	**< 0.001**
£*Hyperuricemia*	10.8%	4.4%	2.05	0.71-5.91	0.176	1.58	0.439

* Lipid profile parameters, folatemia, vitamin B12 and uric acid were adjusted for gender, BMI, cigarette cigarette smoking, alcoholic beverages, diabetes and hypertension; * Hcys was adjusted for gender, BMI, cigarette smoking, alcoholic beverages, diabetes, hypertension, folatemia and vitamin B12; *Diabetes was adjusted for gender, BMI, cigarette smoking, alcoholic beverages, hypertension and dyslipidemia; *Obesity was adjusted for gender, cigarette smoking, alcoholic beverages, hypertension, diabetes and dyslipidemia; *Hypertension was adjusted for gender, cigarette smoking, alcoholic beverages, diabetes and dyslipidemia; \ c-HDL <1.1 mmol/L (in men) and < 0 .9 (in women); £ uric acid: 210-420 µmol/L (in men) and 150-360 µmol/L (in women)

Table 4. Association between bipolar I disorder and cigarette smoking, alcoholic beverages, obesity, diabetes, hypertension, lipid profile parameters, hyperhomocysteinemia, hypofolatemia, hypovitamin B12, and hyperuricemia.

We showed significant association between bipolar I disorder and some cardiovascular risk factors: obesity (33.1% *Vs* 8%, OR = 5.68, IC 95% = 2.94-10.96; p < 0.001), hyperLp(a) (47.7% *Vs* 14.8%, OR = 5.25, IC 95% = 3.04-9.07; p < 0.001), hypertriglyceridemia (53.1% *Vs* 17.7%, OR = 4.10, IC 95% = 2.44-6.90; p < 0.001), hypofolatemia (66.2% *Vs* 36.2%, OR = 3.44, IC 95% = 2.13-5.54; p < 0.001), hyperhomocysteinemia (39.2% *Vs* 18%, OR = 2.80, IC 95% = 1.66-4.72; p < 0.001) and cigarette smoking (52.3% *Vs* 39.4%, OR = 1.68, IC 95% = 1.06-2.66; p = 0,025). After adjustment for potential confounder factors, these associations remained significant (table 4).

Alcoholic beverage, diabetes and hyperuricemia were not significantly associated with this illness but we showed that they were more frequents in patients than controls (13.1% *Vs* 6.9%, p = 0.067; 16.1% *Vs* 9.7%, p = 0.325; 10.8% *Vs* 4.4%, p = 0.439; respectively). Additionally, the risk of diabetes and hyperuricemia were respectively multiplied by 1.5 in patients (16.1% *Vs* 9.7%, OR = 1.60, IC 95% = 0.62-4.12; p = 0.325; 10.8% *Vs* 4.4%, OR = 1.58, IC 95% = 0.49-5.08; p = 0.439) and the risk of alcoholic beverage by two (13.1% *Vs* 6.9%, OR = 2.04, IC 95% = 0.94-4.44; p = 0.067) (table 4).

On the contrary, this disease was not associated with hypertension (5.4% *Vs* 16%, OR = 0.43, IC 95% = 0.14-1.29; p = 0.136) nor with hyperLDL (13.1% *Vs* 26.9%, OR = 0.48, IC 95% = 2.53-7.95; p < 0.001) (table 4).

Fig.1. illustrates the receiver Operating Characteristic (ROC) of three index of atherogenicity as predictive factors of cardiovascular risk.

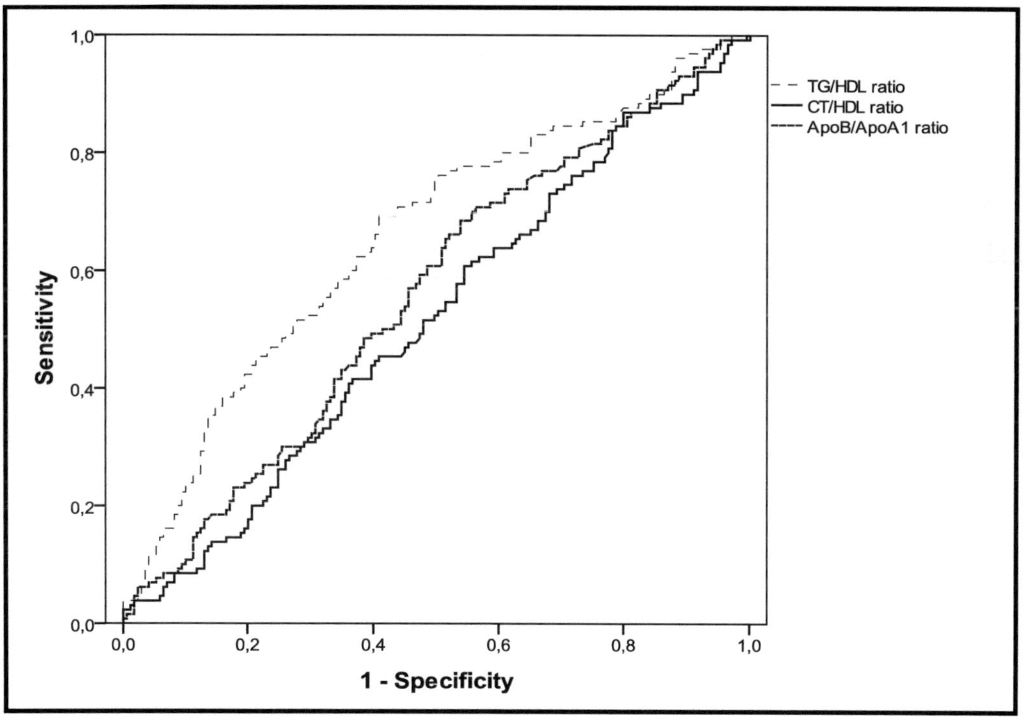

TG: triglycerides; CT: cholesterol

Fig. 1. Receiver Operating Characteristic (ROC) of three index of atherogenicity as predictive factors of cardiovascular risk.

The specificity and sensibility of three index of atherogenicity as predictive factors of cardiovascular risk are shown in table 5.

Parameters	AUC (95% CI)	Cut off	Specificity	Sensibility	p
TG/HDL	0.65 [0.59-0.71]	1.12	0.63	0.62	**$< 10^{-3}$**
CT/HDL	0.52 [0.44-0.57]	3.93	0.53	0.57	0.661
ApoB/ApoA1	0.56 [0.49-0.62]	0.66	0.54	0.55	0.070

TG: triglycerides; CT: cholesterol; AUC; Area under the curve

Table 5. Specificity and sensibility of three index of atherogenicity as predictive factors of cardiovascular risk

Fig. 2. Illustrates the Receiver Operating Characteristic (ROC) of Lp(a) and homocysteine as predictive factors of cardiovascular risk.

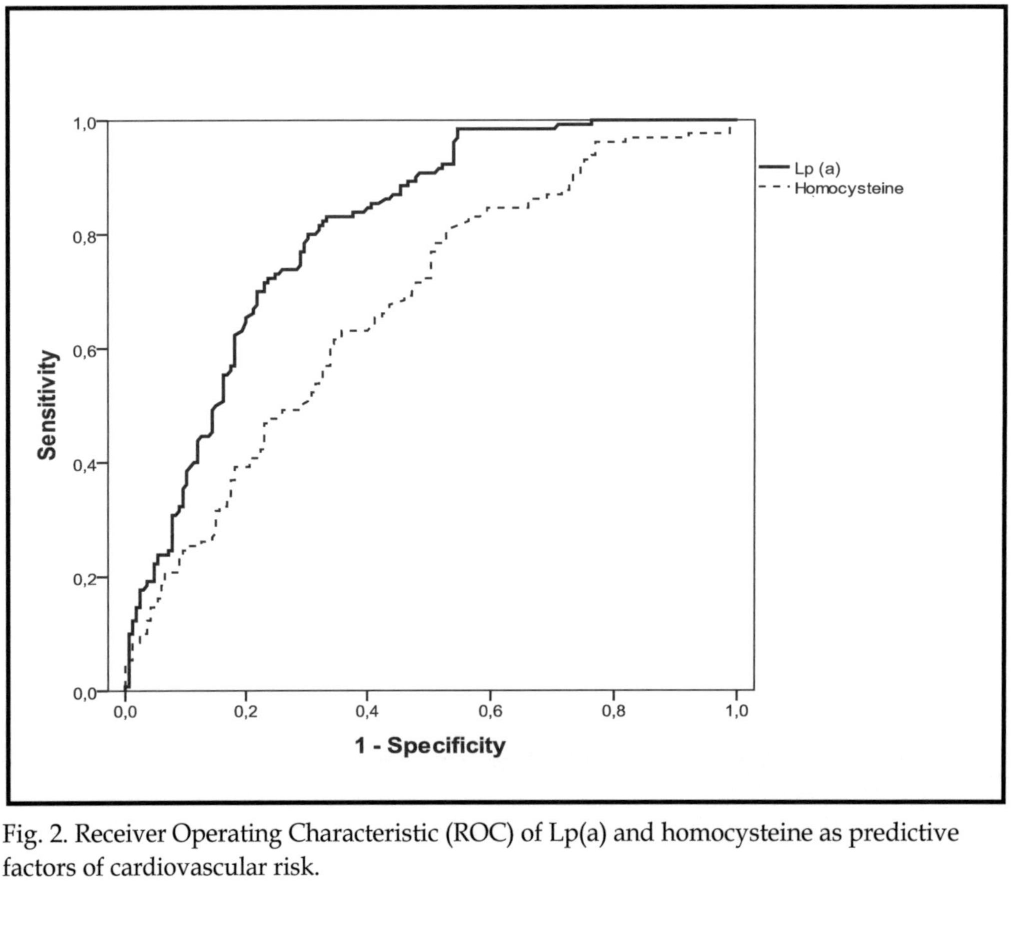

Fig. 2. Receiver Operating Characteristic (ROC) of Lp(a) and homocysteine as predictive factors of cardiovascular risk.

Table 6 reports the specificity and sensibility of Lp(a) and homocysteine as predictive factors of cardiovascular risk.

Parameters	AUC (95% CI)	Cut off	Specificity	Sensibility	p
Lp(a) (mg/L)	0.80 [0.75-0.85]	168	0.75	0.74	$< 10^{-3}$
Homocysteine (µmol/L)	0.52 [0.44-0.57]	13.4	0.60	0.62	$< 10^{-3}$

AUC; Area under the curve

Table 6. Specificity and sensibility of Lp(a) and homocysteine as predictive factors of cardiovascular risk.

TG/HDL ratio and Lp(a) were found as the best predictive factors of cardiovascular risk in terms of sensibility (0.62, 0.74; respectively) and specificity (0.63, 0.75; respectively) at threshold of 1.12 and 168 mg/L, respectively (tables 5, 6; fig 1, 2).
The prevalence of metabolic syndrome (modified NCEP-ATP III) and its profile in bipolar I patients are shown in table 7.

	N	%
Total of the association of 5 criteria	**2**	**5.9**
Diabetes, Obesity, Hypertriglyceridemia, Low c-HDL	1	
Diabetes, Obesity, Low c-HDL, High blood pressure	1	
Diabetes, Hypertriglyceridemia, Low c-HDL, High blood pressure	1	
Total of the association of 4 criteria	**3**	**8.8**
Obesity, Hypertriglyceridemia, Low c-HDL	15	
Diabetes, Low c-HDL, Hypertriglyceridemia	6	
Obesity, Hypertriglyceridemia, Diabetes	4	
Obesity, Hypertriglyceridemia, High blood pressure	2	
Diabetes , High blood pressure, Obesity	1	
Hypertriglyceridemia, Low c-HDL, High blood pressure	1	
Total of the association of 3 criteria	**29**	**85.3**
At least three or more criteria	**34**	**100**

Table 7. Prevalence of metabolic syndrome (modified NCEP-ATP III) and its profile in bipolar I patients.

The prevalence of metabolic syndrome in bipolar I patients was 26.1% (N = 34). The highest prevalence of this syndrome was obtained by the association between obesity, low c-HDL and hypertrilyceridemia (44.1 %) (Table 7).
Table 8 reports the Prevalence of the components of metabolic syndrome in the total sample of bipolar I patients.

Criteria	N (%)
c-HDL < 1.1 mmol/L (men) and < 0 .9 (women)	**77(59.2)**
TG ≥ 1.7 mmol/L	**69(53.1)**
BMI ≥ 28.5 kg/m²	**44 (33.8)**
Fasting blood glucose ≥ 6.1 mmol/L	**21 (16.1)**
Blood pressure ≥ 130/85 mm Hg	**7(5.4)**

Table 8. Prevalence of the components of metabolic syndrome in the total sample (N=130).

The prevalence of individual diagnostic components, in the total sample, was as follows: 59.2% for low c-HDL, 53.1% for hypertriglyceridemia, 33.8% for obesity (BMI ≥ 28.5 kg/m²), 16.1% for high fasting glucose and 5.4% for hypertension (Table 8).
Table 9 reports the characteristics of patients with or without metabolic syndrome.

	With MS [N= 34 (26.1%)]	**Without MS [N= 96 (73.9%)]**	**p values**
Variables	**N (%)**	**N (%)**	
Gender			
Men	21 (24.7)	64 (75.3)	0.60
Women	13 (28.9)	32 (71.1)	
Illness episode			
Depressive	4 (19)	17 (81)	0.651[a]
Euthymic	19 (26)	54 (74)	
Manic	11 (30.5)	25 (69.5)	
Treatment			
Antipsychotics	10 (26.3)	28 (73.7)	0.9574[a]
Mood stabilizers	24 (26.1)	68 (74.9)	
Lithium	4 (33.3)	8 (66.7)	
Valproic acid	17 (26.6)	47 (73.4)	
Carbamazepine	2 (20)	8 (80)	
Lithium and valproic acid	1 (16.7)	5 (83.3)	
	Mean ± SD	**Mean ± SD**	p
***Age** (years)*	40.4 ± 8.8	37.0 ± 12.7	0.11
HOMA-IR	6.0 ± 4.3*	2.4 ± 1.7**	**< 0.001**
***Uric acid** (μmol/L)*	335 ±117	272 ± 92	**< 0.001**

* n = 23 (11 diabetic patients were excluded);
** n = 86 (10 diabetic patients were excluded
[a]Statistical analysis was detected using Fisher's exact test

Table 9. Characteristics of patients with or without metabolic syndrome.

We found that gender was not associated with metabolic syndrome, 24.7% in men and 28.9% in women. As to age, we found that patients with metabolic syndrome were older than metabolic syndrome free patients (40.4 ± 8.8 years *Vs* 37.0 ± 12.7 years), but this difference was not significant (table 9).
Our present data showed that there is no difference in metabolic syndrome prevalence between patients receiving antipsychotic and mood stabilizers treatment. However, we noted that patients treated with lithium had the highest prevalence of metabolic syndrome (table 9).
Our study failed to show any significant association between metabolic syndrome and illness episode, whereas, manic patients had the highest prevalence of this disorder (30.5%) (table 9).
Patients with metabolic syndrome had significantly higher levels of uric acid ($p < 0.001$) than metabolic syndrome free patients (table 9).
Concerning HOMA-IR analysis, after diabetic patients exclusion (n = 21), we noted that patients with metabolic syndrome had significantly higher levels of HOMA-IR ($p < 0.001$) than metabolic syndrome free patients (table 9).

The variations of lipid profile parameters according to the illness episode and therapeutic characteristics of bipolar I patients are shown in table 10.

	Triglycerides (mmol/L)	Cholesterol (mmol/L)	c-HDL (mmol/L)		c-LDL (mmol/L)	Lp (a) (mg/L)	ApoB/Apo A1
			Men	Women			
Patients (n = 130)	1.95 ± 1.55	4.42 ± 0.99	1.04 ± 0.37	1.17 ± 0.36	2.14 ± 1.10	243 ± 223	0.71 ± 0.23
Illness episode							
Depressive (n = 21)	1.95 ± 1.32	4.49 ± 0.96	1.12 ± 0.28	0.99 ± 0.36	2.14 ± 1.09	158 ± 91	0.82 ± 0.41
Euthymic (n = 73)	1.94 ± 1,80	4.53± 0.96	1.05 ± 0.41	1.26 ± 0.33	2.18 ± 1.04	268 ± 242	0.68 ± 0.19
Manic (n = 36)	1.97 ± 1.25	4.14 ± 1.0	0.98 ± 0.32	1.10 ± 0.11	2.08 ± 1.25	240 ± 228	0.70 ± 0.26
Treatment							
Valproic acid (n = 64)	1.78 ± 1.20	4.25 ±1.00	1.05 ± 0.40	1.13 ± 0.24	2.11 ± 1.12	240 ± 232	0.70 ± 0.24
Lithium (n = 12)	1.43 ± 0.95	4.40 ± 0.85	1.10 ± 0.36	0.86 ± 0.49	2.17 ± 0.82	170 ± 93	0.78 ± 0.29
Carbamazepine (n = 10)	2.24 ± 3.25	4.60 ± 1.10	0.97 ± 0.33	1.44 ± 0.40	1.75 ± 0.74	293 ± 221	0.66 ± 0.22
AVP and Li (n =6)	2.33 ± 1.07	3.93 ± 0.40	1.10 ± 0.28	0.79	2.10 ± 1.22	153 ± 69	0.76 ± 0.23
Anti-psychotics (n = 38)	2.26 ± 1.64	4.74 ± 1.00	1.03 ± 0.36	1.26 ± 0.40	2.30 ± 1.23	271 ± 248	0.71 ± 0.30

AVP: valproic acid; Li: lithium

Table 10. Variations of lipid profile parameters according to the illness episode and therapeutic characteristics of bipolar I patients.

Our study failed to show any significant association between lipid profile parameters, illness episode and treatment, while euthymic patients were found to have the highest levels of Lp(a) and depressive patients had the highest levels of ApoB/ApoA1 ratio (table 10). Additionally, we showed that women taking lithium had the lowest c-HDL values and patients taking carbamazepine had the highest values of Lp(a) (table 10).

Table 11 reports the variations of uric acid, homocysteine, folate and vitamin B12 concentrations according to the illness episode and therapeutic characteristics of bipolar I patients.

	Uric acid (µmol/L)		Homocysteine (µmol/L)	Folate (µg/L)	Vitamin B12 (ng/L)
	Men (n = 85)	Women (n = 45)			
Patients (n = 130)	311 ± 99	246 ± 97	15.8 ± 8.9	3.3 ± 0.9	356 ± 198
Illness episode					
Depressive (n = 21)	228 ± 79	205 ± 128	15.2 ± 6.7	3.4 ± 1.3	481 ± 299[a]
Euthymic (n = 73)	309 ± 110	271 ± 95	16.1 ± 10.1	3.4 ± 0.7	322 ± 165
Manic (n = 36)	327 ± 87	217 ± 57	15.5 ± 7.7	3.3 ± 1.2	352 ± 158
Treatment					
Valproic acid (n = 64)	328 ± 91	279 ± 109	16.3 ± 10.0	3.5 ± 0.9	361 ± 91
Lithium (n = 12)	331 ± 79	219 ± 88	17.1 ± 12.7	2.8 ± 0.6	399 ± 79
Carbamazepine (n = 10)	278 ± 160	207± 61	16.9 ± 9.4	3.2 ± 0.8	240 ± 160*
AVP and Li (n = 6)	343 ± 76	288	15.5 ± 2.9	3.0 ± 0.8	518 ± 236*
Antipsychotics (n = 38)	269 ± 96	218 ± 83	14.2 ± 5.9	3.4 ± 1.5	338 ± 233

AVP: valproic acid; Li: lithium; *Carb Vs AVP/Li, $p = 0.04$; [a]$F_{2\text{-}130} = 5.688$, $p = 0.004$

Table 11. Variations of uric acid, homocysteine, folate and vitamin B12 concentrations according to the illness episode and therapeutic characteristics of bipolar I patients.

We found a significant association between vitamin B12 values and illness episode ($F_{2\text{-}130} = 5.688$, $p = 0.004$). Manic patients had lower values of this parameter than depressive patients. Moreover, we showed that vitamin B12 was significantly associated with the therapeutic characteristics. Indeed, patients taking carbamazepine had significantly lower values of this parameter than those taking valproic acid and lithium ($p = 0.04$) (table 11).

In patients, there was no significant change in homocysteine, folate and uric acid values in relation to illness episodes and the treatment, whereas the lowest values of uric acid were seen in depressive patients (both in men and women) compared to manic patients and in men taking antipsychotics and women taking carbamazepine compared to the other groups (table 11).

The distribution of BMI according to the illness episode and therapeutic characteristics is shown in table 12.

Our study failed to show any significant association between the BMI and to the illness episode and, therapeutic characteristics. However, we found that obesity was more frequent in depressive patients than in those with manic episode (38.1% *Vs* 27.8%). In addition, obesity and overweight were more frequent (72% and 52%; respectively) in patients taking valproic acid or lithium (table 12).

BMI (kg/m²) **Characteristics**	**BMI ≥ 30** **n = 43 (%)**	**25 ≤ BMI < 30** **n = 40 (%)**	**BMI** **< 25** **n = 47 (%)**
Illness episode			
Depressive (n = 21)	8 (38.1)	4 (19.1)	9 (42.8)
Euthymic (n = 73)	25 (34.2)	23 (31.5)	25 (34.3)
Manic (n = 36)	10 (27.8)	13 (36.1)	13 (36.1)
Treatment			
Valproic acid (n = 64)	25 (39.1)	17 (26.6)	22 (34.3)
Lithium (n = 12)	6 (50)	4 (33.3)	2 (16.7)
Carbamazepine (n = 10)	2 (20)	5 (50)	3 (30)
AVP and Li (n = 6)	2 (33.3)	3 (50)	1 (16.7)
Antipsychotics (n = 38)	8 (21.1)	11 (28.9)	19 (50)

AVP: valproic acid; Li: lithium

Table 12. Distribution of BMI according to the illness episode and therapeutic characteristics.

4. Discussion

Our study showed that patients had significantly higher levels of triglycerides and Lp(a), and significantly lower levels of ApoA1 than control subjects. Furthermore, bipolar I disorder was showed to have significant association with hyperLp(a) (47.7% *Vs* 14.8%, OR = 4.48, IC 95% = 2.53-7.95; $p < 0.001$) and hypertriglyceridemia (53.1% Vs 17.7%, OR = 3.71, IC 95% = 2.13-6.46; $p < 0.001$).

In patients, the TG/HDL ratio and Lp(a) were found as the best predictive factors of cardiovascular risk in terms of sensibility (0.62, 0.74; respectively) and specificity (0.63, 0.74; respectively) at threshold of 1.12 and 168 mg/L, respectively. These results reflect a high risk of cardiovascular disease and may explain the high rates of morbidity and mortality in this population. Several studies have found mortality rates between 1.5 and 2.5 times higher in bipolar patients than the general population. After suicide and accidents, cardiovascular and all vascular diseases are the leading causes of death in these patients, with standardized mortality ratios ranging from 1.47 to 2.6. (Garcia-Portilla et al., 2009; Sicras et al., 2008).

The exact mechanisms increasing the incidence of cardiovascular risk in bipolar patients remain to be clarified, but they possibly include industrialisation, stress, lack of exercise, dietary lipids (that is, omega-3 fatty acid deficiency), increasing incidence of smoking and alcohol consumption and other factors (Ezzaher et al., 2010). These hypotheses will be, in part, justified later in this study.

Several investigators have been hypothesized that abnormalities in fatty acid composition may play a role in psychiatric disorders (Horrobin & Bennett, 1999). Maes et al. (1996, 1999) reported that patients with major depression had a significantly elevated ratio of ecosapentaenoic acid (EPA; 20: 5n-3)/docosahexaenoic acid (DHA; 22: 6n-3), lower level of EPA and total n-3 Omega-3 polyunsaturated fatty acids, in both serum cholesteryl esters and phospholipids when compared to patients with minor depression and normal controls. Similar findings were revealed in terms of fatty acid compositions of the erythrocyte membrane (Adams et al., 1996; Edwards et al., 1998; Peet et al., 1998; Chiu et al., 2003).

Moreover, many prospective and case-control studies have shown a positive association between serum triglycerides and coronary artery disease risk and demonstrated the importance of fasting triglycerides level as an independent risk factor. A number of clinical trials including the Framingham Heart Study have concluded that a low HDL cholesterol level predicts the risk for coronary artery disease independently of other risk factors. Each 1 mg/dL decrease in HDL cholesterol has been shown to increase risk for coronary artery disease by 2% in men and 3% in women. The Veterans Affairs High-Density Lipoprotein Cholesterol Interventional Trial, investigating the impact of fibrate therapy on cardiovascular risk, demonstrated that 6% increase in HDL cholesterol was associated with a 22% decrease in coronary events (Kabakci et al., 2008). In addition, Lp(a) has been shown to be an independent risk factor for atherosclerosis (Hakim et al., 2008) and has been found to exert a broad variety of pro-atherogenic and pro-thrombotic properties (von Eckardstein et al., 2001). Elevated plasma Lp(a) has been shown also to be associated with premature cardiovascular disease, premature cerebrovascular disease and premature peripheral vascular disease (Valentine et al., 1996).

The underlying mechanism for the altered lipid status in bipolar patients is unclear. A possible explanation might be found in the patient's nutritional status, the decrease in physical activity and the medications used (Ezzaher et al., 2010). Additionally, Chung et al. (2007) reported that bipolar disorder is associated with perturbations in lipid profile which play an important role in the pathophysiology of mood disorders, particularly in bipolar disorders. Indeed, cholesterol is one component of circulating lipoprotein particles that, besides handling cholesterol, carries micronutrients such as vitamins A and E as well as triglycerides and phospholipids. The latter compounds give rise to substrates such as fatty acids and choline, which are used in both the structural lipids of neuronal membranes and intercellular communication. Therefore, higher levels of one or more compounds of lipoprotein particles circulating in the bloodstream may produce subtle but measurable enhancements of mental processes by influencing the supply of fat-soluble micronutrients, specific fatty acids, or structural lipids (Ezzaher et al., 2010).

Our study failed to found any significant association between lipid profile parameters and illness episode, while euthymic patients were found to have the highest levels of Lp(a). Additionally, depressive patients had the highest levels of ApoB/Apo A1 ratio. However, some authors (Sagud et al., 2009) showed that serum cholesterol and LDL values were significantly lower in manic patients and others (Chung et al., 2007) showed that there was no difference in mean serum level of cholesterol or triglycerides among patients with manic, mixed, or depressive episode. These differences could be due to ethnicity and eating habits.

About therapeutic characteristics, any significant association was shown between lipid profile parameters and treatment, while, women taking lithium had the lowest c-HDL values and patients taking carbamazepine had the highest values of Lp(a). The mechanism(s) by which these drugs exert weight gain are not well known, but are presumed to involve increased energy intake (e.g., overeating), decreased energy expenditure (e.g., reduced resting metabolic rate, reduced physical activity, or reduced diet-induced thermogenesis), or a combination of the two (Malhotra & McElroy, 2002).

Additionally, we found that the prevalence of metabolic syndrome was 26.1% among patients, 24.7% in men and 28.8% in women. These prevalences were definitely higher than those reported in the Tunisian general population (13% in men and 18% in women) using a previous criteria (Bouguerra et al., 2006).

Compared with other studies, the prevalence of metabolic syndrome in our patients is included between those in Spanish patients (22.4%), Italian patients (25.3%) and US patients (30%) (Garcia-Portilla et al., 2008; Salvi et al., 2008; Fagiolini et al., 2005). The increasing prevalence of metabolic syndrome is important because it confers greater cardiovascular morbidity and mortality. Prospective observational studies have demonstrated an association between metabolic syndrome and development of type II diabetes (Hanson et al., 2002; Resnick et al., 2003; Klein et al., 2002; Sattar et al., 2003), cardiovascular disease (Lakka et al., 2002; Kip et al., 2004), and stroke (Kurl et al.,2006).

Our study showed that the highest prevalence of metabolic syndrome was obtained by the association between obesity, low c-HDL and hypertriglyceridemia. Moreover, the most individual components of this syndrome, in the total sample of patients, was low c-HDL (59.2%), hypertriglyceridemia (53.1%) and obesity (BMI $\geq$ 28.5 kg/m^2) (33.8%), confirming in part the higher risk of dyslipidemia and obesity in bipolar I patients and in other hand the higher risk of cardiovascular disease in this population.

We found no significant difference in the prevalence of metabolic syndrome among gender and age. This is in line with results reported by Yumru et al., (2007).

We noted that there was no significant change in the prevalence of metabolic syndrome in relation to illness episode; however, manic patients had the highest prevalence. This may explain the high risk of cardiovascular disease in manic patients compared with depressive one (Murray et al., 2009). Additionally, Angst et al. (2002) showed that individuals with bipolar I disorder are at greater risk for cardiovascular mortality than individuals with bipolar II disorder. However, the difference in cardiovascular mortality between the two bipolar subtypes reflects the manic symptom burden, which predicts cardiovascular mortality independently of diagnosis and cardiovascular risk factors at intake. The results suggest that mania, either directly (through factors intrinsic to illness) or indirectly (through other mediators or associated variables), may itself influence cardiovascular disease.

Our study failed to show any significant association between metabolic syndrome and treatment. However, we noted that patients treated with lithium had the highest prevalence of metabolic syndrome. The increased risk to develop metabolic syndrome during treatment with lithium is in part related to its propensity to induce weight gain. According to Casey, lithium has been shown to stimulate appetite and increase calorie intake through different mechanisms.

HOMA-IR is significantly higher in patients with metabolic syndrome than others. This increase in HOMA-IR values reflects an insulin resistance and is associated with two to three fold increases in cardiovascular disease independent of classical risk factors (Toalson et al., 2004). In addition, uric acid levels were significantly higher in patients with metabolic syndrome. According to Vuorinen-Markkola et al. (1994), hyperuricemia forms another consistent feature of the metabolic syndrome what led to the suggestion of uric acid being a new component of the syndrome.

In addition, Chien et al., (2008) reported that metabolic syndrome induces high oxidative stress and the accompanying hyperuricemia worsens this stress. Furthermore, uric acid stimulates vascular smooth muscle proliferation, induces endothelial dysfunction, decreases endothelial nitric oxid production, and consequently, makes peripheral tissue resistant to insulin effects and results in endothelial dysfunction (Chien et al., 2008). High levels of uric acid are associated with increased renal glomerular pressure and sodium reabsorption, enhanced by high insulin concentrations (Alkerwi et al., 2009). In addition, hyperuricemia was associated with insulin resistance markers, including triglycerides, microalbuminuria and impaired glucose tolerance. These disturbances contribute to increase cardiovascular risk (Chien et al., 2008). This insulin- resistance causes steatosis, which is associated with hyper secretion of hepatic enzymes (Fromenty et al., 2004).

In men, uric acid was significantly higher in patients than controls. Additionally, the risk of hyperuricemia in bipolar I patients was approximately multiplied by 1.5 (10.8% *Vs* 4.4%, OR = 1.58, IC 95% = 0.49-5.08; p = 0.439). Many, but not all, epidemiological studies have suggested that high plasma uric acid is a risk factor for cardiovascular diseases. This raised level of plasma uric acid, parallel to an increased risk of cardiovascular diseases, could be either primary or secondary to the underlying causes of the cardiovascular diseases. However, the specific role of plasma uric acid in this constellation remains uncertain, although it may be involved in the platelet adhesiveness, aggregation, or inflammation and it may be implicated in the genesis of hypertension. In contrast, there is some evidence that the increase of plasma uric acid is protective against the cardiovascular diseases, since uric acid acts as an endogenous antioxidant, and the higher plasma uric acid levels found in cardiovascular diseases patients suggest that any protective antioxidant effect of uric acid is hidden by other negative effects in these pathogeneses (Haj mouhamed et al., 2010).

Additionally, Torres et al. (2007), reported that hyperuricemia which implicated in the oxidative stress plays an important role in the pathophysiology of bipolar disorders. The idea that the purinergic system might be involved in bipolar disorder dates back to Kraepelin, who was the first to describe an association between manic symptoms, uric acid excretion, hyperuricemia, and gout. In fact, the purinergic system modulates sleep, motor activity, cognition, attention, behavior, and mood. Even in the absence of a psychiatric diagnosis, individuals with higher uric acid levels are more likely to show higher drive, disinhibition, hyperthymia, or irritable temperament (Lorenzi et al., 2010). Similarly, diseases characterized by purinergic turnover dysfunction and uric acid overproduction (e.g., Lesch-Nyhan syndrome) are associated with impulsive/aggressive behavior, disinhibition, and increased sexual drive (Salvadore et al., 2010).

Among clinical and therapeutic characteristics, we found that there was no significant change in uric acid values in relation to illness episodes and the treatment. This finding is not in agreement with the previous studies that reported that plasma uric acid levels were higher only during the manic phase of bipolar disorder but not during the depressive or euthymic phases (De Berardis et al., 2008). Additionally, lithium was found to low uric acid plasma levels and to have uricosuric effects in mania. Carbamazepine and phenytoin similarly decreased uric acid levels; in contrast, valproate appeared to have the opposite effect. However, it is important to note that the effect of these drugs on uric acid levels in relationship to clinical improvement in patients with bipolar disorder has not been systematically evaluated (Salvadore et al., 2010).

Compared with controls, patients had significantly higher levels of homocysteine and significantly lower levels of folatemia. Additionally, significant associations were showed between bipolar I disorder and hyperhomocysteinemia (39.2% *Vs* 18%, OR = 1.95, IC 95% = 1.04-3.69; $p = 0.038$) and hypofolatemia (66.2% *Vs* 36.2%, OR = 3.69, IC 95% = 2.20-6.19; $p < 0.001$). Homocysteine is an intermediary metabolite of the essential amino acid methionine. Folate and vitamin B12 are required for remethylation of homocysteine to methionine (Hankey & Eikelboom, 1999).

According to Reynolds (2006), hyperhomocysteinaemia has long been identified as a risk factor for vascular disease and the lowering of homocysteine concentrations by the treatment with folic acid, or possibly vitamin B12 and vitamin B6 which might reduce the risk of both cardiovascular and cerebrovascular diseases. Moreover, the association between increased circulating homocysteine concentrations and premature vascular thrombotic events in individuals with hereditary homocystinuria is well established. This process may include platelet activation, smooth muscle cell proliferation, and enhanced leukocyte binding to the endothelium. In recent years, a relationship between milder degrees of hyperhomocysteinaemia and vascular disease has emerged, and this has been the subject of intense research. Hyperhomocysteinemia can be caused by a wide range of disorders, the most important of which are genetic defects of the enzymes involved in homocysteine metabolism and/or deficiencies of their co-factors: folate (former vitamin B9), vitamin B12 and vitamin B6 (Haj mouhamed et al., 2011).

Our study showed a significant association between bipolar I disorder and hyperhomocysteinemia. The exact mechanisms underlying the hyperhomocysteinemia in this disease are not completely understood and controversed among studies. Several hypotheses have been postulated including nutritional folate and vitamin B deficiency, and/or reduced glomerular filtration rate in bipolar patients (Vuksan-Ćusa et al., 2011). En effect, we found a significant association between this disease and hypofolatemia. Furthermore, some authors (Atmaca et al., 2005) showed that at a high concentration, homocysteine is considered to be a neurotoxic substance, causing activation of NMDA (N-methyl D-aspartate) receptors and leading to excitotoxicity. By impairing the neural plasticity and promoting neuronal degeneration, homocysteine could contribute to the pathogenesis of neurodegenerative and psychiatric disorders (Ipcioglu et al., 2008). Additionally, homocysteine is a methyl donor when activated to S-adenosylmethionine. So aberrant DNA methylation due to hyperhomocysteinemia also may be involved in the pathogenesis of bipolar disorder as well as schizophrenia (Mill et al., 2008).

In the other hand, folate appears to influence the synthesis rate of tetrahydrobiopterin, a cofactor in the hydroxylation of phenylalanine and tryptophan, rate-limiting steps in the biosynthesis of dopamine, norepinephrine, and serotonin, neurotransmitters postulated to play a role in the monoamine hypothesis of affective disorders. In addition, methyl tetrahydrofolate has been shown to bind to presynaptic glutamate receptors, where it may

potentially modulate the release of other neurotransmitters, including the monoamines (Atmaca et al., 2005).
Moreover, some studies showed that lower folatemia in patients with psychiatric disorders can be due to their nutritional status (Reif et al., 2005). Indeed, poor appetite as a symptom of bipolar disorder could lead to decreased intake of B vitamins which could then lead to elevated homocysteine concentrations (Tolmunen et al., 2004).
We found a significant association between vitamin B12 values and illness episode. Manic patients had lower values of this parameter than depressive patients. This can be explained by the eating habits of bipolar patients. Indeed, Parikh et al. (2000) found that manic episode is often associated with weight loss.
About therapeutic characteristics, we showed that only vitamin B12 was significantly associated with the medication use. Indeed, patients taking carbamazepine had significantly lower values of this parameter than those taking valproic acid and lithium. These findings are not in agreement with others studies. In fact, Derkes and Westphal (2005) showed that carbamazepine can cause elevated homocysteine concentrations. Although, according to Ozbek et al (2008), homocysteine, folate and vitamin B12 were not related to drug usage. Additionally, Osher et al (2008) reported that there were no significant differences in homocysteine levels between patients receiving versus not receiving lithium, neuroleptic or valproate. However, Sener et al. (2006) suggested that carbamazepine, as enzyme inducer, can directly modulate the activity of different liver enzymes. Liver enzyme induction may cause depletion of the cofactor involved, folic acid, pyridoxal 5′-phosphate and vitamin B12, leading to the alterations in homocysteine status.
Our study showed that bipolar I patients are so much more likely to be smokers than controls (52.3% *Vs* 39.4%, OR = 1.68, IC 95% = 1.06-2.66; $p = 0.025$). An association between smoking and bipolar I disorder has been established and prevalence rates for lifetime and current smoking have been shown to be as high as 82.5% and 68.8% respectively (Lasser et al., 2000). The possible explanations for the high rates of smoking include an increased genetic vulnerability, a greater susceptibility to addiction because of a greater subjective experience of reward or pleasure, or that tobacco helps relieve some of the symptoms related to a behavioural disorder. For example, cigarette smoking may be an attempt to self-medicate symptoms of depression, anxiety, boredom or loneliness. Other possible explanations for continuing to smoke include increased withdrawal symptoms and reduced side effects from psychiatric medication (Williams & Ziedonis, 2004). Additionally, it has been reported that nicotine stimulates the brain to release dopamine, which is associated with pleasurable feelings, and smokers quickly develop regular smoking patterns. Eventually, smokers need increasing levels of nicotine to feel 'normal'. In the other hand, cigarette smoking is known to contribute to many diseases, including cancer, chronic obstructive pulmonary disease, stroke, cardiovascular diseases, and peptic ulcers. Investigators have attempted to elucidate the mechanisms of the pathogenesis associated with cigarette smoking, but the conclusions were not consistent. A basic hypothesis is that free radicals cause oxidative damage to macromolecules such as lipids, proteins, and DNA. Therefore, these radicals play an important role in the pathogenesis of these diseases (Haj mouhamed et al., 2010).
In this study, the prevalence of obesity is higher in patients with bipolar I disorder than in controls. Moreover, the risk of obesity in these patients is approximately multiplied by nine (33.1% *Vs* 8%, OR = 8.69, IC 95% = 3.61-20.87; $p < 0.001$).

In bipolar I patients, the prevalences of obesity and overweight were respectively 33.1 % and 30.7 %. These findings were similar to those reported by Elmslie et al (2000) and Fagiolini et al (2002) (36 % and 32 %). However, higher values were reported by McElroy et al (2004) (44 % and 20 %).

For this population, we found that the prevalence of obesity greatly exceeded that found in controls (12.3%) and in the general population (20%) (Haddad et al., 2006). Obesity in patients with bipolar I disorder thus constitutes a major public health problem and suggests that the development and testing of specific interventions that target the obesity epidemic in this particular population are urgently needed. Bipolar disorder and obesity both have tremendous impact on the physical and mental well-being of affected individuals. Therefore, both illnesses should be treated with a coordinated intensive and multifaceted treatment (Fagiolini et al., 2003).

Moreover, the risk of obesity in these patients is approximately multiplied by nine (33.1% *Vs* 8%, OR = 8.69, IC 95% = 3.61-20.87; $p < 0.001$). This could be one of the missing factors in understanding the relationship between psychiatric disorders and increased cardiovascular risk. In fact, some studies have reported that psychiatric disorders, particularly bipolar disorder, are significantly associated with adverse cardiovascular events and coronary heart disease (Garcia-Portilla et al., 2009). The mechanisms through which obesity leads to coronary heart disease remain hotly debated, but the accumulation, particularly, of visceral fat is widely favoured as the primary mechanism, leading, through the release of fatty acids and other mediators, to insulin resistance, dyslipidaemia, and a pro-inflammatory state. However, obesity in general, and central obesity in particular (ie. excessive visceral intra-abdominal fat) have been under-recognised as risk factors for coronary heart disease in the population, where most attention has been placed on smoking and cholesterol (Pinkney, 2001).

According to Raji et al (2009), the cardiovascular afflictions including obesity, diabetes, hypertension and stroke increase the risk for cognitive decline and dementia, but it is unknown whether these factors, specifically obesity and type 2 diabetes mellitus, are associated with specific patterns of brain atrophy. Obesity and type 2 diabetes mellitus may amplify the risk for dementia by worsening cerebral atrophy even in cognitively intact individuals, raising their vulnerability to future Alzheimer's disease neuropathology.

The same authors, mostly in subjects younger than 65 years, suggest also that increased body tissue fat content (adiposity) is correlated with atrophy in the temporal cortex, frontal lobes, putamen, caudate, precuneus, thalamus, and white matter. It is unknown, but of great interest, whether high tissue fat content, as measured by BMI, is associated with differences in brain structure in cognitively normal elderly (Raji et al., 2009).

Additionally, some studies showed that obesity has psychosocial consequences, including discrimination and stigmatization, which may contribute to the severity of bipolar disorder by negatively impacting patients' general physical health and functioning, quality of life, self-esteem, and psychological well-being. Obese patients have an increased risk of sleep apnea, which causes sleep disruptions and may lead to mood destabilization in patients with bipolar disorder. Obesity may also impact effectiveness of pharmacotherapies by altering the distribution and elimination of medications. Truncal obesity, which is most common, increases the risk of type 2 diabetes mellitus, dyslipidemia, hypertension, stroke, ischemic heart disease, and early death (Cheymol, 2000; Fagiolini et al., 2003; Plante & Winkelman, 2008).

In addition, obesity was more frequent in depressive patients than in those with manic episode (38.1% *Vs* 27.8%). Previous studies reported that patients who had depressive symptomatology were more likely to have excessive caloric and cholesterol intake, to smoke and to be inactive than non-depressed subjects. Another explanation might involve biological mechanisms: it is ascertained that hypothalamic–pituitary- adrenal (HPA) axis dysregulation and high cortisol blood levels lead to increased visceral fat. HPA axis dysregulation has been a common finding in both unipolar and bipolar disorders; recently, some studies reported that increased cortisol blood levels correlated to the amount of intra-abdominal fat in major depression (Maina et al., 2008).

About therapeutic characteristics, we found that obesity and overweight were more frequent (72% and 52%; respectively) in patients taking valproic acid or lithium. These findings are in line with those reported by De Hert et al. (2011). Moreover, Casey et al. (2005) reported that lithium have been shown to stimulate appetite through different mechanisms. The "carbohydrate craving" that is thought to be one of the mechanisms of increased calorie intake in people taking lithium is well known. In addition, it is believed that valproate also stimulates weight gain through a variety of mechanisms, especially the development of insulin resistance and diabetes mellitus type 2. In this line, our study found that this type of diabetes is frequent in patients (16.2%). Additionally, the risk of diabetes is multiplied by 1.5 in patients (16.2% *Vs* 9.7%, OR = 1.60, IC 95% = 0.62-4.12; p = 0.325).

Previous studies suggested that patients with both bipolar disorder and comorbid diabetes have more lifetime psychiatric hospitalizations than patients with bipolar patients without diabetes. The association between these two disorders underscores the importance of screening for diabetes in patients with bipolar illness, particularly because early detection and initiation of treatment to control glycemia may prevent diabetes-related complications. Moreover, other studies have demonstrated cerebrovascular lesions involving small intraparenchymal cerebral vessels and focal infarctions in patients with diabetes. These lesions predominantly occur in areas providing blood supply to the base of the pons, thalamus, and basal ganglia. Diabetes has been implicated as a risk factor for subcortical white-matter lesions observed on magnetic resonance imaging (MRI) scans; similar MRI findings have been noted in patients with bipolar disorder. Cerebral microvascular disease may lead to greater frequency of manic episodes, another reason to minimize diabetes-related complications in patients with comorbid bipolar disorder (Cassidy et al., 1999; Holman et al., 2008).

Alcoholic beverage was not significantly associated with this illness but we showed that it was more frequent in patients than controls (13.1% *Vs* 6.9%, OR = 2.04, IC 95% = 0.94-4.44; p = 0.067). It has been well documented that bipolar disorder and alcoholism commonly co-occur. In fact, the lifetime prevalence of alcohol abuse and drug abuse in people with bipolar disorder are known to be three to nine times more frequent that of the general population (Merikangas et al., 2007; Regier et al., 1990; ten Have et al., 2002).

Additionally, some studies showed that the feelings of depression and anxiety associated with bipolar can be a factor that leads to alcoholism. People with bipolar disorder may use alcohol or other drugs to self medicate these feelings, especially in instances where the person has not been diagnosed. However, alcohol makes the symptoms of bipolar disorder worse. Anyone who shows symptoms of bipolar disorder should seek the advice of medical professionals (Le Strat, 2010).

Some studies have shown that alcohol directly contributes to heart disease and stroke. Heavy drinking raises levels of triglycerides circulating in the bloodstream leading to diabetes and blocked or narrowed arteries that carry blood to the heart. If coronary arteries are clogged with fats, blood cannot flow freely, resulting in heart disease or stroke. Additionally, alcohol directly contributes to heart failure by damaging the heart muscle and arteries. Cardiomyopathy, or an enlargement of the heart muscle, results from long-term alcohol use. An enlarged heart no longer works efficiently and fails to provide enough oxygenated blood to other organs of the body. Furthermore, alcohol is associated with cardiac arrhythmia (irregular heartbeat), sudden cardiac death, stroke and atrial fibrillation (Pearson, 1996).

In our patients, hypertension was not associated with bipolar disorder (5.4% *Vs* 16%, OR = 0.43, IC 95% = 0.14-1.29; p = 0.136). De Heart et al. (2010) explained the decrease of hypertension frequency in individuals with a mental illness by changes in lifestyle of patients such as reducing salt intake.

Several methodological limitations should be considered when interpreting these findings. First, larger sample sizes of groups would be beneficial. Second, our work is a cross-sectional study that does not permit to follow up biological parameters. Third the sample of bipolar patients may not be representative of more heterogeneous populations. Finally, the diagnosis of controls was made by psychiatrists but without formal use of structured instruments to exclude psychiatric disorders in controls.

5. Conclusion

Our results demonstrate that Tunisian bipolar I patients are exposed to higher cardiovascular risk. In fact, they had perturbations in lipid profile: significantly higher values of triglycerides and Lp(a), and significantly lower values of ApoA1, significantly hyperhomocysteinemia and hyperuricemia (in men), significantly hypofolatemia and high prevalence of metabolic syndrome. Obesity, hyperLp(a), hypertriglyceridemia, hypofolatemia, hyperhomocysteinemia and cigarette smoking were the main cardiovascular risk factors associated with bipolar I disorder. Indeed, the risk of obesity was increased approximately for nine once, hyperLp(a), hypertriglyceridemia and hypofolatemia approximately for four once and the other factors approximately for tow once. The TG/HDL ratio and Lp(a) were found as the best predictive factors of cardiovascular risk in terms of sensibility and specificity at threshold of 1.12 and 168 mg/L, respectively.

Our findings noted a significant association between vitamin B12 values and illness episode. Manic patients had lower values of this parameter than depressive patients. Moreover, we showed that vitamin B12 was significantly associated with the therapeutic characteristics. Indeed, patients taking carbamazepine had significantly lower values of this parameter than those taking valproic acid and lithium. Additionally, there was no significant change in homocysteine, folate, uric acid values and metabolic syndrome in relation to illness episode and the treatment, whereas the patients with metabolic syndrome had significant higher levels of HOMA-IR and uric acid than metabolic syndrome free.

Therefore, bipolar I patients require specific care, particularly for lipid profile, vitamin status and weight; the effectiveness of this care will be evaluated during follow-up period Clinicians should track the effects of treatment on physical and the biological parameters, and should facilitate access to appropriate medical care.

6. Acknowledgement

The authors thank the patients and control subjects for their assistance in this study.

7. References

Alkerwi, A.; Boutsen, M.; Vaillant, M.; Barre, J.; Lair, ML.; Albert, A.; Guillaume, M. & Dramaix, M. (2009). Alcohol consumption and the prevalence of metabolic syndrome: A meta-analysis of observational studies. *Atherosclerosis*, 204, 624-635.

American Psychiatric Association. (2004). *Diagnostic and Statistical Manual of Mental Disorders*, 4th edition. American Psychiatric Association,Washington DC.

Angst, F.; Stassen, HH.; Clayton, PJ. & Angst, J. (2002). Mortality of patients with mood disorders: follow-up over 34-38 years. *Journal of Affective Disorders*, 68, 167-181.

Atmaca, M.; Tezcan, E.; Kulolu, M.; Kirtas, O. & Ustunda, B. (2005). Serum folate and homocysteine levels in patients with obsessive-compulsive disorder. *Psychiatry and Clinical Neurosciences*, 59, 616-620.

Bouguerra, R.; Ben Salem, L.; Alberti, H.; Ben Rayana, C.; El Atti, J.; Blouza, S. Gaigi, S.; Achour, A.; Ben Slama, C. & Zouari, B. (2006). Prevalence of metabolic abnormalities in the Tunisian adults: a population based study. *Diabetes & Metabolism*, 32, 215-221.

Casey, DE. (2005). Metabolic issues and cardiovascular disease in patients with psychiatric disorders. *The American Journal of Medicine*, 118, 15-22.

Cassidy, F.; Ahearn, E. & Carroll, BJ. (1999). Elevated frequency of diabetes mellitus in hospitalized manic-depressive patients. *The American Journal of Psychiatry*, 156, 9, 1417-1420.

Cheymol, G. (2000). Effects of obesity on pharmacokinetics implications for drug therapy. *Clinical Pharmacokinetics*, 39,3, 215-231.

Chien, KL.; Hsub, HC.; Lee, YT. & Chen, MF. (2008). Renal function and metabolic syndrme components on cardiovascular and all-cause mortality. *Atherosclerosis*, 197, 860-867.

Chung, KH.; Tsai, SY. & Lee, HC. (2007). Mood symptoms and serum lipids in acute phase of bipolar disorder in Taiwan. *Psychiatry and Clinical Neurosciences*, 61, 428-433.

De Brardis, D.; Conti, CM.; Campanella, D.; Carano, A.; Di Giuseppe, B.; Valchera, A.; Tancredi, L.; Serroni, N.; Pizzorno, AM.; Fulcheri, M.; Gambi, F.; Sepede, G.; Moschetta, FS.; Salerno, RM. & Ferro, FM. (2008). Evaluation of plasma antioxidant levels during different phases of illness in adult patients with bipolar disorder. *Journal of Biological Regulators & Homeostatic Agents*, 22, 195-200.

De Hert, M.; Correll, CU.; Bobes, J.; Cetkovich-Bakmas, M.; Cohen, D.; Asai I.; Detraux J.; Gautam S.; Möller HJ.; Ndetei, DM.; Newcomer, JW.; Uwakwe R. & Leucht S. (2011). Physical illness in patients with severe mental disorders. I. Prevalence, impact of medications and disparities in health care. *World Psychiatry*, 10, 52-77.

De Hert, M.; Dekker, JM.; Wood, D.; Kahl, KG.; Holt, RIG. & Möller, HJ. (2010). Maladie cardiovasculaire et diabète chez les sujets souffrant d'une maladie mentale sévère. Déclaration de position de l'European Psychiatric Association (EPA), soutenue par l'European Association for the study of Diabetes (EASD) et l'European Society of Cardiology (ESC). *European Psychiatry*, in press.

Dierkes, J. & Westphal S. (2005). Effect of drugs on homocysteine concentrations. *Seminars in Vascular Medicine*, 5(2), 124-139.

Elmslie, JL.; Silverstone, JT.; Mann, JL.; Williams, SM. & Romans, SE. (2000). Prevalence of overweight and obesity in bipolar patients. *The Journal of Clinical Psychiatry*, 61, 179-184.

Ezzaher, A.; Haj Mouhamed, D.; Mechri, A.; Neffati, F.; Douki, W.; Gaha, L. & Najjar, MF. (2010). Lower paraoxonase 1 activity in Tunisian bipolar I patients. *Annals of General Psychiatry*, 9, 36.

Fagiolini, A.; Frank, E.; Houck, PR.; Mallinger, AG.; Swartz, HA.; Buysse, DJ.; Ombao H. & Kupfer, DJ. (2002). Prevalence of obesity and weight change during treatment in patients with bipolar I disorder. *The Journal of Clinical Psychiatry*, 63, 528-533.

Fagiolini, A.; Kupfer, DJ.; Houck, PR.; Novick, DM. & Frank, E. (2003). Obesity as a correlate of outcome in patients with bipolar I disorder. *The American Journal of Psychiatry*, 160, 1, 112-117.

Fagiolini, A.; Frank, E.; Scott, JA.; Turkin, S. & Kupfer, DJ. (2005). Metabolic syndrome in bipolar disorder: findings from the bipolar disorder center for Pennsylvanians. *Bipolar Disorders*, 7, 424-430.

Fromenty, B.; Robin, MA.; Igoudjil, A.; Mansouri, A. & Pessayre, D. (2004). The ins and outs of mitochondrial dysfunction in NASH. *Diabetes & Metabolism*, 30, 121-138.

Garcia-Portilla, MP.; Saiz, PA.; Benabarre, A.; Sierra, P.; Perez, J.; Rodriguez, A.; Livianos, L.; Torres, P. & Bobes, J. (2008). The prevalence of metabolic syndrome in patients with bipolar disorder. *Journal of Affective Disorders*, 106, 197-201.

Garcia-Portilla, MP.; Saiz, PA.; Bascaran, MT.; Martinez, S.; Benabarre, A.; Sierra, P.; Torres, P.; Montes, JM.; Bousoño, M. & Bobes, J. (2009). Cardiovascular risk in patients with bipolar disorder. *Journal of Affective Disorders*, 115, 1-7.

Haddad, FG.; Brax, H.; Zein, E. & Abou el Hessen, T. (2006). L'obésité et les pathologies associées dans un centre de soins au Liban. *Journal Médical Libanais*, 54, 152-155.

Haj Mouhamed, D.; Ezzaher, A.; Neffati, F.; Douki, W.; Gaha, L. & Najjar, MF. (2010). Effect of cigarette smoking on plasma uric acid concentrations. *Environmental Health and Preventive Medicine*, 1-6.

Haj Mouhamed, D.; Ezzaher, A.; Neffati, F.; Douki, W. & Najjar, MF. (2011). Effect of cigarette smoking on plasma homocysteine concentrations. *Clinical Chemistry and Laboratory Medicine*, 49, 3, 479-483.

Hakim, NA.; Hafizan, MT.; Baizurah, MH. & Zainal, AA. (2008). Serum lipoprotein(a) levels in patients with atherosclerotic peripheral vascular disease in Hospital Kuala Lumpur. *Asian Journal of Surgery*, 31, 1, 11-15.

Hankey, GJ. & Eikelboom, JW. Homocysteine and vascular disease. (1999). *Lancet*, 354, 407-413.

Hanson, RL.; Imperatore, G.; Bennet, PH. & Knowler, WC. (2002). Components of the "metabolic syndrome" and incidence of type 2 diabetes. *Diabetes*, 51, 3120.

Holman, RR.; Paul, SK.; Bethel, MA.; Matthews, DR. & Neil, HA. (2008). 10-year follow-up of intensive glucose control in type 2 diabetes. *The New England Journal of Medicine*, 359, 15, 1577-1589.

Ipcioglu, OM.; Ozcan, O.; Gultepe, M.; Ates, A.; Basoglu, C. & Cakir, E. (2008). Reduced urinary excretion of homocysteine could be the reason of elevated plasma homocysteine in patients with psychiatric illnesses. *Clinical Biochemistry*, 41, 831-835.

Kabakci, G.; Koylan, N.; Ilerigelen, B.; Kozan, O. & Buyukozturk, K. (2008). Impact of dyslipidemia on cardiovascular risk stratification of hypertensive patients and association of lipid profi le with other cardiovascular risk factors: results from the ICEBERG study. *Journal of Integrated Blood Pressure Control,* 1, 5-13.

Kessler, RC.; Berglund, P.; Demler, O.; Jin, R.; Merikangas, KR. & Walters, EE. (2005). Lifetime prevalence and age-of-onset distributions of DSM-IV disorders in the National Comorbidity Survey Replication. *Archives of General Psychiatry*, 62, 593-602.

Kip, KE.; Marroquin, OC.; Kelley, DE.; Johnson, BD.; Kelsey, SF.; Shaw, LJ.; Rogers, WJ. & Reis, SE. (2004). Clinical importance of obesity versus the metabolic syndrome in cardiovascular risk in women: a report from the Women's Ischemia Syndrome Evaluation (WISE) study. *Circulation,* 109, 706.

Klein, BE.; Klein, R. & Lee, KE. (2002). Components of the metabolic syndrome and risk of cardiovascular disease and diabetes in Beaver Dam. *Diabetes Care,* 25, 1790.

Kurl, S.; Laukkanen, JA.; Niskanen, L.; Laaksonen, D.; Sivenius, J.; Nyyssönen, K. & Salonen, JT. (2006). Metabolic syndrome and the risk of stroke in middle-aged men. *Stroke,* 37, 806-811.

Lakka, HM.; Laaksonen, DE.; Lakka, TA. Niskanen, LK.; Kumpusalo, E.; Tuomilehto, J. & Salonen, JT. (2002). The metabolic syndrome and total cardiovascular disease mortality in middle-aged men. *The Journal of the American Medical Association*, 288, 2709.

Lasser, K.; Boyd, JW.; Woolhandler, S.; Himmelstein, DU.; McCormick, D. & Bor, DH. (2000). Smoking and mental illness: A population-based prevalence study. *The Journal of the American Medical Association*, 284, 2606-2610.

Le Strat, Y. Trouble bipolaire et comorbidités addictives. (2010). *Annales medico-psychologiques*, 168, 584-587.

Lorenzi, TM.; Borba, DL.; Dutra, G. & Lara, DR. (2010). Association of serum uric acid levels with emotional and affective temperaments. *Journal of Affective Disorders,* 121, 161-164.

Maina, G.; Salvi, V.; Vitalucci, A.; D' Ambrosio, V. & Bogetto, F. (2008). Prevalence and correlates of overweight in drug-naïve patients with bipolar disorder. *Journal of Affective Disorders*, 110, 149-155.

Malhotra, S. & McElroy, S. (2002). Medical management of obesity associated with mental disorders. *The Journal of Clinical Psychiatry*, 63, 24-32.

Marmol, F. (2008). Lithium: bipolar disorder and neurodegenerative diseases possible cellular mechanisms of the therapeutic effects of lithium. *Progress in Neuro-Psychopharmacology & Biological Psychiatry*, 32, 1761-1771.

McElroy, SL.; Kotwal, R.; Malhotra, S.; Nelson, EB.; Keck, PE. & Nemeroff, CB. (2004). Are mood disorders and obesity related a review for the mental health professional. *The Journal of Clinical Psychiatry*, 65, 634-651.

Merikangas, KR.; Akiskal, HS.; Angst, J.; Greenberg, PE.; Hirschfeld, RM.; Petukhova, M. & Kessler, RC. (2007). Lifetime and 12-month prevalence of bipolar spectrum disorder in the national comorbidity survey replication. *Archives of General Psychiatry*, 64, 543-552.

Mill J, Tang T, Kaminsky Z.; KhareT.; Yazdanpanah, S.; Bouchard, L.; Jia, P.; Assadzadeh, A.; Flanagan, J.; Schumacher, A.; Wang SC. & Petronis, A. (2008). Epigenomic profiling reveals DNA-methylation changes associated with major psychosis. *The American Journal of Human Genetics*, 82, 696-711.

Muntoni, S.; Atzori, L.; Mereu, R.; Manca, A.; Satta, G.; Gentilini, A.; Bianco, P.; Baule, A.; Baule, GM. & Muntoni, S. (2009). Risk factors for cardiovascular disease in Sardinia from 1978 to 2001: A comparative study with Italian mainland. *The European Journal of Internal Medicine*, 20, 373-377.

Murray, DP.; Weiner, M.; Prabhakar, M. & Fiedorowicz, JG. (2009). Mania and mortality: why the excess cardiovascular risk in bipolar disorder?. *Current Psychiatry Reports*, 11, 475- 480.

National Cholesterol Education Program (NCEP). (2002). Expert panel on detection, evaluation, and treatment of high blood cholesterol in adults (Adult Treatment Panel III). Third Report of the National Cholesterol Education Program (NCEP). Expert panel on detection, evaluation, and treatment of high blood cholesterol in adults (Adult Treatment Panel III) final report. *Circulation*, 106, 3143-3421.

Osher, Y.; Bersudsky Y.; Silver H.; Sela, BA. & Belmaker, RH. (2008). Neuropsychological correlates of homocysteine levels in euthymic bipolar patients. *Journal of Affective Disorders*, 105, 229-233.

Ozbek, Z.; Kucukali, CI.; Ozkok, E.; Orhan, N.; Aydin, M.; Kilic, G.; Sazci, A. & Kara, I. (2008). Effect of the methylenetetrahydrofolate reductase gene polymorphisms on homocysteine, folate and vitamin B12 in patients with bipolar disorder and relatives. *Progress in Neuro-Psychopharmacology & Biological Psychiatry*, 32: 1331-1337.

Ozdemir, A.; Yalinbas, B.; Selamet, U.; Eres, M.; Turkmen, F.; Kumbasar, F.; Murat, B.; Keskin, AT. & Barut, Y. (2007). The effect of hepatitis C virus infection on insulin resistance in chronic haemodialysis patients. *Yonsei Medical Journal* , 48, 274-280.

Parikh, S.; Parker, C.; Cooke, R.; Krüger, S.; McIntyre, R.; Kusznir, A.; Bartha, C.; Ashton, L.; Damianakis, M.; Mancini, D. & Zetes-Zanatta, L. (2000). *Le trouble bipolaire. Guide d'information*, Camh, Ontario, Canada.

Pearson, TA. (1996). Alcohol and heart disease. *Circulation*, 94, 3023-3025.

Pinkney, J. (2001). Implications of obesity for diabetes and coronary heart disease in clinical practice. *British Journal of Diabetes & Vascular Disease*, 1, 103-106.

Plante, DT. & Winkelman, JW. (2008). Sleep disturbance in bipolar disorder: therapeutic implications. *The American Journal of Psychiatry*, 165, 7, 830-843.

Regier, DA.; Farmer, ME.; Rae, DS.; Keith, SJ.; Judd, LL. & Goodwin, FK. (1990). Comorbidity of mental disorders with alcohol and other drug abuse. Results from the Epidemiologic Catchment Area (ECA) study. *The Journal of the American Medical Association*, 264, 2511-2518.

Reif, A.; Pfuhlmann, B. & Lesch, KP. (2005). Homocysteinemia as well as methylenetetrahydrofolate reductase polymorphism are associated with affective psychoses. *Progress in Neuro-Psychopharmacology & Biological Psychiatry,* 29: 1162-1168.

Resnick, HE.; Jones, K.; Ruotolo, G.; Jain, AK.; Henderson, J.; Lu, W. & Howard, BV. (2003). Insulin resistance, the metabolic syndrome, and risk of incident cardiovascular disease in nondiabetic American Indians: the Strong Heart study. *Diabetes Care,* 26, 861.

Revicki, DA.; Matza, LS.; Flood, E. & Lloyd, A. (2005). Bipolar disorder and health-related quality of life: review of burden of disease and clinical trials. *Pharmacoeconomics,* 23, 6, 583-594.

Reynolds, E. (2006). Vitamin B12, folic acid and the nervous system. *Lancet Neurol*ogy, 5, 949-960.

Sagud, M.; Mihaljevic-Peles, A.; Pivac, N.; Jakovljevic, M. & Muck-Seler, D. (2007). Platelet serotonin and serum lipids in psychotic mania. *Journal of Affective Disorders,* 61, 428-433.

Salvadore, G.; Viale, CI.; Luckenbaugh, DA.; Zanatto, V.; Portela, LV.; Souza, DO.; Zarate, CA. & Machado-Vieira, R. (2010). Increased uric acid levels in drug-naïve subjects with bipolar disorder during a first manic episode. *Progress in Neuro-Psychopharmacology & Biological Psychiatry,* 34, 819-821.

Salvi, V.; Albert, U.; Chiarle, A.; Soreca, I.; Bogetto, F. & Maina, G. (2008). Metabolic syndrome in Italian patients with bipolar disorder. *General Hospital Psychiatry,* 30, 318-323.

Sattar, N.; Gaw, A.; Scherbakova, O.; Ford, I.; O'Reilly, DSJ.; Haffner, SM.; Isles, C.; Macfarlane, PW.; Packard, CJ.; Cobbe, SM. & Shepherd, J. (2003). Metabolic syndrome with and without C-reactive protein as a predictor of coronary heart disease and diabetes in the West of Scotland Coronary Prevention Study. *Circulation,* 108, 414.

Sener, U.; Zorlu, Y.; Karaguzel, O.; Ozdamar, O.; Coker, I. & Topbas, M. (2006). Effects of common anti-epileptic drug monotherapy on serum levels of homocysteine, Vitamin B12, folic acid and Vitamin B6. *Seizure,* 15, 79-85.

Sicras, A.; Rejas, J.; Navarro, R.; Serrat, J. & Blanca, M. (2008). Metabolic syndrome in bipolar disorder: a cross-sectional assessment of a Health Management Organization database. *Bipolar Disord*ers, 10, 1-10.

Simon, GE. (2003). Social and economic burden of mood disorders. *Biological Psychiatry,* 54, 208-215.

Ten Have, M.; Vollebergh, W.; Bijl, R. & Nolen, WA. (2002). Bipolar disorder in the general population in the Netherlands (prevalence, consequences and care utilisation): data from the Netherlands Mental Health Survey and Incidence Study (NEMESIS). *Journal of Affective Disorders,* 68, 203-213.

Toalson, P., Ahmed, S., Hardy, T. & Kabinoff, G. (2004). The metabolic syndrome in patients with severe mental illnesses. *Primary care companion to the Journal of clinical psychiatry,* 6, 152-158.

Tolmunen, T.; Hintikka, J.; Voutilainen, S.; Ruusunen, A.; Alfthan, G.; Nyyssönen, K.; Viinama¨ki, H.; Kaplan, GA. & Salonen, JT. (2004). Association between depressive symptoms and serum concentrations of homocysteine in men: a population study[1-3]. *The American Journal of Clinical Nutrition*, 80, 1574-1578.

Torres, IJ.; Boudreau, VG. & Yatham, LN. (2007). Neuropsychological functioning in euthymic bipolar disorder: a meta-analysis. *Acta psychiatrica Scandinavica. Supplementum*, 434, 17-26.

Valentine, RJ.; Kaplan, HS.; Green, R.; Jacobsen, DW.; Myers, SI. & Clagett, GP. (1996). Lipoprotein (a), homocysteine, and hypercoagulable states in young men with premature peripheral on arthrosclerosis: A prospective controlled analysis. *Journal of Vascular* Surgery, 23, 53-63.

von Eckardstein, A.; Schulte, H.; Cullen, P. & Assmann, G. (2001). Lipoprotein(a) further increases the risk of coronary events in men with high global cardiovascular risk. *Journal of the American College of Cardiology*, 37, 2, 434-439.

Vuksan-Ćusa, B.; Jakovljević, M.; Sagud, M.; Mihaljević Peleš, A.; Marčinko, D.; Topić, R.; Mihaljević, S. & Sertić, J. (2011). Metabolic syndrome and serum homocysteine in patients with bipolar disorder and schizophrenia treated with second generation antipsychotics. *Psychiatry Research*, 189(1), 21-25.

Vuorinen-Markkola, H. & Yki-Jarvinen, H. (1994). Hyperuricemia and insulin resistance. *The Journal of Clinical Endocrinology & Metabolism*, 78, 25-29.

Williams, JM. & Ziedonis, D. (2004). Addressing tobacco among individuals with a mental illness or an addiction. *Addictive Behaviors*, 29, 1067-1083.

Wittchen, HU.; Mühlig, S. & Pezawas, L. (2003). Natural course and burden of bipolar disorders. *International Journal of Neuropsychopharmacology*, 6, 145-154.

Woods, SW. (2000). The economic burden of bipolar disease. *Journal of Clinical Psychiatry*, 61, 38- 41.

World Health Organisation. (1997). *Obesity: Preventing and Managing the Global Epidemic (publication WHO/NÛT/NCD/98.1)*, Geneva, Switzerland.

Yumru, M.; Savas, HA.; Kurt, E.; Kaya, MC.; Salek, S.; Savas, E. Oral, ET. & Atagun, I. (2007). Atypical antipsychotics related metabolic syndrome in bipolar patients. *Journal of Affective Disorders*, 98, 247-252.

Wyatt, RJ. & Henter, I. (1995). An economic evaluation of manic-depressive illness-1991. *Social Psychiatry and Psychiatric Epidemiology*, 30, 213-219.

Edwards, R.; Peet, M.; Shay, J. & Horrobin, D. (1998). Omega-3 polyunsatu- rated fatty acid levels in the diet and in red blood cell membranes of depressed patients. *Journal of Affective Disorders*, 48, 149-155.

Peet, M.; Murphy, B.; Shay, J. & Horrobin, DF. (1998). Depletion of omega-3 fatty acid levels in red blood cell membranes of depressive patients. *Biological Psychiatry*, 43, 315-319.

Maes, M.; Smith, R.; Christophe, A.; Cosyns, P.; Desnyder, R. & Meltzer, HJ. (1996). Fatty acid composition in major depression: decreased omega 3 fractions in cholesteryl esters and increased C20:4 omega 6/C20:5 omega 3 ratio in cholesteryl esters and phospholipids. *Journal of Affective Disorders*, 38, 35-46.

Maes, M.; Christophe, A.; Delanghe, J.; Altamura, C.; Neels, H. & Meltzer, HT. (1999). Lowered omega-3 polyunsaturated fatty acids in serum phospholipids and cholesteryl esters of depressed patients. *Psychiatry Research*, 85, 275-291.

Chiu, CC.; Huang, SY.; Suc, KP.; Luc, ML.; Huanga, MC.; Chen, CC. & Shen, WW. (2003). Polyunsaturated fatty acid deficit in patients with bipolar mania. *European Neuropsychopharmacology*, 13, 99-103.

17

Dyslipidemia and Mental Illness

D. Saravane
Head of Department Medicine and Specialists
Ville-Evrard Hospital Neuilly/Marne
France

1. Introduction

Almost most mental illness, such as schizophrenia, bipolar disorder, and depression are associated with undue medical morbidity and mortality. It represents a major health problem, with 20 to 30 years shorter lifetime mortality are primarily due to premature cardiovascular disease (myocardial infarction, stroke...). The cardiovascular events are strongly linked to non modifiable risk factors such as age, gender, personal and/or family history, but also to crucial modifiable risk factors, such as overweight and obesity, dyslipidemia, diabetes, hypertension and smoking.

Although these classical risk factors exist in the general population epidemiological studies suggest that patients with severe mental illness have an increased prevalence of these risk factors.

Another point is the causes of increased metabolic and cardiovascular risk in this population are related to poverty, poor diet, sedentary and compared to the general population. The increased morbidity and mortality limited behaviour access to medical care, but also to the use of psychotropic medication. Over recent years it has become apparent that antipsychotic drugs can have a negative impact on some of the modifiable risk factors.

2. Epidemiological studies

Results of most research on the physical health of people with mental health illness suggest the morbidity and the mortality from certain physical disease is high in these populations. Patients with schizophrenia are a medically vulnerable population due to underdiagnosed medical problems, and minimal or not utilization of primary care services. Not only there is increased medical morbidity among these patients, there is also increased mortality.

Medical comorbidity in patients with bipolar disorder, is associated with an intensification of bipolar depressive symptoms and other indices of bipolar severity, as well as premature mortality. Somatic health issues remain underrecognized and suboptimally treated.

2.1 Mortality

An increasing number of studies have found higher rates of mortality in schizophrenia patients due to natural causes (Mortensen & Juel, 1993; Ruschena et al, 1998). Such increased rates of mortality due to natural causes highlight the failure to detect and manage physical health conditions in this group. In meta-analysis deaths due to natural causes accounted for

59% of the excess mortality in schizophrenia (Brown, 1997). Respiratory and cardiovascular diseases are the most common causes of natural death. The standard mortality ratio (SMR) for respiratory disease was 226 (95%CI, 209-244) and for cardiovascular disease 110 (95%CI, 105-115) (Brown, 1997). However, another study found an SMR of 1.78 for men and 0.86 for women with schizophrenia for ischemic heart disease (Lawrence et al, 2003). Analysis of standardized mortality ratios for deaths from natural causes showed an increased risk of death in patients with a wide range of psychiatric conditions, including substance misuse, schizophrenia, bipolar disorder and unipolar depression. The Standardized mortality ratios (SMR) showed that in schizophrenia it is 1.57 for all cause mortality, and cardiovascular and cancer deaths accounted for the largest number of deaths with SMRs of 1.04 and 1.00 respectively (Harris & Barraclough, 1998). Depression confers a 24% increased risk of dying within the next 6 years (Wulsin, 2000). A study published through the Centers for Disease Control and Prevention (CDC) compared the mortality of public mental health patients in 8 states with the mortality of the states' general population, for 1997 through 2000. In all the study states, mental health had a higher risk of death than the general population and died at much younger ages compared with their cohorts. In all states studied, cardiac disease was found to be the leading cause of death in mentally ill patients. And this population had lost decades of potential years of life, with average exceeding 25 years (Colton & Manderscheid, 2006).

Another indicator of the medical care is avoidable mortality. These indicators are calculated by selecting the number of avoidable causes of death considered amenable to health care (Rustein et al, 1976). A follow-up study of 30045 psychiatric in-patients born between 1912-1970 was conducted to specifically address avoidable mortality. The standardized rate ratios (SRR) for male patients with schizophrenia are 3.74 (95%CI, 2.38-5.89) and 3.99 (95%CI, 2.47-6.44) for females (Ringback Weitoft et al, 1998).

2.2 Morbidity

A study list some of the common physical conditions found in people with psychosis. These include diabetes, hyperlipidemia, cardiovascular disease, obesity, malignant neoplasms, HIV/AIDS, hepatitis, osteoporosis, hyperprolactinemia, irritable bowel syndrome and helicobacter pylori infection (Lambert et al, 2003). The prevalence of physical illness in medically screened chronic psychiatric samples has been variously reported to be 12-53% (Lyketsos et al, 2002). Another study estimate that 35% of psychiatric patients have undiagnosed physical disorder (Felker et al, 1996).Some studies have attempted to establish whether medical comorbidity exacerbates patient' psychiatric condition (Bartsch et al, 1998).

Not only do patients with mental illness die of natural causes at high rate, when medical conditions occur, these patients are much more likely to underdiagnosed and undertreated. Several studies have shown that the detection rate of physical illness among patient with mental illness is very poor. A study estimated that 45% of patients in California's public mental-health system had physical disease and, of these, 47% were undetected by the treating physician (Koran, 1989). Another study of psychiatric clinic patients revealed remarkably similar findings: 43% of patients had physical illnesses and, of these, 48% had not been diagnosed by the referring doctor, non-psychiatrist physicians had missed 33% and psychiatrists had missed 50% (Koranyi, 1979). Hall et al found that 46% of patients admitted to a research ward had an unrecognized physical illness that either caused or exacerbated

their psychiatric illness; 80% had physical illnesses requiring treatment, and 4% had precancerous conditions or illnesses (Hall et al, 1981).
Research indicates that 25% to 80% of patients with schizophrenia and other mental illness have a serious medical comorbidity, yet less than half of these medical conditions are diagnosed (Cradock-O'Leary et al, 2002).

3. Causes of poor physical health in mental illness

A number of reasons exist to explain the poor detection of physical health problems in patient with mental illness. Some patients are unaware of any physical health problems, usually a consequence of cognitive deficits associated with their mental illness (Goldman, 1999). Often there is a reluctance to seek medical help and when it sought patient with mental health find it difficult to describe their problems to a medical practitioner, or present with atypical medical symptoms. Patient with schizophrenia have been shown to have a high tolerance for pain and subsequently are less likely to report this symptom (Dworkin, 1994). Another complexity concerns the effects of psychiatric illness on perceived physical health. For example, depression can lead to an increase in perceived physical symptoms and worsening of subjective health outcomes.
The management of medical conditions is a complex and problematic issue, arising largely because of the separation of medical and psychiatric health care services. The stigma of mental illness is one obvious barrier preventing psychiatric patients from receiving adequate physical health care, as some physicians may be uncomfortable in working with this patient. Another concern is managing physical conditions where patients that have an increased prevalence with psychiatric illness and where there is a general lack of treatment compliance. The challenging task of managing physical illness with this patient requires skill, patience and experience as patients often present late with complications. (Table 1)

System-Related Barriers
Lack of insurance coverage
Lack of access to health care
Stigmatization by health care providers
Lack of understanding of benefits of preventive services by health care workers
Lack of integration of medical and mental health systems
Patients-Barriers
Poverty
Non compliance
Pour communication skills
Denials of illness Related

Table 1. Barriers to health care for patients with mental illness. Adapted from Goldman.

3.1 Lifestyle risk factors

In recent years, there is a growing concern about physical illness in patients with mental illnesses, specifically the risk of cardiovascular disease. Those patients are more likely to be overweight, to smoke, to have hypertension, hyperglycemia or diabetes, and dyslipidemia (Table 2).

	Estimated prevalence, % (RR)	
Modifiable risk factors	Schizophrenia	Bipolar disorder
Overweight	45–55% (1,5–2)	21–49% (1-2)
Smoking	50–80% (2-3)	54-68% (2-3)
Diabetes	10-15% (2)	8-17% (1,5-2)
Hypertension	19-58% (2-3)	35-61% (2-3)
Dyslipidemia	25-69% (≤5)	25-38% (≤3)
Metabolic syndrome	37-63% (2-3)	30-49% (1,5-2)

Table 2. Estimation prevalence and relative risk 5 (RR) of modifiable cardiovascular disease risk factors in schizophrenia and bipolar disorder compared to the general population. Adapted from Correll, 2007

3.1.1 Obesity

Excessive body weight increases the risk of morbidity from number conditions, including hypertension, dyslipidemia, type II diabetes, coronary heart disease. Excess abdominal fat is associated with dyslipidemia, hypertension and glucose intolerance. Risk of comorbid diseases has been shown to rise as BMI increases above 25 kg/m2. In psychiatric practice, weight gain is a long recognized and commonly encountered problem. A study of patients with schizophrenia reported 51% of males and 59% of females to be clinically obese, compared with 33% of people with other psychiatric disorders. This study provided an estimate of mean weight gain in patients who received standard doses of antipsychotics over 10-week period. The mean increases were 4.45 kg with clozapine, 4.15 with olanzapine, 2.92 kg with sertindole, 2.10 kg with risperidone, and 0.04 kg with ziprasidone (Allison & Casey, 2001). It is important to note that substantial weight gain is associated with both atypical (eg, clozapine, olanzapine) and conventional (eg, thioridazine, chlorpromazine) antipsychotics.

3.1.2 Smoking

The prevalence of smoking greatly exceeds that in the general population (Table 1) Heavy cigarette smoking is intimately associated with schizophrenia and it may have implications for the underlying neurobiology of the disease. Smoking is a good example of how behavior and treatment interact to increase morbidity at a number of levels. It is a risk factor for respiratory and ischemic heart disease and stroke. Cigarette smoking induces hepatic microsomal enzymes, which increase the metabolism of psychotropic medication, reducing plasma levels of antipsychotics notably olanzapine and clozapine. It may influence the patient's behavior and the treatment outcome. Therefore smokers usually require greater levels of antipsychotic medication than non-smokers to achieve similar blood levels.

3.1.3 Diabetes

It is another risk factor for coronary atherosclerosis that is associated with metabolic abnormalities that result in changes in the transport, composition and metabolism of lipoproteins.

3.1.4 Hypertension

Is a cardiovascular risk factor as it produces structural changes within the arteries. The seq uel of hypertension are greatly affected by comorbidities such as dyslipidemia, smoking, diabetes, lack of physical activity, sodium intake, and stress.

Other risk factors are attributable to unhealthy lifestyle, including social scale such as unemployment, poorer financial standing, poor diet and sedentary behaviour.
Concerning diet, a study (Mc Creadle, 2003) examined in detail the dietary intake of 102 people with schizophrenia in Scotland. Their fruit and vegetable consumption averaged 16 portions per week, less than half the recommended intake.
Brown et al, 1999 and Mc Creadle, 2003 found that patients with schizophrenia tended to take only small amounts of exercice. Factors such as features of the illness, sedative medication and lack of opportunity and general motivation may be relevant.

3.2 Medication

Psychotropic medication is associated with a host of physical complications and side effects. Old antipsychotic medication was associated with neurologic side effects, including involuntary movement disorders, such as akathisia, parkinsonism, tardive dyskinisia. New antipsychotics are more commonly use. Despite the low propensity of new antipsychotics towards extra pyramidal side effects other adverse effects associated with them include excessive weight gain, metabolic disturbances. Medical conditions attributed to the use of typical and atypical antipsychotic medication include diabetes, hyperlipidemia, and cardiovascular disease: specifically hypertension and cardiac arrhythmias, obesity (Meyer, 2002; Davidson, 2002).

4. The metabolic syndrome

Much attention has been focused on the metabolic syndrome which brings together a series of abnormal clinical and metabolic findings which are predictive of cardiovascular risk. The most commonly used definition for the metabolic syndrome are the Adult Treatment Panel III (ATP III) of the National Cholesterol Education Program (NCEP), (Jama, 2001) and the adapted ATP-III-A proposed by the American to Heart Association following the American Diabetes Association lowering of the threshold for impaired fasting glucose 100mg/dl. (Quindy et al, 2005 ; Alberti et al, 2006).
Another recent definition, by the International Diabetes Federation (Alberti et al, 2006; Sarafidis &, Nilsson, 2006) stressed the importance of waist circumference, using ethnic/race specific criteria (Table 3).

	ATP III 3 out of 5 criteria required	ATP III A 3 out of 5 criteria required	IDF waist + 2 criteria required
Waist (cm)	M>102, F>88	M>102, F>88	M≥94,F≥80
Blood pressure	≥130/85*	≥130/85*	≥130/85*
HDL cholesterol (mg/dl)	M<40, F<50	M<40,F<50	M<40,F<50
Triglycerides (mg/dl)	≥150	≥150	≥150
Fasting glucose (mg/dl)	≥110**	≥100**	≥100**

*or treated with antihypertensive medication
**or treated with insulin or hypoglycemic medication

Table 3. Definitions of metabolic syndrome: The metabolic syndrome has been shown to be an important risk factor for the development of both type 2 diabetes and cardiovascular disease.

In the study, the clinical Antipsychotic Trials of Intervention Effectiveness (CATIE), one third of patients met the NCEP criteria for metabolic syndrome at baseline (Mc Eoy et al, 2005 ; Meyer et al, 2005).
And from this study, 88% of patients with dyslipidemia were not receiving treatment, as were 62% of the hypertensive patients and 38% those with diabetes (Nasrallah et al, 2006). The presence of the metabolic syndrome increases the risk for the distribution of fat within the body is a key factor. Abdominal fat distribution, particularly visceral adiposity, increases the risk of dyslipidemia, glucose intolerance, and cardiovascular disease. Multiple organ systems are affected, including adipose, muscle, hepatic, nervous, and adrenal tissues, and the most important site of impact is the vasculature. The concept of insulin resistance is central to the metabolic syndrome. Insulin resistance is a major contributor to glucose intolerance, and the lipoprotein abnormalities seen in the metabolic syndrome are also predictable, at least in part, from the known effects of insulin to inhibit lipolysis in adipocytes. With resistance to insulin, unchecked lipolysis leads to increased delivery of free fatty acids to the liver for triglyceride synthesis and packaging into very low-density lipoprotein (VLDL) particles. Higher VLDL levels contribute to lower HDL levels because of the reciprocal exchanges between these lipoproteins mediated by cholesterol ester transfer protein. Is has been shown that blood pressure is related to insulin resistance independent of differences in age, gender, and degree of obesity(Zavaroni et al,1992). Visceral obesity is the primary determinant of insulin resistance and, as such, represents the fundamental pathophysiologic change leading to the metabolic syndrome. The risk of insulin resistance increases with adiposity, particularly the amount of visceral adiposity. Insulin resistance is associated with impaired glucose control, increase plasma triglycerides, reduced high-density lipoprotein (HDL) cholesterol, increased blood pressure, increased risk of blood clotting, and increases in markers of inflammation, all which are associated with an increase risk for cardiovascular disease. Thus, markers of insulin resistance, such as elevated fasting plasma Triglycerides, can be a key point for monitoring and evaluating a patient's risk.

5. Effects of antipsychotics treatment

Antipsychotic treatment is associated with metabolic side effects that include various degrees of weight gain, dyslipidemia and susceptibility to type 2 diabetes (Newcomer, 2005).
Elevated blood lipids, particularly triglycerides, are associated with some typical antipsychotic agents. Shortly after their introduction, phenothiazines were found to elevate serum triglyceride and total cholesterol levels. Then much was written on the effects of specific atypical drugs on lipid profiles. Both clozapine and olanzapine have been shown to cause significant hypertriglyceridemia compared with typicals. Studies have also reported a significant association between weight gain and triglyceride change for patients under atypical antipsychotic therapy (Meyer, 2001).
The atypical antipsychotics vary in their propensity to induce weight gain (Table 4): clozapine and olanzapine produce the most weight gain, quetiapine and risperidone produce intermediate weight gain, and ziprasidone and aripiprazole produce the least weight gain (Allison et al, 1999; American Diabetes Association [ADA], 2004). The differences in weight gain associated with these agents reflect their order of risk for insulin resistance, glucoregulatory dysfunction, and dyslipidemia (Haupt & Newcomer 2002; ADA, 2004).

Antipsychotic	Weight	Risk for diabetes	Worsening lipid proli B
Clozapine	+++	+	+
Olanzapine	+++	+	+
Risperidone	++	D	D
Quetiapine	++	D	D
Ziprasidone	+/-	-	-
Aripiprazole	+/-	-	-

[a]Adapted with the permission from the American Diabetes Association Abbreviation:
D = discrepant results
Symbols: + = increased effect, - = no effect

Table 4. Atypical antipsychotic drugs and metabolic disturbances[a]

Metabolic disturbances related to atypical antipsychotics may result from a direct alteration of insulin sensitivity and/or insulin secretion. Antipsychotic affinity at both histamine and muscarinie acetylcholine receptors correlates with weight gain and metabolic liability (Matsui-Sakata, 2005) and impaired parasympathic regulation of β all activity may contribute to metabolic risk (Silvestre &-Prous, 2005). Certain antipsychotic agents may directly impair glucose transporter function. Direct attenuation of glucose transporter function by antipsychotic agents would result in elevations in circulating glucose and a compensatory hypersecretion of insulin, which overtime may further reduce insulin sensitivity, triggering the cascade of events leading to metabolic syndrome and type 2 diabetes (Dwyer & Donohoe, 2003).

Some antipsychotic drugs increase appetite and this leads to adiposity. Affinity of the antipsychotic drugs for histamine-1 (H1) receptors closely correlates with weight-gaining potential and appears to involve H1 receptor-linked activation of hypothalamic AMP-kinase. Also, 5-HT2C receptor antagonism may contribute to weight gain. The H1 and 5HT2C blocking effects of antipsychotic medications may interfere with leptin-mediated appetite suppression (Reynolds,2006; Matsui-Sakata et al,2005).

Adiposity alone does not explain the potential side effects of atypical antipsychotic medications. Animal and human studies describe the adverse effect of clozapine and olanzapine on insulin and glucose metabolism (Hasnain & Vieweg, 2008). Significant insulin resistance has also been documented in non-obese patients receiving clozapine or olanzapine versus those receiving risperidone (Henderson et al, 2006). Diminished or inefficient insulin release from pancreatic beta cells as well peripheral insulin resistance may underlie the diabetogenic effect of some antipsychotic medications. Blocking muscarinic type 3 and 5-HT1A receptors may be a factor to diminished pancreatic beta-cells responsiveness and blocking 5HT2A receptor may suppress glucose uptake in muscle (Nasrallah, 2008). Some antipsychotic medications may impair and/or alter the action of insulin on adipocytes leading to progressive lipid accumulation (Vestri et al, 2007). The impaired effect of insulin on adipocytes may explain weight gain independent dyslipidemia (De leon et al, 2007, Birkenaes et al, 2008).

Another study examine whether patients taking selective serotonin reuptake inhibitors (SSRIs) are more likely to have elements of the metabolic syndrome compared with those taking no psychotropic drugs. Patients taking SSRIs had a significantly increased prevalence of obesity, abdominal fat, and hypercholesterolemia. The associations with this factors were significant after adjustment for age, gender , and several covariates. The individuals SSRIs might display differences in their side effect profile, the study performed analysis of the various SSRIs. Paroxetine was strongly associated with general and abdominal obesity but not with hypercholesterolemia, whereas citalopram was associated with neither obesity nor dyslipidemia. Patients taking sertraline, fluoxetine, or fluvoxamine, SSRIs treatment was significantly associated with abdominal obesity and with hypercholesterolemia. SSRIs induce transcriptional activation of cholesterol and fatty acid biosynthesis. The lipogenic effect could represent a common mechanism for explaining in part the lipid disturbances (Reader et al, 2006).

Weight gain is a major side effect of the main mood stabilizers. Chronic treatment with lithium is associated with increased weight, reaching more than 10kg in 20% of patients (Garland et al, 1998).Valproic acid leads to unequivocal weight gain. Lamotrigene, another anticonvulsant that acts as a mood stabilizer, is not associated with significant weight gain (Zimmermann et al, 2003).

With regard to mood stabilizers, additional factors could be involved. An insulin-like action cause by lithium at the treatment stage could increase fat deposition. In addition, edema secondary to sodium retention and subclinical hypothyroidism also contribute to weight gain (Garland et al, 1998). The mechanism by which the valproic acid causes weight gain is still little explored; an action in the sense of inhibiting oxidation of fatty acids might be involved (Isojärvi et al, 1998).

Studies are not in accordance. A controlled study, with children undergoing anticonvulsant treatment, did not find significant changes in HDL and triglycerides levels associated with use of carbamazepine or valproic acid. But, in the group taking carbamazepine, there were was significant increase in total cholesterol levels (Fanzoni et al, 1992).

Another study assessed 101 patients undergoing anticonvulsant therapy for at least 3 months. Compared with controls paired for gender and age, patients taking valproic acid presented significantly lower total cholesterol and LDL levels; patients taking carbamazepine presented significantly increased HDL and apolipoprotein A levels (Calandre et al, 1991).

6. Screening and monitoring

Identification of treatable pathology in a high-risk population, that is, screening for diabetes, dyslipidemia, hypertension is important and facilitates preventive strategies and early diagnosis. Another goal is to track metabolic disturbance in relation to antipsychotic treatment. Dyslipidemia is a general term that defines an increase in the serum concentration of various lipoproteins. Lipoproteins are usually classified into three major categories:

- Low-density lipoproteins (LDLs) are cholesterol-rich particles whose concentration is directly correlated with the risk of myocardial infarction and death.
- Very-low-density lipoproteins (VLDLs) are triglyceride-rich particles whose concentration is strongly correlated with the level of insulin resistance and inversely proportional to the serum concentration of high-density lipoproteins (HDLs).
- HDL particles are antiatherogenic lipid particles, and high serum levels of HDL are protective against coronary artery disease.

6.1 Screening

In the general population, lipid screening with a fasting lipid profile (total chol, LDL, HDL and triglyceride) is recommended for all adults aged 20 years and older, repeteated every 5 years in asymptomatic individuals (Expert Panel on Detection, Evaluation and Treatment, of High Blood Cholesterol in Adults, 2001). Adequate fasting, about 10 to 12 hours is necessary to obtain valid LDL and triglyceride levels-Target LDL levels are determined by a Framingham assessment based on age, sex, chol, HDL, systolic blood pressure, and smoking status (Wilson et al, 1998). Patients on antipsychotic treatment frequently have a metabolic dyslipidemia with elevations of triglyceride and reduced HDL (Cohn et al, 2004), along with associated features of the metabolic syndrome. Some SSRIs induced metabolic disturbance particularly hypercholesterolemia.

Treatment of metabolic dyslipidemia is a secondary goal for intervention following achievement of LDL targets. Clinical trials show that LDL-lowering therapy reduces risk for coronary heart disease (CHD). For these reasons, ATP III continues to identify elevated LDL cholesterol as the primary goal of cholesterol-lowering therapy. Those with diabetes or established cardiovascular disease are considered high risk and are treated to the most stringent LDL targets. Risk determinants in addition to LDL cholesterol include the presence or absence of CHD, other clinical forms of atherosclerotic disease , and the major risk factors other than LDL. Other major risk factors are cigarette smoking, hypertension, low HDL cholesterol, family history of premature CHD, diabetes and age. These major risks are commonly observed in patients with mental illness.

A variety of medical conditions and drugs can exacerbate hyperlipidemias. Elevations of the serum LDL cholesterol level can occur in response to hypothyroidism and nephrotic syndrome. Hypertriglyceridemia and decreased HDL levels are commonly seen with insulin resistance, diabetes, and the metabolic syndrome. This fact is usually seen in patients with mental illness. Individuals are characterized by their coronary risk profile according to the National Cholesterol Education Program Adult Treatment Panel III guidelines, as shown in Table 5.

Lipoprotein and serum concentration	Status
Low-density lipoprotein (LDL) cholesterol) (primary target of therapy)	
<100 mg/dl	Optimal
100-129mg/dl	Near optimal
130-159 mg/dl	Borderline high
≥160 mg/dl	High
Total cholesterol	
<200 mg/dl	Desired
200-239 mg/dl	Borderline high
≥ 240 mg/dl	High
HDL cholesterol	
<40	Low
≥60	High

Table 5. ATP III Classification of LDL, Total, and HDL Cholesterol (mg/dL)

6.2 Monitoring

To monitor for antipsychotic - associated metabolic disturbances, patients should be assessed before antipsychotic treatment is initiated. The results of such an assessment can also influence antipsychotic choice, particularly when patients have existing metabolic pathology or elevated risk factors. The frequency of subsequent assessments is different as it is reflected in the various antipsychotic monitoring guidelines: Mount Sinai (Chobarian et al, 2003), Australia (Lambert et al, 2004) ADA-APA(ADA,2004) Belgium (De Nayer, 2005), United Kingdom (Expert Consensus Meeting, 2004), Canada (Canadian Diabetes Association, 2005), France (Saravane et al, 2009) (Table 6).To summarize these recommendations, there are many aeras of general agreement about the importance of baseline monitoring before starting treatment and that patients should be followed more closely for the first 3 to 4 months of treatment, with subsequent ongoing reevaluation. The utility of the following tests and measures was emphasized: fasting plasma glucose, fasting lipid profile, weight and height, waist circumference, and blood pressure.

A recent study characterizes associations between the combined warnings and recommendations and baseline metabolic testing and Second-Generation Antipsychotic Drugs (SGA). A total of 109451 patients receiving Medicaid who began taking SGA was compared to a control cohort of 203527 patients who began taking albuterol but did nor receive antipsychotic medication. The main outcome measures was the monthly rates of baseline serum glucose and lipid testing for SGA-treated and propensity-matched albuterol-treated patients and monthly share of new prescriptions for each SGA drug. In a Medicaid-receiving patients, baseline glucose and lipid testing for SGA was infrequent and showed little change following the monitoring recommendations. Initial testing rates for SGA-treated patients were low: glucose, 27%; lipids, 10%. The warning was not associated with an increase in glucose testing among SGA-treated patients and was associated with only a marginal increase in lipid testing rates: 1.7%; P=. 02.(Morrato, 2010).

The important question is given the risks in patients with mental illness, how should they be monitored and how should they be treated?

Current studies indicate that patients with mental illness do not receive adequate evaluation and effective treatment of their cardio-metabolic problems. Effective communication between the primary care physician and the psychiatrist is very important for the mentally ill because of their impaired capacity to care for themselves. Such communication will improve monitoring, help early detection of metabolic disorders, and limit duplication of clinical or laboratory workup. Monitoring for metabolic side effects is primarily the responsibility of the physician prescribing antipsychotic medication and in most cases that would be a psychiatrist.

If the primary care physician observes that the patient is being prescribed such drugs without being monitored effectively, he/she should discuss this with the psychiatrist. The psychiatrist may not have the expertise to manage any abnormalities that are detected and in such situations the primary care physician will most likely take over both monitoring and management. Liaison should extend to any healthcare professionals involved in the care of patients with mental illness.

Given the serious health risks, patients taking antipsychotic drugs should receive appropriate baseline screening and ongoing monitoring.

	Mount Sinaï	Australia	ADA-APA	Belgium	UK	Canada	France
	Patients to monitor						
	Schizophrenia any antipsychotic	All patients any antipsychotic	All patients SGA	Schizophrenia SGA	Schizophrenia any antipsychotic	Schizophrenia	All patients any antipsychotic
Fasting Plasma Glucose (FPG)	x	x	x	x	x	x	x
Random glucose		x			x		
Hba1c	If FPG not feasible				x		
OGTT						Follow up	
Lipids	x	x	x	x		x	x
Weight	x	x	x	x		x	x
Height	x	x	x	x		x	x
Waist circumference	x	x	x	x		x	x
Hip		x					x
Family and medical history	x	x	x	x		x	x
Ethnicity	x	x		x			
Tobacco				x			
Diet activity		x		x		x	
Signs and symptoms of diabetes	x		x	x	x	x	x
ECG							x
Blood pressure		x	x	x		x	x

Table 6. Recommended guidelines to monitor and initial workup.

6.2.1 Baseline monitoring

The recommendations are that baseline screening measures be obtained before or as soon as clinically feasible after, the initiation of any antipsychotic medication. We have to consider ethnicity, dietary habits, physical activity, support system, smoking, and alcohol and drug abuse. Keep in mind that psychotropic medications other than antipsychotic drugs such as some antidepressants and mood stabilizers may link to weight gain. The baseline assessments include:

- Personal and family history of obesity, diabetes, dyslipidemia, hypertension or cardiovascular disease
- Weight and height, so that BMI can be calculated
- Waist circumference at the level of the umbilicus
- Blood pressure
- Fasting plasma glucose
- Fasting lipid profile

If any abnormalities are identified, first, patients should be informed of their condition and supported in making lifestyle changes to adopt a healthier diet and increase physical activity. Psychiatrists should not hesitate to refer the patient to the appropriate health care professional or specialist knowledgeable about these disorders.

Even for patients free of metabolic disorders, monitor potential risk factors. Weight gain may not be dose-dependent and patients with low body mass index at baseline may be particularly vulnerable to weight gain. Glucose and lipid metabolism abnormalities may occur without weight gain.

6.2.2 Follow-up monitoring

The patient's weight should be reassessed at 4, 8, and 12 weeks after initiating or changing SGA therapy and quarterly thereafter at the time of routine visits. If a patient gains > 5% of his or her initial weight at any time during therapy, one should consider switching the medication. When switching, consideration should be given to all aspects of the individual's condition, the comparative risks and benefits of changing medications, and the individual's response to medication in managing the primary symptoms of the mental illness. In some cases, cost and availability may also be a consideration.

Fasting plasma glucose, lipid profile, and blood pressure should also be assessed 3 months after initiation of medication. Thereafter, blood pressure, plasma glucose values, lipid profile should be obtained annually or more frequently in those who have a higher baseline risk for the development of diabetes, dyslipidemia or hypertension.

7. Treatment

With all the risk factors and in the case of dyslipidemia and to reduce the global mortality of patients with mental illness we should consider lipid goal of therapy for these patients. The benefits and risks of different therapeutic agents used in the treatment of dyslipidemia and its comorbidities should be considered in the context of the patient's psychiatric condition and treatment.

7.1 Drugs

ATP III recommends a multifaceted lifestyle approach to reduce risk for coronary heart disease (CHD). This approach is designated therapeutic lifestyle changes (TLC). Some patients whose short-term or long-term risk for CHD is high will require LDL-lowering drugs in addition to TLC. When drugs are prescribed, attention to TLC should always be maintained and reinforced. Available drugs are:

- HMG-CoA reductase inhibitors: statins, their side effects are myopathy and increased liver enzymes
- Bile acid sequestrants , their side effects including gastrointestinal distress, constipation and decreased absorption of some drugs
- Nicotinic acid side effects are essentially flushing, hyperglycemia, hyperuricemia (gout), upper gastrointestinal distress and hepatotoxicity
- Fibric acids, with their side effects including dyspepsia, gallstones, myopathy, unexplained non-CHD deaths in WHO study

All these drugs reduced major coronary events, CHD deaths but we have to be carefull with their side effects and contraindications when prescribing these drugs.
Beyond the underlying risk factor, therapies directed against the lipid and nonlipid risk factors of the metabolic syndrome will reduce CHD risk.
The management of dyslipidemia in mental health is defined, as recommended by the Consensus Development Conference on Antipsychotic Drugs and Obesity and Diabetes by:
The lifestyle interventions with diet, increased physical activity and smoking cessation. They are the firs-line treatments to decrease the risk for cardiovascular disease in patient with metabolic syndrome.

7.2 Diet

Interventions that address nutrition and weight management should become a routine part of psychiatric care. Patients with mental illness did not know the components of a healthy diet. The healthy eating behavior includes:

- Cutting down fast food
- Increased healthy food items like fruits, vegetables, fish and decreased high glycemic index food items and monounsaturated fats
- Decreased processed fat free food
- Consume 4-6, but small meals
- Minimizing intake of soft drinks with sugar and with artificial sweetener

The lifestyle changes should be gradual and adapted individually for each patient. There are various educational and psychosocial programs that address the issues of health and wellness exist, like ' The Healthy Living' program (Vreeland, 2007; Hoffmann et al, 2006).

7.3 Physical activity

Patients who developed psychosis are more likely to be physically inactive (OR=3.3,95% CI 1.4-7.9) and to have poor cardio respiratory fitness (OR=2.2, 95% CI 0.6-7.8) compared with those who did not develop psychosis (Koivukangas et al, 2010). Modern guidelines on managing the physical health risks associated with schizophrenia include a recommendation about the importance of physical activity levels and fitness. This recommendation includes:

- To advise patients to engage at least 30 minutes of moderately vigorous activity on most days of the week
- Reduce sedentary behaviors such as TV watching, video/computer games
- Treating/reducing sedation and extra pyramidal effects of medications

Some studies showed that physical activity, with and without diet, resulted in modest weight loss, reduction of blood pressure and decreases in fasting plasma concentrations of glucose and insulin (Vancampfort et al, 2009).

7.4 Medication

In the general population there are many studies evaluating the impact of lipid lowering in primary and secondary prevention of coronary heart disease and stroke, but there are some concerns about its value in primary prevention, especially in vulnerable population (Vrecer et al, 2003).

Whether a low or lowered serum cholesterol level is associated with harm has been the subject of debate for a long time; ever since the unexpected finding of an increased risk of noncardiovascular mortality in early trials of lipid-lowering therapy. Subsequent research has generated conflicting evidence regarding the relation between cholesterol and violent behavior, mental illness , with positive studies imputing alterations in central serotoninergic activity as a potential underlying mechanism. A case-control study studied a cohort of 94441 individuals, 458 had newly diagnosed depression and 105 had a recorded diagnosis of suicide risk. Compared with matched control subjects, and even after adjustment for potential confounders, neither dyslipidemia nor its treatment was associated with an increase risk of depression. Similarly, no association was found between treatment and suicide risk. (Yang, 2003).

A 3-month study demonstrated that statins prescribed to patients with schizophrenia and severe dyslipidemia whilst taking antipsychotic medication led to a significant improvement in lipid profiles (Hanssens et, 2007). An earlier study with rosuvastatin proved effective in managing dyslipidemia in schizophrenic patients on antipsychotics. This study showed improvement in lipid profiles but not benefits in terms of high-density lipoprotein, waist measurement, BMI or glucose homeostasis (De Hert et al, 2006).

This last study supports the view that statins can be safely used in the short term to control abnormal lipids levels. However, there are no long-term data on its impact on either relapse or all-cause mortality, and again this is a priority for research.

The presence of metabolic syndrome is an indication for more aggressive lipid-lowering measures. Medications that raise HDL, nicotinic acid or fibrates, may be particularly beneficial in patients with metabolic syndrome, but they have not been as widely studied as medications that lower LDL-cholesterol in patients with mental illness.

The preferred initial management is still very much a lifestyle modification approach including exercise and diet.

8. Conclusion

Despite the availability of published clinical guidelines, patients with mental illness receiving medications remain vulnerable to the cardio-metabolic complications of these drugs. Implementation of a coordinated metabolic monitoring and management program for patient with mental illness will require a review of current practice and the introduction of new procedures, both of which will require time and effort on the part of the health care community.

Involvement of patient with mental illness in their treatment program will require the provision of information about their condition and medication and the development of approaches that empower, encourage, and support patients in their decisions on treatment and well-being.

The evaluation of new therapies should include detailed assessments of physical health and future risk estimates in addition to standard psychiatric outcomes. Psychiatrists have to arrange the appropriate examination and investigation of patients at risk of developing

significant physical morbidity, working very closely with general practitioners and with other specialists when appropriate. We have to weight up the risk of metabolic disturbance and its potential impact on future cardiovascular risk when selecting an antipsychotic drug. We have to take a careful medical history and be prepared to monitor weight and other metabolic risk, such as glucose and lipid profile. The lipid area is significantly understudied in patients taking antipsychotic medications. Lipids may be more important than diabetes because dyslipidemia appears to occur at a higher prevalence in this patient population. Lipid levels are a significant problem because physicians are seeing hypertriglyceridemia. Knowing what we know about what causes and contributes to cardiovascular disease, we are obliged to play detective and figure out why psychiatric patients are dying sooner and more often of cardiovascular disease than the general population.
The big challenge for all is to ensure that the physical health of patients with mental illness is given the priority it deserves, helping them to face their future with the lowest possible morbidity and mortality odds stacked against them.

9. References

Alberti KGMM, Zimmet P, Shaw J. (2006). Metabolic syndrome - a new world - wide definition. A consensus statement from the International Diabetes Federation. Diabetic 25: 469–80

Allison DB, Metore JL, HEO M et al. (1999). Antipsychotic-induced weight gain: a comprehensive research synthesis. Am J Psychiatry, 156: 1686-1696

Allison DB, Casey De (2001); Antipsychotic–induced weight gain: a review of the literature. J Clin Psychiatry 6é (Suppl 7): 22-31

American Diabetes Association; American Psychiatric Association; American Association of Clinical Endocrinologists; North American Association for the Study of Obesity. Consensus development conference on antipsychotic drugs and obesity and diabetes care (2004); 27: 596-601. Available at: http//care. Diabetejournals.org/cgi/reprint/27/2/596

American Diabetes Association, American Psychiatric Association, American Association of Clinical Endocrinologists; North American Association for the Study of Obesity. Consensus development conference on antipsychotic drugs and obesity and diabetes care. Diabetes Care (2004); 27: 596-601

Bartsch DA, Shen DL, Feinberg LE et al (1990). Screening CMHC out patients for physical illness. Hospital and Community Psychiatry 41: 786-790

Birkenaes AB, Birkeland Ja, Engh JA et al (2008). Dyslipidemia independent of body mass in antipsychotic-treated patients under real-life conditions; J Clin Psychopharmacol 28: 132-137

Brown S. (1997). Excess mortality of schizophrenia A meta - analysis. Br J. Psychiatry; 171: 502–8

Calandre EP, Rodriguez-Lopez C, Blasquez A et al, (1991). Serum lipids, lipoproteins and apolipoprotein A and B in epileptic patients treated with valproic acid and carbamazepine or Phenobarbital. Acta Neurol Scand, 83(4): 250-253

Cohn T, Prud'homme D, Streiner D et al. (2004)Characterizing coronary heart disease risk in chronic schizophrenia: high prevalence of the metabolic syndrome. Can J Psychiary, 49: 753-60

Colton CW, Manderscheid RW (2006). Congruencies in increased mortality rates, year of potential life lost, and causes of death among public mental health clients in eight states. Prev Chronic Dis, 3: A42

Consensus development conference on antipsychotic drugs and obesity and diabetes (2004) J Clin Psychiatry 65(2): 267-272

Correl CV. (2007) Balancing efficacy and safety in treatment with antipsychotics. CNS Spectr; 12 (suppl, 17) : 12–20

Canadian Diabetes Association. (2005) Positision paper: antipsychotic medications and associated risk of weight gain and diabetes. Canadian Journal of Diabetes 29:111-2

Chobanian AV, Bakris GL, Black HR, Cushman WC, Green LA, Izzo JL Jr, and others. (2003) Seventh report of the Joint National Committee on Prevenion, Detection, Evaluation, and Treatment of High Blood Pressure. Hypertension 42: 1206-52.

Cradock-O'Leary J, Young AS, Yano EM, et al (2002). Use of general medical services by VA patients psychiatric disorders. Psychiatr Serv 53: 874-878

Davidson M (2002). Risk of cardiovascular disease and sudden death in schizophrenia. J Clin Psychiatry 63 (Suppl 9): 5-11

De Hert M,Kalnicka D, van Winkel R et al. (2006). Treatment with rosuvastatin for severe dyslipidemia in patients with schizophrenia and schizoaffective disorder. J Clin Psychiatry 67/1889-96.

De Leon J, Susce MT, Johnson M et al (2007). A clinical study of the association of antipsychotics with hyperlipidemia Schizophr Res 92 : 95-102

De Nayer A, De Hert M, Scheem A, Van Gaal L, Peuskens J. (2005) Belgian consensus on metabolic problems associated with atypical antipsychotics. International Journal of Psychiatry in Clinical Pratice 9:130-7

Dworkin R (1994). Pain insensitivity in schizophrenia: A neglected phenomenon and some implications. Schizophrenia Bulletin 20: 235-248

Dwyer DS, Donohoe D: (2003) Induction of hyperglycemia in mice with atypical antipsychotic drugs that inhibit glucose uptake. 75:255-260

Expert Panel on Detection and Evaluation of Treatment of High Blood Cholesterol in Adults. Executive summary of the third report of the National Cholesterol Education Program (NCEP) expert panel on detection, evaluation and treatment of high blood cholesterol in adults (Adult Treatment Panel III)(2001). JAMA, 285: 2486-97

Expert Group. "Schizophrenia and Diabetes 2003" Expert Consensus Meeting. (2004) Dublin, 3-4 October 2003: consensus summary. Br J Psychiatry Suppl 47:S112-4

Fanzoni E, Govoni M, D'Addato S et al (1991). Total cholesterol, high-density lipoprotein cholesterol, and triglycerides in children receiving antiepileptic drugs. Epilepsia, 33(5): 932-935

Felker B, Yazel JJ, Short D (1996). Mortality and medical comorbidity among psychiatric patients. A review. Psychiatric Services 47: 1356-1363

Garland EJ, Remick RA, Zis AP: (1998) Weight gain with antidepressants and lithium. J Clin Psychopharmocol, 8(5): 323-330

Goldman L (1999). Medical illness in patients with schizophrenia Journal of Clinical Psychiatry, Suppl 21, vol 60 pp 10-15

Grundy SM, Cleeman JL, Daniels SR et al (2005). Diagnosis and management of the metabolic syndrome: an American Heart Association/National Heart, Lung and Blood

Institute Scientific Statement. Circulation, 112: 2735-52

Hall RC, Gardner ER, Popkin MK et al; (1981) Unrecognized physical illness prompting psychiatric admission: a prospective study. Am J Psychiatry 138: 629-635

Hanssens L, De Hert M, van Winkel R et al. (2007) Pharmacological treatment of severe dyslipidaemia in patients with schizophrenia. Int J Clin Psychopharnacol; 22:43-9

Harris EC, Barraclough B (1998). Excess mortality of mental disorder . British Journal of Psychiatry 173: 11-53

Henderson DC, Copeland PM, Borba CP et al (2006). Glucose metabolism in patients with schizophrenia treated with olanzapine or quetiapine: a frequently sampled intravenous glucose tolerance test and minimal model analysis. J Clin Psychiatry 67: 789-797.

Hoffmann VP, Bushe C, Meyers AL et al (2008). A wellness intervention program for patients with mental illness:self-reported outcomes. J Clin Psychiatry 10(4): 329-331

Isojärvi JL, Rättyä J, Myllylä VV et al (1998). Valproate, lamitrogene, and insulin-mediated risks in women with epilepsy. Ann Neurol, 43(4): 446-451

Koran LM, Sox HC Jr, Marton KI et al (1989). Medical evaluation of psychiatric patients. Results in a state mental health system. Arch Gen Psychiatry 46: 733-740

Koranyi EK (1979). Morbidity and rate of undiagnosed physical illnesses in a psychiatric clinic population. Arch Gen Psychiatry 36: 414-419

Koivukangas J, Tammelin T, Kaakinen M et al (2010). Physical activity and fitness in adolescents at risk for psychosis within the Northern Finland 1986 Birth Cohort. Schizophr Res 116: 152-158

Lambert TJR, Velakoulis D, Pantelis C (2003).Medical comorbidity in schizophrenia. Medical Journal of Australia 178, Suppl 5: 567-570

Lambert TJ, Chapman LH. (Aust 2004) Diabetes, psychotic disorders and antipsychotic therapy: a consensus statement Med J 181:544-8

Lawrence D, Holman C, Jablensky A et al (2003). Death rate from ischemic heart disease in Western Australian psychiatric patients 1980-1998; British Journal of Psychiatry 182: 31-36

Lyketsos C, Dunn G, Kaminsky M et al (2002). Medical comorbidity in psychiatric inpatients. Relation to clinical outcomes and hospital length of stay Psychosomatics 43: 24-30

Matsui-Sakata A, Ohtani H, Sawada Y/ (2005) Receptor occupancy-based analysis of the contribution of various receptors to antipsychotic-induced weight gain and diabetes mellitus. Drug Metab Pharmacokinet 27:398-378

Mc Creadle RG (2003). Diet, smoking and cardiovascular risk in people with schizophrenia. Descriptive study. British Journal of Psychiatry, 183, 534-539

Mc Evoy JP, Meyer JM, Goff et al (2005). Prevalence of the metabolic syndrome in patients with schizophrenia: baseline results from the Clinical Antipsychotic Trials of Intervention Effectiveness (CATIE) schizophrenia trial and comparison with national estimates from NHANES III, schizophr Res, 80: 19–32

Meyer JM, Nasrallah HA, Mc Evoy JP et al (2005). The clinical Antipsychotic Trials of Intervention Effectiveness (CATIE) Schizophrenia Trial: clinical comparison of subgroups with and without the metabolic syndrome Shizophr Res, 80: 9–18

Meyer JM (2001). Effects of typical Antipsychotics on weight and serum lipid levels. J. Clin Psychiatry, 62 (suppl 27), 27–34

Morrato EH, Druss B, Hartung DM et al (2010). Metabolic testing in 3 states Medicaid programs after FDA warnings and ADA/APA recommendations for second-generation antipsychotic drugs Arch Gen Psychiatry, vol 67(1): 17-25

Mortensen P , Juel K (1993). Mortality and causes of death in first admitted schizophrenic patients. British Journal of Psychiatry 163: 183-189

Newcomer J. (2005) Second-generation (atypical) antipsychotics and metabolic effects : a comprehensive literature review? CNS Drugs, 19

Nasrallah HA (2008). Atypical antipsychotic-induced metabolic side effects: insights from receptor-binding profiles. Mol Psychiatry 13: 27-35

Nasralah HA, Meyer JM, Goff DC et al. (2006). Low rates of treatment for hypertention, dyslipidemia and diabetes in schizophrenia: data from the CATIE schizophrenia trial sample at baseline. Schizophr RES 86: 15-22

Reynolds GP, Hill MJ, Kirk SI (2006). The 5-HT2C receptor and antipsychotic induced weight gain-mechanisms and genetics, J. Psychopharmacol, 20: 15-18

Ringback Weitoft G, Gullberg A, Rosen M (1998). Avoidable mortality among psychiatric patients. Social Psychiatry and Psychiatric Epidemiology 33: 430-437

Rushena D, Mullen P, Burgess P, et al (1998). Sudden death in psychiatric patients. British Journal of Psychiatry 173: 331-336

Rutstein D, Berenberg W, Chalmers T et al (1976). Measuring the quality of medical care. A clinical method. New England Journal of Medecine 294: 582-588

Saravane D, B. Feve, Frances Y et al (2009). Drawing up guidelines for the attendance of physical health of patients with severe mental illness. L'Encéphale, 35: 330–339

Sarafidis PA, Nilsson PM (2006). The metabolic syndrome: a glance at its history. J Hypertension, 24: 621 – 626

Silvestre JS, Prous J: (2005) Research on adverse drug events, I: muscarinic M3 receptor binding affinity could predict the risk antipsychotics to induce type 2 diabetes. Methods Find Exp Clin Pharmacol 27:289-304

Vancampfort D, Knapen J, De Hert M et al (2009). Cardiometabolic effects of physical activity interventions for people with schizophrenia. Phys Ther Rev 14: 388-398

Vestri HS, Maianu L, Moellering DR et al (2007). Atypical antipsychotic drugs directly impair insulin action in adipocytes: effects on glucose transport, lipogenesis, and antilipolysis, Neuropsychopharmacology 32: 765-772

Vrecer M, Turk S, Drinovec J et al (2003). Use of statin in primary and secondary prevention of coronary heart disease and ischemic stroke. Meta-analysis of randomized trials. Int J Clin Pharmacol Ther 41: 567-577

Vreeland B (2007). Behavioral changes in patients with mental illness. J Clin Psychiatry 68 (Suppl 4): 8-13

Wilson PW, D'Agostini RB, Levy D et al (1998). Prediction of coronary heart disease using risk factor categories. Circulation 97: 1837-1847

Wulsin LR (2000). Does depression kills? Arch Intern Med 160: 1731-1732

Yang CC, Jick SS, Jick H (2003). Lipid-lowering drugs and the risk of depression and suicidal behavior. Arch Intern Med 163: 1926-1932

Zimmermann U, Kraus T, Himmerisch H et al (2003). Epidemiology, implications and mechanisms underlying drug-induced weight gain in psychiatric patients. J Psychiatr Res, 37(3): 193-220

18

Dyslipidemia Induced by Stress

Fernanda Klein Marcondes[1], Vander José das Neves[1], Rafaela Costa[1], Andrea Sanches[1], Tatiana Sousa Cunha[1,2], Maria José Costa Sampaio Moura[3], Ana Paula Tanno[4] and Dulce Elena Casarini[5*]

1. Introduction

The pioneering work of Hans Selye (1936) led to the use of the word "stress" in a biological context gaining popularity world-wide. Stress is as an organic response to stressors that can be aversive stimuli or unknown situations capable of compromising homeostasis. During the stress reaction, the sympathetic nervous system and hypothalamic-pituitary-adrenal axis are stimulated. Consequently, serum concentrations of classical stress hormones, namely catecholamines and glucocorticoids, are increased and act on cells and tissues inducing adaptive changes in order to protect the organism and allow its survival. In addition, the stress reaction can also modulate immune system activities and the secretion of other hormones (gonadotrophins, estrogen, testosterone, thyroid, angiotensins).

Considering that organic homeostatic systems are subject to frequent environmental and internal variations, Sterling and Eyer (1988) proposed the term alostasis to describe the adaptative processes that actively maintain stability through physiological changes.

The terms eustress and efficient allostasis describe facile adaptation, such as a quick peak stress response to mobilize energy to deal with an acute stressor, and a rapid return to baseline, when the stressor terminates. On the other hand, distress or allostatic load refers to an imbalance in systems that promote adaptation (Epel, 2009; Korte et al., 2005). This imbalance can simply be the result of too much repeated stress, but it can also be the result of adaptative systems that are out of balance and fail to shut-off or, alternatively, systems that fail to return to normal (Epel, 2009). Therefore the shut-off of the stress response is particularly important, because, when systems do not shut off in time, they can cause damage or promote pathology (McEwen, 1998).

The classical stress hormones, glucocorticoids (cortisol) and catecholamines (epinephrine and norepinephrine), are catabolic and modulate the breakdown of glycogen, triglycerides and proteins into molecules that can be rapidly metabolized in order to generate energy (Black, 2002). These responses enable energy substrates to be directed to organs and tissues

*[1]Department of Physiological Sciences, Piracicaba Dental School, University of Campinas, Piracicaba, Brazil
[2]Science and Technology Institute, Federal University of São Paulo, São José dos Campos, Brazil
[3]Life Sciences Center, Pontifical Catholic University of Campinas, Campinas, Brazil
[4]Division of Pharmacy, Faculty of Americana, Americana, Brazil
[5]Department of Medicine, Federal University of São Paulo, São Paulo, Brazil

with the greatest demand during the stress reaction, and support the fight or flight reaction to a stressor.

During acute stress, there is a rapid and transient increase in blood concentrations of total cholesterol, low-density lipoprotein (LDL), apoprotein B, triglycerides, and free fatty acids (Stoney, 2007). This increase persists as along as the stressor is maintained (Black, 2002), and disappears in stress-free periods (Stoney et al., 1999). In chronic stress situations, it has been shown that dyslipidemia is maintained and may persist even after the stressor is no longer present (Neves et al., 2009).

2. Dyslipidemia induced by stress: Physiological mechanisms

Many studies have shown the effect of stress on lipid metabolism. Stress associated with a major disaster, such as an earthquake or loss of job and income is associated with increased total cholesterol, LDL, and triglycerides in the bloodstream (Stoney, 2007). The perception of increased stress during a period of high workload is associated with elevated cholesterol in the bloodstream and ingestion of foods that increase cholesterol (McCann et al., 1990). Acute psychological stress in healthy men and women reduces the clearance rate of exogenous fat (Stoney et al., 2002). Chronic psychological stress increased the plasma cholesterol level in medical students (O'Donnell et al., 1987). In a more recent study, Yoo et al., 2011, showed high prevalence of hypercholesterolemia in stressed female law enforcement officers in comparison with the general female population. Moreover, elevated basal cortisol concentrations and lower circadian cortisol variability can induce dyslipidemia in patients with depressive and anxiety disorders (Venn et al., 2009; Vogelzangs et al., 2007). These patients presented hypercortisolism, increased serum levels of total cholesterol, LDL, and triglycerides and decreased serum levels of HDL (Venn et al., 2009).

In animal studies, it has been shown that electric shock stress increases plasma cholesterol concentrations (Berger et al., 1980), and unpredictable immobilization stress decreases HDL, increases blood LDL, and very-low-density lipoprotein (VLDL) concentrations in rats (Bryant et al., 1988). Chronic mild unpredictable stress increases triglycerides, total cholesterol, VLDL, and LDL concentrations in the bloodstream of stressed rats compared with control rats and this effect was observed 15 days after the stress protocol had ended (Neves et al., 2009).

The stressful modern lifestyle exerts a strong influence on lipid metabolism (Black, 2002) and may transform adaptative responses to pathophysiological changes. Acute increases in blood lipids are necessary for the individual to survive and adapt to the stressor. However prolonged changes in lipid metabolism induced by chronic stress can result in cardiovascular diseases such as atherosclerosis, coronary heart disease, and stroke (Brindley et al., 1993).

The negative effects of sustained stress-induced dyslipidemia are related to a bidirectional relationship between stress hormones and insulin. Catecholamines directly stimulate free fatty acid and glycerol secretion in the bloodstream from fat depots, a process that may result from increased blood flow through adipose tissue or from adipose-β_2 adrenoceptor stimulation (Stoney, 2007). Stress-induced high glucocorticoid concentration exerts a permissive effect on these lipolytic actions of catecholamines (Brindley et al., 1993). Since insulin regulates triglyceride synthesis and hepatic VLDL production, insulin resistance results in unregulated triglyceride synthesis and VLDL production (Stoney, 2007) and triglycerides are secreted by the liver in large quantities within the VLDL particles (Black, 2003). Therefore both catecholamines and glucocorticoids antagonize the actions of insulin, contributing to insulin resistance (Kyrou & Tsigos, 2009; Lafontan & Langin, 2009).

Moreover, hyperinsulinemia acts centrally to stimulate sympathetic nervous system activity, resulting in increased secretion of catecholamines (Black, 2003), and the absence of satisfactory insulin action facilitates the actions of cortisol and glucagon, which in turn stimulate phosphatidate phosphohydrolase activity to synthesize hepatic triglyceride (Brindley et al., 1993).

The cortisol also induces apoprotein B (apo B) secretion from the liver in the proportion of one apo B molecule per VLDL particle (Brindley et al., 1993), consequently increasing the VLDL concentrations in the bloodstream. As each VLDL particle is metabolized to intermediate-density lipoprotein (IDL) or LDL, the action of the cortisol that stimulates apo B secretion also results in increased LDL particles in the blood. Furthermore, in the presence of stress-induced insulin resistance, high levels of glucocorticoids suppress the hepatic LDL receptors, which delay LDL clearance (Stoney, 2007).

Contributing to all these processes, it has been shown that perilipin, which coats the surface of lipid droplets to restrict lipase access to the triglyceride core within the droplet, may suffer phosphorylation and/or down-regulation by glucocorticoid action, thereby facilitating the lipolysis of triglycerides in fatty acids and glycerol (Xu et al., 2001). This sets off a vicious cycle, leading to more and more triglycerides being produced by the liver and secreted in VLDL particles, as a result of the stimulation of glucocorticoids and fatty acids.

In addition, norepinephrine and cortisol inhibit lipoprotein lipase activity, leading to diminished triglyceride clearance, decrease in HDL concentration, and increase in VLDL, IDL, and LDL concentrations in the bloodstream (Stoney, 2007). Norepinephrine also diminishes hepatic triglyceride lipase activity, which in turn promotes high concentrations of lipoproteins rich in triglycerides in the blood (Stoney, 2007).

In the context of stress-induced dyslipidemia, changes in food ingestion must also be considered. During acute stress, transient dyslipidemia and food intake inhibition are mediated by β-adrenergic activation and increased hypothalmic corticotrophin releasing hormone (CRH) levels which act as catabolic signals. On the other hand, chronic activation of the hypothalamic-pituitary-adrenal axis has been associated with overeating and obesity (Dallman et al., 2004; Nishitani & Sakakibara, 2006). Many studies have supported this relationship. Lemieux & Coe, 1995, related that approximately 50% of women with posttraumatic stress disorder as a result of childhood sexual abuse were overweight, and also showed high concentrations of norepinephrine, epinephrine, and dopamine in urine. Changes in sleep-wake cycles associated with stress, resulting in sleep loss, induce decreased leptin levels, increased ghrelin levels, and increased hunger and appetite (Pejovic et al., 2010; Spiegel et al., 2004). In addition, the parent's lifestyle can influence metabolism, and individuals exposed to maternal stress during intrauterine life can exhibit deregulation of body weight control mechanisms and blood lipid profile (De Moura, 2008). The relationship between excessive glucocorticoids and visceral fat accumulation has also been discussed by Björntorp & Rosmond, 1999.

Thus, the typical response to chronic stress is not by way of avoiding food but by increasing the intake of sugar- and fat-rich comfort foods, which make people feel better

(Stoney, 2007; Torres & Nowson, 2007). Dallman et al., 2003, suggested that people or animals eat comfort food in an attempt to reduce activity in the 'chronic stress-response network' with its attendant anxiety. They suggested the following mechanism: first, in the periphery, glucocorticoids stimulate accretion of mesenteric energy stores; second, as the abdominal energy-generated (unidentified) signal increases, the negative input to catecholaminergic cells in the nucleus tractus solitarius reduces the synthesis of enzymes required for norepinephrine synthesis; third, the decreased noradrenergic signal to the hypothalamic paraventricular nucleus (PVN), in turn, decreases CRH synthesis and secretion. Thus, there is a powerful metabolic feedback control of CRH in the PVN, which may indirectly decrease glucocorticoid-action in the central nucleus of the amygdala; and thereby control anxiety (Korte et al., 2005). Consequently, all these mechanisms can lead to obesity and dyslipidemia due to overeating. In addition, it has been proposed that when chronic stress, to which animals and humans cannot easily adapt, is combined with high-fat high-sugar diets, it stimulates the sympathetic nerves to upregulate the expression of neuropeptide Y, an adrenergic cotransmitter and stress mediator. Stress and hypercaloric diets also increase glucocorticoid concentration in visceral fat, which in turn upregulates the expression of neuropeptide Y and its receptor Y2R, resulting in fat growth, hyperinsulinemia and hyperlipidemia (Bartolomucci et al., 2009; Kuo et al., 2008).

Some studies have also shown that glucocorticoid actions in the target tissues depend not only on circulating hormone levels, but also on intracellular glucocorticoid receptors and activities of both 11β-Hydroxysteroid dehydrogenase type 1 (11β-HSD1) and 2 (Bose et al., 2009). The effects of glucocorticoid are enhanced by the enzyme 11β-HSD1 in the stromal cells of visceral fat, since this enzyme catalyzes the conversion of inactive cortisone to active glucocorticoid in local tissue. It has been shown that transgenic knockout mice, which overexpress 11β-HSD1 in adipose tissue, present accumulation of visceral adipose tissue, hypertension, dyslipidemia and glucose intolerance (Masuzaki et al., 2001; Masuzaki & Flier, 2003). Therefore 11β-HSD1 plays an important role in the development of metabolic disease associated with stress (Bose et al., 2009; Walker & Stewart, 2003).

In addition, cytokines such as interleukin 6 (IL-6), tumor necrosis factor (TNF)-α, and leptin released from fatty cells also contribute to dyslipidemia induced by stress. IL-6 increases the activity of 11β-HSD1 with consequent expansion of visceral fat. TNF-α induces lipolysis in adipose tissue. Both IL-6 and TNF-α decrease lipoprotein lipase activity, contributing to the increase in triglyceride levels induced by stress (Black, 2003). Moreover, TNF-α induces insulin resistance because it depresses insulin receptor activity (Yudkin et al., 2000). TNF-α also induces IL-6 synthesis, and stimulates leptin synthesis, which acts centrally to decrease appetite and increase thermogenesis to decrease fat storage (Black, 2003). Leptin increases the activity of sympathetic nervous system centrally (Mohamed-Ali et al., 1998), which in turn stimulates increased release of TNF-α and IL-6 from adipocytes (Black, 2003). This sympathetic nervous system hyperactivity induced by high levels of leptin in the bloodstream would provide an additional effect of catecholamines on the genesis of insulin resistance and dyslipidemia associated with stress in obese individuals.

Therefore, dyslipidemia induced by stress involves complex interactions among stress hormones, insulin, adipose tissue metabolism and cytokines. Figure 1 indicates the physiological mechanisms of dyslipidemia induced by stress.

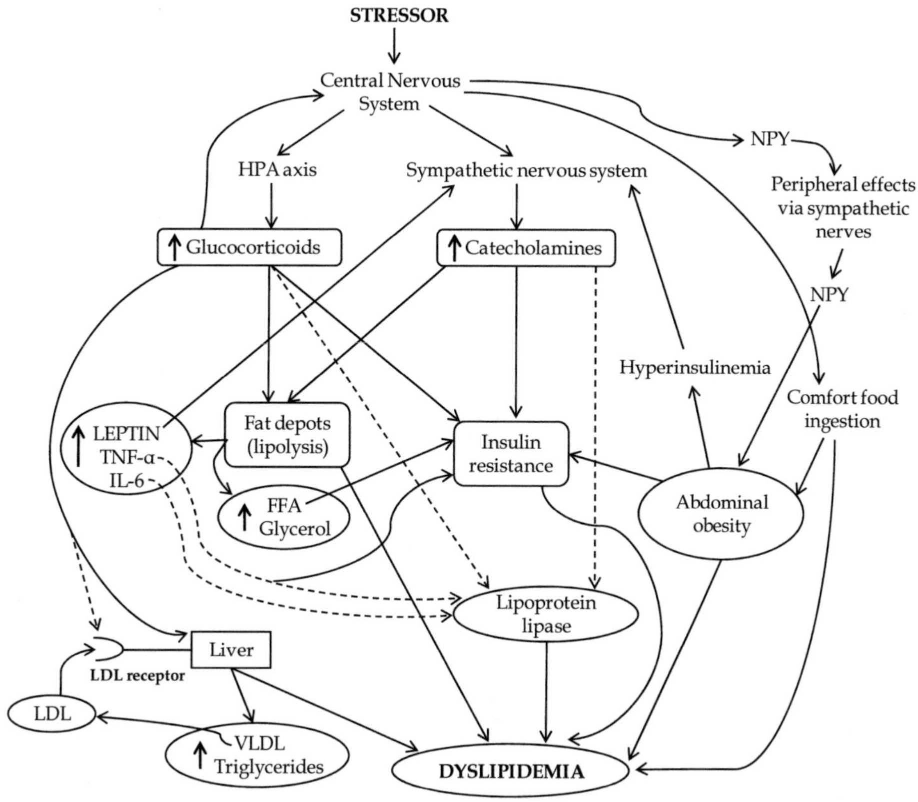

Fig. 1. Schematic representation of physiological mechanisms of dyslipidemia induced by stress. Hypothalamic-pituitary-adrenal axis (HPA), low-density lipoprotein (LDL), very-low-density lipoprotein (VLDL), free fatty acids (FFA), neuropeptide Y (NPY), tumor necrosis factor (TNF-α), interleukin 6 (IL-6). Solid arrows show stimulatory effects; dashed arrows indicate inhibitory effects.

3. Stress, dyslipidemia and atherosclerosis: Putative mechanisms

Atherogenic dyslipidemia is a major underlying cause of the development of atherosclerosis, which is an inflammatory disease (Mullick et al., 2006; Sheril et al., 2009). Since the stress-induced atherogenic lipid profile potentiates the effects of dietary and genetic factors in atherogenesis (Brindley et al., 1993), stress has been recognized as a risk factor for atherosclerosis (Kyrou & Tsigos, 2009; Shively et al., 2009). However, despite the association between dyslipidemia and atherosclerosis, many individuals develop severe atherosclerotic lesions associated with low serum lipid concentration, and others develop far more severe atherosclerosis than would be expected on the basis of a modest elevation of serum lipids (Kaplan et al., 1983). In this context, other effects of stress, not related specifically to dyslipidemia, are also involved in atherogenesis (Bierhaus et al., 2003; Gu et al., 2009) and approximately 40% of cases without known causal factor, have been attributed to stressful situations (Black, 2002).

The atherogenic effects of stress include changes in nitric oxide (NO) and cytokine production, vascular smooth muscle mitogenesis, occurrence of insulin resistance, neuropeptide Y (NPY) actions and modulation of the renin-angiotensin system activity. These effects are directly and indirectly related to stress-induced dyslipidemia, as will be pointed out below.

The healthy endothelium provides a smooth barrier that limits the activation of proinflammatory factors, blocks the transfer of Apo-B 100-containing atherogenic lipid particles into subendothelial space, inhibits the release of chemokines and cytokines, and prevents platelet and monocyte adhesion to the vascular wall (Cersosimo & DeFronzo, 2006). A high amount of NO is produced by endothelial nitric oxide synthase (eNOS). It is a vasodilator, has antithrombogenic properties, is an inhibitor of smooth muscle cell proliferation and of leukocyte- and monocyte-adhesion (Badimón & Martínez-González, 2002; Sudano et al., 2006). Decrease in NO bioavailability is a key feature of endothelial dysfunction resulting in lower responses to vasodilator agents (Codoñer-Franch et al., 2011), and represents an early stage of atherosclerosis (Badimón & Martínez-González, 2002). Endothelial dysfunction contributes to the development and progression of atherosclerosis by favoring coagulation, inflammatory cell adhesion, imbalance between vasoconstriction and vasodilation, and by enhancing transendothelial transport of atherogenic particles (Cersosimo & DeFronzo, 2006).

High stress-induced glucocorticoid levels reduce the expression of guanosine triphosphate cyclohydrolase 1 messenger ribonucleic acid (mRNA), necessary for tetrahydrobiopterin cofactor (BH_4) synthesis, which stabilizes eNOS (Mitchell et al., 2004). If BH_4 levels decrease, endothelial eNOS becomes uncoupled and transfers electrons to molecular oxygen generating superoxide anions (Rizzo et al., 2009), which react avidly with NO to form peroxynitrites (Förstermann & Münzel, 2006), resulting in diminished NO bioavailability, and favoring the traffic of oxidized lipids across the endothelium. Associated with this injurious effect of glucorticoids, the high LDL levels induced by stress also decrease eNOS mRNA expression (Liao et al., 1995).

Considering dyslipidemia induced by stress, it has been reported that before structural changes appear, chronic elevations of cholesterol in the bloodstream are frequently associated with impaired endothelium-dependent NO production due to increased interaction between caveolin and eNOS (Feron et al., 1999). Caveolin proteins are expressed in the majority of the cell types that play a role in atherogenesis, including endothelial cells, macrophages, and smooth muscle cells (Frank & Lisanti, 2004). High levels of LDL-cholesterol increase the caveolin concentration in endothelial cells (Feron et al., 1999), strengthen the calveolin-eNOS complex, and reduce the interaction between Ca^{2+}-calmodulin and eNOS. These effects decrease eNOS translocation from caveolae to the cytoplasm and considerably diminish NO production (Feron et al., 1999; Frank & Lisanti, 2004). In addition, lipid peroxidation induced by stress also impairs nitric oxide production (NO), stimulates inflammatory response, and increases the traffic of inflammatory molecules and oxidized LDL to sub-endothelial space, leading to vascular endothelial dysfunction (Black, 2002; Black, 2003; Black & Garbutt, 2002; Rizzo et al., 2009).

Insulin resistance is also involved in the atherogenic effects of stress. Insulin stimulates NO production by the endothelium (Muniyappa & Quon, 2007). During chronic stress cortisol-induced insulin resistance (Black, 2002; Kyrou & Tsigos, 2009) decreases this effect, and endothelial dysfunction may occur. In addition, insulin resistance is associated with inhibition of the phosphatidylinositol 3-kinase pathway and over-stimulation of the mitogen-activated protein kinase pathway in endothelial cells. Impairment of the phosphatidylinositol 3-kinase pathway reduces eNOS activity, and accentuates free fatty acid-evoked oxidative stress. These effects decrease NO bioavailability and promote an imbalance between vasoconstriction and vasodilation (Cersosim & DeFronzo, 2006; Muniyappa & Quon, 2007) predisposing the individual to atherosclerosis and arterial hypertension. In addition insulin resistance increases the reactive oxygen species, reducing eNOS activity (Muniyappa et al., 2008).

Morphological changes in blood vessels are also associated with atherosclerosis. The increase in intima media thickness (IMT) in the carotid artery has been used as a marker of target organ damage in human hypertension (Sierra & de la Sierra, 2008). In experimental studies, the IMT of the aorta observed in stressed rats (Okruhlicová et al., 2008) was related to the atherogenic effects of stress. In healthy blood vessels, NO produced by the endothelium maintains the mitogenic quiescence of smooth muscle cells. Decreased NO bioavailability induced by stress-related glucocorticoid levels or -insulin resistance results in the loss of this effect and consequently vessel wall hypertrophy may occur (Costa & Assreuy, 2005). In fact, it has been observed that rats submitted to chronic mild unpredictable stress presented higher IMT and lower relaxation response to acetylcholine in the thoracic aorta, in comparison with non stressed animals. These effects were observed 15 days after the end of the stress protocol and were associated with insulin resistance and dyslipidemia. However, in this study, the dyslipidemia induced by the hypercaloric diet alone, did not promote morphological or functional changes in the thoracic aorta, or insulin resistance evidencing the role of stress in pro-atherogenic effects (Neves et al., 2011).

NPY, a hormone known as orexigenic peptide, may also be involved in the atherogenic effects of stress. Some stressors such as cold and aggression, increase the release of NPY from sympathetic nerves (Kuo et al., 2007). The peripheral actions of NPY are stimulatory, synergizing with glucocorticoids and catecholamines to potentiate the stress response. It causes prolonged vasoconstriction, potentiating the effect of norepinephrine, induces hyperlipidemia, and vascular remodeling via smooth muscle cell proliferation, in addition to stimulating monocyte migration and activation (Kuo et al., 2007). NPY upregulates its Y2 receptors in a glucocorticoid-dependent manner in abdominal fat, consequently leading to abdominal obesity, hyperinsulinemia and dyslipidemia (Kuo et al., 2008). In blood vessels, Y1 and Y5 receptor activation promotes pro-atherogenic responses (Zukowska, 2005).

In addition to all the above-mentioned mechanisms, the inflammatory process also forms part of the stress response (Black, 2003), and is pathophysiologically linked to atherosclerosis (van Oostrom et al., 2004). In the atherogenic process, the high level of catecholamines induced by stress stimulates endothelial permeability to the traffic of oxidized LDL. Once trapped in the endothelium of an artery, LDL can undergo progressive oxidation, cross the endothelial barrier, and be internalized by macrophages expressing scavenger receptors, leading to lipid peroxide formation and accumulation of cholesterol esters, culminating in foam cells formation (Ross, 1999; Singh & Mehta, 2003). Oxidized LDL upregulates the expression of adhesion molecules and secretion of chemokines, which contributes to the recruitment of circulating monocytes and leukocytes (Cersosimo & DeFronzo, 2006; Steinberg, 2002). One of the initial steps in the formation of atherosclerosis is the adhesion of monocytes to the endothelium, their entry into sub-endothelial space, followed by their differentiation into macrophages (Lamharzi et al., 2004). These cells are then responsible for taking up LDL and other particles, thereby starting the atherogenesis process (Lamharzi et al., 2004). In foam cell formation, the macrophages in the endothelial space also have VLDL receptors, which bind the apolipoprotein (apo) E-containing lipoproteins, including VLDL, intermediate density lipoprotein, and β-migrating VLDL. The LDL-receptor-related protein in macrophages is also capable of binding apo E-containing lipoproteins, lipoprotein lipase, and lipoprotein lipase-triglyceride-rich lipoprotein complex (Nakazato, 1996), leading to a sequence in the development of atherosclerosis.

In addition, high levels of free fatty acids also may amplify monocyte inflammation via toll-like receptors in the presence of high glucose levels (Dasu & Jialal, 2011). Lamharzi et al., 2004, showed that free fatty acids in concert with glucose stimulate machrophage proliferation involving glucose-dependent oxidation of LDL in atherosclerotic lesions. Toll like receptors are expressed by machrophages in murine and human lipid-rich atherosclerotic plaques and upregulated by oxidized LDL (Xu et al., 2001). Recently Gu et al., 2009, showed the importance of toll-like receptor 4 in atherosclerosis induced by chronic mild stress in aortas from apolipoprotein-E-knockout-mice. Toll-like receptor 4 is present in T cells, monocytes, and macrophages, and is a key signaling receptor of innate immunity. Toll-like receptor 4 plays an important role in atherogenesis because it recognizes pathogen-associated molecular patterns and activates inflammatory cells via the nuclear factor kB (NF-kB) pathway (Bierhaus et al., 2003; Gu et al., 2009). During the stress reaction, glucocorticoids and catecholamines can induce cytokine production by endothelial cells and macrophages (Black, 2003; Chae et al., 2001) and activation of the NF-kB pathway leads to the synthesis of the following proinflammatory chemokines: interleukin 1-β, inteleukin 6, TNF-α, monocyte chemoattractant protein-1, intercellular adhesion molecule-1. Interleukin 1-β and inteleukin 6 influences smooth muscle cell proliferation and/or migration (Gu et al., 2009), and inhibits eNOS activity (Muniyappa et al., 2008). TNF-α increases endothelin-1 secretion, decreases NO production in endothelial cells, inducing vasoconstriction (Muniyappa & Quon, 2007), and can induce interleukin 6 production (Black, 2003). Monocyte chemoattractant protein-1 is correlated with neointimal proliferation and plays a role in the transition from the stable state of lesion to the more complex state of atherosclerosis (Tellez et al., 2011). Intercellular adhesion molecule-1 may contribute to accelerating atherosclerosis in insulin-resistant states (Muniyappa et al., 2008). Hypertriglyceridemia associated with stress may also increase NF-kB, consequently activating proinflammatory molecules (Fitch et al., 2011).

In addition, the accumulation of macrophages may also be associated with increased plasma concentration of C-reactive protein (CRP) (Ross, 1999). CRP is the principal down-stream mediator of inflammatory acute phase response, which is primarily derived via interleukin 6-dependent hepatic biosynthesis (Pradhan et al., 2001). CRP interacts with oxidized LDL to form proatherogenic oxidized LDL/CRP complexes, perpetuating vascular inflammation, triggering an autoimmune response, and accelerating atherogenesis (Matsuura et al., 2009; Sitia et al., 2010).

Activation of the renin-angiotensin system (RAS) by stress also plays a role in the pathogenesis of endothelial dysfunction, hypertension and atherosclerosis. Lipid accumulation in blood vessels enhances the expression of RAS components, which in turn stimulates accumulation of oxidized LDL in blood vessels (Singh & Mehta, 2003). Activation of the angiotensin II-type 1 receptor (AT_1R) leads to vasoconstriction and neurohumoral activation, and is associated with reduced NO bioavailability, vascular cell apoptosis, increased oxidized LDL receptor expression, and proinflammatory cytokine production (Sitia et al., 2010). According Nickening et al., 1999, LDL-cholesterol can accumulate in vascular smooth muscle cells, and this effect is mediated via AT_1R. Angiotensin II increases LDL uptake by arterial wall macrophages (Keidar et al., 1994). Angiotensin II binds LDL and the angiotensin II-modified LDL is taken up by macrophages via scavenger receptors, leading to cellular cholesterol accumulation (Keidar et al., 1996). In atherogenic dyslipidemia, hypercholesterolemia increases AT_1R density and its functional responsiveness to vasoconstrictors, whereas the administration of statins reduces AT_1R expression and deregulates its functions. Moreover, the localization of angiotensin-converting enzyme in atherosclerotic lesions suggests a capacity for local generation of angiotensin II and proinflammatory substances (Sitia et al., 2010). There is also evidence that hypercholesterolemia increases plasma angiotensinogen and angiotensin peptide production (Sitia et al., 2010), and that AT_1R antagonism improves hypercholesterolemia-associated endothelial dysfunction, resulting in an anti-atherosclerotic effect (Taguchi et al., 2011).

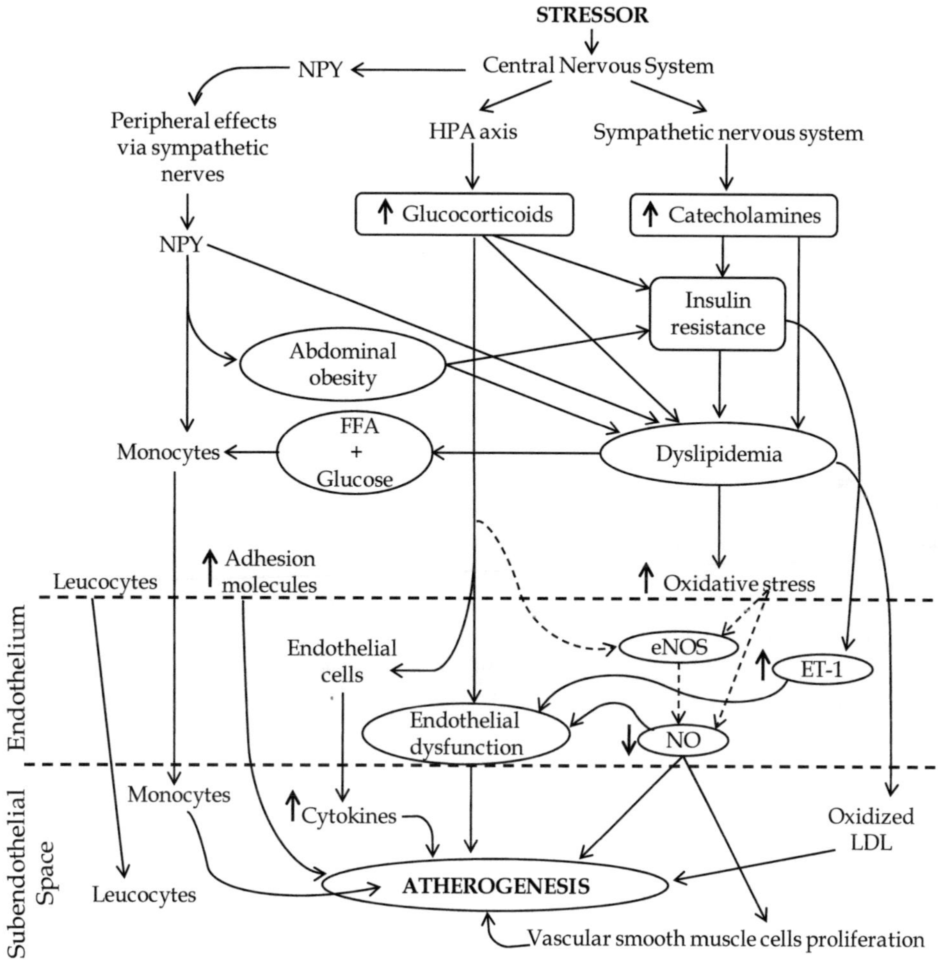

Fig. 2. Schematic representation of putative mechanisms involved in the relations between among stress, dyslipidemia, and atherosclerosis. Hypothalamic-pituitary-adrenal axis (HPA), neuropeptide Y (NPY), low-density lipoprotein (LDL), very-low-density lipoprotein (VLDL), free fatty acids (FFA), endothelial nitric oxide synthase (eNOS), nitric oxide (NO), endothelin 1 (ET-1). Solid arrows show stimulatory effects; dashed arrows indicate inhibitory effects.

Atherosclerosis is an inflammatory disease and stress contributes to its development. Therefore, if we can block or minimize the stress components that directly or indirectly induce atherogenesis, it will be possible to preserve the protective components of vascular function and structure, thereby developing new preventive and therapeutic possibilities. Figure 2 illustrates the putative mechanisms of the relations between stress, dyslipidemia, and atherosclerosis.

4. Reduction of dyslipidemia induced by stress: Physical exercise and nutritional intervention

The role of stress in the etiology of chronic degenerative diseases is increasingly recognized (Gerber & Pühse, 2009; Holmes et al., 2010; Tsatsoulis & Fountoulakis, 2006; Yin et al., 2005). Moreover, it has been reported that obese people have an exaggerated response to stress, which may further increase the risk of weight gain, leading to the development of insulin resistance, hyperlipidemia, diabetes mellitus, hypertension and atherosclerosis in both men and women. This burden of chronic degenerative diseases is strongly influenced by several lifestyle factors, including the way an individual perceives a stressful situation, i.e., "mental fitness" and also his/her general physical condition or "physical fitness" (McEwen, 1998).
Tsatsoulis & Fountoulakis, 2006, demonstrated that stress-mediated allostatic load, in the presence of physical inactivity, is associated with an increased risk of mental and physical illness, and direct evidence for this notion has been provided by several studies. A strong inverse association between physical activity and the metabolic syndrome has been demonstrated, and several years ago this association was shown to be much steeper in unfit individuals (Kriska et al., 1993; Lindgärde & Saltin, 1981). Evidence for this view was also provided by the MacArthur studies of successful aging based on a large cohort of elderly men and women (Seeman et al., 1997), showing that subjects with low levels of physical and mental fitness had higher prevalence of cardiometabolic disease when compared with those with high fitness levels. Moreover, a strong association between physical inactivity, excessive food consumption, high-fat diet and increasing incidence of insulin resistance, Type 2 diabetes, (Hawley, 2004; Steanovv et al., 2011), development of obesity (Venables & Jeukendrup, 2009; Vessby, 2000) and depression (Win et al., 2011) has also been described in the literature. Considering that stress, physical inactivity, and aging (associated with declining physical activity and metabolic rate, coupled with an energy intake not matched to the declining need), in addition to a high-fat diet, are the very features of our current lifestyle, the incidence of this "stress-induced/exercise deficient" phenotype is becoming increasingly prevalent in modern society (Davy et al., 1996, Hawley, 2004, Poehlman et al., 1995, Schiut et al., 1998, Tsatsoulis & Fountoulakis, 2006).
Based on the above mentioned findings, it is reasonable to assume that physical inactivity may potentiate the stress-related allostatic load and comorbidities, since the energy substrate that is mobilized during stress is not oxidized but is stored in visceral fat depots. This adaptation creates a vicious cycle, in which perceived stress is also associated with decreased participation in several health behaviors including exercise, social behaviors, stress management/rest, and safety/environmental behaviors, as shown by Padden et al., 2011, in the study on health behavior of military spouses during deployment separation. In this context, physical exercise practiced as a non-pharmacological alternative, either with or without the association of pharmacological therapies, is very important, and a great deal of attention should be given to the barriers imposed, especially by mood disorders, including depression. Individuals in this

condition are at disadvantage, since most of the time they lack the energy and motivation to exercise, and this overwhelming feeling of lethargy seems very difficult to shift (Chaput et al., 2011). In this situation, when psychological stress is not accompanied by physical activity (such as the fight or flight reaction) and by effective use and fast clearance of free fatty acids, triggered by stimulation of the sympathetic nervous system, these are converted into triglycerides by the liver and then circulate in the blood within the VLDL (Howard et al., 1993). In fact, this maladaptative situation can lead to the development of dyslipidemia, reflected by elevated plasma triglyceride and reduced HDL concentration, overproduction of VLDL-apolipoprotein (apo) B-100, decreased catabolism of apoB containing particles, and increased catabolism of HDL apoA-I particles (Watts et al., 2008; Watts et al., 2009).

While physical inactivity may potentiate the stress-induced allostatic load, there is accumulating evidence suggesting that the adoption of an active lifestyle, including exercise training, may play a protective role in stress system dysregulation, reducing vulnerability to stress, and possibly delaying or preventing the future development of comorbidities, such as dyslipidemia, hypertension and insulin resistance (Roberts & Barnard, 2005; Tsatsoulis & Fountoulakis, 2006). In addition, physical activity may induce favorable changes in traditional and emerging coronary heart disease biomarkers among individuals with, or at high risk of coronary heart disease (Chainani-Wu et al., 2011). Assuming that the stress response is a neuroendocrine mechanism that occurs in anticipation of physical action, it is reasonable to assume that physical activity should provide the vehicle to prevent or combat the somatic and emotional consequences of stress. Thus, physical activity may promote physical and psychological benefits that are involved in both the indirect action of exercise in reducing stress, and a direct effect on various metabolic functions of the body (McMurray & Hanckney, 2005).

The first rationale for using exercise as a stress reduction strategy was based on the cross-stressor adaptation, a promising hypothesis first presented in the 1990s (Sothmann et al., 1996), which has not received strong support since the publication of recent meta-analyses (Forcier et al., 2006; Hamer et al., 2006; Jackson & Dishman, 2006). According to Chaput et al., 2011, the key question now is whether physical activity, which seems to modulate the level of stress, may interact in the relationship between stress and obesity. Different possible mechanisms have been proposed, suggesting that exercise training might protect against stress induced obesity. Regular exercise has been demonstrated to have positive effects on plasma lipid and lipoprotein profiles (Durstine et al., 2002) and these results may have a significant independent effect on HDL cholesterol (Thompson et al., 1988). During physical activity, exercise increases lipid oxidation and lipolysis to ensure an adequate oxygen supply (McMurray & Hanckney, 2005), increases the ability of muscle tissue to take up and oxidize nonesterified fatty acids, and increases muscle lipoprotein lipase activity (Eriksson et al., 1997). Although studies indicate that exercise training changes gene expression in adipose tissue in different ways, affecting some types of adipose tissue more than others (Company et al., 2010), the lowering of plasma triglycerides proves the effects of exercise on VLDL kinetics. Moreover, it is important to highlight that a single 90-min bout of whole body resistance exercise (Tsekouras et al., 2009) or 2h of cycling (Magkos et al., 2006) was proven to be enough to decrease fasting plasma VLDL-triglyceride concentrations by increasing VLDL-triglyceride removal from plasma. These results may be due to the increase in blood flow and hepatic insulin sensitivity associated with an increase in lipoprotein lipase activity.

In addition to its possible direct effect modulating the stress response, exercise training improves insulin sensitivity, which might counteract the insulin resistance state produced by chronic hypercortisolemia (Tsatsoulis & Fountoulakis, 2006). Insulin secretion could then be reduced, and thereby, its deleterious impact on energy intake may be diminished. Moreover, exercise training improves glucose tolerance among non-diabetic, non-obese subjects with hypertriglyceridemia (Lampman & Schteingart, 1991) and enhances the oxidative capacity of skeletal muscle (Tsatsoulis & Fountoulakis, 2006). Together, these beneficial adaptations could prevent stress-induced fat deposition by routing the energy mobilized in response to the stressor toward oxidation rather than storage.

Apart from the protective effects of exercise on the physical and metabolic aspects related to stress, a number of psychological and cognitive benefits have also been reported in the literature. These include improvements in depression and anxiety scores and general improvement in mood, cognitive functioning (Callaghan, 2004; Tsatsoulis & Fountoulakis, 2006), well-being and self esteem, leading to a decrease in body fat, triglycerides, LDL/HDL cholesterol ratio in stressed patients (De Geus & Stubbe, 2007). Physical activity can improve mental health by reducing depressive symptoms in young men (McGale et al., 2011) and in patients with metabolic syndrome (Rubenfire et al., 2011). Moreover exercise induces the elevation of circulating brain derived neurotrophic factor, which is known to improve the health and survival of nerve cells, suggesting that exercise influences brain health (Yarrow et al., 2010). Using animal models, exercise has also been shown to induce antidepressant responses (Greenwood et al., 2003). In rats, swimming exercise induces a remission of anhedonic symptoms suggesting that exercise training might induce biological alterations similar to those provided by antidepressant drugs. In addition, exercise plays an important role in hippocampal protection from damage caused by exposure to glucocorticoids (Sigwalt et al., 2011). In this context, physical activity was able to stimulate the proliferation of hippocampal cells (Ehninger & Kempermann, 2003), promote alterations in synaptic plasticity, neurogenesis and synaptogenesis (Castrén, 2005), and may also be linked to increased levels of brain testosterone (Mukai et al., 2006).

Another beneficial effect of exercise is related to feeding behavior. Stressful situations have been shown to affect feeding behavior (Wallis & Hetherington, 2009) that result in increased energy intake through the stimulation provided by ingesting palatable foods that may serve as feedback signals that reduce the perception and discomfort of stress, thereby contributing to the development of dyslipidemia and obesity (Dallman et al., 2005). Moreover glucorticoids are associated with high neuropeptide Y secretion, which has an orexigenic activity and increases the intake of sugar- and fat-rich- comfort foods (Kuo et al., 2008) and can lead to a state of leptin resistance and elevated levels of this hormone (Zakrzewska et al., 1997). In this context, it has been demonstrated that physical activity has the potential to modulate appetite control by improving the sensitivity of the physiological satiety signalling system, by adjusting macronutrient preferences or food choices and by altering the hedonic response to food (Blundell et al., 2003). Indeed, dietary modification, associated with physical activity has been shown to exert significantly favorable effects on the treatment and prevention of stress-induced comorbidities, improving glycemia, blood pressure, body weight, fat distribution, and lipid profile, which in turn suggest that chronic degenerative diseases are largely preventable (Dagogo et al., 2010). Although exercise cannot change total cholesterol and LDL-cholesterol unless dietary fat intake is reduced, this result may be dependent on the amount of energy expenditure during exercise (Durstine et al., 2002). Furthermore, depending on the time that the exercise is performed (before or after ingestion of fatty foods), its acute responses related to improvement in lipoprotein metabolism may be different (Hashimoto et al., 2011). In a review of several studies realized by Leon & Sanchez

2001, one of proposals evaluated was the effects of aerobic exercise training on blood lipids and the relationship between these effects and diet. The results showed that majority of physically active individuals had an increase in HDL cholesterol, but this could be changed if there was a concomitant reduction in fat intake. The association between low-fat diet and exercise reduces LDL and HDL-cholesterol levels. Furthermore, reductions in total cholesterol, LDL-cholesterol and triglyceride levels were less frequently observed. As regards body weight loss, there was considerable variability between the groups, ranging from 7.2 Kg in the group that was not exposed to dietary intervention to 17.9 Kg in the group that underwent dietary intervention. In addition, Rubenfire et al., 2011, demonstrated that the association between changes in diet and exercise was effective in reducing cardiovascular risk in patients with metabolic syndrome. In this study, the nutritional component was based on a Mediterranean food pattern, and all the participants were provided with the information needed to optimize their nutritional choices in order to improve blood lipid and glucose levels, decrease body weight and blood pressure, and decrease insulin resistance (Rubenfire et al., 2011). It has also been proposed that high-fiber diets protect against obesity and cardiovascular disease by lowering insulin levels (Ludwig et al., 1999). In obese men, the implementation of a high-fiber and low-fat diet associated with regular physical activity resulted in significant reductions in inflammation and dyslipidemia by reducing serum lipids, insulin, oxidative stress, leukocyte-endothelial interactions (Roberts & Barnard, 2005).

Dietary fat influences glucose and lipid metabolism by altering cell membrane function, enzyme activity, insulin signaling, and gene expression (Risérus et al., 2009; Yamazaki et al., 2011) and dietary fructose consumption appears to induce dyslipidemia, obesity (Stanhope et al., 2009) and hypertension (Cunha et al., 2007; Farah et al., 2006). A combination of social stress and high-fat diet resulted in a significant imbalance in lipid regulation associated with changes in the expression of hepatic genes, responsible for its regulation (Chuang et al., 2010). Therefore, clinical strategies based on low fat and sugar intake associated with increase in physical exercise have been used, and have contributed to reducing the risks of developing coronary and metabolic diseases.

5. Conclusion

Dyslipidemia induced by stress is part of the body's response to cope with stressors. The mobilization of lipids, glucose and proteins, allows the organs and tissues to maintain homeostasis and adapt to the stressor. Any deficiency in the activation of this mobilization of energetic fuels can compromise the survival of the individual. Therefore, the increase in blood lipids induced by stress is adaptive and it should return to normal levels when the stressor ends. However, when the stressor is maintained over a long period, the dyslipidemia induced by stress persists and may have deleterious effects, contributing to the occurrence of insulin resistance, obesity, hypertension and atherosclerosis. Considering that physical inactivity may potentiate these effects, the association of physical exercise and control of hypercaloric food consumption have been used in the treatment of dyslipidemia. Knowledge about the physiological mechanisms involved in the adaptive role of transient dyslipidemia induced by acute stress, and in the deleterious effects of sustained dyslipidemia induced by chronic stress is very important in the improvement and development of preventive and therapeutic approaches because in modern society we are continuously exposed to stressors.

6. Acknowledgment

The authors thank Margery Galbraith for English editing.

7. References

Badimón, L. & Martínez-González J. (2002). Endothelium and vascular protection: an update. *Revista española de cardiología,* Vol.55, No.1 (January 2002), pp. 17-26, ISSN 0300-8932.

Bartolomucci, A.; Cabassi, A.; Govoni, P.; Ceresini, G.; Cero, C.; Berra, D.; Dadomo, H.; Franceschini, P.; Dell'Omo, G.; Parmigiani, S. & Palanza, P. (2009). Metabolic consequences and vulnerability to diet-induced obesity in male mice under chronic social stress. *PloS one [electronic resource].* Vol.4, No.1, (January 2009), pii. e4331, ISSN 1932-6203 online.

Berger, D.F.; Starzec, J.J.; Mason, E.B. & DeVito, W. (1980). The effects of differential psychological stress on plasma cholesterol levels in rats. *Psychosomatic medicine,* Vol.42, No.5, (September 1980), pp.481-492, ISSN 0033-3174.

Bierhaus, A.; Wolf, J.; Andrassy, M.; Rohleder, N.; Humpert, P.M.; Petrov, D.; Ferstl, R.; von Eynatten, M.; Wendt, T.; Rudofsky, G.; Joswig, M.; Morcos, M.; Schwaninger, M.; McEwen, B.; Kirschbaum, C. & Nawroth, P.P. (2002). A mechanism converting psychosocial stress into mononuclear cell activation. *Proceedings of the National Academy of Sciences of the United States of America,* Vol.100, No.4, (February 2003), pp. 1920-1925, ISSN 0027-8424.

Björntorp, P. & Rosmond, R. (1999). Hypothalamic origin of the metabolic syndrome X. *Annals of the New York Academy of Sciences,* Vol.892, (November 1999), pp. 297-307, ISSN 0077-8923.

Black, P.H. (2002). Stress and the inflammatory response: a review of neurogenic inflammation. *Brain, behavior, and immunity,* Vol.16, No.6, (December 2002), pp. 622-653, ISSN 0889-1591.

Black, P.H. (2003). The inflammatory response is an integral part of the stress response: Implications for atherosclerosis, insulin resistance, type II diabetes and metabolic syndrome X. *Brain, behavior, and immunity,* Vol.17, No.5, (October 2003), pp. 350-364, ISSN 0889-1591.

Black, P.H. & Garbutt, L.D. (2002). Stress, inflammation and cardiovascular disease. *Journal of psychosomatic research,* Vol.52, No.1, (January 2002), pp. 1-23, ISSN 0022-3999.

Blundell, J.E.; Stubbs, R.J.; Hughes, D.A.; Whybrow, S. & King, N.A. (2003). Cross talk between physical activity and appetite control: does physical activity stimulate appetite? *The Proceedings of the Nutrition Society,* Vol.62, No.3, (August 2003), pp. 651-661, ISSN 0029-6651.

Bose, M.; Oliván, B. & Laferrère, B. (2009). Stress and obesity: the role of the hypothalamic-pituitary-adrenal axis in metabolic disease. *Current opinion in endocrinology, diabetes, and obesity,* Vol.16, No.5, (October 2009), pp. 340-346, ISSN 1752-296X.

Brindley, D.N.; McCann, B.S.; Niaura, R.; Stoney, C.M. & Suarez, E.C. (1993). Stress and lipoprotein metabolism: modulators and mechanisms. *Metabolism: clinical and experimental,* Vol.42, No.9 Suppl 1, (September 1993), pp. 3-15, ISSN 0026-0495.

Bryant, H.U; Story, J.A. & Yim G.K. (1988). Assessment of endogenous opioid mediation in stress-induced hypercholesterolemia in the rat. *Psychosomatic medicine,* Vol.50, No.6, (November-December 1988), pp. 576-585, ISSN 0033-3174.

Callaghan, P. (2004). Exercise: a neglected intervention in mental health care? *Journal of psychiatric and mental health nursing*, Vol.11, No.4, (August 2004), pp. 476-483, ISSN 1351-0126.

Castrén, E. (2005). Is mood chemistry? *Nature reviews. Neuroscience*, Vol.6, No.3, (March 2005), pp. 241-246, ISSN 1471-003X.

Cersosimo, E. & DeFronzo, R.A. (2006). Insulin resistance and endothelial dysfunction: the road map to cardiovascular diseases. 2006. Diabetes/metabolism research and reviews, Vol.22, No.6, (November/December 2006), pp. 423-436, ISSN 1520-7552.

Chae, C.U.; Lee, R.T.; Rifai, N. & Ridker, P.M. (2001). Blood pressure and inflammation in apparently healthy men. *Hypertension*, Vol.38, No.3, (September 2001), pp. 399-403, ISSN 0194-911X.

Chainani-Wu, N.; Weidner, G.; Purnell, D.M.; Frenda, S.; Merritt-Worden, T.; Pischke, C.; Campo, R.; Kemp, C.; Kersh E.S. & Ornish, D. (2011). Changes in Emerging Cardiac Biomarkers After an Intensive Lifestyle Intervention. *The American journal of cardiology*, Epub ahead of print, doi:10.1016/j.amjcard.2011.03.077, ISSN 1879-1913.

Chaput, J.P.; Klingenberg, L.; Rosenkilde, M.; Gilbert, J.A.; Tremblay, A. & Sjödin, A. (2010). Physical activity plays an important role in body weight regulation. *Journal of obesity [electronic resource]*, Vol.2011 (2011), pii. 360257, ISSN 2090-0716 on line, ISSN 2090-0708 print.

Chuang, J.C.; Cui, H.; Mason, BL.; Mahgoub, M.; Bookout, A.L.; Yu, H.G.; Perello, M.; Elmquist, J.K.; Repa, J.J.; Zigman, J.M. & Lutter, M. (2010). Chronic social defeat stress disrupts regulation of lipid synthesis. *Journal of lipid research*, Vol.51, No.6, (June 2010), pp. 1344-1353, ISSN 0022-2275.

Codoñer-Franch, P.; Tavárez-Alonso, S.; Murria-Estal, R.; Megías-Vericat, J.; Tortajada-Girbés, M. & Alonso-Iglesias, E. (2011). *Nitric oxide production is increased in severely obese children and related to markers of oxidative stress and inflammation.* Atherosclerosis, Vol.215, No.2, (April 2011), pp. 475-480, ISSN 0021-9150.

Company, J.M.; Booth, F.W.; Laughlin, M.H.; Arce-Esquivel, A.A.; Sacks, H.S.; Bahouth, S.W. & Fain, J.N. (2010). Epicardial fat gene expression after aerobic exercise training in pigs with coronary atherosclerosis: relationship to visceral and subcutaneous fat. *Journal of applied physiology*, Vo.109, No.6, (December 2010), pp. 1904-1912, ISSN 8750-7587.

Costa, R.S. & Assreuy J. (2005). Multiple potassium channels mediate nitric oxide-induced inhibition of rat vascular smooth muscle cell proliferation. *Nitric oxide: biology and chemistry/official journal of the Nitric Oxide Society*, Vol.13, No.2, (September 2005), pp. 145-51, ISSN 1089-8603.

Cunha, T.S.; Farah, V.; Paulini, J.; Pazzine, M.; Elased, K.M.; Marcondes, F.K.; Irigoyen, M.C.; De Angelis, K.; Mirkin, L.D. & Morris, M. (2007). Relationship between renal and cardiovascular changes in a murine model of glucose intolerance. *Regulatory peptides*, Vol.139, No.1-3, (March 2007), pp. 1-4, ISSN 0167-0115.

Dagogo-Jack, S.; Egbuonu, N. & Edeoga, C. (2010). Principles and practice of nonpharmacological interventions to reduce cardiometabolic risk. *Medical principles and practice: international journal of the Kuwait University, Health Science Centre*, Vol.19, No.3, (March 2010), pp. 167-175, ISSN 1011-7571.

Dallman, M.F.; La Fleur, S.E.; Pecoraro, N.; Gomez, F.; Houshyar, H. & Akana, S.F. (2004). Minireview: Glucocorticoids - food intake, abdominal obesity, and wealthy nations in 2004. *Endocrinology*, Vol.145, No.6, (June 2004), pp. 2633-2638, ISSN 0013-7227.

Dallman, M.F.; Pecoraro, N.; Akana, S.F.; La Fleur, S.E.; Gomez, F.; Houshyar, H.; Bell, M.E.; Bhatnagar, S.; Laugero, K.D. & Manalo, S. (2003). Chronic stress and obesity: a new view of "comfort food". *Proceedings of the National Academy of Sciences of the United States of America,* Vol.100, No.20, (September 2003), pp. 11696-11701, ISSN 0027-8424.

Dallman, M.F.; Pecoraro, N.C. & la Fleur, S.E. (2005). Chronic stress and comfort foods: self-medication and abdominal obesity. *Brain, behavior, and immunity,* Vo.19, No.4 (July 2005), pp. 275-280. ISSN 0889-1591.

Dasu, M.R. & Jialal, I. (2010). Free fatty acids in the presence of high glucose amplify monocyte inflammation via Toll-like receptors. American *journal of physiology. Endocrinology and metabolism,* Vol. 300, No.1, (January 2011), pp. E145-154, ISSN 1522-1555 online, ISSN 0193-1849 print.

Davy, K.P.; Evans, S.L.; Stevenson, E.T. & Seals, D.R. (1996). Adiposity and regional body fat distribution in physically active young and middle age women. *International journal of obesity and related metabolic disorders: journal of the International Association for the Study of Obesity,* Vol.20, No.8, (August 1996), pp. 777-783, ISSN 0307-0565.

De Geus, E.J.C. & Stubbe, J.H. (2007). Aerobic exercise and stress reduction, In: *Encyclopedia of Stress,* pp. 73-78, George Fink (editor), ELSEVIER, ISBN 978-0-12-088503-9, San Diego, CA - USA.

De Moura, E.G.; Lisboa, P.C. & Passos, M.C. (2008). Neonatal programming of neuroimmunomodulation-role of adipocytokines and neuropeptides. *Neuroimmunomodulation,* Vol.15, No.3, (October 2008), pp.176-188, ISSN 1021-7401.

Durstine, J.L.; Grandjean, P.W.; Cox, C.A. & Thompson, P.D. (2002). Lipids, lipoproteins, and exercise. *Journal of cardiopulmonary rehabilitation,* Vol.22, No.6, (November/December 2002), pp. 385-398, ISSN 0883-9212.

Dzubur Kulenović, A.; Kucukalić, A. & Malec, D. (2008). Changes in plasma lipid concentrations and risk of coronary artery disease in army veterans suffering from chronic posttraumatic stress disorder. *Croatian medical journal,* Vol.49, No.4, (August 2008), pp. 506-514, ISSN 0353-9504.

Ehninger, D. & Kempermann, G. (2003). Regional effects of wheel running and environmental enrichment on cell genesis and microglia proliferation in the adult murine neocortex. *Cerebral Cortex,* Vol.13, No.8, (August 2003), pp. 845-851, ISSN 1047-3211.

Epel E.S. (2009). Psychological and metabolic stress: a recipe for accelerated cellular aging? *Hormones (Athens),* Vol.8, No.1, (January-March 2009), pp. 7-22, ISSN 1109-3099.

Eriksson, J.; Taimela, S. & Koivisto, V.A. (1997). Exercise and the metabolic syndrome. *Diabetologia,* Vol.40, No.2, (February 1997), pp. 125-135, ISSN 0012-186X.

Farah, V.; Elased, K.M.; Chen, Y.; Key, M.P.; Cunha, T.S.; Irigoyen, M.C. & Morris, M. (2006). Nocturnal hypertension in mice consuming a high fructose diet. *Autonomic neuroscience: basic & clinical.* Vol.130, No.1-2, (December 2006), pp. 41-50, ISSN 1566-0702.

Feron, O.; Dessy, C.; Moniotte, S.; Desager, J.P. & Balligand, J.L. (1999). Hypercholesterolemia decreases nitric oxide production by promoting the interaction of caveolin and endothelial nitric oxide synthase. *The Journal of clinical investigation,* Vol.103, No.6, (March 1999), pp. 897-905, ISSN 0021-9738.

Fitch, K.V.; Stavrou, E.; Looby, S.E.; Hemphill, L.; Jaff, M.R. & Grinspoon, S.K. (2011). Associations of cardiovascular risk factors with two surrogate markers of subclinical atherosclerosis: Endothelial function and carotid intima media thickness. *Atherosclerosis,* Epub ahead of print, doi: 10.1016/j.atherosclerosis. 2011.04.009, (April 2011), ISSN 0021-9150.

Forcier, K.; Stroud, L.R.; Papandonatos, G.D.; Hitsman, B.; Reiches, M.; Krishnamoorthy, J. & Niaura, R. (2006). Links between physical fitness and cardiovascular reactivity and recovery to psychological stressors: a meta-analysis. *Health psychology: official journal of the Division of Health Psychology, American Psychological Association,* Vol.25, No.6, (November 2006), pp. 723–739, ISSN 0278-6133.

Förstermann, U. & Münzel, T. (2006). Endothelial nitric oxide synthase in vascular disease: from marvel to menace. *Circulation,* Vol.113, No.13, (April 2006), pp. 1708-1714, ISSN 0009-7322.

Frank, P.G. & Lisanti, M.P. (2004). Caveolin-1 and caveolae in atherosclerosis: differential roles in fatty streak formation and neointimal hyperplasia. *Current opinion in lipidology,* Vol.15, No.5, (October 2004), pp. 523-529, ISSN 0957-9672.

Gerber, M. & Pühse, U. (2009). Review article: do exercise and fitness protect against stress-induced health complaints? A review of the literature. *Scandinavian journal of public health,* Vol.37, No.8, (November 2009), pp. 801-819, ISSN 1403-4948.

Greenwood, B.N.; Foley, T.E.; Day, H.E.; Campisi, J.; Hammack, S.H.; Campeau, S.; Maier, S.F. & Fleshner, M. (2003) Freewheel running prevents learned helplessness/behavioral depression: role of dorsal raphe serotonergic neurons. *The Journal of neuroscience: the official journal of the Society for Neuroscience,* Vol.23, No.7, (April 2003), pp. 2889–2898, ISSN 0270-6474.

Gu, H.; Tang, C.; Peng, K.; Sun, H. & Yang, Y. (2009). Effects of chronic mild stress on the development of atherosclerosis and expression of toll-like receptor 4 signaling pathway in adolescent apolipoprotein E knockout mice. *Journal of biomedicine & biotechnology,* Vol.2009, (August 2009), pp. 1-13, ISSN 1110-7243.

Hamer, M.; Taylor, A. & Steptoe, A. (2005). The effect of acute aerobic exercise on stress related blood pressure responses: a systematic review and meta-analysis. *Biological psychology,* Vol.71, No.2, (2006), pp. 183-190, ISSN 1873-6246 online, ISSN 0301-0511 print.

Hawley, J.A. (2004). Exercise as a therapeutic intervention for the prevention and treatment of insulin resistance. *Diabetes/metabolism research and reviews,* Vol.20, No.5, (Sepember/October 2004), pp. 383–393, ISSN 1520-7552.

Hashimoto, S.; Ootani, K.; Hayashi, S. & Naito, M. (2011). Acute Effects of Shortly Pre-Versus Postprandial Aerobic Exercise on Postprandial Lipoprotein Metabolism in Healthy but Sedentary Young Women. *Journal of atherosclerosis and thrombosis,* Epub ahead of print, doi: 10.5551/jat.8482 (June 2011), ISSN 1880-3873.

Holmes, M.E.; Ekkekakis, P. & Eisenmann, J.C. (2009). The physical activity, stress and metabolic syndrome triangle: a guide to unfamiliar territory for the obesity researcher. *Obesity reviews: an official journal of the International Association for the Study of Obesity,* Vol.11, No.7, (July 2010), pp. 492-507, ISSN 1467-789X online, 1467-7881 print.

Howard, B.V. (1993). Insulin, insulin resistance, and dyslipidemia. *Annals of the New York Academy of Sciences,* Vol.683, (June 1993), pp. 1-8, ISSN 1749-6632.

Jackson, E.M. & Dishman, R.K. (2006). Cardiorespiratory fitness and laboratory stress: a meta-regression analysis. *Psychophysiology,* Vol.43, No.1, (January 2006), pp. 57–72, ISSN 0048-5772.

Kaplan, J.R.; Manuck, S.B.; Clarkson, T.F.; Lusso, F.M.; Taub, D.M. & Miller, E.W. (1983). Social stress and atherosclerosis in normocholesterolemic monkeys. *Science,* Vol.220, No.4598, (May 1983), pp. 733-735, ISSN 0036-8075.

Keidar, S.; Kaplan, M.; Shapira, C.; Brook, J.G. & Aviran, M. (1994). Low density lipoprotein isolated from patients with essential hypertension exhibits increased propensity for oxidation and enhanced uptake by macrophages: a possible role for angiotensin II. *Atherosclerosis,* Vol.107, No.71, (May 1994), pp. 71-84, ISSN 0021-9150.

Keidar, S.; Kaplan, M. & Aviram, M. (1996). Angiotensin II-modified LDL is taken up by macrophages via the scavenger receptor, leading to cellular cholesterol accumulation. *Arteriosclerosis, thrombosis, and vascular biology,* Vol.16, No.1, (January 1996), pp.97-105, ISSN 1079-5642.

Korte, S.M.; Koolhaas, J.M.; Wingfield, J.C. & McEwen, B.S. (2004). The Darwinian concept of stress: benefits of allostasis and costs of allostatic load and the trade-offs in health and disease. *Neuroscience and behavioral reviews,* Vol.29, No.1, (February 2005), pp. 3–38, ISSN 1873-7528 online, ISSN 0149-7634 print.

Kriska, A.M.; LaPorte, R.E.; Pettitt, D.J.; Charles, M.A.; Nelson, R.G.; Kuller, L.H.; Bennett, P.H. & Knowler, W.C. (1993). The association of physical activity with obesity, fat distribution and glucose intolerance in Pima Indians. *Diabetologia,* Vol.36, No.9, (September 1993), pp. 863-869, ISSN 0012-186X.

Kuo, L.E.; Abe, K. & Zukowska, Z. (2007). Stress, NPY and vascular remodeling: Implications for stress-related diseases. *Peptides,* Vo.28, No.2 (February 2007), pp. 435-440, ISSN 0196-9781.

Kuo, L.E.; Czarnecka, M.; Kitlinska, J.B.; Tilan, J.U.; Kvetnanský, R. & Zukowska, Z. (2008). Chronic stress, combined with a high-fat/high-sugar diet, shifts sympathetic signaling toward neuropeptide Y and leads to obesity and the metabolic syndrome. *Annals of the New York Academy of Sciences,* Vol.1148, (December 2008), pp. 232–237. ISSN 0077-8923.

Kyrou, I & Tsigos, C. (2009). Stress hormones: physiological stress and regulation of metabolism. *Current opinion in pharmacology,* Vol.9, No.6, (December 2009), pp. 787-793, ISSN 1471-4892.

Lafontan, M. & Langin, D. (2009). Lipolysis and lipid mobilization in human adipose tissue. Progress in lipid research, Vol.48, No.5, (September 2009), pp. 275-297, ISSN 0163-7827.

Lamharzi, N.; Renard, C.B.; Kramer, F.; Pennathur, S.; Heinecke, J.W.; Chait, A. & Bornfeldt, K.E. (2004). Hyperlipidemia in concert with hyperglycemia stimulates the proliferation of macrophages in atherosclerotic lesions: potential role of glucose-oxidized LDL. *Diabetes,* Vol.53, No.12, (December 2004), pp. 3217-3225, ISSN 0012-1797.

Lampman, R.M. & Schteingart, D.E. (1991). Effects of exercise training on glucose control, lipid metabolism, and insulin sensitivity in hypertriglyceridemia and non-insulin dependent diabetes mellitus. *Medicine and science in sports and sxercise,* Vol.23, No.6, (June 1991), pp. 703-712, ISSN: 0195-9131.

Lemieux, A.M. & Coe, C.L. (1995). Abuse-related posttraumatic stress disorders: evidence for chronic neuroendocrine activation in women. *Psychosomatic medicine,* Vol. 57, No.2, (March/April 1995), pp.105-115, ISSN 0033-3174.

Leon, A.S. & Sanchez, O.A. (2001). Response of blood lipids to exercise training alone or combined with dietary intervention. *Medicine and science in sports and exercise,* Vol.33, No.6, (June 2001), pp. S502-S515, ISSN 0195-9131.

Liao, J.K.; Shin, W.S.; Lee, W.Y. & Clark, S.L. (1995). Oxidized low-density lipoprotein decreases the expression of endothelial nitric oxide synthase. *The Journal of biological chemistry,* Vol.270, No.1, (January 1995), pp. 319-324, ISSN 0021-9258.

Lindgärde, F. & Saltin, B. (1981). Daily physical activity, work capacity and glucose tolerance in lean and obese normoglycaemic middle-aged men. *Diabetologia,* Vol.20, No.2, (February 1981), pp. 134-138, ISSN 0012-186X.

Ludwig, D.S.; Pereira, M.A.; Kroenke, C.H.; Hilner, J.E.; Van Horn, L.; Slattery, M.L. & Jacobs, D.R. Jr. (1999). Dietary fiber, weight gain, and cardiovascular disease risk factors in young adults. JAMA, Vol.282, No.16, (October 1999), pp. 1539-1546, ISSN 0098-7484.

Magkos, F.; Wright, D.C.; Patterson, B.W.; Mohammed, B.S. & Mittendorfer, B. (2005). Lipid metabolism response to a single, prolonged bout of endurance exercise in healthy young men. *American journal of physiology. Endocrinology and metabolism,* Vol.290, No.2, (February 2006), pp. E355-E362. ISSN 1522-1555 online, 0193-1849 print.

Masuzaki, H. & Flier JS. (2003). Tissue-specific glucocorticoid reactivating enzyme, 11 beta-hydroxysteroid dehydrogenase type 1 (11 beta-HSD1)--a promising drug target for the treatment of metabolic syndrome. *Current drug targets. Immune, endocrine and metabolic disorders,* Vol.3, No.4, (December 2003), pp. 255-262, ISSN 1568-0088.

Masuzaki, H.; Paterson, J.; Shinyama, H.; Morton, N.M.; Mullins, J.J.; Seckl, J.R. & Flier, J.S. (2001). A transgenic model of visceral obesity and the metabolic syndrome. *Science,* Vol.294, No.5549, (December 2001), pp. 2166-2170, ISSN 0036-8075.

Matsuura, E.; Kobayashi, K.; Matsunami, Y.; Shen, L.; Quan, N.; Makarova, M.; Suchkov, S.V.; Ayada, K.; Oguma, K. & Lopez, L.R. (2009). Autoimmunity, infectious immunity, and atherosclerosis. *Journal of clinical immunology,* Vol.29, No.6, (November 2009), pp. 714-721, ISSN 0271-9142.

McEwen, B.S. (1998). Protective and damaging effects of stress mediators: central role of the brain. *Dialogues in clinical neuroscience,* Vol.8, No.4, (2006), pp. 367-381, ISSN 1294-8322.

McCann, B.S.; Warnick, G.R. & Knopp, R.H. (1990). Changes in plasma lipids and dietary intake accompanying shifts in perceived workload and stress. *Psychosomatic medicine,* Vol.52, No.1, (January/February 1990), pp. 97-108, ISSN 0033-3174.

McGale, N.; McArdle, S. & Gaffney, P. (2011). Exploring the effectiveness of an integrated exercise/CBT intervention for young men's mental health. *British journal of health psychology,* Vol.16, No.3, (September 2011), pp.457-471, ISSN 1359-107X.

McMurray, R.G. & Hackney, A.C. (2005). Interactions of metabolic hormones, adipose tissue and exercise. *Sports medicine,* Vol.35, No.5, (2005), pp. 393-412, ISSN 0112-1642.

Mitchell, B.M.; Dorrance, A.M.; Mack, E.A. & Webb, R.C. (2004). Glucocorticoids decrease GTP cyclohydrolase and tetrahydro-biopterin-dependent vasorelaxation through glucocorticoid receptors. *Journal of cardiovascular pharmacology,* Vol.43, No.1, (January 2004), pp. 8-13, ISSN 0160-2446.

Mohamed-Ali, V.; Pinkney, J.H. & Coppack, S.W. (1998). Adipose tissue as an endocrine and paracrine organ. *International journal of obesity and related metabolic disorders: journal of the International Association for the Study of Obesity,* Vol.22, No.12, (December 1998), pp. 1145-1158, ISSN 0307-0565.

Mukai, H.; Tsurugizawa, T.; Ogiue-Ikeda, M.; Murakami, G.; Hojo, Y.; Ishii, H.; Kimoto, T. & Kawato, S. (2006). Local neurosteroid production in the hippocampus: influence on synaptic plasticity of memory. *Neuroendocrinology,* Vol.84, No.4, (2006), pp. 255-263, ISSN: 0028-3835.

Mullick, A.E.; Tobias, P.S. & Curtiss, L.K. (2006). Toll-like receptors and atherosclerosis: key contributors in disease and health? *Immunologic research,* Vol.34, No.3, (2006), pp. 193-209, ISSN 0257-277X.

Muniyappa, R. & Quon, M.J. (2007).Insulin action and insulin resistance in vascular endothelium. *Current opinion in clinical nutrition and metabolic care,* Vol.10, No.4, (July 2007), pp. 523-530, ISSN 1363-1950.

Muniyappa, R.; Iantorno, M. & Quon, M.J. (2008). An integrated view of insulin resistance and endothelial dysfunction. *Endocrinology and metabolism clinics of North America,* Vol.37, No.3, (September 2008), pp. 685-711, ISSN 0889-8529.

Nakazato, K.; Ishibashi, T.; Shindo, J.; Shiomi, M. & Maruyama, Y. (1996). Expression of very low density lipoprotein receptor mRNA in rabbit atherosclerotic lesions. *The American journal of pathology,* Vol.149, No.6, (December 1996), pp. 1831-1838, ISSN 0002-9440.

Neves, V.J.; Moura, M.J.C.S.; Almeida, B.S.; Costa, R.; Sanches, A.; Ferreira, R.; Tamascia, M.L.; Romani, E.A.O.; Novaes, P.D. & Marcondes, F.K. (2011). Chronic stress, but not hypercaloric diet, impairs vascular function in rats. *Stress: the international journal on the biology of stress,* (2011), Epub ahead of print, doi:10.3109/10253890.2011.601369, ISSN 1025-3890.

Neves, V.J.; Moura, M.J.C.S.; Tamascia, M.L.; Ferreira, R.; Silva, N.S.; Costa, R.; Montemor, P.L.; Narvaes, E.A.O.; Bernardes, C.F.; Novaes, P.D. & Marcondes, F.K. (2009). Proatherosclerotic effects of chronic stress in male rats: Altered phenylephrine sensitivity and nitric oxide synthase activity of aorta and circulating lipids. *Stress: the international journal on the biology of stress,* Vol.12, No.4, (July 2009), pp. 320-327, ISSN 1025-3890.

Nickenig, G.; Bäumer, A.T.; Temur, Y.; Kebben, D.; Jockenhövel, F. & Böhm, M. (1999). Statin-sensitive dysregulated AT1 receptor function and density in hypercholesterolemic men. *Circulation,* Vol.100, No.21, (November 1999), pp. 2131-2134, ISSN 0009-7322.

Nishitani, N. & Sakakibara, H. (2005). Relationship of obesity to job stress and eating behavior in male Japanese workers. International journal of obesity : journal of the International Association for the Study of Obesity, Vol.30, No.3, (March 2006), pp. 528-533, ISSN 1476-5497 online, ISSN 0307-0565 print.

O'Donnell, L.; O'Meara, N.; Owens, D.; Johnson, A.; Collins, P. & Tomkin, G. (1987). Plasma catecholamines and lipoproteins in chronic psychological stress. *Journal of the Royal Society of Medicine,* Vol.80, No.6, (June 1987), pp. 339-342, ISSN 0141-0768.

Okruhlicová, L; Dlugosová, K.; Mitasíková, M. & Bernátová, I. (2008). Ultrastructural characteristics of aortic endothelial cells in borderline hypertensive rats exposed to chronic social stress. *Physiological research/Academia Scientiarum Bohemoslovaca,* Vol.57, Suppl.2, (March 2008), pp. S31-37, ISSN 0862-8408.

Padden, D.L.; Connors, R.A. & Agazio, J.G. (2011). Determinants of health-promoting behaviors in military spouses during deployment separation. *Military medicine,* Vol.176, No.1, (January 2011), pp.26-34, ISSN: 0026-4075.

Pejovic, S.; Vgontzas, A.N.; Basta, M.; Tsaoussoglou, M.; Zoumakis, E.; Vgontzas, A.; Bixler, E.O. & Chrousos, G.P. (2010). Leptin and hunger levels in young healthy adults after one night of sleep loss. Journal of sleep research, Vol.19, No.4, (December 2010), pp. 552-558, ISSN 0962-1105.

Poehlman, E.T.; Toth, M.J.; Bunyard, L.B.; Gardner, A.W.; Donaldson, K.E.; Colman, E.; Fonong, T. & Ades, P.A. (1995). Physiological predictors of increasing total and central adiposity in aging men and women. *Archives of internal medicine,* Vol.155, No.22, (December 1995), pp. 2443-2448, ISSN 0003-9926.

Pradhan, A.D.; Manson, J.E.; Rifai, N.; Buring, J.E.& Ridker, P.M. (2001).C-reactive protein, interleukin 6, and risk of developing type 2 diabetes mellitus. *JAMA,* Vol.286, No.3, (July 2001), pp. 327-334, ISSN 0098-7484.

Risérus, U.; Willett, W.C. & Hu, F.B. (2008). Dietary fats and prevention of type 2 diabetes. *Progress in lipid research,* Vol.48, No.1, (January 2009), pp. 44-51, ISSN 1873-2194 online, 0163-7827 print.

Rizzo, M.; Kotur-Stevuljevic, J.; Berneis, K.; Spinas, G.; Rini, G.B.; Jelic-Ivanovic, Z.; Spasojevic-Kalimanovska, V. & Vekic, J. (2009). Atherogenic dyslipidemia and oxidative stress: a new look. *Translational research: the journal of laboratory and clinical medicine,* Vol.153, No.5, (May 2009), pp. 217-223. ISSN 1931-5244.

Roberts, C.K. & Barnard, R.J. (2005). Effects of exercise and diet on chronic disease. *Journal of applied physiology,* Vol.98, No.1, (January 2005), pp. 3-30, ISSN: 8750-7587.

Ross, R. (1999). Atherosclerosis--an inflammatory disease. *The New England journal of medicine,* Vol.340, No.2, (January 1999), pp. 115-126, ISSN. 0028-4793.

Rubenfire, M.; Mollo, L.; Krishnan, S.; Finkel, S.; Weintraub, M.; Gracik, T.; Kohn, D. & Oral, E.A. (2011). The Metabolic Fitness Program: Lifestyle modification for the metabolic syndrome using the resources of cardiac rehabilitation. *Journal of cardiopulmonary rehabilitation and prevention,* Epub ahead of print doi: 10.1097/HCR. 0b013e318220a7eb, (July 2011), ISSN 1932-751X.

Schuit, A.J.; Schouten, E.G.; Miles, TP.; Evans, W.J.; Saris, W.H.M. & Kok, F.J. (1998). The effect of six months training on weight, body fatness and serum lipids in apparently healthy elderly Dutch men and women International. *International journal of obesity and related metabolic disorders: journal of the International Association for the Study of Obesity,* Vol.22, No.9, (September 1998), pp. 847-853, ISSN 0307-0565.

Seeman, T.E.; Singer, B.H.; Rowe, J.W.; Horwitz, R.I. & McEwen, B.S. (1997). Price of adaptation--allostatic load and its health consequences. MacArthur studies of successful aging. *Archives of internal medicine,* Vol.157, No.19, (October 1997), pp. 2259-2268, ISSN 0003-9926.

Selye, H. (1936). A syndrome produced by diverse nocuous agents. *Nature,* Vol.138, (July 1936), p.32, ISSN 1476-4687.

Sheril, A.; Jeyakumar, S.M.; Jayashree, T.; Giridharan, N.V. & Vajreswari A. (2008). Impact of feeding polyunsaturated fatty acids on cholesterol metabolism of dyslipidemic obese rats of WNIN/GR-Ob strain. *Atherosclerosis,* Vol.204, No.1, (May 2009), pp.136-140, ISSN 1879-1484 online, ISSN 0021-9150 print.

Shively, C.A.; Register, T.C. & Clarkson, T.B. (2009). Social stress, visceral obesity, and coronary artery atherosclerosis: product of a primate adaptation. American journal of primatology, Vol.71, No.9, (September 2009), pp. 742-751, ISSN 0275-2565.

Sierra, C. & de la Sierra, A. (2008). Early detection and management of the high-risk patient with elevated blood pressure. *Vascular health and risk management,* Vol.4, No.2, (April 2008), pp. 289-296, ISSN 1176-6344.

Sigwalt, A.R.; Budde, H.; Helmich, I.; Glaser, V.; Ghisoni, K.; Lanza, S.; Cadore, E.L.; Lhullier, F.L.; F de Bem A.; Hohl, A.; J de Matos, F.; de Oliveira, P.A.; S Prediger, R.D.; A Guglielmo, L.G. & Latini, A. (2011). Molecular aspects involved in swimming exercise training reducing anhedonia in a rat model of depression. *Neuroscience,* Epub ahead of print, doi:10.1016/j.physletb.2003.10.071, (June 2011), ISSN 1873-7544.

Singh, B.M. & Mehta, J.L. (2003). Interactions between the renin-angiotensin system and dyslipidemia: relevance in the therapy of hypertension and coronary heart disease. *Archives of internal medicine,* Vol.163, No.11, (June 2003), pp. 1296-1304, ISSN 0003-992

Sitia, S.; Tomasoni, L.; Atzeni, F.; Ambrosio, G.; Cordiano, C.; Catapano, A.; Tramontana, S.; Perticone, F.; Naccarato, P.; Camici, P.; Picano, E.; Cortigiani, L.; Bevilacqua, M.; Milazzo, L.; Cusi, D.; Barlassina, C.; Sarzi-Puttini, P. & Turiel, M. (2010). From endothelial dysfunction to atherosclerosis. *Autoimmunity reviews,* Vol.9, No.12, (October 2010), pp. 830-834, ISSN 1568-9972.

Sothmann, M.S.; Buckworth, J.; Claytor, R.P.; Cox, R.H.; White-Welkley, J.E. & Dishman, R.K. (1996). Exercise training and the cross-stressor adaptation hypothesis. *Exercise and sport science reviews,* Vol.24, (1996), pp. 267-287, ISSN 0091-6331.

Spiegel, K.; Tasali, E.; Penev, P. & Van Cauter E. (2004). Brief communication: Sleep curtailment in healthy young men is associated with decreased leptin levels, elevated ghrelin levels, and increased hunger and appetite. *Annals of internal medicine,* Vol. 141, No.11, (December 2004), pp. 846-850, ISSN 0003-4819.

Stanhope, K.L.; Schwarz, J.M.; Keim, N.L.; Griffen, S.C.; Bremer, A.A.; Graham, J.L.; Hatcher, B.; Cox, C.L.; Dyachenko, A.; Zhang, W.; McGahan, J.P.; Seibert, A.; Krauss, R.M.; Chiu, S.; Schaefer, E.J.; Ai, M.; Otokozawa, S.; Nakajima, K.; Nakano, T.; Beysen, C.; Hellerstein, M.K.; Berglund, L. & Havel, P.J. (2009). Consuming fructose-sweetened, not glucose-sweetened, beverages increases visceral adiposity and lipids and decreases insulin sensitivity in overweight/obese humans. *The journal of Clinical Investigation,* Vol.119, No.5, (May 2009), pp. 1322-1334, ISSN 0021-9738.

Steanovv, T.S.; Vekova, A.M.; Kurktschiev, D.P. & Temelkova-Kurktschiev, T.S. (2011). Relationship of physical activity and eating behaviour with obesity and type 2 diabetes mellitus: Sofia Lifestyle (SLS) study. *Folia Medica,* Vol.53, No.1, (January/March 2011), pp. 11-18, ISSN 0204-8043.

Steinberg, D. (2002). Atherogenesis in perspective: hypercholesterolemia and inflammation as partners in crime. *Nature medicine,* Vol.8, No.11, (November 2002), pp. 1211-1217, ISSN 1078-8956.

Sterling, P. & Eyer, J. (1988). Allostasis: a new paradigm to explain arousal pathology. In: *Handbook of Life Stress, Cognition and Health,* Fisher, S. & Reason, J (editors), pp. 629-649, JOHN WILEY & SONS, ISBN-10: 0471912697/ISBN-13: 978-0471912699, New York - USA.

Stoney, C.M. (2007). Cholesterol and Lipoproteins, In: *Encyclopedia of Stress,* George Fink (editor), pp. 478-483, ELSEVIER, ISBN 978-0-12-088503-9, San Diego, CA - USA.

Stoney, C.M.; Niaura, R.; Bausserman, L. & Matacin, M. (1999). Lipid reactivity to stress: I. Comparison of chronic and acute stress responses in middle-aged airline pilots. *Health psychology : official journal of the Division of Health Psychology, American Psychological Association,* Vol.18, No.3, (May 1999), pp. 241-250, ISSN 0278-6133.

Stoney, C.M.; West, S.G.; Hughes, J.W.; Lentino, L.M.; Finney, M.L.; Falko, J. & Bausserman, L. (2002). Acute psychological stress reduces plasma triglyceride clearance. *Psychophysiology,* Vol.39, No.1, (January 2002), pp. 80-85, ISSN 0048-5772.

Sudano, I.; Spieker, L.E.; Hermann, F.; Flammer, A.; Corti, R.; Noll, G. & Lüscher, T.F. (2006). Protection of endothelial function: targets for nutritional and pharmacological interventions. *Journal of cardiovascular pharmacology,* Vol.47, No.2, (June 2006), pp. S136-S150, ISSN 0160-2446.

Taguchi, I.; Inoue, T.; Kikuchi, M.; Toyoda, S.; Arikawa, T.; Abe, S. & Node, K. (2011). Pleiotropic effects of ARB on dyslipidemia. *Current vascular pharmacology,* Vol.9, No.2, (March 2011), pp. 129-135, ISSN 1570-1611.

Tellez, A.; Schuster, D.S.; Alviar, C.; López-Berenstein, G.; Sanguino, A.; Ballantyne, C.; Perrard, X.Y.; Schulz, D.G.; Rousselle, S.; Kaluza, G.L. & Granada, J.F. (2011). Intramural coronary lipid injection induces atheromatous lesions expressing proinflammatory chemokines: implications for the development of a porcine model of atherosclerosis. *Cardiovascular revascularization medicine: including molecular interventions,* Epub ahead of print, doi:10.1016/j.carrev.2011.03.007, (May 2011), ISSN 1878-0938.

Thompson, P.D.; Cullinane, E.M.; Sady, S.P.; Flynn, M.M.; Bernier, D.N.; Kantor, M.A.; Saritelli, A.L. & Herbert, P.N. (1988). Modest changes in high-density lipoprotein concentration and metabolism with prolonged exercise training. *Circulation,* Vol.78, No.1, (July 1988), pp. 25-34, ISSN 0009-7322.

Torres, S.J. & Nowson, C.A. (2007). Relationship between stress, eating behavior, and obesity. *Nutrition,* Vol.23, No.11-12, (November/December 2007), pp. 887-894, ISSN 0899-9007.

Tsatsoulis, A. & Fountoulakis, S. (2006). The protective role of exercise on stress system dysregulation and comorbidities. . *Annals of the New York Academy of Sciences,* Vol.1083 (November 2006), pp. 196-213, ISSN 0077-8923.

Tsekouras, Y.E.; Magkos, F.; Prentzas, K.I.; Basioukas, K.N.; Matsama, S.G.; Yanni, A.E.; Kavouras, S.A. & Sidossis, L.S. (2009). A single bout of whole-body resistance exercise augments basal VLDL-triacylglycerol removal from plasma in healthy untrained men. *Clinical science,* Vol.116, No.2, (January 2009), pp. 147-156, ISSN 0143-5221.

van Oostrom, A.J.; van Wijk, J. & Cabezas, M.C. (2004). Lipaemia, inflammation and atherosclerosis: novel opportunities in the understanding and treatment of atherosclerosis. *Drugs,* Vol.64, No.2 (2004), pp. 19-41, 0012-6667.

Veen, G.; Giltay, E.J.; DeRijk, R.H.; van Vliet, I.M.; van Pelt, J. & Zitman, F.G. (2009). Salivary cortisol, serum lipids, and adiposity in patients with depressive and anxiety disorders. *Metabolism: clinical and experimental,* Vol.58, No.6, (June 2009), pp. 821-827, ISSN 0026-0495.

Venables, M.C. & Jeukendrup, A.E. (2009). Physical inactivity and obesity: links with insulin resistance and type 2 diabetes mellitus. *Diabetes/metabolism research and reviews,* Vol.25, No.1, (September 2009), pp. S18-S23, ISSN 1520-7552.

Vessby, B. (2000). Dietary fat and insulin action in humans. *The British journal of nutrition,* Vol.83, No.1, (March 2000), pp. S91-S96, ISSN 0007-1145.

Vogelzangs, N.; Suthers, K.; Ferrucci, L.; Simonsick, E.M.; Ble, A.; Schrager, M.; Bandinelli, S.; Lauretani, F.; Giannelli, S.V. & Penninx, B.W. (2007). Hypercortisolemic depression is associated with the metabolic syndrome in late-life. *Psychoneuroendocrinology,* Vol.32, No.2, (February 2007), pp.151-159, ISSN 0306-4530.

Walker, E.A. & Stewart, P.M. (2003). 11beta-hydroxysteroid dehydrogenase: unexpected connections. *Trends in endocrinology and metabolism: TEM,* Vol.14, No.7, (September 2003), pp.334-339, ISSN 1043-2760.

Wallis, D.J. & Hetherington M.M. (2008). Emotions and eating: Self-reported and experimentally induced changes in food intake under stress. *Appetite,* Vol.52, No.2, (April 2009), pp. 355-362, ISSN 1095-8304 online, 0195-6663 print.

Watts, G.F.; Barrett, P.H.R. & Chan, D.C. (2008). HDL metabolism in context: looking on the bright side. *Current opinion in lipidology,* Vol.19, No.4, (August 2008), pp. 395-404, ISSN 0957-9672.

Watts, G.F.; Ooi, E.M.M. & Chan, D.C. (2009). Therapeutic regulation of apoB100 metabolism in insulin resistance in vivo. *Pharmacology & therapeutics,* Vol.123, No.3, (September 2009), pp. 281–291, ISSN: 0163-7258.

Win, S.; Parakh, K.; Eze-Nliam, C.M.; Gottdiener, J.S.; Kop, W.J. & Ziegelstein, R.C. (2011). Depressive symptoms, physical inactivity and risk of cardiovascular mortality in older adults: the Cardiovascular Health Study. *Heart: official journal of the British Cardiac Society,* Vol.97, No.6, (March 2011), pp. 500-505, ISSN 1355-6037.

Xu, C.; He, J.; Jiang., H.; Zu, L.; Zhai, W.; Pu, S. & Xu, G. (2009). Direct effect of glucocorticoids on lipolysis in adipocytes. *Molecular endocrinology,* Vol.23, No.8, (May 2009), pp. 1161-1170, ISSN 0888-8809.

Xu, X.H.; Shah, P.K.; Faure, E.; Equils, O.; Thomas, L.; Fishbein, M.C.; Luthringer, D.; Xu, X.P.; Rajavashisth, T.B.; Yano, J.; Kaul, S. & Arditi, M. (2001). Toll-like receptor-4 is expressed by macrophages in murine and human lipid-rich atherosclerotic plaques and upregulated by oxidized LDL. *Circulation,* Vol.104, No.25 (December 2001), pp. 3103-3108, ISSN 0009-7322.

Yamazaki, Y.; Hashizume, T.; Morioka, H.; Sadamitsu, S.; Ikari, A.; Miwa, M. & Sugatani, J. (2011). Diet-induced lipid accumulation in liver enhances ATP-binding cassette transporter g5/g8 expression at bile canaliculi. *Drug metabism and pharmacokinetics,* Epub ahead of print, doi:10.2133/dmpk.DMPK-11-RG-025, (May 2011), ISSN 1880-0920.

Yarrow, J.F.; White, L.J.; McCoy, S.C. & Borst, S.E. (2010). Training augments resistance exercise induced elevation of circulating brain derived neurotrophic factor (BDNF). *Neuroscience letters,* Vol.479, No.2, (July 2010), pp. 161-165, ISSN 0304-3940.

Yin, Z.; Davis, C.L.; Moore, J.B. & Treiber, F.A. (2005). Physical activity buffers the effects of chronic stress on adiposity in youth. *Annals of behavioral medicine: a* publication *of the Society of Behavioral Medicine,* Vol.29, No.1, (February 2005), pp. 29-36, ISSN 0883-6612.

Yoo, H. & Franke, W.D. (2010). Stress and cardiovascular disease risk in female law enforcement officers. *International archives of occupational and environmental health,* Vol.84, No.3, (March 2011), pp. 279-286, ISSN 1432-1246 online, ISSN 0340-0131 print.

Yudkin, J.S.; Kumari, M.; Humphries, S.E. & Mohamed-Ali, V. (2000). Inflammation, obesity, stress and coronary heart disease: is interleukin-6 the link? *Atherosclerosis,* Vol.148, No.2, (Februery 2000), pp. 209-214, ISSN 0021-9150.

Zakrzewska, K.E.; Cusin, I.; Sainsbury, A.; Rohner-Jeanrenaud, F. & Jeanrenaud, B. (1997). Glucocorticoids as counterregulatory hormones of leptin: toward an understanding of leptin resistance. *Diabetes,* Vol.46, No.4, (April 1997), pp. 717-719, ISSN 0012-1797.

Zukowska, Z. (2005). Atherosclerosis and angiogenesis: what do nerves have to do with it? *Pharmacological reports: PR.* Vol.57, Supplement, (June 2005), pp. 229-234, ISSN 1734-1140.

19

Cholesterol and Triglycerides Metabolism Disorder in Malignant Hemopathies

Romeo-Gabriel Mihăilă
"Lucian Blaga" University of Sibiu
Romania

1. Introduction

The aim of this chapter is to achieve a synthesis of the major studies existing in the literature on correlations between lipid metabolism and malignant hemopathies. We will expose the fundamental research data and their impact on clinical treatment. The purpose of this review is to help the clinicians to understand better the pathological disorders of the lipid metabolism and use the existing therapeutic arsenal to improve the treatment outcomes. The research and the recognition of the presence of dyslipidemia is useful, as well as monitoring them during oncological therapy. The treatment of dyslipidemia may not be only an option when a patient with malignant hemopathy has acquired multidrug resistance. It can contribute to reversing this resistance, but it can also have adverse effects that must be recognized, followed and treated.

There are numerous studies in literature, but the connection between blood levels of various lipid fractions and hematologic malignancies is still unknown (Cvetkovic et al., 2009). Various epidemiological studies have found that between blood lipids and various neoplastic diseases there are correlations, thus the question is whether in the pathogenesis of cancer are not involved various lipid disorders (Moschovi M et al., 2004). At the same time it is believed that in patients with metabolic syndrome (MS), blood lipid levels may have correlations with the risk of cancer (Ulmer H et al., 2009).

2. The lipid profile evolution under cancer treatment

Cvetkovic & al. studied 47 patients with malignant non-Hodgkin's lymphoma (NHL) and found that before the treatment, compared with patients in the control group, blood levels of phospholipids, cholesterol (CH) and high density lipoprotein-cholesterol (HDL-cholesterol) had significantly lower values. After chemotherapy (3 or 6 cycles) the blood lipid levels reached even lower values in patients where the disease progressed, as opposed to those who achieved complete remission or whose disease was stationary, cases in which lipids increased progressively. (Cvetkovic et al., 2009).

In an other study conducted in Poland on the lipid levels of 238 patients with different hematological malignant diseases Kuliszkiewicz-Janus M et al. found that HDL-cholesterol values were significantly different from those of patients in the control group when the disease was in active phase, but in the remission phase the difference was statistically significant only in patients with NHL and acute leukemia (Kuliszkiewicz-Janus et al., 2008).

In a health investigation conducted on 156,153 subjects, with 5079 incident cancers in men and 4738 cancers in women, and a mean of 10.6 years of survey, there was an inverse association between serum triglyceride (TG) levels and NHL (2). But in the study conducted by Kuliszkiewicz-Janus M et al., the TG value increased in the active disease period in all the hematological malignancies besides NHL (Kuliszkiewicz-Janus et al., 2008).

Mihăilă R and al. made a cross-sectional research on all the patients with chronic lymphocytic leukemia (CLL) existing in a county department of hematology and a group of volunteer subjects from the medical staff with no malignant pathology. They found an augmentation of TG values in the patients with CLL ($p < 0.00001$), an argument for a possible link between the MS and chronic lymphoproliferations. Hypercholesterolemia present in the patients with CLL from the above study may have consequences regarding the multiple drug resistance, subject to further future study. (Mihăilă et al., 2010)

Nearly all the children with ALL when diagnosed and during chemotherapy revealed a predictable model of serum dyslipidemia that consisted of very low levels of HDL-cholesterol, and elevated TG, and low-density lipoprotein cholesterol (LDL-cholesterol), that regained normal values during the remission period (Moschovi et al., 2004).

In patients with secondary hemophagocytic syndrome an augmentation of TG was observed when diagnosed or during the disease period and TG values decreased when the disease improved under treatment (Okamoto et al., 2009). In patients with aggressive T cell lymphoma, fasting TG level was higher in those with hemophagocytic syndrome group than in the patients who had no hemophagocytic syndrome (Tong et al., 2008).

3. The consequences of treatments with antineoplastic drugs

In children with acute lymphoblastic leukemia (ALL), treated with asparaginase dyslipidemia was frequently observed (Cohen et al., 2010).

A child heterozygote for apolipoprotein E 3/4 and with ALL who received pegasparaginase, presented an important aumentation of serum TG value, which normalized after continuous insulin infusion (Lawson et al., 2011). Another patient with a heterozygote type of familial lipoprotein lipase defect syndrome developed an important increase of serum TG value that was treated by three plasma exchanges with frozen plasma (Nakagawa et al., 2008).

An adult patient with ALL also had an acute pancreatitis because of an important hypertriglyceridemia that appeared after asparaginase administration (Kfoury-Baz et al., 2008), as well as a 10 years old boy who had been previously treated with asparaginase and corticosteroids (Ridola et al., 2008), both successfully treated by plasmapheresis sessions (Kfoury-Baz et al., 2008; Ridola et al., 2008).

In a group of children and adolescent patients recently diagnosed with ALL during treatment a progresive increase of serum CH values to 274+/-124 mg/dl was observed. In this group of patients the average value of TG during tratment was 459+/-526 mg/dl. Two patients had hypertriglyceridemia-related complications: a thrombosis of saggital sinus and an infarct of the left frontal lobe. The observed dyslipidemia disappeared in all children after the asparaginase administration (Cohen et al., 2010).

A prospective study assessed the lipid levels in children with ALL. At diagnosis, there was a significantly low level of total CH and HDL-cholesterol and at the same time a high level of TG. The patients were treated with the ALLIC 2002 protocol (including L-asparaginase), during which the values of total CH and HDL-cholesterol augmented, but they still remained lower than for the control group. The main serum TG level was significantly higher as compared to that of witnesses (Zalewska-Szewczyk et al., 2008).

A retrospective analysis showed that imatinib mesylate, used for the treatment of patients with chronic myeloid leukemia, led to a diminishing of serum CH and TG values (Franceschino et al., 2008). In a Romanian patient with chronic myeloid leukemia who received usual-dose of imatinib mesylate, a rapid and sustained normalization of serum CH, TG, low- and high-density lipoproteins and glucose values was found (Gologan et al., 2009).

In some types of leukemia it was found that Kit receptor tyrosine kinase is overexpressed in a pathological manner, also that CH depletion was able to prevent Kit-mediated activation of the phosphatidylinositol 3-kinase downstream target Akt, which inhibits cell proliferation (Jahn et al., 2007).

The treatment of cutaneous lymphomas with T cells using bexarotene can produce a serum TG augmentation, as in the three cases reported. The treatment with fenofibrate is recommended, but if adverse effects occure or a statin is needed to reduce hypertriglyceridemia, omega-3 fatty acids may be a therapeutic solution during the bexarotene administration. (Musolino et al., 2009)

4. Is the metabolic syndrome a risk factor for some malignant hemopathies?

The main risk factors for excess weight and obesity are high caloric diet and sedentary lifestyle. A study conducted in a county hospital in Transylvania examined the presence of MS in all 56 patients with NHL existing in its records and a control group of 64 consecutive patients with non-cancerous diseases in the same hospital (control group). Patients with NHL had significantly more frequently arterial hypertension, significantly higher body mass index values, and a significantly higher number of components of the MS as compared to those of the control group. This observation advocates the idea that excess weight may be a risk factor for this type of neoplasia. (Mihăilă et al., 2009)

In a group of 170 non-Hispanic white pediatric cancer survivors, among males, body adiposity was more important in survivors than in witnesses, as was trunk fat. The survivors had higher values of CH, TG, LDL-cholesterol than the witnesses, and the first watched TV more hours than controls (Miller TL et al., 2010). It was observed that the young survivors of ALL, disease which they had in their childhood, especially those who received cranial radiotherapy, are likely to develop hyperlipidemia, insulin resistance, obesity, arterial hypertension and even MS soon after the treatment (Trimis et al., 2007).

After an average period of 37 months after the end of type ALL-BFM 90 chemotherapy protocol, out of 52 patients almost half were overweight, nearly 6% - obese, more than half had at least one risk factor for MS, and about 6% had MS (Kourti et al., 2005).

It was found that the consequences of treatment performed for ALL during childhood may become manifest when subjects reach adulthood. Cranial irradiation favors more the appearance of MS: 60% of those who had been so treated had at least two of the five components of MS when they become adults, and only 20% of those who had not been irradiated. The pathogenetic mechanism that explains the metabolic effects of cranial irradiation implies growth hormone (GH) deficiency, lower level of insulin-like growth factor 1, fasting hyperinsulinemia, abdominal obesity and hyperlipidemia, especially in women (Gurney et al., 2006). In another study, ALL survivors who received cranial irradiation developed more frequently MS than those nonirradiated (23% towards 7%), probably because of higher prevalence of excess weight and arterial hypertension (van Waas et al., 2010).

In a study conducted on a group of 184 adults who had ALL in their childhood, the overall prevalence of MS has been even higher - 9.2%. Peripheral stem cell allografts after total body irradiation favored the occurrence of hypertriglyceridemia, low HDL-cholesterol and increased fasting glucose level (Oudin et al., 2011).

In Sweden a group of adults was analysed; they survived after ALL during childhood and were submitted to radio-and chemotherapy. Those who received treatment for 5 years with GH compared with those not treated so for 8 years, showed significant changes in HDL-cholesterol, glucose and apolipoprotein B / apolipoprotein A1 ratio, and MS was significantly less frequent. (Follin et al., 2010)

Another study conducted in Sweden on adults who had childhood leukemia, found an augmentation of total body fat, especially of trunk adiposity and an evolution towards an unfavorable lipid spectrum. These observations were correlated with low levels of endocrine secretion of GH, a consequence of previous cranial irradiation. (Jarfelt et al., 2005)

An interesting combination of diseases was described in a 54 years old woman: after being diagnosed with chronic neutrophilic leukemia a liver biopsy was made. The histopathological diagnosis was of nonalcoholic steatohepatitis (NASH) with neutrophilic infiltrate. The authors consider that the leukemia cells that infiltrated the liver contributed to the emergence of NASH. The administration of cytosine arabinoside contributed to a significant decrease in fat degeneration. (Yoshida et al., 2004)

There are few studies on the metabolism of chylomicrons in patients with cancer. The study of a group of patients with Hodgkin and nonHodgkin lymphoma, as compared to a healthy control group, led to the observation that after an intravenous administration of a chylomicron-like emulsion, the levels of CH, TG and VLDL were significantly higher in patients with lymphoma because of the profound disturbance of the chylomicrons lipolysis and their removal deficit. (Gonçalves et al., 2003)

A very interesting observation was achieved in a line of promyelocytic leukemia NB4 cells: the administration of peroxisome proliferator-activated receptor gamma ligands was able not only to induce differentiation but also to favor lipogenesis in NB4 cells. This fact suggests a close link between differentiation and lipogenesis process in human myeloid cells thus stimulated. (Yasugi et al., 2006).

5. Cholesterol metabolism disorder

It is known that cell membranes contain lipid rafts, belonging to CH-rich microdomains. These components of the cell membrane are involved in intracellular signal transduction processes mediated by the receptor and in the self-renewal of ES cells. (Lee et al., 2010) The administration of methyl-beta-cyclodextrin, that is a CH-sequestering agent useful for the lipid raft destruction, is able to restore the activity of large conductance background K(+) channels. This favors the activation by stretch. (Nam et al., 2007) The depletion of CH from the cell membranes leads to lipid rafts destruction, that are responsible for bloking the translocation of leukemia inhibitory factor receptor and gp 130 (Port et al., 2007).

A group of Russian researchers studied the role of membrane CH in a line of human leukaemia K562 cells regarding the regulation of mechanosensitive cation channels activated by stretch. They consider that the above-mentioned suppression of this channel activation in leukemia cell line by methyl-beta-cyclodextrin is produced by F-actin rearrangement due to lipid raft destruction. (Morachevskaya et al., 2007)

In the regulation of lipid and CH metabolism liver X receptors are also involved, they are nuclear receptors. They can modulate the proliferation and survival of both normal and malignant B and T lymphocytes. (Geyeregger et al., 2009)

The correlation between increasing CH in lipid domains and the possible cancerosus cell transformation is very interesting (Ajith et al., 2008). It is believed that CH is important for cell proliferation, because low serum CH values may be the result of high cellular CH need of cancerous cells. Low serum CH values correlate with elevated levels of CH in lymphocytes. Evidence of low levels of CH in the culture medium is due to the development of lymphoma cells, which would consume more CH for their own proliferation. The experimental administration of mevastatin in vitro, which inhibits CH synthesis, did not determine a significant variation of the concentration of CH in the culture medium, while cell growth diminished. (Pugliese et al., 2010)

Low serum CH levels are also frequently found in acute leukemia patients. These patients have significantly lower serum values of CH, HDL-cholesterol, and LDL-cholesterol. A possible explanation for the low levels of HDL-cholesterol in the patients with acute leukemia could be an increased expression of a possible selective site for HDL-cholesteryl ester. (Gonçalves et al., 2005)

Malignant, proliferative cells have an intense metabolism of CH, while decreased intake of CH is responsible for decreasing cell proliferation. In a human line of promyelocytic HL-60 cells, an inhibition of cell cycle progression from G2 phase can be obtained by an enzymatic inhibition of CH synthesis at a stage before 7-dehydrocholesterol production. Drugs such as zaragozic acid or SKF 104976 can induce the expression of antigen 11c, a cluster of differentiation. These products have a comparable action to all-trans retinoic acid, which induces monocyte differentiation. (Sánchez-Martín et al., 2007)

Chronic lymphocytic leukemia (CLL) is a heterogenous malignant hemopathy. In these patients, in the presence of UM-IGHV, which is a negative prognostic factor, there are increased levels of CH and lactate and low levels of glycerol and 3-hydroxybutyrate. (MacIntyre et al., 2010)

CD5 antigen is responsible for CH synthesis and even for adipogenesis. It is known that malignant cells from CLL are undergoing a process of continuous stimulation due to CD5 activation and cell survival. (Gary-Gouy et al., 2007) A continuous activation of an antiapoptotic pathway explains the CLL cells survival. Apolipoprotein E4-very low density lipoproteins is responsible for the high level of apoptosis in CLL cells. Lipoprotein lipase is the enzyme that metabolizes very low density lipoproteins to low-density lipoprotein. It was observed that an increase of lipoprotein lipase mRNA levels is present in CLL patients with shorter survival. (Weinberg et al., 2008)

CH synthesis is also increased in patients with T-ALL who are glucocorticoid resistant (Beesley et al., 2009).

The growth of a promyelocytic leukemia cell line - HL-60 can be experimentally supressed by sodium cholesteryl sulfate, cholesteryl bromide, and cholesteryl-5alpha. The first two are responsible for the cell arrest in S and G2/M phases, and the last product - in the G2/M phase. (Ishimaru et al., 2008)

It was found that in xenotransplanted severely combined immunodeficient mice the most abundant bone marrow CH amounts are located in leukemia-rich sites. In vitro, in leukemic cells CH is able to stimulate FLT-1 expression and VEGF production. Human leukemic cells from patients with AML are significantly richer in CH than normal cells and this CH augmentation represents a marker of aggressive evolution. (Casalou et al., 2011)

6. Experimental and clinical observations on cholesterol metabolism disorder

ABCA1 and ApoA-I are responsible for the efflux of CH in human monocyte leukemia cell line derived foam cells. This decrease of the concentration of CH can be enhanced by administration of rosiglitazone. (Lü et al., 2010) Animals fed on alternate days have showed lower incidence of lymphomas, after tumor inoculation have had higher survival, and some types of cells have proliferated more slowly. It seems that this diet in humans would favor increased levels of HDL-cholesterol and lower those of triacylglycerol. (Varady et al., 2007)
It was found that ether phospholipid edelfosine is able to accumulate and selectively destroy mantle cell lymphoma and CLL cells, underlining the importance of the action on lipid rafts and Fas/CD95 for the therapy of these lymphoproliferations. CH depletion is involved in lipid raft disruption and in the diminishing of drug captation. (Mollinedo et al., 2010)
Some clinical observations on the presence of dyslipidemia in patients with malignant hemopathies are presented in Table 1.

Author	Disease	Dyslipidemia
Inamoto et al., 2005	ALL + cholestasis from graft versus host disease	hypercholesterolemia
Lim et al., 2007	NHL	serum HDL-cholesterol decrease
Gokhale et al., 2007	NHL	serum total CH level was significantly higher in patients who completed the treatment for NHL than in those who completed ALL therapy
Garg et al., 2011	intravascular large B cell lymphoma	low serum levels of HDL-cholesterol
Helman et al., 2011	MALT + obesity	hypercholesterolemia

MALT = mucosa-associated lymphoid tissue lymphoma

Table 1. Examples of dyslipidemia in patients with malignant hemopathies.

7. The cholesterol and the treatment with anti-CD20 monoclonal antibodies

It has been noted that the loss of CH is responsible for the decrease in the number of sites that can fix some monoclonal antibodies, including CD20. CH depletion or Shiga-like toxin binding have been causes of disruption of CD20 localization, but not of CD77 in lipid rafts. (Jarvis et al., 2007)
DXL625 is an anti-CD20 monoclonal antibody, capable of causing independently in vitro apoptosis of a lymphoma B cells line. This apoptosis is inhibited by the loss of membrane CH or of chelation of extracellular calcium, fact that underlines the role of lipid raft and calcium in this process. (Bingaman et al., 2010)
Many lymphoproliferations with B cells have indication of treatment with rituximab, an anti-CD20 antibody. The inhibitor therapeutic effect of rituximab occurs at the same time as the decrease of CH deposits from lipid rafts, with decreased B-cell receptor relocation to lipid rafts structures, and with the disruption of the expression of BCR immunoglobulin, lowering it. (Kheirallah et al., 2010)

The first monoclonal antibody that was approved for the treatment of B-cell lymphoproliferative malignancies was rituxan, a chimeric monoclonal anti-CD20 antibody.
It has been observed that the monoclonal antibody attachment to CD20 produces a redistribution of these antigens to lipid rafts, which are specialized membrane microdomains. If rituxan is not used, the CD20 antigen affinity to lipid rafts is small. Intracellular calcium entry and apoptosis have been completely eliminated experimentally by extracting CH, which has led to the destruction of the integrity of lipid raft structures and to the dissociation of CD20 antigen from a fraction that is resistant to Triton X-100. From this it results that for the activation of caspase induced by CD20- lipid rafts appear to have an essential role. (Janas et al., 2005)
In multidrug resistance two populations of P-glycoprotein (P-gp) are involved. One is located in the membrane regions that are resistant to detergent; it has optimal P-gp ATPase activity; the verapamil can activate it and the orthovanadate can inhibit it almost entirely. The other population is located in another part of the membrane; it has less activity than P-gp ATPase of the first population; the verapamil can inhibit it, and its sensitivity to the orthovanadate is less. The first population of Pgp is surrounded by deposits of CH that may have the role to stimulate the P-gp ATPase activity, but the CH near the second population of Pgp does not seem to have such a role. (Barakat et al., 2005)
Rituximab induced apoptosis may be diminished by depletion of membrane deposits of CH, which does not allow the association to the detergent-insoluble lipid rafts of the antigen hypercrosslinked CD20. Under the action of rituximab, the antibody-bound CD20, found in lipid rafts in a high-affinity structure, activates src family kinases, interfering with the signal-transmission mechanism, which it inhibits. (Unruh et al., 2005)
Besides their CH-lowering effects, statins have pleiotropic effects, including the antileukemic ones observed in vitro and in vivo (Sassano et al., 2009), but they disrupt the binding (Winiarska et al., 2008) and the antitumour activity of rituximab (Ennishi et al., 2010), as a consequence of the changing of the antigen CD20 conformation (Ennishi et al., 2010; Winiarska et al., 2008). Statins interfere with the detection of CD20 as well as the antilymphomatous function of the rituximab (Winiarska et al., 2008). But in a study that analyzed the progression-free survival in 3 years and overall survival in a group of patients with diffuse large B-cell lymphoma, including some patients who were taking statins, it was found that there were no statistically significant differences, fact that advocates the idea that statins used in clinical treatment do not alter the prognosis of patients with diffuse large B-cell lymphoma under R-CHOP treatment. (Ennishi et al., 2010)

8. Statins as adjuvant treatment in malignant hemopathies

After chemotherapy, the blasts of acute myeloid leukemia (AML) respond by increasing cellular content of CH, which increases resistance to treatment. (Kornblau et al., 2007) Statins are pharmacologic inhibitors of 3-hydroxy-3-methylglutaryl-CoA reductase (HMG-CoA reductase) - the regulatory enzyme of CH synthesis (Nonaka et al., 2009; Sassano et al., 2007). In vitro, they block HMG-CoA reductase and by this they contribute to restore sensitivity to chemotherapy. (Kornblau et al., 2007) HMG-CoA regulates not only the synthesis of CH but also that of the higher isoprenoids, as geranylgeranyl pyrophosphate (Fuchs et al., 2008). By the inhibition of the prenylation processes, in vitro, statins reduce cellular proliferation and stimulate apoptosis of cancerous cells (Nonaka et al., 2009; Sassano et al., 2007). It was found that simvastatin inhibits geranylgeranylation processes of small

GTPases Rab5B and Rac1 in certain leukemic cells (for example, adult T-cell leukemia). (Nonaka et al., 2009)

The excessive proliferation inhibition induced by simvastatin results from the induction of apoptosis, cell cycle arrest in phase G2 / M, and accumulation of p21 protein. Simvastatin is able to remove resistance to apoptosis that occurs during treatment with bortezomib, by reducing geranylgeranyl pyrophosphate synthesis and cell survival mechanism dependant on this. (Fuchs et al., 2008) In IgM secreting cell lines and cells from Waldenstrom macroglobulinaemia, simvastatin showed antiproliferative and cytotoxic effects and stimulated the apoptosis. Simvastatin had a synergistic effect with bortezomib, dexamethasone and fludarabine by augmenting their cytotoxicity. (Moreau et al., 2008).

A group of 23 patients with lymphoproliferative diseases, for which statins had not been contraindicated, was treated for 3 days with simvastatin at a dose of 120 mg/day. Serum CH level and that of total lipids decreased significantly ($p<0.001$ and, respectively, $p = 0.016$). Serum ALT decreased unsignificantly, while that of AST increased, the growth was close to the statistical significance limit, but was not higher than the upper normal level. Flowcytometric dosage of annexine V showed that simvastatin induced early and late apoptosis increase ($p = 0.007$, respectively, $p = 0.003$). By its effect on apoptosis, simvastatin could be an adjuvant treatment for patients with lymphoproliferative disorders. (Mihăilă et al., 2009)

By their CH-lowering effect, statins are promising drugs for the treatment of lymphomas (63 Winiarska et al., 2008). A female patient suffering from NHL with large B-cells whose primary location was the mammary gland had hypercholesterolemia, hypertriglyceridemia and was hypertensive. During the treatment with R-CHOP and radiotherapy that followed (30 Gy), she received lovastatin (20 mg/day) and verapamil. After the first 30 days of treatment, both CH and TG were normalized, and after the whole treatment, the patient has been in complete remission that persists today. (Mihăilă et al, 2008) Lovastatin was administered to the patient not only because she was dyslipidemic, but also because the literature claims that the drug is useful in malignant lymphomas, leukemias and multiple myeloma by its pleiotropic effects. In 1998 the first article about a farnesyltransferase inhibitor (L-744, 832) was published, inhibitor that proved to be effective in mice with mammary carcinomas and lymphomas (Mangues et al., 1998). Lovastatin acts by inhibition of geranylgeranylation, followed by reduction of intracellular signaling mechanisms, which results in reduction of time and dose-dependency of the viability of lymphoma cells in vitro. This is the result of apoptosis stimulation as well as of the decrease of lymphoma cells proliferation, the latter by induction of G1 arrest in cell cycle (van de Donk et al., 2003).

In a rat lymphoma model lovastatin administration during radiotherapy led to cell cycle arrest in different phases, which justified the continuation of the treatment with this drug in the female patient during radiotherapy; the experimental model mentioned, the combination of lovastatin with radiotherapy resulted in a synergistic action (Rozados et al., 2005, as cited in Mihăilă et al., 2008). Lovastatin administration did not preclude the response to polychemoterapy that included rituximab. In fact, although it is only one case, the experimental findings do not always overlap with clinical outcomes. The authors consider that the combination of lovastatin with verapamil favored the response to anticancer treatment and prevented the possible multidrug resistance (Mihăilă et al., 2008). The combination of lovastatin + R-CHOP did not lead to adverse effects. Six years after the end of therapy, the patient is still in complete remission.

In a cell line of acute promyelocytic leukemia (NB4) atorvastatin and fluvastatin showed to be potent stimulators of cell differentiation and apoptosis (Sassano et al., 2007). When to the treatment with idarubicin and high-dose cytarabine of patients with AML pravastatin was added, CR / CRp was observed in 11 of 15 new patients, out of which 8 of 10 had unfavorable cytogenetics, and 9 of 22 patients who received rescue medication that pravastatin did not influence the length of neutropenia, of thrombocytopenia or of the toxicity of chemotherapy. (Kornblau et al., 2007)

Statins are active also in acute promyelocytic leukemia cells, where they augment the antileukemic response that depends on all-trans retinoic acid (ATRA). The c-Jun NH_2-terminal kinase pathway is required for leukemic cells differentiation induced by statins. Statins also intervene in modulating ATRA-dependent transcription. This was revealed by the selective expression of a large number of genes (400) when atorvastatin was administered together with ATRA. (Sassano et al., 2009) This drug combination could be a solution for reversing the ATRA-resistance of leukemic cells (Sassano et al., 2007).

Unlike the subgroup of normal and AML cells CD34 (-), the CD34 (+) is more sensitive to lovastatin. Both populations of cells were strongly inhibited when lovastatin was added to chemotherapy. Leukemic cell samples from different patients with AML had heterogeneous sensitivity to lovastatin. Fifty percent of the patients with unfavorable treatment response had cytogenetic examination with poor prognosis and significantly more blasts in the peripheral blood. (de Jonge-Peeters et al., 2009)

It was observed that high expression of CXCR4 correlates with a shorter survival time of patients with AML. In some models of cancer hypoxia it leads to the increase of CXCR4. On the other hand, increased $pO_{(2)}$ causes depletion of CH, which alters lipid rafts and leads to structural changes, which result in increased rejection of CXCR4 microparticles. (Fiegl et al., 2009) Atorvastatin administred in doses of 16 mg/kg body wt showed to be effective in the inhibition of ascites tumor growth and induced apoptosis of a cell line of Daltons' Lymphoma Ascites that was transplanted into mice (Ajith et al., 2008).

In vitro, simvastatin induced apoptosis of CLL cells, found in short term culture and contributed to lower BCL-2/BAX report; it was found that its effect of apoptosis induction is tumor-specific and does not affect normal lymphocytes. The association of simvastatin with fludarabine or cladribine synergistically induces DNA damages, and these lead to apoptosis. The proportion of cells found in apoptosis induced by simvastatin +/- chemotherapy was not correlated with the expression of negative prognostic markers of the disease (ZAP-70 and CD38) or its stage in the RAI classification. (Podhorecka et al., 2010)

The interaction of adhesion molecules, with fundamental role in cellular interaction processes, including those concerning EBV-transformed B cells is blocked by some statins. These drugs also inhibit intracellular activation of NF-kappaB and contribute to the emergence of transformed B-cell apoptosis. In mice with severe combined immune deficiency, simvastatin caused delayed emergence of the lymphomas induced by EBV. (Cohen et al., 2005)

Both the simvastatin and the tipifarnib have cytotoxic effect on AML cell lines and their associated administration has a synergistic effect. This combination administered to CD34(+) AML cells resulted in the increase of the inhibitory effect only on normally responsive AML cells; however, the combination administred to CD34(-) AML cells had augmented inhibitory effect in all cells. (van der Weide et al., 2009)

It was observed that statins are able to decrease the expression of BCL-2, an antiapoptotic molecule, favoring the appearance of apoptosis of CD4(+) CD28(null) T cells - a T aggressive and long-lasting lymphocyte subpopulation, which can infiltrate the atheromatous plaques, contributing to the their destabilization, which facilitates the instalation of major coronary accidents. (Link et al., 2011)

9. ABC transporters and cholesterol homeostasis

In many neoplastic diseases, increased expression of proteins on which depends the multidrug resistance correlates with the presence of refractory disease. A small proportion of AML leukemia cells is responsible for the tumor proliferation and expansion. These are leukemic stem cells, primitive cells, which are frequently in a quiescent state. When they leave the quiescent state and progress along the cell cycle, these cells are characterized by the ability of self-renewal and express some ATP-binding cassette (ABC) transporters. It was observed that when some ABC transporters have a high expression in leukemia cells, the prognosis of patients with AML is reserved as the response to treatment is inadequate. (de Jonge-Peeters et al., 2007)

The most studied transporter is the P-glycoprotein transporter (P-gp) - an ABC transporter responsible for unidirectional transmembrane translocation of the substrate (Gayet et al., 2005). P-gp is frequently involved in the emergence of multidrug resistance during chemotherapy (Shu & Liu, 2007). The multidrug resistance gene encodes this membrane transporter. Not only P-gp occurs in CH homeostasis at the cellular level, but also the synthesis of CH and CH-esters affects ATP-ase (Bucher et al., 2007) and the transmembrane transport by P-gp (Bucher et al., 2007; Shu & Liu, 2007). The lipid structure of the cell membranes also depends on the P-gp function (Dos Santos et al., 2007).

The ATP-ase activity of P-gp is controlled linearly by CH of the membrane structure. On the other hand, the decrease of membrane CH correlates with the non-linear decrease of the daunorubicin efflux induced by P-gp. An effective way to raise awareness of ALL CEM resistant to chemotherapy cells consists of partial depletion of the CH from cell membrane structure, that lowers the daunorubicin efflux by P-gp. (Gayet et al., 2005)

CH is able to increase basal activity of P-gp ATP-ase and increase P-gp sensitivity to progesterone and verapamil, modulators of this transporter. (Bucher et al., 2007) LDL-cholesterol can enlarge P-gp expression. In an experiment conducted in vitro, HMG-CoA reductase inhibitors were added to a primitive leukemia cells line (KG1a) and the observation was that lovastatin caused a decrease of 26% of P-gp expression, and pravastatin - a decrease of 16 %. (Connelly-Smith et al., 2007) But the CH derived from LDL was also able to restore sensitivity to chemotherapy of a human lymphoblastic leukemia cell line. It seems that the mechanism explaining this return is the restoration of the membrane CH and the reducing of the P-gp-associated ATPase to the same level. (Shu & Liu, 2007) The changes of the membrane CH quantity may be responsible for P-gp inhibition. It was observed that disassembly of lipid rafts can be produced both by the decrease of the CH content and by its increase. For a normal capacity of P-gp transport it is necessary to maintain accurate properties of membrane structures known as lipid raft. (Dos Santos et al., 2007)

In a clinical trial involving patients with CLL the P-gp expression of lymphocytes from peripheral blood was determined flowcytometricaly. Those patients whose lymphocytes expressed P-gp were treated for 6 days with 80 mg lovastatin daily, then a new sample of peripheral blood was examined flowcytometricaly. Lymphocytes of six of the 27 studied patients expressed P-gp; about 20% of them were positive. Following the administration of lovastatin only 7.33% of them also expressed P-gp ($p = 0.016$). Compared to the proportion of positive lymphocytes at baseline, the decline was of 63.35%. During the study, CH decreased statistically significantly, with 20.43%. There was no observation of the appearance of possible drug adverse effects. In conclusion, the 6 days therapy with lovastatin was able to reduce significantly the CH and the number of lymphocytes in the membranes where P-gp is expressed, so that this statin could contribute through its pleiotropic effects to reduce multidrug resistance, especially when it is followed by chemotherapy. (Mihăilă et al., 2010)

This drug efflux pump can be inhibited by verapamil, too, the research made in vitro proved that it can reduce multidrug resistance. In such a study conducted in two patients with leukemic lymphoma resistant to treatment, verapamil was able to increase the intracellular amount of doxorubicin (Tidefelt et al., 1994).

It was found that verapamil was able to overcome the P-gp - mediated resistance to doxorubicin and vincristine in a canine cell line of B cell lymphoma (GL-1) (Uozurmi et al., 2005, as cited in Mihăilă et al., 2008). These experimental findings were not confirmed by parallel administration of chemosensitizer verapamil to chemotherapy (cyclophosphamide, doxorubicin, vincristine, and dexamethasone) in patients with medium and high level NHL found in advanced stages. This drug combination did not increase the therapeutic response and did not extend the survival in these patients as compared to those treated only with the mentioned chemotherapy (without verapamil) (Gaynor et al., 2001, as cited in Mihăilă et al., 2008), but it cannot be excluded that it could be effective in some patients who develop multidrug resistance. But, in metastatic breast carcinoma that has become resistant to anthracyclines verapamil has showed that it is able to increase the survival of patients (Belpomme et al., 2000, as cited in Mihăilă et al., 2008). In the case of the patient described above with hypertension and primary mammary NHL, the evolution has been favorable under the combination of verapamil to chemo- and radiotherapy, that has resulted in a event-free survival of 6 years (up to the present day) (Mihăilă et al., 2008).

In another study, 45 patients with proliferative haematological disorders were included in one of the following two groups: A - those who had hypertension and who received verapamil + chemotherapy, and B - those with normal blood pressure, who received only chemotherapy. Group A included 7 patients with chronic lymphoproliferations and 2 with chronic myleoproliferations; under treatment, both systolic and diastolic pressure decreased significantly in all patients in the group. Initially the serum CH level was higher than in the patients in group B ($p = 0.004$), while other biological tests did not vary significantly between group A and B. No adverse effects were observed during the study. The fact that the initial blood CH was higher in in patients in group A suggests that malignant cells of patients in group B captured more blood CH that contributed to their proliferation. Although the average survival was not significantly different between group A and B, in group A there were more patients with stable disease (77.78% versus 44.44% - $p<0.0001$) while in group B more patients had progressive disease (30.56 % versus 11.11% - $p<0.0001$). The deaths due to progressive disease were significantly more numerous in group B. The authors consider that verapamil is useful not only because of its antihypertensive effect, but also due to its pleiotropic effects through which it could influence the evolution of neoplasia by inhibiting P-gp function and the efflux of drugs from lymphoma or leukemia cells. (Mihăilă et al., 2008)

10. Conclusions

Various epidemiological studies have found that between blood lipids and various neoplastic diseases there are some correlations.

Some authors found that in patients with newly diagnosed NHL the blood levels of CH, phospholipids and HDL-cholesterol had lower values than those of controls and the values of CH increased progressively after chemotherapy if the disease reached complete remission or was stationary, unlike those with disease progression, that their blood lipid levels were even lower.

Nearly all the children with ALL when diagnosed and during chemotherapy revealed a predictable model of serum dyslipidemia that consisted of very low levels of HDL-cholesterol, and elevated TG, and LDL-cholesterol, that regained normal values during the remission period.

In children with ALL, treated with asparaginase, hypertriglyceridemia was frequently observed and it can be cause of acute pancreatitis and thrombosis.

Imatinib mesylate, used for the treatment of patients with chronic myeloid leukemia, led to a diminishing of serum CH and TG values and CH depletion can inhibit cell proliferation.

The young survivors of ALL, disease which they had in their childhood, especially those who received cranial radiotherapy, are likely to develop hyperlipidemia, insulin resistance, obesity, arterial hypertension and even MS soon after the treatment.

Cranial irradiation favors more the appearance of MS by GH deficiency, lower level of insulin-like growth factor 1, fasting hyperinsulinemia, abdominal obesity and hyperlipidemia, especially in women.

It is believed that CH is important for cell proliferation, because low serum CH values may be the result of high cellular CH need of cancerous cells. Low serum CH values correlate with elevated levels of CH in lymphocytes. Malignant, proliferative cells have an intense metabolism of CH, while decreased intake of CH is responsible for decreasing cell proliferation.

An increase of lipoprotein lipase mRNA levels is present in CLL patients with shorter survival.

CD5 antigen is responsible for CH synthesis and even for adipogenesis. It is known that malignant cells from CLL are undergoing a process of continuous stimulation due to CD5 activation and cell survival.

The loss of CH is responsible for the decrease in the number of sites that can fix some monoclonal antibodies, including CD20. Statins interfere with the detection of CD20 antigen as well as the antilymphomatous function of the rituximab, but this effect was not showed in some clinical studies.

Statins reduce cellular proliferation and stimulate apoptosis of cancerous cells. By their pleiotropic effects, statins can be useful in the treatment of different diseases, like NHL, CLL, multiple myeloma and AML, as adjuvant therapy.

The association of simvastatin with fludarabine or cladribine synergistically induces DNA damages, and these lead to apoptosis.

Statins are active also in acute promyelocytic leukemia cells, where they augment the antileukemic response that depends on all-trans retinoic acid.

The ATP-ase activity of P-gp, frequently involved in the emergence of multidrug resistance during chemotherapy, is controlled linearly by CH of the membrane structure. The changes of the membrane CH quantity may be responsible for P-gp inhibition.

This drug efflux pump can be inhibited by statins and verapamil.
By their pleiotropic effects, statins are useful not only for dyslipidemia treatment, but also in antineoplastic therapy.

11. Acknowledgment

I am deeply grateful to my teacher - Melinda Erzse - who was kind to check the English text and make the appropriate corrections.

12. References

Ajith, T.A.; Anu, V., & Riji, T. (2008). Antitumor and apoptosis promoting properties of atorvastatin, an inhibitor of HMG-CoA reductase, against Dalton's Lymphoma Ascites tumor in mice. *J Exp Ther Oncol*. Vol.7, No.4, (October-December 2008), pp.291-298, ISSN: 1359-4117.

Barakat, S.; Gayet, L., Dayan, G., Labialle, S., Lazar, A., Oleinikov, V., Coleman, A.W., & Baggetto, L.G. (2005). Multidrug-resistant cancer cells contain two populations of P-glycoprotein with differently stimulated P-gp ATPase activities: evidence from atomic force microscopy and biochemical analysis. *Biochem J*. Vol.388, Pt.2, (June 2005), pp.563-571.

Beesley, A.H.; Firth, M.J., Ford. J., Weller, R.E., Freitas, J.R., Perera, K.U., & Kees, U.R. (2009). Glucocorticoid resistance in T-lineage acute lymphoblastic leukaemia is associated with a proliferative metabolism. *Br J Cancer*. Vol.16, No.100(12), (June 2009), pp.1926-1936.

Bingaman, M.G.; Basu, G.D., Golding, T.C., Chong, S.K., Lassen, A.J., Kindt, T.J., & Lipinski C.A. (2010). The autophilic anti-CD20 antibody DXL625 displays enhanced potency due to lipid raft-dependent induction of apoptosis. *Anticancer Drugs*. 2010 Jun; Vol.21, No.5, (June 2010), pp.532-542.

Bucher, K.; Belli, S., Wunderli-Allenspach, H., & Krämer, S.D. (2007). P- glycoprotein in proteoliposomes with low residual detergent: the effects of cholesterol. *Pharm Res*. Vol.24, No.11, (November 2007), pp.1993-2004.

Casalou, C.; Costa, A., Carvalho, T., Gomes, A.L., Zhu, Z., Wu, Y., & Dias, S. (2011). Cholesterol Regulates VEGFR-1 (FLT-1) Expression and Signaling in Acute Leukemia Cells. *Mol Cancer Res*. Vol.9, No.2, (February 2011), pp.215-224.

Cohen, H.; Bielorai, B., Harats, D., Toren, A., & Pinhas-Hamiel, O. (2010). Conservative treatment of L-asparaginase-associated lipid abnormalities in children with acute lymphoblastic leukemia. *Pediatr Blood Cancer*. Vol.54, No.5, (May 2010), pp.703-706.

Cohen, J.I. (2005). HMG CoA reductase inhibitors (statins) to treat Epstein-Barr virus- driven lymphoma. *Br J Cancer*. Vol.92, No.9, (May 2005), pp.1593-1598.

Connelly-Smith, L.; Pattinson, J., Grundy, M., Shang, S., Seedhouse, C., Russell, N., & Pallis, M. (2007). P-glycoprotein is downregulated in KG1a-primitive leukemia cells by LDL cholesterol deprivation and by HMG-CoA reductase inhibitors. *Exp Hematol*. Vol.35, No.12, (December 2007), pp.1793-1800.

Cvetkovic, Z.; Cvetkovic, B., Petrovic, M., Ranic, M., Debeljak-Martarcic, J., Vucic, V., & Glibetic, M. (2009). Lipid profile as a prognostic factor in cancer patients. *J BUON*. Vol.4, No.3, (July-September 2009), pp.501-506.

de Jonge-Peeters, S.D.; Kuipers, F., de Vries, E.G., & Vellenga, E. (2007). ABC transporter expression in hematopoietic stem cells and the role in AML drug resistance. *Crit Rev Oncol Hematol*. Vol.62, No.3, (June 2007), pp.214-226.

de Jonge-Peeters, S.D.; van der Weide, K., Kuipers, F., Sluiter, W.J., de Vries, E.G., & Vellenga, E. (2009). Variability in responsiveness to lovastatin of the primitive CD34+ AML subfraction compared to normal CD34+ cells. *Ann Hematol*. Vol.88, No.6, (June 2009), pp.573-580.

Dos Santos, S.M.; Weber, C.C., Franke, C., Müller, W.E., & Eckert, G.P. (2007). Cholesterol: Coupling between membrane microenvironment and ABC transporter activity. *Biochem Biophys Res Commun*. Vol.354, No.1, (March 2007), pp.216-221.

Ennishi, D.; Asai, H., Maeda, Y., Shinagawa, K., Ikeda, K., Yokoyama, M., Terui, Y., Takeuchi, K., Yoshino, T., Matsuo, K., Hatake, K., & Tanimoto, M. (2010). Statin-independent prognosis of patients with diffuse large B-cell lymphoma receiving rituximab plus CHOP therapy. *Ann Oncol*. Vol.21, No.6, (June 2010), pp.1217-221.

Fiegl, M.; Samudio, I., Clise-Dwyer, K., Burks, J.K., Mnjoyan, Z., & Andreeff, M. (2009). CXCR4 expression and biologic activity in acute myeloid leukemia are dependent on oxygen partial pressure. *Blood*. Vol.113, No.7, (February 2009), pp.1504- 1512.

Follin, C.; Thilén, U., Osterberg, K., Björk, J., & Erfurth, E.M. (2010). Cardiovascular risk, cardiac function, physical activity, and quality of life with and without long-term growth hormone therapy in adult survivors of childhood acute lymphoblastic leukemia. *J Clin Endocrinol Metab*. Vol.95, No.8, (August 2010), pp.3726-3735.

Franceschino, A.; Tornaghi, L., Benemacher, V., Assouline, S., & Gambacorti-Passerini, C. (2008). Alterations in creatine kinase, phosphate and lipid values in patients with chronic myeloid leukemia during treatment with imatinib. *Haematologica*. Vol.93, No.2, (February 2008), pp.317-318.

Fuchs, D.; Berges, C., Opelz, G., Daniel, V., & Naujokat, C. (2008). HMG-CoA reductase inhibitor simvastatin overcomes bortezomib-induced apoptosis resistance by disrupting a geranylgeranyl pyrophosphate-dependent survival pathway. *Biochem Biophys Res Commun*. Vol.374, No.2, (September 2008), pp.309-314.

Garg, A.; Hosfield, E.M., & Brickner, L. (2011). Disseminated intravascular large B cell lymphoma with slowly decreasing high-density lipoprotein cholesterol. South Med J. Vol.104, No.1, (January 2011), pp.53-56.

Gary-Gouy, H.; Sainz-Perez, A., Marteau, J.B., Marfaing-Koka, A., Delic, J., Merle-Beral, H., Galanaud, P., & Dalloul, A. (2007). Natural phosphorylation of CD5 in chronic lymphocytic leukemia B cells and analysis of CD5-regulated genes in a B cell line suggest a role for CD5 in malignant phenotype. *J Immunol*. Vol.179, No.7, (October 2007), pp.4335-4344.

Gayet, L.; Dayan, G., Barakat, S., Labialle, S., Michaud, M., Cogne, S., Mazane, A., Coleman, A.W., Rigal, D., & Baggetto, L.G. (2005). Control of P-glycoprotein activity by membrane cholesterol amounts and their relation to multidrug resistance in human CEM leukemia cells. *Biochemistry*. Vol.44, No.11, (March 2005), pp.4499- 4509.

Geyeregger, R.; Shehata, M., Zeyda, M., Kiefer, F.W., Stuhlmeier, K.M., Porpaczy, E., Zlabinger, G.J., Jäger, U., & Stulnig, T.M. (2009). Liver X receptors interfere with cytokine-induced proliferation and cell survival in normal and leukemic lymphocytes. *J Leukoc Biol*. Vol.86, No.5, (November 2009), pp.1039-1048.

Gokhale, C.D.; Udipi, S.A., Ambaye, R.Y., Pai, S.K., & Advani, S.H. (2007). Post-therapy profile of serum total cholesterol, retinol and zinc in pediatric acute lymphoblastic leukemia and non-Hodgkin's lymphoma. *J Am Coll Nutr*. Vol.26, No.1, (February 2007), pp.49-56.

Gologan, R.; Constantinescu, G., Georgescu, D., Ostroveanu, D., Vasilache, D., Dobrea, C., Iancu., D., & Popov, V. (2009). Hypolipemiant besides antileukemic effect of imatinib mesylate. *Leuk Res*. Vol.33, No.9, (September 2009), pp.1285-1287.

Gonçalves, R.P.; Hungria, V.T., Chiattone, C.S., Pozzi, D.B., & Maranhão, R.C. (2003). Metabolism of chylomicron-like emulsions in patients with Hodgkin's and with non-Hodgkin's lymphoma. *Leuk Res*. Vol.27, No.2, (February 2003), pp.147-153.

Gonçalves, R.P.; Rodrigues, D.G., & Maranhão, R.C. (2005). Uptake of high density lipoprotein (HDL) cholesteryl esters by human acute leukemia cells. *Leuk Res*. Vol.29, No.8, (August 2005), pp.955-959.

Gurney, J.G.; Ness, K.K., Sibley, S.D., O'Leary, M., Dengel, D.R., Lee, J.M., Youngren, N.M., Glasser, S.P., & Baker, K.S. (2006). Metabolic syndrome and growth hormone deficiency in adult survivors of childhood acute lymphoblastic leukemia. *Cancer*. Vol.107, No.6, (September 2006), pp.1303-1312.

Helman, R.; Teixeira, P.P., Mendes, C.J., Szegö, T., & Hamerschlak, N. (2011). Gastric MALT Lymphoma and Grade II Obesity: Gastric Bypass Surgery as a Therapeutic Option. *Obes Surg*. Vol.21, No.3, (March 2011), pp.407-409.

Inamoto, Y.; Teramoto, T., Shirai, K., Tsukamoto, H., Sanda, T., Miyamura, K., Yamamori, I., Hirabayashi, N., & Kodera, Y. (2005). Severe hypercholesterolemia associated with decreased hepatic triglyceride lipase activity and pseudohyponatremia in patients after allogeneic stem cell transplantation. Int J *Hematol*. Vol.82, No.4, (November 2005), pp.362-366.

Ishimaru, C.; Yonezawa, Y., Kuriyama, I., Nishida, M., Yoshida, H., & Mizushina, Y. (2008). Inhibitory effects of cholesterol derivatives on DNA polymerase and topoisomerase activities, and human cancer cell growth. *Lipids*. Vol.43, No.4, (April 2008), pp.373-382.

Jahn, T.; Leifheit, E., Gooch, S., Sindhu, S., & Weinberg, K. (2007). Lipid rafts are required for Kit survival and proliferation signals. *Blood*. 2007 Vol.110, No.6, (September 2007), pp.1739-1747.

Janas, E.; Priest, R., Wilde, J.I., White, J.H., & Malhotra, R. (2005). Rituxan (anti-CD20 antibody)-induced translocation of CD20 into lipid rafts is crucial for calcium influx and apoptosis. *Clin Exp Immunol*. Vol.139, No.3, (March 2005), pp.439-46.

Jarfelt, M.; Lannering, B., Bosaeus, I., Johannsson, G., & Bjarnason, R. (2005). Body composition in young adult survivors of childhood acute lymphoblastic leukaemia. *Eur J Endocrinol*. Vol.153, No.1, (July 2005), pp.81-89.

Jarvis, R.M.; Chamba, A., Holder, M.J., Challa, A., Smith, D.C., Hodgkin, M.N., Lord, J.M., & Gordon, J. (2007). Dynamic interplay between the neutral glycosphingolipid CD77/Gb3 and the therapeutic antibody target CD20 within the lipid bilayer of model B lymphoma cells. *Biochem Biophys Res Commun*. 2007 Vol.355, No.4, (April 2007), pp.944-949.

Kfoury-Baz, E.M.; Nassar, R.A., Tanios, R.F., Otrock, Z.K., Youssef, A.M., Albany, C., Bazarbachi, A., & Salem, Z.M. (2008). Plasmapheresis in asparaginase-induced hypertriglyceridemia. *Transfusion.* Vol.48, No.6, (June 2008), pp.1227-1230. Kheirallah, S.; Caron, P., Gross, E., Quillet-Mary, A., Bertrand-Michel, J., Fournié, J.J., Laurent, G., & Bezombes, C. (2010). Rituximab inhibits B-cell receptor signaling. *Blood.* Vol.115, No.5, (February 2010), pp.985-994.

Kornblau, S.M.; Banker, D.E., Stirewalt, D., Shen, D., Lemker, E., Verstovsek, S., Estrov, Z., Faderl, S., Cortes, J., Beran, M., Jackson, C.E., Chen, W., Estey, E., & Appelbaum, FR. (2007). Blockade of adaptive defensive changes in cholesterol uptake and synthesis in AML by the addition of pravastatin to idarubicin + high- dose Ara-C: a phase 1 study. *Blood.* Vol.109, No.7, (April 2007), pp.2999-3006. Kourti, M.; Tragiannidis, A., Makedou, A., Papageorgiou, T., Rousso, I., & Athanassiadou, F. (2005). Metabolic syndrome in children and adolescents with acute lymphoblastic leukemia after the completion of chemotherapy. *J Pediatr Hematol Oncol.* Vol.27, No.9, (September 2005), pp.499-501.

Kuliszkiewicz-Janus, M.; Małecki, R., & Mohamed, A.S. (2008). Lipid changes occuring in the course of hematological cancers. *Cell Mol Biol Lett.* Vol.13, No.3, (September 2008), pp.465-474, ISSN 1689-1392.

Lawson, E.B.; Gottschalk, M., & Schiff, D.E. (2011). Insulin infusion to treat severe hypertriglyceridemia associated with pegaspargase therapy: a case report. *J Pediatr Hematol Oncol.* Vol.33, No.2, (March 2011), pp.e83-86.

Lee, M.Y.; Ryu, J.M., Lee, S.H., Park, J.H., & Han, H.J. (2010). Lipid rafts play an important role for maintenance of embryonic stem cell self-renewal. *J Lipid Res.* Vol.51, No.8, (August 2010), pp.2082-2089.

Lim, U.; Gayles, T., Katki, H.A., Stolzenberg-Solomon, R., Weinstein, S.J., Pietinen, P., Taylor, P.R., Virtamo, J., & Albanes, D. (2007). Serum high-density lipoprotein cholesterol and risk of non-Hodgkin lymphoma. *Cancer Res.* Vol.67, No.11, (June 2007), pp.5569-5574.

Link, A.; Selejan, S., Hewera, L., Walter, F., Nickenig, G., & Böhm, M. (2011). Rosuvastatin induces apoptosis in CD4(+)CD28 (null) T cells in patients with acute coronary syndromes. *Clin Res Cardiol.* Vol.100, No.2, (February 2011), pp.147- 158.

Lü, Z.; Gou, L.P., Chen, L., Xie, B., & Qin, J. (2010). [Effect of lovastatin and rosiglitazone on cholesterol reverse transportation in foam cell]. *Zhonghua Nei Ke Za Zhi.* Vol.49, No.8, (August 2010), pp.696-699.

MacIntyre, D.A.; Jiménez, B., Lewintre, E.J., Martín, C.R., Schäfer, H., Ballesteros, CG., Mayans, J.R., Spraul, M., García-Conde, J., & Pineda-Lucena, A. (2010). Serum metabolome analysis by 1H-NMR reveals differences between chronic lymphocytic leukaemia molecular subgroups. *Leukemia.* Vol.24, No.4, (April 2010), pp.788-797.

Mangues, R.; Corral, T., Kohl, N.E., Symmans, W.F., Lu, S., Malumbres, M., Gibles, J.B., Oliff, A., & Pellicer, A. (1998). Antitumor effect of a farnesyl protein transferase inhibitor in mammary and lymphoid tumors overexpressing N-ras in transgenic mice. *Cancer Res.* Vol.58, (March 1998), pp.1253-1259.

Mihăilă, R.; Rezi, E.C., Cătană, A., Flucuş, O., Deac, M., & Mihăilă, R. (June 2008). Can Verapamil influence the evolution of the malignant haemopathies? The 13th Congress of the European Hematology Association, Copenhagen, Denmark, June, 12-15, 2008; In: *Haematologica – the Hematology Journal.* Abstract Book: 518, ISSN 0390-6078.

Mihăilă, R.; Rezi, E.C., & Deac, M. (2008). Primary mammary non-Hodgkin malignant lymphoma. *Archives of the Balkan Medical Union*, Vol.43, No.4, (December 2008), pp.289-292, ISSN 0041-6940.

Mihăilă, R.; Mocanu, L., Rezi, E.C., Cătană, A., Flucuş, O., Bera, L., Mihăilă, R., & Deac, M. (June 2009). The role of simvastatin in inducing apoptosis at patients with malignant haemopathies. The 14th Congress of the European Hematology Association, Berlin, June 4-7, 2009; In: *Haematologica – the Hematology Journal*. Abstract Book: 1194, ISSN 0390-6078.

Mihăilă, R.; Rezi, E.C., Isăilă, R., Boca, G., Mihăilă, R., & Deac, M. (June 2009). Is obesity a risk factor for nonHodgkin malignant lymphomas? The 14th Congress of the European Hematology Association, Berlin, June 4-7, 2009. In: *Haematologica – the Hematology Journal*, 2010, S2; Abstract Book: 1725, ISSN 0390-6078.

Mihăilă, R.; Cocişiu, G., Bera, L., Cătană, A., Flucuş, O., Rezi, E.C., Mihăilă, R., & Ciută, D. (June 2010). Study concerning the association between chronic lymphocytic leukemia and dyslipidemia. The 15th Congress of the European Hematology Association, Barcelona, Spain, June 10-13, 2010. In *Haematologica – the Hematology Journal*, 2010, S2; Abstract Book: 526-527, ISSN 0390-6078.

Mihăilă, R.; Mocanu, L., Cocişiu, G., Ciută, D., & Mihăilă, R. (2010). Effect of lovastatin on multidrug resistance to patients with chronic lymphocytic leukemia. *Archives of the Balkan Medical Union*, Vol.45, No.3, (September 2010), pp. 186-188. ISSN 0041-6940

Miller, T.L.; Lipsitz, S.R., Lopez-Mitnik, G., Hinkle, A.S., Constine, L.S., Adams, M.J., French, C., Proukou, C., Rovitelli, A., & Lipshultz, S.E. (2010). Characteristics and determinants of adiposity in pediatric cancer survivors. *Cancer Epidemiol Biomarkers Prev*. Vol.19, No.8, (August 2010), pp.2013-2022.

Mollinedo, F.; de la Iglesia-Vicente, J., Gajate, C., Estella-Hermoso de Mendoza, A., Villa-Pulgarin, J.A., de Frias, M., Roué, G., Gil, J., Colomer, D., Campanero, M.A., & Blanco- Prieto, M.J. (2010). In vitro and In vivo selective antitumor activity of Edelfosine against mantle cell lymphoma and chronic lymphocytic leukemia involving lipid rafts. *Clin Cancer Res*. Vol.16, No.7, (April 2010), pp.2046-2054, ISSN: 1557-3265.

Morachevskaya, E.; Sudarikova, A., & Negulyaev, Y. (2007). Mechanosensitive channel activity and F-actin organization in cholesterol-depleted human leukaemia cells. *Cell Biol Int*. Vol.31, No.4, (April 2007), pp.374-381.

Moreau, A.S.; Jia, X., Patterson, C.J., Roccaro, A.M., Xu, L., Sacco, A., O'Connor, K., Soumerai, J., Ngo, H.T., Hatjiharissi, E., Hunter, Z.R., Ciccarelli, B., Manning, R., Ghobrial, I.M., Leleu, X., & Treon, S.P. (2008). The HMG-CoA inhibitor, simvastatin, triggers in vitro anti-tumour effect and decreases IgM secretion in Waldenstrom macroglobulinaemia. *Br J Haematol*. Vol.142, No.5, (September 2008), pp.775-785.

Moschovi, M.; Trimis, G., Apostolakou, F, Papassotiriou, I., & Tzortzatou-Stathopoulou, F. (2004). Serum lipid alterations in acute lymphoblastic leukemia of childhood. *J Pediatr Hematol Oncol*. Vol.26, No.5, (May 2004), pp.289-293.

Musolino, A.; Panebianco, M., Zendri, E., Santini, M., Di Nuzzo, S., & Ardizzoni, A. (2009). Hypertriglyceridaemia with bexarotene in cutaneous T cell lymphoma: the role of omega-3 fatty acids. *Br J Haematol*. Vol.145, No.1, (April 2009), pp.84-86.

Nakagawa, M.; Kimura, S., Fujimoto, K., Atumi, H., Imura, J., Chikazawa, Y., Imamura, H., Okuyama, H., Yamaya, H., Fukushima, T., Nakagawa, A., Asaka, M., & Yokoyama, H. (2008). A case report of an adult with severe hyperlipidemia during acute lymphocytic leukemia induction therapy successfully treated with plasmapheresis. *Ther Apher Dial*. Vol.12, No.6, (December 2008), pp.509-513.

Nam, J.H.; Lee, H.S., Nguyen, Y.H., Kang, T.M., Lee, S.W., Kim, H.Y, Kim, S.J., Earm, Y.E., & Kim, S.J. (2007). Mechanosensitive activation of K+ channel via phospholipase C-induced depletion of phosphatidylinositol 4,5-bisphosphate in B lymphocytes. *J Physiol*. Vol.582, No.3, (August 2007), pp.977-990.

Nonaka, M.; Uota, S., Saitoh, Y., Takahashi, M., Sugimoto, H., Amet, T., Arai, A., Miura, O., Yamamoto, N., & Yamaoka, S. (2009). Role for protein geranylgeranylation in adult T-cell leukemia cell survival. *Exp Cell Res*. 2009 Jan 15; Vol.315, No.2, (January 2009), pp.141-150.

Okamoto, M.; Yamaguchi, H., Isobe, Y., Yokose, N., Mizuki, T., Tajika, K., Gomi, S., Hamaguchi, H., Inokuchi, K., Oshimi, K., & Dan, K. (2009). Analysis of triglyceride value in the diagnosis and treatment response of secondary hemophagocytic syndrome. *Intern Med*. Vol.48, No.10, (October 2009), pp.775-781, ISSN: 1349-7235

Oudin, C.; Simeoni, M.C., Sirvent, N., Contet, A., Begu-Le Corroller, A., Bordigoni, P., Curtillet C, Poirée M, Thuret I, Play B, Carazza Massot M, Chastagner P, Chambost H, Auquier, P., & Michel, G. (2011). Prevalence and risk factors of the metabolic syndrome in adult survivors of childhood leukemia. *Blood*. Vol.117, No.17, (April 2011), pp.4442-4448.

Podhorecka, M.; Halicka, D., Klimek, P., Kowal, M., Chocholska, S., & Dmoszynska, A. (2011). Simvastatin and purine analogs have a synergic effect on apoptosis of chronic lymphocytic leukemia cells. *Ann Hematol*. Vol.89, No.11, (November 2010), pp.1115-1124.

Port, M.D.; Gibson, R.M., Nathanson, N.M. (2007). Differential stimulation-induced receptor localization in lipid rafts for interleukin-6 family cytokines signaling through the gp130/leukemia inhibitory factor receptor complex. *J Neurochem*. Vol.101, No.3, (May 2007), pp.782-793.

Pugliese, L.; Bernardini, I., Pacifico, N., Peverini, M., Damaskopoulou, E., Cataldi, S., & Albi, E. (2010). Severe hypocholesterolaemia is often neglected in haematological malignancies. *Eur J Cancer*. Vol.46, No.9, (June 2010), pp.1735-1743.

Ridola, V.; Buonuomo, P.S., Maurizi, P., Putzulu, R., Annunziata, M.L, Pietrini, D., & Riccardi, R. (2008). Severe acute hypertriglyceridemia during acute lymphoblastic leukemia induction successfully treated with plasmapheresis. *Pediatr Blood Cancer*. Vol.50, No.2, (February 2008), pp.378-380.

Sánchez-Martín, C.C.; Dávalos, A., Martín-Sánchez, C., de la Peña, G., Fernández-Hernando, C., & Lasunción, M.A. (2007). Cholesterol starvation induces differentiation of human leukemia HL-60 cells. *Cancer Res*. Vol.67, No.7, (April 2007), pp.3379-3386.

Sassano, A.; Katsoulidis, E., Antico, G., Altman, J.K., Redig, A.J., Minucci, S., Tallman, M.S., & Platanias, L.C. (2007). Suppressive effects of statins on acute promyelocytic leukemia cells. *Cancer Res*. Vol.67, No.9, (May 2007), pp.4524-4532.

Sassano, A.; Lo Iacono, M., Antico, G., Jordan, A., Uddin, S., Calogero, R.A., & Platanias, L.C. (2009). Regulation of leukemic cell differentiation and retinoid-induced gene expression by statins. *Mol Cancer Ther*. Vol.8, No.3, (March 2009), pp.615-625.

Shu, Y. & Liu, H. (2007). Reversal of P-glycoprotein-mediated multidrug resistance by cholesterol derived from low density lipoprotein in a vinblastine-resistant human lymphoblastic leukemia cell line. *Biochem Cell Biol.* Vol.85, No.5, (October 2007), pp.638-646.

Tidefelt, U.; Juliusson, G., Elmhorn-Rosenborg, A., Peterson, C., & Paul, C. (1994). Increased intracellular concentrations of doxorubicin in resistant lymphoma cells in vivo by concomitant therapy with verapamil and cyclosporin A. *Eur J Haematol.* Vol.52, (May 1994), pp.276-282, ISSN 1600-0609

Tong, H.; Ren, Y., Liu, H., Xiao, F., Mai, W., Meng, H., Qian, W., Huang, J., Mao, L., Tong, Y., Wang, L., Qian, J., & Jin, J. (2008). Clinical characteristics of T-cell lymphoma associated with hemophagocytic syndrome: comparison of T-cell lymphoma with and without hemophagocytic syndrome. *Leuk Lymphoma.* Vol.49, No.1, (January 2008), pp.81-87.

Trimis, G.; Moschovi, M., Papassotiriou, I., Chrousos, G., & Tzortzatou-Stathopoulou, F. (2007). Early indicators of dysmetabolic syndrome in young survivors of acute lymphoblastic leukemia in childhood as a target for preventing disease. *J Pediatr Hematol Oncol.* Vol.29, No.5, (May 2007), pp.309-314.

Ulmer, H.; Borena, W., Rapp, K., Klenk, J., Strasak, A., Diem, G., Concin, H., & Nagel, G. (2009). Serum triglyceride concentrations and cancer risk in a large cohort study in Austria. *Br J Cancer.* Vol.101, No.7, (October 2009), pp.1202-1206.

Unruh, T.L.; Li, H., Mutch, C.M., Shariat, N., Grigoriou, L., Sanyal, R., Brown, C.B., & Deans, J.P. (2005). Cholesterol depletion inhibits src family kinase-dependent calcium mobilization and apoptosis induced by rituximab crosslinking. *Immunology.* Vol.116, No.2, (October 2005), pp.223-232.

van de Donk, N.W.; Schotte, D., Kamphuis, M.M., van Marion, A.M., van Kessel, B., Bloem, A.C., & Lokhorst, H.M. (2003). Protein geranylgeranylation is critical for the regulation of survival and proliferation of lymphoma tumor cells. *Clin Cancer Res.* Vol.9, (November 2003), pp.5735-5748, ISSN: 1557-3265

van der Weide, K.; de Jonge-Peeters, S.D., Kuipers, F., de Vries, E.G., & Vellenga, E. (2009). Combining simvastatin with the farnesyltransferase inhibitor tipifarnib results in an enhanced cytotoxic effect in a subset of primary CD34+ acute myeloid leukemia samples. *Clin Cancer Res.* Vol.15, No.9, (May 2009), pp.3076-3083.

van Waas, M.; Neggers, S.J., Pieters, R., & van den Heuvel-Eibrink, M.M. (2010). Components of the metabolic syndrome in 500 adult long-term survivors of childhood cancer. *Ann Oncol.* Vol.21, No.5, (May 2010), pp.1121-1126, ISSN 1569-8041

Varady, K.A. & Hellerstein, M.K. (2007). Alternate-day fasting and chronic disease prevention: a review of human and animal trials. *Am J Clin Nutr.* Vol.86, No.1, (July 2007), pp.7-13.

Weinberg, J.B.; Volkheimer, A.D., Mihovilovic, M., Jiang, N., Chen, Y., Bond, K., Moore, J.O., Gockerman, J.P., Diehl, L.F., de Castro, C.M., Rizzieri, D.A., Levesque, M.C., Dekroon, R., & Strittmatter, W.J. (December 2008). Apolipoprotein E genotype as a determinant of survival in chronic lymphocytic leukemia. *Leukemia.* 2008 Dec; Vol.22, No.12, (December 2008), pp.2184-2192.

Winiarska, M.; Bil, J., Wilczek, E., Wilczynski, G.M., Lekka, M., Engelberts, P.J., Mackus, W.J., Gorska, E., Bojarski, L., Stoklosa, T., Nowis, D., Kurzaj, Z., Makowski, M., Glodkowska, E., Issat, T., Mrowka, P., Lasek, W., Dabrowska-Iwanicka, A., Basak, G.W., Wasik, M., Warzocha, K., Sinski, M., Gaciong, Z., Jakobisiak, M., Parren, P.W., & Golab, J. (2008). Statins impair antitumor effects of rituximab by inducing conformational changes of CD20. *PLoS Med.* Vol.5, No.3, (March 2008). Pp.e64.

Yasugi, E.; Horiuchi, A., Uemura, I., Okuma, E., Nakatsu, M., Saeki, K., Kamisaka, Y., Kagechika, H., Yasuda, K., & Yuo, A. (2006). Peroxisome proliferator-activated receptor gamma ligands stimulate myeloid differentiation and lipogenensis in human leukemia NB4 cells. *Dev Growth Differ.* Vol.48, No.3, (April 2006), pp.177-188.

Yoshida, C.; Kojima, H., Iijima, T., Katsura, Y., Shimizu, S., Suzukawa, K., Mukai, H.Y., Hasegawa, Y., Abei, M., & Nagasawa, T. (2004). Association of non-alcoholic steatohepatitis (NASH) with chronic neutrophilic leukemia. *Eur J Haematol.* Vol.72, No.3, (March 2007), pp.225-228.

Zalewska-Szewczyk, B.; Matusiak, I., Wyka, K., Trelińska, J., Stolarska, M., & Młynarski, W. (2008). [Changes in the lipid profile in children with acute lymphoblastic leukaemia - the influence of the disease and its treatment]. *Med Wieku Rozwoj.* Vol.12, No.4, Pt.2, (October-December 2008), pp.1035-1040.

20

Lipids in the Pathogenesis of Benign Prostatic Hyperplasia: Emerging Connections

Ajit Vikram and Poduri Ramarao
Central University of Punjab
India

1. Introduction

Benign prostatic hyperplasia (BPH) is a common melody of the aging men characterized by noncancerous enlargement of the prostate gland and is often associated with lower urinary tract symptoms (LUTS) (Berry et al., 1984). Approximately, 60 percent of men aged over 50 years have histological evidence of BPH and, after the age of 70, the proportion increases to 80 percent (Berry et al., 1984). It is a chronic, progressive and highly prevalent disease, clinically manifests as LUTS, posing a socioeconomic burden to the patients (Saigal and Joyce, 2005). Recently, Stranne et al., reported that one-third of the Swedish male population aged over 50 years have LUTS, which is often associated with BPH (Stranne et al., 2009). BPH is rarely fatal, but affects the quality of life, and if left untreated, serious life-threatening complications may arise. Prostatic growth and development are governed by the genetic (Sanda et al., 1994), hormonal (Marker et al., 2003) and dietary factors (Bravi et al., 2006). Although, its etiology is not well understood, several theories have been proposed to explain the pathogenesis of BPH (Alberto et al., 2009; Bosch, 1991; Srinivasan et al., 1995). Augmented steroidal signaling and mesenchymal-epithelial interactions are required for the normal as well as pathological growth of the prostate gland (Marker et al., 2003). However, current literature indicates that apart from steroids, peptides and lipids are also playing a crucial role in the pathogenesis of BPH (Cai et al., 2001; Culig et al., 1996; Escobar et al., 2009; Kaplan-Lefko et al., 2008; Rahman et al., 2007; Rick et al., 2011; Story, 1995; Vikram and Jena, 2011a; Vikram et al., 2010c). Even if the effects of peptides and lipids on the growth of the gland is milder as compared to that of steroids, chronic change in their levels either due to dietary habit or genetic predispositions can significantly contribute to the initiation and/or progression of the disease over a period of time. Existing clinical/epidemiological and preclinical studies provide convincing evidence for the association between insulin-resistance, metabolic disorder and type 2 diabetes with the BPH (Francisco and Francois, 2010; Vikram et al., 2010a; Wang and Olumi, 2011). Previous experimental studies in our laboratory suggested that insulin-resistance associated secondary rise in the plasma insulin level plays a central role in the prostatic enlargement (Vikram and Jena, 2011b; Vikram et al., 2010a; b; 2011a; Vikram et al., 2010c; Vikram et al., 2011b). Other peptides such as insulin-like growth factor-I (IGF-I), IGF-I binding proteins (IGFBPs), growth hormone (GH), transforming growth factor-β (TGF-β) family proteins are reported to have important implications in the prostatic growth (Culig et al., 1996; Ikeda et al., 2000; Rick et al., 2011; Vikram et al., 2010c). However, information on the role of lipids in the prostatic growth is scarce and there is a need of further research in this area. Nevertheless, existing in-vitro, in-vivo and clinical/epidemiological studies suggests that apart from contributing to the development of insulin-resistance and secondary hyperinsulinemia, lipids has a direct role in the normal prostatic growth and pathogenesis of the BPH.

2. Role of lipids in transcriptional regulation

Lipids are conventionally known as an important constituent of the biological membranes and as a signaling molecule in the cytoplasm. The presence of lipids in the nucleus and identification of phosphotidylinositol (PtdIns)-4-kinse activity in the preparation that were enriched in nuclear membranes (Smith and Wells, 1983a; b), and identification of PtdIns-4-phosphate and PtdIns-4,5-bisphosphate that were differentially metabolized from lipids in the cytoplasm provided early evidence for the nuclear lipid signaling (Irvine, 2003). A recent study by Lee et al., explores the nuclear activities of lipids, showing that dilauroyl phosphotidlycholine controls transcriptional program through nuclear-receptor dependent pathway (Ingraham, 2011; Lee et al., 2011). The study was of particular interest as phosphotidylcholine reversed some of the consequences of high-fat diet feeding (Lee et al., 2011), which is known to promote the cellular proliferation, contractility and overall enlargement of the prostate in rodents (Vikram et al., 2010c). The nuclear signaling and transcriptional regulation by lipids implies that targeting nuclear lipid signaling might be of value in finding the answers for the diseases associated with dietary habit and sedentary lifestyle such as insulin-resistance, type 2 diabetes, several cancers and BPH.

3. Insulin-resistance and BPH

The main function of insulin includes regulation of glucose uptake, glycogenesis and tight control of the plasma glucose level (Vikram and Jena, 2010). Insulin-resistance is a condition in which normal level of insulin elicits subnormal response. It is a condition which is associated with a group of disorders such as obesity, dyslipidemia, elevated fasting glucose level, hyperinsulinemia and hypertension. In addition to the type 2 diabetes and cardiovascular diseases, patients with insulin-resistance syndrome are at higher risk of BPH (Kasturi et al., 2006). Possible implications of the diabetes, insulin-resistance and insulin-resistance associated disorders in the pathogenesis of BPH have been previously reviewed, and interested readers are encouraged to read the concerned articles for more information (Vikram et al., 2010a; Wang and Olumi, 2011).

4. Fatty acids, dietary fat and BPH

Strong appetite for the sugar, fat, and salt might have been adaptive for our ancestors, as they had very little access to sweet, fatty and salty foods. We have inherited these appetites and have easy access to these foods. As a consequence many of us suffer from obesity, high blood level of lipids, insulin-resistance, diabetes, hypertension, heart disease, several types of cancer and other aging-related disorders, including BPH. Sedentary lifestyle and fat-rich diets are considered as major contributor to the rise in the incidences of metabolic disorders. Over the past 60 years in USA, the ratio of dietary intake of ω-6-FA verses ω-3-FA has increased from 2:1 to 25:1 (Simopoulos, 1999), and animal fat is a major source of ω-6-FAs which has been found to be associated with the higher risk of LUTS and BPH (Maserejian et al., 2009; Suzuki et al., 2002). Considering the rise in the incidence of LUTS/BPH in the obese and insulin-resistant individuals, it becomes increasingly important to understand the role of lipids in the pathogenesis of disease.

4.1 Evidence from in-vitro experiments

Limited information is available on the direct role of fatty acids (FAs) in the growth of normal and benign prostatic cells, as most of the studies have been conducted on the prostate cancer cell lines. However, cancer cell lines studies have indicative value for the potential effects of these FAs, as like prostate cancer, BPH is also associated with the pathological increase in the cell proliferation. A recent report indicating dominant uptake of FAs by the prostate cells [non-malignant (RWPE-1) as well as malignant (LnCaP and PC-3)] suggests their important role in the growth and development of the gland (Liu et al., 2010). Pandalai et al., reported growth promoting effects of ω-6-FAs on the rat non metastatic epithelial cell lines (EPYP1 & EPYP2), rat metastatic cell line (Met-Ly-Lu), and human metastatic prostate cancer cells (PC-3, LnCaP & TSU) (Pandalai et al., 1996). Arachidonic acid, a ω-6-FA treatment led to accelerated growth of the PC-3 cells in-vitro (Ghosh and Myers, 1997). Further, Rose et al., reported concentration-dependent stimulation of PC-3 cells by the linolenic acid (ω-6-FA) and inhibition with the eicosapentanoic acid and docosahexanoic acid (ω-3-FAs) (Rose and Connolly, 1991). Further, long term eicosapentanoic acid treatment has been found to inhibit the metastatic activities of the PC-3 cells (Rose and Connolly, 1991). Recently, we investigated the effects of the serum of high-fat diet-fed (saturated animal fat-lard) rats on the growth of PC-3 cells, and a significant acceleration in the growth was observed (Vikram and Jena, 2011a). The serum characteristics of these rats indicated a rise in the glucose, triglyceride, cholesterol and insulin levels. Although, rise in the insulin level appears to be the primary cause for the accelerated growth of the cells owing to the mitogenic effects of the hormone, the possibility of direct growth promoting effects of lipids cannot be denied. Taken together, these studies suggest that at least ω-6-FAs have a growth stimulating effects on the prostatic cells, and thus represent a potential risk factor for BPH.

4.2 Evidence from in-vivo experiments

The study by Cai et al., provided first evidence for the prostatic growth promoting effects of dietary fat in rats (Cai et al., 2001). Similarly, Rahman et al., observed enlargement of the ventral prostate and increased expression of alpha-adrenergic receptors in the hyperlipidemic rats (Rahman et al., 2007). Further, inclusion of the saturated animal fat (lard) in the diet induced prostatic enlargement and changed the expression of androgen receptor and peroxysome proliferator activated receptor γ (PPARγ) (Escobar et al., 2009). Polyunsaturated FAs are ligands for the PPARγ, which is involved in the regulation of cell differentiation and proliferation (Morales-Garcia et al., 2011; Parast et al., 2009), and therefore appears to represent a possible link between diet and prostatic growth (Escobar et al., 2009). Prostatic atrophy and increased apoptosis in the hypoinsulinemic rats (induced by selective β-cell toxins, either streptozotocin or alloxan) further supports the view that insulin plays a central role in the prostatic growth and development (Arcolino et al., 2010; Ikeda et al., 2000; Suthagar et al., 2009; Vikram et al., 2011b; Vikram et al., 2008; Yono et al., 2008;

Yono et al., 2005). Increased cell proliferation and enlargement of ventral prostate in rats kept on the diet rich in saturated fat was observed (Vikram et al., 2010b; 2011a; Vikram et al., 2010c). Interestingly, pioglitazone (a synthetic PPARγ receptor agonist) treatment led to decreased cell proliferation, increased apoptosis and restoration of prostatic weight in the diet-induced insulin-resistant rats (Vikram et al., 2010b; Vikram et al., 2010c). This observation can be explained on the basis of the restoration of insulin-sensitivity and secondary hyperinsulinemia as pioglitazone is known to improve the insulin-sensitivity (Vikram and Jena, 2010). Further, increased oxidative stress and incidence of prostatic adenocarcinoma and hyperplasia was observed in the rats kept on high-cholesterol diet for long time (80 - 100 weeks) (Homma et al., 2004). Increased expression of NADPH oxidase subunits, activation of NF-kB signaling and decreased expression of glutathione peroxidase 3 clearly indicated the increased oxidative stress and activation of inflammatory response in ventral prostate of the HFD-fed rats (Sekine et al., 2011; Vykhovanets et al., 2011). Inflammation has been greatly implicated as a risk factor for the development of BPH (Abdel-Meguid et al., 2009; Chughtai et al.; Donnell, 2011; Kim et al., 2011a; Wang et al., 2008). Despite a marginal decrease in the weight of the prostate in ACI/seg rats an significant increase in the expression of 5-α-reductase 2 mRNA level was observed in the high-fat diet-fed rats (Cai et al., 2006). Based on these evidences from animal studies it appears that (i) insulin-resistance associated secondary hyperinsulinemia, (ii) activation of PPARγ signaling by FAs and (iii) increased prostatic inflammation are the important nodes for further investigative studies.

4.3 Evidence from clinical/epidemiological studies

Presence of dyslipidemia in the BPH patients is a frequently noted condition under clinical setups (Nandeesha et al., 2006). High level of total cholesterol, LDL-cholesterol, triglyceride, decreased level of HDL-cholesterol increases the risk of BPH, and cholesterol-lowering medication may reduce the risk (Moyad and Lowe, 2008). Yang et al., compared FA profiles in the serum of patients with prostate cancer and BPH and proposed that polyunsaturated FAs have certain relation with BPH and prostate cancer (Yang et al., 1999). Higher serum LDL is associated with greater risk of BPH (Parsons et al., 2008), and physical activity, which is known to decrease the serum lipid level is associated with the decreased risk for BPH (Parsons and Kashefi, 2008). Hyperlipidemia is closely associated with the obesity, higher body mass index (BMI), and these parameters show a positive correlation with the BPH (Dahle et al., 2002; Hammarsten and Hogstedt, 1999; Hammarsten et al., 1998; Parsons et al., 2006; Parsons et al., 2009). Kim et al., reported that the patients with more BMI tend to have larger prostate volume and higher International Prostate Symptom Score (Kim et al., 2011b). Several studies indicate that obesity and sedentary lifestyle substantially increases the risk for BPH (Dahle et al., 2002; Parsons, 2011; Parsons et al., 2006; Parsons et al., 2009). Recently, it has been reported that the central obesity is a better predictor of LUTS (Kim et al.; Lee et al., 2009). In a health professionals follow up study a moderate association between FAs intake and risk of BPH was observed (Suzuki et al., 2002). A cross-sectional study of 1545 men aged 30-79 years in the Boston Area Community Health Study the associations between dietary intakes of total energy, carbohydrates, protein, fat, cholesterol and LUTS in men was examined (Maserejian et al., 2009). Results indicated that high-energy intake was associated with higher LUTS symptoms and the storage symptoms increased with the higher fat intake

(Maserejian et al., 2009). Further, Kristal et al., reported significant increase in the symptomatic BPH with higher total fat intake and polyunsaturated fats, and showed a significant decrease in the symptomatic BPH with high-protein intake and alcohol consumption (Kristal et al., 2008). Leptin and adiponectin are closely associated with the obesity, and effort has been made to identify the relationship, if any, between these mediators and the risk of BPH. Although, no association has been observed between plasma leptin level and BPH (Hoon Kim et al., 2008; Lagiou et al., 1998), high plasma adiponectin concentrations were found to be associated with the reduced risk of symptomatic BPH (Schenk et al., 2009). Few independent studies indicate that obesity is associated with hyperinsulinemia, which in turn promotes the prostatic growth and risk for BPH (Becker et al., 2009; Kogai et al., 2008; Vogeser et al., 2009). In contrast, few reports argue that, obesity is associated with increased estrogen/androgen ratio and sympathetic activity, both individually hypothesized to promote the development of BPH (Giovannucci et al., 1994). Obesity can augment prostatic growth either by (i) promoting the development of insulin-resistance and secondary hyperinsulinemia or by (ii) increasing the estrogen/androgen ratio. In contrast, isolated report indicates an inverse association between obesity and BPH owing to reduced testosterone level in the obese people (Zucchetto et al., 2005). However, further studies investigating the relationship between plasma FAs level, obesity, BMI and prostatic growth are needed to shed light on the pathogenesis of BPH. Although, systematic clinical studies have not been performed to evaluate the effect of lifestyle modifications on the BPH outcomes, number of studies supports the view that heart-healthy lifestyle changes would have beneficial effect on the prostatic health and will eventually improve the quality of life of patients.

5. Emerging mechanistic connections

5.1 Autotaxin-lysophosphatidic acid pathway

Lysophophatidic acid (LPA) is a small water soluble phospholipid, which binds to its G-protein coupled receptors and activates several downstream signaling pathways (Berdichevets et al., 2010; Rancoule et al., 2011). It is primarily produced by the activity of the phospholipase autotaxin (ATX) (Van Meeteren and Moolenaar, 2007). Excessive fat intake is associated with adiposity, development of insulin-resistance and obesity, and these conditions are known to increase the expression of ATX, and therefore the LPA levels (Ferry et al., 2003). Recent study indicating the expression of LPA-related molecules in the prostate (Zeng et al., 2009) suggests that LPA might have an important role in the normal prostatic growth and pathogenesis of the BPH (Sakamoto et al., 2004). Kulkarni et al., proposed ATX-LPA axis as a possible link between excessive dietary fat intake and prostatic hyperplasia (Kulkarni and Getzenberg, 2009). LPA is involved in the inflammatory responses and experimental studies indicating increased oxidative stress and NF-kB activation in the ventral prostate of high-fat diet-fed rodents (Sekine et al., 2011; Vykhovanets et al., 2011), which are known to develop prostatic enlargement (Vikram et al., 2010b; 2011a; Vikram et al., 2010c) supports the hypothesis. Further, clinical studies indicate that systemic inflammation or lower level of soluble receptors that bind to the inflammatory cytokines increase the BPH risk (Schenk et al., 2010). The pharmacological inhibitors of ATX such as S32826 (Ferry et al., 2008) and ongoing efforts of medicinal chemists (North et al., 2010; North et al., 2009; Parrill and Baker, 2010) in this direction might provide an answer to therapeutic management of the BPH.

5.2 PPARγ signaling

PPARs are ligand activated transcription factors, which includes polyunsaturated FAs, eicosanoids, prostaglandins, docosahexaenoic acid, thiozolidinediones, and non-steroidal anti-inflammatory drugs. A recent study by Jiang et al., showed that conditional prostatic epithelial knockout of PPARγ resulted in the inflammation and focal hyperplasia which developed into prostatic intraepithelial neoplasia (Jiang et al.). Increased expression of PPARγ and overall enlargement of the prostate was observed in the rats kept on diet rich in saturated fat (Escobar et al., 2009). We also observed increased cell proliferation and prostatic enlargement in rodents kept on high-fat diet (Vikram et al., 2010b; 2011a; Vikram et al., 2010c). Moreover, pioglitazone (a PPARγ agonist) treatment restored prostate size in these rats (Vikram et al., 2010b; Vikram et al., 2010c). A recent study indicating the dominant uptake of FAs (as compared to glucose) by the malignant as well as non-malignant prostatic cells (Liu et al., 2010) underlines the possible role of PPARγ in the prostatic growth and development. These findings suggest that PPARγ represents a potential link between dietary fat and prostatic growth. However, further studies are needed to characterize its role in the normal and pathological growth of the prostate.

5.3 Hyperinsulinemia: Altered insulin/IGF signaling

Hyperinsulinemia generally develops as a compensatory response to the decreased insulin mediated actions under the insulin-resistant conditions (McKeehan et al., 1984). Experimental (Cai et al., 2001; Escobar et al., 2009; Rahman et al., 2007; Vikram et al., 2010a; b; 2011a; Vikram et al., 2010c) and clinical/epidemiological (Hammarsten et al., 2009; Hammarsten and Hogstedt, 2001; Nandeesha et al., 2006) studies indicate that the hyperinsulinemia is an independent contributor to the prostatic cell proliferation and pathogenesis of the BPH. Further, hyperinsulinemic condition can contribute to the augmented prostatic growth by several ways such as (i) increasing the serum level of IGF-I (Chokkalingam et al., 2002; Nam et al., 1997), (ii) possibility of the binding of insulin with the IGF-I receptor (IGF-IR) under the hyperinsulinemic conditions and (iii) binding of IGF-I to the insulin receptor (IR) (Belfiore and Frasca, 2008; Li et al., 2005). Further, IR has two isoforms, A and B, the former is having metabolic as well as mitogenic effects while B is mainly concerned with the metabolic effects. IR isoforms exhibit difference in the binding affinities to the ligand(s) and downstream signaling cascade (Giudice et al., 2011; Kosaki et al., 1995; Leibiger et al., 2001; Sciacca et al., 2003; Uhles et al., 2003; Vogt et al., 1991). IGF-II binds to the IR-A and mediates its growth promoting effects but not with IR-B (Frasca et al., 1999; Morrione et al., 1997). This means that insulin, IGF-I and IGF-II competes to bind with the IR-A, while only insulin binds with the IR-B. The hybrid receptors, IR-A/IR-B and IR/IGF-I further complicates the molecular diversification of the insulin signaling system. IR-A/IR-B hybrid receptors were found to bind to both insulin and IGF-II and therefore, resemble IR-A homodimers rather IR-B homodimers (Blanquart et al., 2008). The IR/IGF-IR hybrid receptors (Pandini et al., 2002; Soos et al., 1990) are activated by both insulin as well as IGF-I, but the IGF-I effect is predominant, and it resembles IGF-1R homodimers rather IR homodimers (Langlois et al., 1995). The IGF and insulin signaling system has been summarized in figure 1. Prostate is known to have both isoforms of the IR (Cox et al., 2009). Experimental studies investigating the effect of dietary habits (particularly dietary fat) on the expression of IR isoforms and signaling kinetics might provide valuable insight in the understanding of the pathogenesis of the BPH under the insulin-resistant, obese and diabetic conditions.

5.4 Estrogen/androgen ratio

Androgen deprivation leads to rapid apoptosis of the luminal secretory cells and atrophy of the prostate gland (Ikeda et al., 2000; Vikram et al., 2010c; Vikram et al., 2008). However, with the re-administration of the androgens prostate regains its normal size, and is capable of more than 15 rounds of the regression / regeneration cycle (Wang et al., 2009). Further, administration of either estrogen or dihydrotestosterone leads to hyperproliferation and induction of prostatic hyperplasia in the experimental animals. These simple experiments highlights the crucial role of steroidal hormones in the growth and development of the gland. Aromatase is a CYP450 enzyme which irreversibly converts testosterone to the estradiol, and obesity is associated with increased aromatase activity (Subbaramaiah et al., 2011). Increased aromatase activity in the obese people may lead to rise in the estrogen/androgen ratio and hence the susceptibility for developing BPH. These aspects have been recently reviewed by Nicholson et al., and readers are encouraged to read the review (Nicholson and Ricke, 2011).

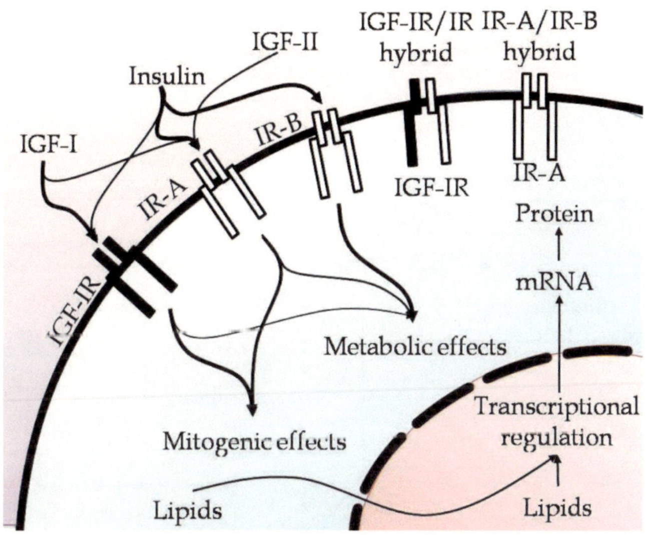

Fig. 1. The IGF and insulin receptor signaling system. To avoid confusion, the binding affinity of the ligands and relative effects of hybrid receptors (metabolic and mitogenic) are not depicted in the figure. However, the IGF-IR/IR hybrid resembles IGF-IR homodimer and IR-A/IR-B resembles IR-A homodimers. Lipids are involved in nuclear signaling and can influence transcriptional regulation and thus growth and differentiation. IGF-I/II; insulin-like growth factor-I/II, IGF-IR; insulin-like growth factor-I receptor, IR-A/B; insuln receptor isoform-A/B.

6. Summary

BPH is a highly prevalent condition of prostate in the aging men population. The worldwide increase in the prevalence of BPH has been thought to be associated with obesity and lifestyle changes such as excessive intake of fat-rich diet and physical inactivity. Considering the changing dietary habits and rising incidences of BPH, it becomes increasingly important to delineate the precise roles of lipids in the normal as well as pathological growth of the prostate. Although, experimental and clinical/epidemiological studies suggest that these conditions contribute to the pathogenesis of both insulin-resistance and BPH, the direct role of lipids in the pathogenesis of prostatic enlargement is far from complete understanding. Role of lipids in the progression of insulin-resistance and other disorders and indirect effect on the prostatic growth owing to compensatory rise in the plasma insulin level is essentially correct, but what has emerged is that the lipids might have a direct influence on the normal as well as pathological growth of the prostate.

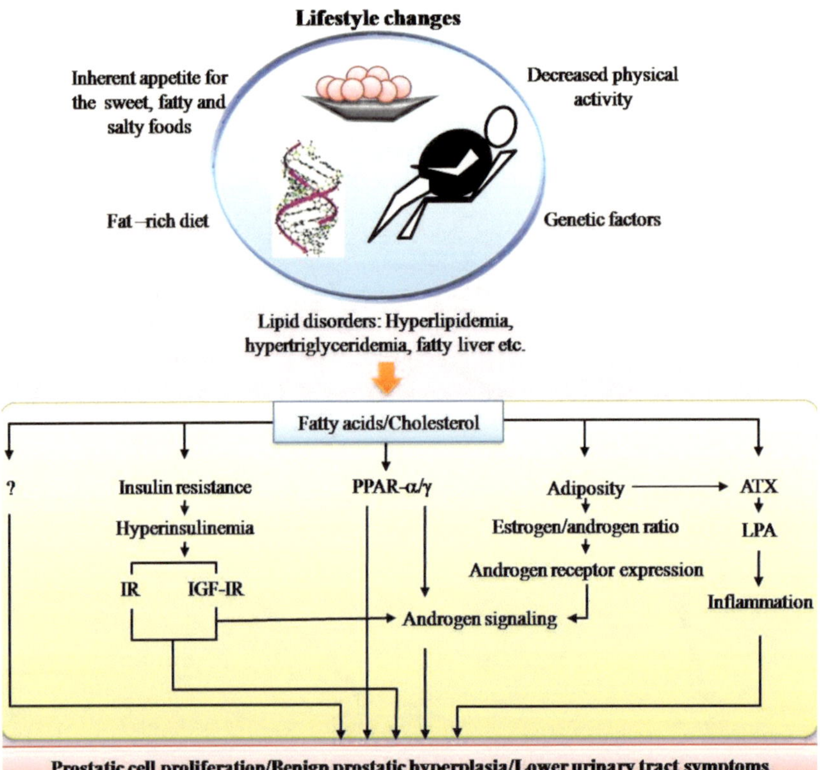

Fig. 2. Modern lifestyle associated changes including increased consumption of fat-rich diets and decreased physical activities contributes to the development of lipid-disorders and obesity. The present illustration demonstrates the possible influence of these factors on the prostatic growth and development. IR; insulin receptor, IGF-IR; insulin-like growth factor-1 receptor, PPAR-α/γ; peroxisome-proliferator activated receptor alpha/gamma, ATX; autotaxin, LPA, lysophosphatidic acid.

7. Conclusion

In addition to the genetic factors, environmental factors such as physical inactivity and excessive intake of dietary fat contribute to the increased incidence of lipid-disorders and obesity worldwide. These factors directly as well as indirectly promote the prostatic growth and contractility of the prostate gland, and represent important risk factors for the development of symptomatic LUTS / BPH (Fig. 2). ATX-LPA axis, PPARγ signaling, hyperinsulinemia/IGF signaling and steroidal signaling are the emerging mechanisms which explains the association between dietary fat intake, obesity and BPH. However, further mechanistic as well as epidemiology based studies are required to delineate the role of lipids in the pathogenesis of BPH. Future research to investigate the direct effect of different types of FAs on the prostatic growth and isoforms specific characterization of insulin and IGF-IR signaling in response to dietary habit is warranted.

8. Acknowledgements

We are thankful to the Central University of Punjab (CUP), Bathinda, Punjab 151 001, India for providing necessary resources to complete the review work.

9. References

Abdel-Meguid, T.A., Mosli, H.A., Al-Maghrabi, J.A., 2009. Prostate inflammation. Association with benign prostatic hyperplasia and prostate cancer. *Saudi Med J*, 30, 1563-1567.

Alberto, B., Umberto, C., Nazareno, S., Andrea, G., Andrea, S., Marco, B., Manuela, T., Valerio, D.G., Giorgio, G., Patrizio, R., Francesco, M., 2009. Benign prostatic hyperplasia and Its aetiologies. *Eur Urol Suppl*, 8, 865-871.

Arcolino, F.O., Ribeiro, D.L., Gobbo, M.G., Taboga, S.R., Goes, R.M., 2010. Proliferation and apoptotic rates and increased frequency of p63-positive cells in the prostate acinar epithelium of alloxan-induced diabetic rats. *Int J Exp Pathol*, 91, 144-154.

Becker, S., Dossus, L., Kaaks, R., 2009. Obesity related hyperinsulinaemia and hyperglycaemia and cancer development. *Arch Physiol Biochem*, 115, 86-96.

Belfiore, A., Frasca, F., 2008. IGF and insulin receptor signaling in breast cancer. *J Mammary Gland Biol Neoplasia*, 13, 381-406.

Berdichevets, I.N., Tyazhelova, T.V., Shimshilashvili Kh, R., Rogaev, E.I., 2010. Lysophosphatidic acid is a lipid mediator with wide range of biological activities. Biosynthetic pathways and mechanism of action. *Biochemistry*, 75, 1088-1097.

Berry, S.J., Coffey, D.S., Walsh, P.C., Ewing, L.L., 1984. The development of human benign prostatic hyperplasia with age. *J Urol*, 132, 474-479.

Blanquart, C., Achi, J., Issad, T., 2008. Characterization of IRA/IRB hybrid insulin receptors using bioluminescence resonance energy transfer. *Biochem Pharmacol*, 76, 873-883.

Bosch, R.J., 1991. Pathogenesis of benign prostatic hyperplasia. *Eur Urol*, 20, 27-30.

Bravi, F., Bosetti, C., Dal Maso, L., Talamini, R., Montella, M., Negri, E., Ramazzotti, V., Franceschi, S., La Vecchia, C., 2006. Macronutrients, fatty acids, cholesterol, and risk of benign prostatic hyperplasia. *Urology*, 67, 1205-1211.

Cai, L.Q., Imperato-McGinley, J., Zhu, Y.S., 2006. Regulation of prostate 5alpha-reductase-2 gene expression and prostate weight by dietary fat and caloric intake in the rat. *Prostate*, 66, 738-748.

Cai, X., Haleem, R., Oram, S., Cyriac, J., Jiang, F., Grayhack, J.T., Kozlowski, J.M., Wang, Z., 2001. High fat diet increases the weight of rat ventral prostate. *Prostate*, 49, 1-8.

Chokkalingam, A.P., Gao, Y.T., Deng, J., Stanczyk, F.Z., Sesterhenn, I.A., Mostofi, F.K., Fraumeni, J.F., Jr., Hsing, A.W., 2002. Insulin-like growth factors and risk of benign prostatic hyperplasia. *Prostate*, 52, 98-105.

Chughtai, B., Lee, R., Te, A., Kaplan, S., Inflammation and benign prostatic hyperplasia: clinical implications. *Curr Urol Rep*, 12, 274-277.

Cox, M.E., Gleave, M.E., Zakikhani, M., Bell, R.H., Piura, E., Vickers, E., Cunningham, M., Larsson, O., Fazli, L., Pollak, M., 2009. Insulin receptor expression by human prostate cancers. *Prostate*, 69, 33-40.

Culig, Z., Hobisch, A., Cronauer, M.V., Radmayr, C., Hittmair, A., Zhang, J., Thurnher, M., Bartsch, G., Klocker, H., 1996. Regulation of prostatic growth and function by peptide growth factors. *Prostate*, 28, 392-405.

Dahle, S.E., Chokkalingam, A.P., Gao, Y.T., Deng, J., Stanczyk, F.Z., Hsing, A.W., 2002. Body size and serum levels of insulin and leptin in relation to the risk of benign prostatic hyperplasia. *J Urol*, 168, 599-604.

Donnell, R.F., 2011. Benign prostate hyperplasia: a review of the year's progress from bench to clinic. *Curr Opin Urol*, 21, 22-26.

Escobar, E.L., Gomes-Marcondes, M.C., Carvalho, H.F., 2009. Dietary fatty acid quality affects AR and PPARgamma levels and prostate growth. *Prostate*, 69, 548-558.

Ferry, G., Moulharat, N., Pradere, J.P., Desos, P., Try, A., Genton, A., Giganti, A., Beucher-Gaudin, M., Lonchampt, M., Bertrand, M., Saulnier-Blache, J.S., Tucker, G.C., Cordi, A., Boutin, J.A., 2008. S32826, a nanomolar inhibitor of autotaxin: discovery, synthesis and applications as a pharmacological tool. *J Pharmacol Exp Ther*, 327, 809-819.

Ferry, G., Tellier, E., Try, A., Gres, S., Naime, I., Simon, M.F., Rodriguez, M., Boucher, J., Tack, I., Gesta, S., Chomarat, P., Dieu, M., Raes, M., Galizzi, J.P., Valet, P., Boutin, J.A., Saulnier-Blache, J.S., 2003. Autotaxin is released from adipocytes, catalyzes lysophosphatidic acid synthesis, and activates preadipocyte proliferation. Up-regulated expression with adipocyte differentiation and obesity. *J Biol Chem*, 278, 18162-18169.

Francisco, C., Francois, D., 2010. New concepts and pathophysiology of lower urinary tract symptoms in men. *Eur Urol Suppl*, 9, 472-476.

Frasca, F., Pandini, G., Scalia, P., Sciacca, L., Mineo, R., Costantino, A., Goldfine, I.D., Belfiore, A., Vigneri, R., 1999. Insulin receptor isoform A, a newly recognized, high-affinity insulin-like growth factor II receptor in fetal and cancer cells. *Mol Cell Biol*, 19, 3278-3288.

Ghosh, J., Myers, C.E., 1997. Arachidonic acid stimulates prostate cancer cell growth: critical role of 5-lipoxygenase. *Biochem Biophy Res Commun*, 235, 418-423.

Giovannucci, E., Rimm, E.B., Chute, C.G., Kawachi, I., Colditz, G.A., Stampfer, M.J., Willett, W.C., 1994. Obesity and benign prostatic hyperplasia. *Am J Epidemiol*, 140, 989-1002.

Giudice, J., Leskow, F.C., Arndt-Jovin, D.J., Jovin, T.M., Jares-Erijman, E.A., 2011. Differential endocytosis and signaling dynamics of insulin receptor variants IR-A and IR-B. *J Cell Sci*, 124, 801-811.

Hammarsten, J., Damber, J.E., Karlsson, M., Knutson, T., Ljunggren, O., Ohlsson, C., Peeker, R., Smith, U., Mellstrom, D., 2009. Insulin and free oestradiol are independent risk factors for benign prostatic hyperplasia. *Prostate Cancer Prostatic Dis*, 12, 160-165.

Hammarsten, J., Hogstedt, B., 1999. Clinical, anthropometric, metabolic and insulin profile of men with fast annual growth rates of benign prostatic hyperplasia. *Blood Press*, 8, 29-36.

Hammarsten, J., Hogstedt, B., 2001. Hyperinsulinaemia as a risk factor for developing benign prostatic hyperplasia. *Eur Urol*, 39, 151-158.

Hammarsten, J., Hogstedt, B., Holthuis, N., Mellstrom, D., 1998. Components of the metabolic syndrome-risk factors for the development of benign prostatic hyperplasia. *Prostate cancer and prostatic dis*, 1, 157-162.

Homma, Y., Kondo, Y., Kaneko, M., Kitamura, T., Nyou, W.T., Yanagisawa, M., Yamamoto, Y., Kakizoe, T., 2004. Promotion of carcinogenesis and oxidative stress by dietary cholesterol in rat prostate. *Carcinogenesis*, 25, 1011-1014.

Hoon Kim, J., Lee, S.Y., Myung, S.C., Kim, Y.S., Kim, T.H., Kim, M.K., 2008. Clinical significance of the leptin and leptin receptor expressions in prostate tissues. *Asian J Androl*, 10, 923-928.

Ikeda, K., Wada, Y., Foster, H.E., Jr., Wang, Z., Weiss, R.M., Latifpour, J., 2000. Experimental diabetes-induced regression of the rat prostate is associated with an increased expression of transforming growth factor-beta. *J Urol*, 164, 180-185.

Ingraham, H.A., 2011. Metabolism: A lipid for fat disorders. *Nature*, 474, 455-456.

Irvine, R.F., 2003. Nuclear lipid signalling. *Nat Rev Mol Cell Biol*, 4, 349-360.

Jiang, M., Fernandez, S., Jerome, W.G., He, Y., Yu, X., Cai, H., Boone, B., Yi, Y., Magnuson, M.A., Roy-Burman, P., Matusik, R.J., Shappell, S.B., Hayward, S.W., Disruption of PPARgamma signaling results in mouse prostatic intraepithelial neoplasia involving active autophagy. *Cell Death Differ*, 17, 469-481.

Kaplan-Lefko, P.J., Sutherland, B.W., Evangelou, A.I., Hadsell, D.L., Barrios, R.J., Foster, B.A., Demayo, F., Greenberg, N.M., 2008. Enforced epithelial expression of IGF-1 causes hyperplastic prostate growth while negative selection is requisite for spontaneous metastogenesis. *Oncogene*, 27, 2868-2876.

Kasturi, S., Russell, S., McVary, K.T., 2006. Metabolic syndrome and lower urinary tract symptoms secondary to benign prostatic hyperplasia. *Curr Urol Rep*, 7, 288-292.

Kim, B.H., Kim, C.I., Chang, H.S., Choe, M.S., Jung, H.R., Kim, D.Y., Park, C.H., 2011a. Cyclooxygenase-2 overexpression in chronic inflammation associated with benign prostatic hyperplasia: is it related to apoptosis and angiogenesis of prostate cancer? *Korean J Urol*, 52, 253-259.

Kim, G.W., Doo, S.W., Yang, W.J., Song, Y.S., 2010. Effects of obesity on prostate volume and lower urinary tract symptoms in korean men. *Korean J Urol*, 51, 344-347.

Kim, J.M., Song, P.H., Kim, H.T., Moon, K.H., 2011b. Effect of obesity on prostate-specific antigen, prostate volume, and international prostate symptom score in patients with benign prostatic hyperplasia. *Korean J Urol*, 52, 401-405.

Kogai, M.A., Lutov, U.V., Selyatitskaya, V.G., 2008. Hormonal and biochemical parameters of metabolic syndrome in male patients with body weight excess and obesity. *Bull Exp Biol Med*, 146, 806-808.

Kosaki, A., Pillay, T.S., Xu, L., Webster, N.J., 1995. The B isoform of the insulin receptor signals more efficiently than the A isoform in HepG2 cells. *J Biol Chem*, 270, 20816-20823.

Kristal, A.R., Arnold, K.B., Schenk, J.M., Neuhouser, M.L., Goodman, P., Penson, D.F., Thompson, I.M., 2008. Dietary patterns, supplement use, and the risk of symptomatic benign prostatic hyperplasia: results from the prostate cancer prevention trial. *Am J Epidemiol*, 167, 925-934.

Kulkarni, P., Getzenberg, R.H., 2009. High-fat diet, obesity and prostate disease: the ATX-LPA axis? *Nat Clin Pract Urol*, 6, 128-131.

Lagiou, P., Signorello, L.B., Trichopoulos, D., Tzonou, A., Trichopoulou, A., Mantzoros, C.S., 1998. Leptin in relation to prostate cancer and benign prostatic hyperplasia. *Int J Cancer*, 76, 25-28.

Langlois, W.J., Sasaoka, T., Yip, C.C., Olefsky, J.M., 1995. Functional characterization of hybrid receptors composed of a truncated insulin receptor and wild type insulin-like growth factor 1 or insulin receptors. *Endocrinology*, 136, 1978-1986.

Lee, J.M., Lee, Y.K., Mamrosh, J.L., Busby, S.A., Griffin, P.R., Pathak, M.C., Ortlund, E.A., Moore, D.D., 2011. A nuclear-receptor-dependent phosphatidylcholine pathway with antidiabetic effects. *Nature*, 474, 506-510.

Lee, S.H., Kim, J.C., Lee, J.Y., Kim, J.H., Oh, C.Y., Lee, S.W., Yoo, S.J., Chung, B.H., 2009. Effects of obesity on lower urinary tract symptoms in Korean BPH patients. *Asian J Androl*. 11, 663-668.

Leibiger, B., Leibiger, I.B., Moede, T., Kemper, S., Kulkarni, R.N., Kahn, C.R., de Vargas, L.M., Berggren, P.O., 2001. Selective insulin signaling through A and B insulin receptors regulates transcription of insulin and glucokinase genes in pancreatic beta cells. *Mol Cell*, 7, 559-570.

Li, G., Barrett, E.J., Wang, H., Chai, W., Liu, Z., 2005. Insulin at physiological concentrations selectively activates insulin but not insulin-like growth factor I (IGF-I) or insulin/IGF-I hybrid receptors in endothelial cells. *Endocrinology*, 146, 4690-4696.

Liu, Y., Zuckier, L.S., Ghesani, N.V., 2010. Dominant uptake of fatty acid over glucose by prostate cells: a potential new diagnostic and therapeutic approach. *Anticancer Res*, 30, 369-374.

Marker, P.C., Donjacour, A.A., Dahiya, R., Cunha, G.R., 2003. Hormonal, cellular, and molecular control of prostatic development. *Dev Biol*, 253, 165-174.

Maserejian, N.N., Giovannucci, E.L., McKinlay, J.B., 2009. Dietary macronutrients, cholesterol, and sodium and lower urinary tract symptoms in men. *Eur Urol*, 55, 1179-1189.

McKeehan, W.L., Adams, P.S., Rosser, M.P., 1984. Direct mitogenic effects of insulin, epidermal growth factor, glucocorticoid, cholera toxin, unknown pituitary factors and possibly prolactin, but not androgen, on normal rat prostate epithelial cells in serum-free, primary cell culture. *Cancer Res*, 44, 1998-2010.

Morales-Garcia, J.A., Luna-Medina, R., Alfaro-Cervello, C., Cortes-Canteli, M., Santos, A., Garcia-Verdugo, J.M., Perez-Castillo, A., 2011. Peroxisome proliferator-activated receptor gamma ligands regulate neural stem cell proliferation and differentiation in vitro and in vivo. *Glia*, 59, 293-307.

Morrione, A., Valentinis, B., Xu, S.Q., Yumet, G., Louvi, A., Efstratiadis, A., Baserga, R., 1997. Insulin-like growth factor II stimulates cell proliferation through the insulin receptor. *Proc Natl Acad Sci U S A*, 94, 3777-3782.

Moyad, M.A., Lowe, F.C., 2008. Educating patients about lifestyle modifications for prostate health. *Am J Med*, 121, S34-42.

Nam, S.Y., Lee, E.J., Kim, K.R., Cha, B.S., Song, Y.D., Lim, S.K., Lee, H.C., Huh, K.B., 1997. Effect of obesity on total and free insulin-like growth factor (IGF)-1, and their relationship to IGF-binding protein (BP)-1, IGFBP-2, IGFBP-3, insulin, and growth hormone. *Int J Obes Relat Metab Disord*, 21, 355-359.

Nandeesha, H., Koner, B.C., Dorairajan, L.N., Sen, S.K., 2006. Hyperinsulinemia and dyslipidemia in non-diabetic benign prostatic hyperplasia. *Clin Chim Acta*, 370, 89-93.

Nicholson, T.M., Ricke, W.A., 2011. Androgens and estrogens in benign prostatic hyperplasia: Past, present and future. *Differentiation*, (In-press).

North, E.J., Howard, A.L., Wanjala, I.W., Pham, T.C., Baker, D.L., Parrill, A.L., 2010. Pharmacophore development and application toward the identification of novel, small-molecule autotaxin inhibitors. *J Med Chem*, 53, 3095-3105.

North, E.J., Osborne, D.A., Bridson, P.K., Baker, D.L., Parrill, A.L., 2009. Autotaxin structure-activity relationships revealed through lysophosphatidylcholine analogs. *Bioorg Med Chem*, 17, 3433-3442.

Pandalai, P.K., Pilat, M.J., Yamazaki, K., Naik, H., Pienta, K.J., 1996. The effects of omega-3 and omega-6 fatty acids on in vitro prostate cancer growth. *Anticancer Res*, 16, 815-820.

Pandini, G., Frasca, F., Mineo, R., Sciacca, L., Vigneri, R., Belfiore, A., 2002. Insulin/insulin-like growth factor I hybrid receptors have different biological characteristics depending on the insulin receptor isoform involved. *J Biol Chem*, 277, 39684-39695.

Parast, M.M., Yu, H., Ciric, A., Salata, M.W., Davis, V., Milstone, D.S., 2009. PPARgamma regulates trophoblast proliferation and promotes labyrinthine trilineage differentiation. *PLoS One*, 4, e8055.

Parrill, A.L., Baker, D.L., 2010. Autotaxin inhibitors: a perspective on initial medicinal chemistry efforts. *Expert Opin Ther Pat*, 20, 1619-1625.

Parsons, J.K., 2011. Lifestyle factors, benign prostatic hyperplasia, and lower urinary tract symptoms. *Curr Opin Urol*, 21, 1-4.

Parsons, J.K., Bergstrom, J., Barrett-Connor, E., 2008. Lipids, lipoproteins and the risk of benign prostatic hyperplasia in community-dwelling men. *BJU Int*, 101, 313-318.

Parsons, J.K., Carter, H.B., Partin, A.W., Windham, B.G., Metter, E.J., Ferrucci, L., Landis, P., Platz, E.A., 2006. Metabolic factors associated with benign prostatic hyperplasia. *J Clin Endocrinol Metab*, 91, 2562-2568.

Parsons, J.K., Kashefi, C., 2008. Physical activity, benign prostatic hyperplasia, and lower urinary tract symptoms. *Eur Urol*, 53, 1228-1235.

Parsons, J.K., Sarma, A.V., McVary, K., Wei, J.T., 2009. Obesity and benign prostatic hyperplasia: clinical connections, emerging etiological paradigms and future directions. *J Urol*, 182, S27-31.

Rahman, N.U., Phonsombat, S., Bochinski, D., Carrion, R.E., Nunes, L., Lue, T.F., 2007. An animal model to study lower urinary tract symptoms and erectile dysfunction: the hyperlipidaemic rat. *BJU Int*, 100, 658-663.

Rancoule, C., Pradere, J.P., Gonzalez, J., Klein, J., Valet, P., Bascands, J.L., Schanstra, J.P., Saulnier-Blache, J.S., 2011. Lysophosphatidic acid-1-receptor targeting agents for fibrosis. *Expert Opin Investig Drugs*, 20, 657-667.

Rick, F.G., Schally, A.V., Block, N.L., Nadji, M., Szepeshazi, K., Zarandi, M., Vidaurre, I., Perez, R., Halmos, G., Szalontay, L., 2011. Antagonists of growth hormone-releasing hormone (GHRH) reduce prostate size in experimental benign prostatic hyperplasia. *Proc Natl Acad Sci U S A*, 108, 3755-3760.

Rose, D.P., Connolly, J.M., 1991. Effects of fatty acids and eicosanoid synthesis inhibitors on the growth of two human prostate cancer cell lines. *Prostate*, 18, 243-254.

Saigal, C.S., Joyce, G., 2005. Economic costs of benign prostatic hyperplasia in the private sector. *J Urol*, 173, 1309-1313.

Sakamoto, S., Yokoyama, M., Zhang, X., Prakash, K., Nagao, K., Hatanaka, T., Getzenberg, R.H., Kakehi, Y., 2004. Increased expression of CYR61, an extracellular matrix signaling protein, in human benign prostatic hyperplasia and its regulation by lysophosphatidic acid. *Endocrinology*, 145, 2929-2940.

Sanda, M.G., Beaty, T.H., Stutzman, R.E., Childs, B., Walsh, P.C., 1994. Genetic susceptibility of benign prostatic hyperplasia. *J Urol*, 152, 115-119.

Schenk, J.M., Kristal, A.R., Neuhouser, M.L., Tangen, C.M., White, E., Lin, D.W., Kratz, M., Thompson, I.M., 2010. Biomarkers of systemic inflammation and risk of incident, symptomatic benign prostatic hyperplasia: results from the prostate cancer prevention trial. *Am J Epidemiol*, 171, 571-582.

Schenk, J.M., Kristal, A.R., Neuhouser, M.L., Tangen, C.M., White, E., Lin, D.W., Thompson, I.M., 2009. Serum adiponectin, C-peptide and leptin and risk of symptomatic benign prostatic hyperplasia: results from the Prostate Cancer Prevention Trial. *Prostate*, 69, 1303-1311.

Sciacca, L., Prisco, M., Wu, A., Belfiore, A., Vigneri, R., Baserga, R., 2003. Signaling differences from the A and B isoforms of the insulin receptor (IR) in 32D cells in the presence or absence of IR substrate-1. *Endocrinology*, 144, 2650-2658.

Sekine, Y., Osei-Hwedieh, D., Matsuda, K., Raghavachari, N., Liu, D., Furuya, Y., Koike, H., Suzuki, K., Remaley, A.T., 2011. High fat diet reduces the expression of glutathione peroxidase 3 in mouse prostate. *Prostate*, (In-Press).

Simopoulos, A.P., 1999. Essential fatty acids in health and chronic disease. *Am J Clin Nutr*, 70, 560S-569S.

Smith, C.D., Wells, W.W., 1983a. Phosphorylation of rat liver nuclear envelopes. I. Characterization of in vitro protein phosphorylation. *J Biol Chem*, 258, 9360-9367.

Smith, C.D., Wells, W.W., 1983b. Phosphorylation of rat liver nuclear envelopes. II. Characterization of in vitro lipid phosphorylation. *J Biol Chem*, 258, 9368-9373.

Soos, M.A., Whittaker, J., Lammers, R., Ullrich, A., Siddle, K., 1990. Receptors for insulin and insulin-like growth factor-I can form hybrid dimers. Characterisation of hybrid receptors in transfected cells. *Biochem J*, 270, 383-390.

Srinivasan, G., Campbell, E., Bashirelahi, N., 1995. Androgen, estrogen, and progesterone receptors in normal and aging prostates. *Microsc Res Tech*, 30, 293-304.

Story, M.T., 1995. Regulation of prostate growth by fibroblast growth factors. *World J Urol*, 13, 297-305.

Stranne, J., Damber, J.E., Fall, M., Hammarsten, J., Knutson, T., Peeker, R., 2009. One-third of the Swedish male population over 50 years of age suffers from lower urinary tract symptoms. *Scandinavian J Urol Nephrol*, 43, 199-205.

Subbaramaiah, K., Howe, L.R., Bhardwaj, P., Du, B., Gravaghi, C., Yantiss, R.K., Zhou, X.K., Blaho, V.A., Hla, T., Yang, P., Kopelovich, L., Hudis, C.A., Dannenberg, A.J., 2011. Obesity is associated with inflammation and elevated aromatase expression in the mouse mammary gland. *Cancer Prev Res (Phila)*, 4, 329-346.

Suthagar, E., Soudamani, S., Yuvaraj, S., Ismail Khan, A., Aruldhas, M.M., Balasubramanian, K., 2009. Effects of streptozotocin (STZ)-induced diabetes and insulin replacement on rat ventral prostate. *Biomed Pharmacother*, 63, 43-50.

Suzuki, S., Platz, E.A., Kawachi, I., Willett, W.C., Giovannucci, E., 2002. Intakes of energy and macronutrients and the risk of benign prostatic hyperplasia. *Am J Clin Nutr*, 75, 689-697.

Uhles, S., Moede, T., Leibiger, B., Berggren, P.O., Leibiger, I.B., 2003. Isoform-specific insulin receptor signaling involves different plasma membrane domains. *J Cell Biol*, 163, 1327-1337.

Van Meeteren, L.A., Moolenaar, W.H., 2007. Regulation and biological activities of the autotaxin-LPA axis. *Prog Lipid Res*, 46, 145-160.

Vikram, A., Jena, G., 2010. S961, an insulin receptor antagonist causes hyperinsulinemia, insulin-resistance and depletion of energy stores in rats. *Biochem Biophy Res Commun*, 398, 260-265.

Vikram, A., Jena, G., 2011a. Diet-induced hyperinsulinemia accelerates growth of human androgen independent PC-3 cells. *Nut Cancer*, (In-Press).

Vikram, A., Jena, G., 2011b. Role of insulin and testosterone in prostatic growth: who is doing what? *Med Hypotheses*, 76, 474-478.

Vikram, A., Jena, G., Ramarao, P., 2010a. Insulin-resistance and benign prostatic hyperplasia: the connection. *Eur J Pharmacol*, 641, 75-81.

Vikram, A., Jena, G., Ramarao, P., 2010b. Pioglitazone attenuates prostatic enlargement in diet-induced insulin-resistant rats by altering lipid distribution and hyperinsulinaemia. *Brit J Pharmacol*, 161, 1708-1721.

Vikram, A., Jena, G., Ramarao, P., 2011a. Insulin-resistance reduces botulinum neurotoxin-type A induced prostatic atrophy and apoptosis in rats. *Eur J Pharmacol*, 650, 356-363.

Vikram, A., Jena, G.B., Ramarao, P., 2010c. Increased cell proliferation and contractility of prostate in insulin resistant rats: linking hyperinsulinemia with benign prostate hyperplasia. *Prostate*, 70, 79-89.

Vikram, A., Kushwaha, S., Jena, G.B., 2011b. Relative influence of testosterone and insulin in the regulation of prostatic cell proliferation and growth. *Steroids*, 76, 416-423.

Vikram, A., Tripathi, D.N., Ramarao, P., Jena, G.B., 2008. Intervention of D-glucose ameliorates the toxicity of streptozotocin in accessory sex organs of rat. *Toxicol Appl Pharmacol*, 226, 84-93.

Vogeser, M., Schwandt, P., Haas, G.M., Broedl, U.C., Lehrke, M., Parhofer, K.G., 2009. BMI and hyperinsulinemia in children. *Clin Biochem*, 42, 1427-1430.

Vogt, B., Carrascosa, J.M., Ermel, B., Ullrich, A., Haring, H.U., 1991. The two isotypes of the human insulin receptor (HIR-A and HIR-B) follow different internalization kinetics. *Biochem Biophy Res Commun*, 177, 1013-1018.

Vykhovanets, E.V., Shankar, E., Vykhovanets, O.V., Shukla, S., Gupta, S., 2011. High-fat diet increases NF-kappaB signaling in the prostate of reporter mice. *Prostate*, 71, 147-156.

Wang, L., Yang, J.R., Yang, L.Y., Liu, Z.T., 2008. Chronic inflammation in benign prostatic hyperplasia: implications for therapy. *Med Hypotheses*, 70, 1021-1023.

Wang, X., Kruithof-de Julio, M., Economides, K.D., Walker, D., Yu, H., Halili, M.V., Hu, Y.P., Price, S.M., Abate-Shen, C., Shen, M.M., 2009. A luminal epithelial stem cell that is a cell of origin for prostate cancer. *Nature*, 461, 495-500.

Wang, Z., Olumi, A.F., 2011. Diabetes, growth hormone-insulin-like growth factor pathways and association to benign prostatic hyperplasia. *Differentiation*, (In-Press).

Yang, Y.J., Lee, S.H., Hong, S.J., Chung, B.C., 1999. Comparison of fatty acid profiles in the serum of patients with prostate cancer and benign prostatic hyperplasia. *Clin Biochem*, 32, 405-409.

Yono, M., Mane, S.M., Lin, A., Weiss, R.M., Latifpour, J., 2008. Differential effects of diabetes induced by streptozotocin and that develops spontaneously on prostate growth in Bio Breeding (BB) rats. *Life Sci*, 83, 192-197.

Yono, M., Pouresmail, M., Takahashi, W., Flanagan, J.F., Weiss, R.M., Latifpour, J., 2005. Effect of insulin treatment on tissue size of the genitourinary tract in BB rats with spontaneously developed and streptozotocin-induced diabetes. *Naunyn Schmiedebergs Arch Pharmacol*, 372, 251-255.

Zeng, Y., Kakehi, Y., Nouh, M.A., Tsunemori, H., Sugimoto, M., Wu, X.X., 2009. Gene expression profiles of lysophosphatidic acid-related molecules in the prostate: relevance to prostate cancer and benign hyperplasia. *Prostate*, 69, 283-292.

Zucchetto, A., Tavani, A., Dal Maso, L., Gallus, S., Negri, E., Talamini, R., Franceschi, S., Montella, M., La Vecchia, C., 2005. History of weight and obesity through life and risk of benign prostatic hyperplasia. *Int J Obes*, 29, 798-803.

21

Dyslipidemia in Patients with Lipodystrophy in the Use of Antiretroviral Therapy

Rosana Libonati, Cláudia Dutra, Leonardo Barbosa, Sandro Oliveira, Paulo Lisbôa and Marcus Libonati
Tropical Medicine Center, Federal University of the Pará, Pará Brasil

1. Introduction

Dyslipidemia is a change in serum lipids levels, which is associated with increased risk of cardiovascular events when are found elevated (American Heart Association, 2002, Sposito et al., 2007). Before introduction of antiretroviral therapy (HAART), patients with acquired immunodeficiency syndrome (AIDS) developed a dyslipidemia characterized by isolated elevation of triglycerides (TG) and decrease in total cholesterol (TC) and its fractions (Gkrania-Klotsas & Klotsas, 2007; Mulligan, 2003). With the advent of HAART, especially with the use of protease inhibitors (PI), this situation changed to a lipid profile with elevated TG, TC, lipoproteins of very low and low density (VLDL-C and LDL-C) and decrease in high density lipoprotein (HDL-C), leaving these patients at risk for developing diabetes, hypertension and other complications (Chen et al., 2002; Furtado et al., 2007; Garg, 2000; Gkrania-Klotsas & Klotsas, 2007; Kotler, 2008; Mulligan, 2003; Sattler, 2008; Segarra-Newnham, 2002; Schering & Tovar, 2006; Yu et al., 2005).
Studies estimate that the prevalence of dyslipidemia in patients with HIV (Human Immunodeficiency Virus) during use of antiretroviral therapy can vary from 33% to 82% and may be influenced by several factors including study type, sample type and time of HAART (Gkrania-Klotsas & Klotsas, 2007; Schering & Tovar, 2006; Yu et al., 2005).

2. HIV lipodystrophy syndrome

According to UNAIDS and World Health Organization (WHO) (2009) there was a large increase in the prevalence of HIV carriers in the world, reaching 33.4 million in 2008, value explained by the maintenance of annual incidence and the increase of the survival (Lihn et al. 2003; Mallewa et al., 2008). However, was noted a illness pattern change of these patients which ever left to be affected by a clinical feature characteristic of opportunistic diseases to develop HIV lipodystrophy syndrome (HIVLS) (Kramer et al., 2009; Ministry of Health of Brazil, 2008; Samaras et al., 2009; Stankov & Behrens, 2010).
Body composition abnormalities have been reported in 40-50% of HIV-positive outpatients. This proportion is higher in patients receiving antiretroviral therapy. The rate of lipodystrophy can be high depending on the characteristics of the cohort (sex, age and possibly race), the type and duration of antiretroviral therapy (Grinspoon & Carr, 2005).

The HIVLS presents three distinct forms according to distribution pattern: lipoatrophy, with fat loss in limbs, face and buttocks; lipohypertrophy, with localized increase of abdominal, breast and dorsocervical subcutaneous cellular tissue, besides visceral deposit and lipoma formation; and the mixed form with signs of both syndromes earlier (Sattler, 2008; Mello et al., 2008) (Figure 1).

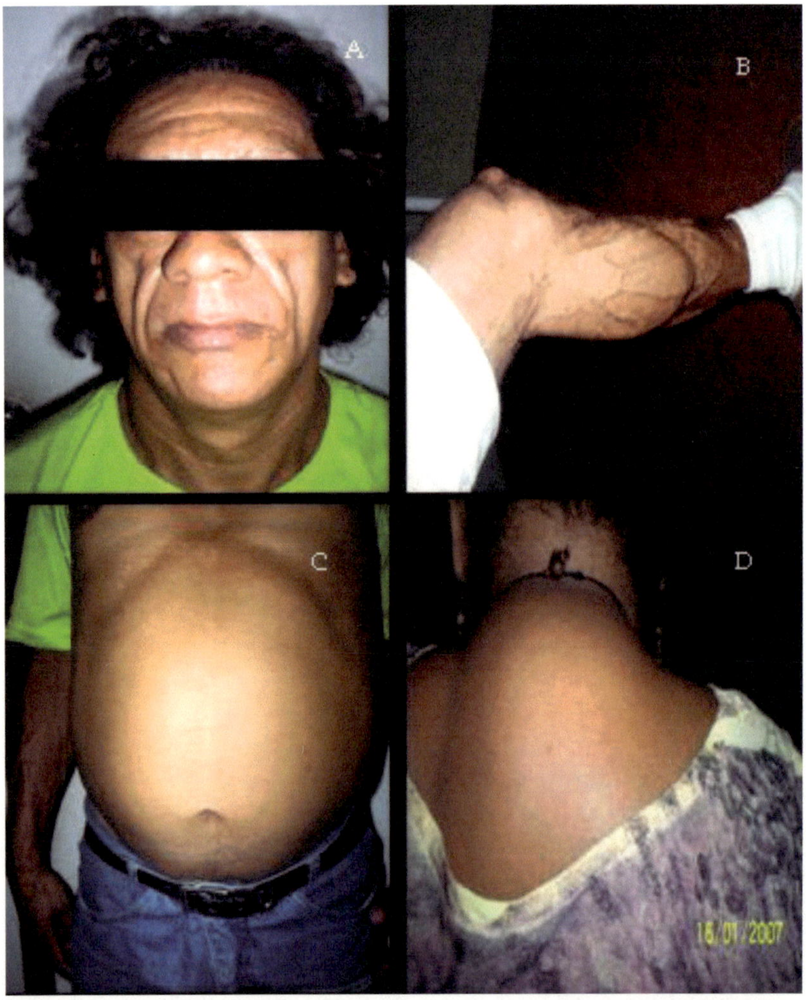

Legend: A) facial lipoatrophy with facial furrows accentuated, bony prominence, and loss of Bichat's fat (malar fat). B) Lipoatrophy of the lower limbs with prominent veins. C) Visceral lipohypertrophy, with increased waist circumference and little subcutaneous tissue. D) Dorsocervical lipohypertrophy. Photos of the collection of Dr. Rosana Libonati.

Fig. 1. Morphological changes in HIV patients with lipodystrophy syndrome, Pará, Brazil.

In addition to fat distribution alterations, metabolic changes are expressed as a mixed dyslipidemia with hypertriglyceridemia, total hypercholesterolemia, low density lipoprotein (LDL-C) elevation, reduction of high density lipoprotein (HDL-C), besides the induction of insulin resistance culminating in establishment of type II diabetes (Furtado et.,

2007; Chen et al., 2002; Garg, 2000; Sattler, 2008, Yu et al., 2005). The changes in the concentrations of plasma lipids are more observed in patients receiving protease inhibitors (PI) (Yu et al., 2005).

Prospective studies investigating body composition in patients starting HAART for the first time have showed increases in fat during the initial months of treatment, followed by a progressive declining in the following three years. In one study, the decline was estimated at 14% per year in white men who received treatment regimens containing zidovudine/lamivudine or stavudine/lamivudine plus protease inhibitor or non-nucleoside reverse transcriptase inhibitor. In contrast, trunk fat increases initially and then remains stable for two or three years, resulting in relative central adiposity. These changes are clinically evident in 20 to 35% of patients after about 12 to 24 months of combination antiretroviral therapy (Grinspoon & Carr, 2005).

The type, duration and current use or not of antiretroviral therapy are strongly associated with the lipoatrophy severity. Therapy based on two nucleoside analogue reverse transcriptase inhibitors and one protease inhibitor has strong association with severe lipoatrophy (Mallon et al., 2003).

Now, the mechanism by which the protease inhibitor causes lipodystrophy remains unknown. Several protease inhibitors prevent preadipocytes differentiation and mild to moderate apoptosis in subcutaneous adipose tissue. Adipose tissue of patients with lipodystrophy has reduced expression of mRNA of several key factors involved in adipogenesis, including Sterol regulatory element binding protein (SREBP1c) and Peroxisome proliferator-activated receptor gamma (PPARγ). *In vitro* studies have shown that protease inhibitors can inhibit lipogenesis and adipocyte differentiation, stimulate lipolysis and prevent nuclear localization of SREBP-1c (Garg, 2000; Grinspoon & Carr, 2005).

The nucleoside analog more strongly associated with lipoatrophy is stavudine, particularly when used in combination with didanosine. Lipoatrophy associated with nucleoside analogue may be due in part by mitochondrial injury caused by inhibition of the mitochondrial DNA polymerase γ within adipocyte and mitochondrial DNA depletion, although the extent and specificity of this effect remains unknown. The nucleoside analogue can inhibit adipogenesis and adipocyte differentiation, promote lipolysis and exert synergistic toxic effect with protease inhibitors *in vitro* and *in vivo* (Grinspoon & Carr, 2005).

In nine studies assessing risk factors for lipoatrophy, were statistically significant more common duration and exposure to thymidine analogues, most commonly stavudine (d4T) (6/9), age (5/9), markers of disease severity (CD4/HIV RNA) (5/9), duration of therapy (3/9) and Caucasian (3/9). A prospective nonrandomized study in 40 HIV-positive patients starting antiretroviral therapy for the first time resulted after an average of 96 weeks, using multivariate analysis, that treatment with d4T is an independent factor for lipoatrophy (Lichtenstein, 2005).

In eight studies assessing lipohypertrophy, the most significant risk factors were duration of therapy (3/8), a marker of disease severity (3/8), age (3/8) and protease inhibitor use (4/8). An additional study evaluating 2258 HIV-positive patients evaluated change in adipose tissue for both gender. Logistic regression showed that men have a significantly lower adjusted risk than women have (OR: 0.47, CI 95%: from 0.38 to 0.58) and a significantly lower risk of lipohypertrophy and mixed redistribution, while the risk of lipoatrophy was similar between genders. Therefore, a rigorous multivariate analysis controlling for numerous variables reveals multiple risk factors, suggesting that the pathogenic mechanism

for fat redistribution seems to be the result of complex interactions between host, disease and drugs factors (Lichtenstein, 2005).
As for the diagnosis of HIVLS, there is not one standard pattern used to subjective body changes mentioned by the patients, anthropometric measurements and metabolic changes demonstrated in fasting laboratory tests (Diehl et al., 2008). Other tests that assist in conducting the HIVLS patients are: bone densitometry, for the investigation of osteopenia/osteoporosis; Dual-emission X-ray absorptiometry (DEXA), which allows an analysis of body composition, especially fat in the limbs, Computed Tomography, to observe presence of visceral fat deposits, and upper abdominal ultrasound for hepatic steatosis assessment (Mallon et al., 2003).
Therefore, the main consequences of HIVLS are increased cardiovascular risk and consequent development of hypertension, diabetes mellitus, atheromatous disease, stroke, myocardial infarction (Kramer et al., 2009). Psychological disorders as well as, like stress and low self-esteem by stigmatizing body changes (Santos et al., 2005; Seidl & Machado, 2008), which not cease to be risk factor for these events already mentioned by activation of sympathetic and glucocorticoids systems, and neuropeptide Y production potentiating the metabolic changes (Licht et al., 2010; Rasmusson et al., 2010).

3. Pathophysiology of dyslipidemia secondary to antiretroviral therapy

Since the implementation of antiretroviral therapy (HAART), in the 90s of last century, the treatment of AIDS has increased the mean life expectancy of HIV-infected population. Until then seen as a death sentence in a matter of short time, the disease have been faced like chronic, and with more optimism. However, despite a decrease in morbidity and mortality, HAART led to a problem that has become a major challenge that patients with AIDS must control: dyslipidemia (Cahn et al., 2010).
The dyslipidemia associated with HAART has been characteristic of elevated total cholesterol (TC), low-density lipoprotein (LDL-C) and triglycerides (TG), in addition to decreased high-density lipoprotein (HDL-C), which results in increased predisposition to the development of hypertension, insulin resistance, diabetes mellitus and cardiovascular complications. There are evidences that cardiovascular manifestations proportions in HIV-infected patients on HAART are higher than in general population (Almeida et al., 2009). This does not mean that the occurrence of dyslipidemia has emerged only with the implementation of antiretroviral drugs to treat AIDS. Before the existence of HAART had been reported lipid profile changes with high levels of triglycerides and low rate of VLDL-C and HDL-C (Sprinz et al., 2010; Grunfeld et al., 1992).
Several studies investigate ways of relating to HAART the effects of dyslipidemia like type of drug used by the patient and how the treatment regimen it has been implemented, but is still lacking a precise explanation for the lipid profile origin. Protease inhibitors (PI) are associated with dyslipidemia and insulin resistance for a considerable time, specifically ritonavir, and a variety of hypotheses (albeit not conclusive) it is presented to explain this association (Noor, 2007; Dubé et al., 2003).
One proposed mechanism to emergence of dyslipidemia is the lipoprotein lipase inhibition by PI, responsible for LDL-C increased, due to difficulty in capturing chylomicrons, resulting in lower hepatic clearance of triglycerides (Sprinz et al., 2010, as cited in Carr & Mooser, 2001). Another hypothesis is that PI has the ability to inhibit steps in lipid metabolism by binding to cellular retinoic acid binding protein type 1 (CRABP-1) and

related protein receptor LDR-c, resulting in hyperlipidemia by higher release of lipids in the circulation. More specifically, the PI on CRABP-1 receptor leads to a reduction of 9-cis retinoic acid and dimerization with the receptor activated by peroxisome proliferator-activated receptor gamma (PPAR-γ), which is involved both in apoptosis of adipocytes and in differentiation between these two. (Sprinz et al., 2010; Carr et al., 1998). A third theory, restricted to ritonavir, antiretroviral therapy suggests it increases the activity of sterol regulatory element binding protein 1 (SREBP-1c), increasing lipogenesis, the rate of VLDL-C and apolipoprotein B liver. Thus, the increase in triglycerides caused by ritonavir that could be related to elevation in hepatic lipoprotein, inhibiting degradation mediated by apolipoprotein B and SREBP-1c in liver (Riddle et al., 2001; Liang et al., 2001).

As regard the insulin resistance promoted by PI, this class of antiretroviral drugs has been related to inhibition of GLUT-4 in the transmembrane transport of glucose, leading to reduced glucose uptake mediated by insulin in peripheral tissue (skeletal muscle and adipocytes), which can lead the modification of lipid levels (Noor, 2007). The fact that some patients had a clinical and laboratory profile more or less flowered depending on the effects that PI has on the lipids metabolism may be related to genetics, suggesting that certain people are more prone to PI effects through manifestation of certain genes so far not identified (Shahmanesh et al., 2001).

With regard to nucleoside reverse transcriptase inhibitors (NRTIs), it is speculated that can lead to reduced synthesis of mitochondrial DNA, leading to decreased oxidative phosphorylation, resulting in subcutaneous adipocyte apoptosis, dyslipidemia, and increased insulin resistance (Maagaard & Kvale, 2009). The reverse transcriptase inhibitor non-nucleoside (NNRTI), particularly Efavirenz, are also related to the onset of metabolic disorders, including dyslipidemia - but they have lower participation. When compared to patients receiving Nevirapine, patients who make use of Efavirenz have higher levels of triglycerides and HDL-C (Sprinz et al., 2010, as cited in Carr et al., 1998).

The type of antiretroviral used in HAART case amends significantly the lipid profile of patient it might be replaced. However, make use of a change in medication or combination of drugs (a strategy that appears more practical than prescription of lipid, at least at first glance) does not always result in improving lipid metabolism, considering the dyslipidemia in HIV infection is related to a multifactorial framework (Sprinz et al., 2010).

Although there are doubts considering the mechanisms linked to development of dyslipidemia in patients receiving HAART, and about assumptions not fully understood, this is still the most effective treatment in patients with AIDS and should not be proscribed for patients. To minimize risks that dyslipidemia implies to health, we recommend the same precautions, both dietary and behavioral (avoiding a sedentary lifestyle) and drug (statins/fibrates) for the general population. The use of fibrates is primarily indicated for reduction of hypertriglyceridemia, while statins are used to reverse the hypercholesterolemia. However, must be careful in prescribing of statins, since there is risk of drug interactions with HAART (Sprinz et al., 2010).

4. Treatment of dyslipidemia secondary to antiretroviral therapy

Hyperlipidemia is a major risk factor for developing of atherosclerosis. Epidemiological studies in adults show a direct association between high levels of total cholesterol and LDL and the incidence of mortality and morbidity in coronary artery disease (CAD) and is LDL-C a predictor of CAD risk at any age, besides low HDL and *diabetes mellitus* (Giddings, 1999).

Dyslipidemia in HIV infection is related to a multifactorial framework (Sprinz et al., 2010), so treatment should be done with non-pharmacological and pharmacological measures.

4.1 Hypercholesterolemia
4.1.1 Non-pharmacologic therapy

The HIV-infected patients with dyslipidemia they should be screened before using those drugs as therapy, with the implementation of the change of lifestyle of these patients through diet, exercise, tobacco control, diabetes mellitus and hypertension (Dubé et al., 2003). In one study, the diet associated with exercise in 11% reduced cholesterol levels of patients infected with HIV (Henry et al., 1998). In another study showed that diet accompanied by resistance exercise at least three times a week reduced the cholesterol level by 18% and triglycerides by 25% (Jones et al., 2001).

The first measure to be taken will always be non-pharmacologic therapy, unless there is urgent need for intervention, as patients at high risk for coronary artery disease (obesity, diabetes, family history of cardiovascular disease) and extremely high levels of LDL-C greater than 220 mg / dL (Dubé et al., 2003).

4.1.2 Pharmacological therapy

The pharmacological treatment for dyslipidemia it is performed with HMG-CoA reductase inhibitors, or statins, are the main representatives of pravastatin and atorvastatin groups. They have been used extensively in clinical practice as first-line treatment for hypercholesterolemia in the general population and in HIV-infected patients, promoting reduction of cardiovascular risk in patients without no history of coronary artery disease and of progression of coronary artery stenosis with decrease of cardiovascular events recurrence, working in primary and secondary, respectively (Dube et al., 2003).

In one study, patients with altered levels of total cholesterol (TC) and triglycerides (TG), using pravastatin 20 mg/day occurring 19% decrease in the level of TC and 37% in the level of TG (Baldini et al., 2000). In another study, diet was associated with therapy with pravastatin 40 mg/day in patients with TC levels greater than 240 mg/dL, indicating a 17% decline in the levels of TC and 19% in the level of LDL-C (Moyle, 2001). Therefore, Palacios et al., in 2002, analyzing a group of patients with TC levels greater than 240 mg/dL under atorvastatin 10 mg/day was found a 27% decrease in the level of TC, 41% of TG and 37% in the LDL-C.

Thus, statins are the first choice in the treatment of elevated LDL-C (> 220 mg / dL) and patients with high total cholesterol associated with hypertriglyceridemia (TG between 200 to 500 mg/dL), initial dose may be used 20-40 mg of pravastatin or atorvastatin 10 mg monitoring possible liver toxicity with laboratory tests (Dube et al., 2003). Protease inhibitors and non-nucleoside inhibitors of reverse transcriptase enzyme use in its metabolism the cytochrome P450 pathway (Smith et al., 2001), the same route used by simvastatin, lovastatin and atorvastatin, then the first two are proscribed to patients under antiretroviral therapy and the latter can be used with caution.

Fibrates are used as second choice in the treatment of hypercholesterolemia. In patients with normal TG and elevated LDL-C levels, a slight decrease in LDL-C ranging from 5 to 20% in the studies carried out. Therefore, the therapeutic fibrates use should be reserved for treatment of hypertriglyceridemia (TG> 500 mg/dL) in these patients (Dube et al., 2003).

4.2 Hypertriglyceridemia

4.2.1 Non-pharmacologic therapy

The non-pharmacologic therapy should be first applied to all patients with hypertriglyceridemia, through modification of lifestyle; diet should be instituted to reduce fat intake, weight reduction, reduction or elimination of alcohol intake, smoking cessation control of hyperglycemia and diabetes with insulin sensitizers such as metformin. In studies, it has been found that diets associated with exercise and resistance training promotes decrease of 21% and 27%, respectively, TG levels in HIV-infected patients (Henry et al., 1998; Yarashesky et al., 2001).

Patients who demonstrate extreme elevations in TG level (> 1000 mg / dL) and with a history of pancreatitis should be treated associating pharmacologic and non-pharmacologic therapy (Dube et al., 2003).

4.2.2 Pharmacologic therapy

Drug therapy should be instituted in all patients with TG levels greater than 500 mg/dL with the introduction of Gemfibrozil with starting dose of 600 mg half an hour before meals (lunch and dinner) or fibrates at a dose 54 to 160 mg/day (Dube et al., 2003). In a study carried out in patients with TG levels higher than 400 mg/dL using fibrate dose of 200 mg/day was observed 14% and 54% decrease of TC and TG levels, respectively (Palácios et al., 2002). Therefore, in another study, patients with TG levels higher than 266 mg/dL, using Gemfibrozil 600 mg/day associated with diet, evolved with a reduction of TG values in 18% (Miller et al., 2002).

The use of statins in general is not recommended for the treatment of hypertriglyceridemia (TG> 500 mg / dL) alone, is recommended when triglyceride levels are between 200 to 500 mg/dL associated with increased total cholesterol (Dubé et al., 2003).

5. Experience of the assistance service of metabolic diseases secondary to antiretroviral therapy for patients with dyslipidemia

Assistance Service of Metabolic Diseases Secondary to Antiretroviral Therapy (HAART) of the João de Barros Barreto University Hospital (HUJBB), Brazilian national reference in transmissible infectious diseases and AIDS, actually, assist about 99 HIV carriers' patients with lipodystrophy syndrome. Into this service, the authors develop a Project titled Lipodystrophy and Antiretroviral Therapy, financed by The State of Pará Research Foundation (FAPESPA), Research Program for the Unified Health System (PPSUS). One of the Project's purposes was the implantation of the lipodystrophy ambulatory care.

The HUJBB lipodystrophy ambulatory care works with team composed by an endocrinologist, a nutrition doctoral student, two medicine M.Sc students, four medical undergraduate students. The medical accompaniment is performed once a week. In the first service is diagnosed the clinical form of lipodystrophy and requested the proper tests (total cholesterol, HDL, LDL, triglycerides, fasting glucose test, oral glucose tolerance, insulin, abdominal ultrasonography to hepatic steatosis diagnostic and computed tomography for evaluation of visceral lipohypertrophy and electrocardiogram). The first patient's return is around 45 days and subsequently every three months for medical accompaniment. Each medical consultation is also performed medical history, measurement of blood pressure, heart auscultation, anthropometric evaluation (measurements of weight, height, skin folds) and bioimpedance. In addition, if need be the patient is referred to other professionals of the multidisciplinary team HUJBB.

Of the accompanied patients with lipodystrophy syndrome in this ambulatory care, 77% (n = 77) have dyslipidemia and presents the following profile: 67.9% were male, mean age of 44.5 years, average time of HIV infection of 8, 3 years, average time of use of antiretroviral therapy for 6.9 years and body mass index of 24.5 kg/m[2]. Regarding risk factors, it is observed that 18.2% are smokers, 40.3% alcoholics, 71.4% sedentary and 45.5% had hepatic steatosis. Regarding the classification of nutritional status (WHO, 1995) 58.4% are eutrophic, thin 6.5% and 35.1% overweight/obesity. Among the co morbidities studied, it appears that 24.7% and 21.1% are hypertensive and diabetics, respectively. When stratifying the lipodystrophy syndrome, according to the clinical manifestations, 35.1%, 10.4% and 54.5% of patients had lipoatrophy, hypertrophy and mixed syndrome, respectively. Concerning average serum lipid levels, there is high levels blood of cholesterol and triglycerides, low HDL-C, and LDL-C within the normal range. In regard to dyslipidemia classification (Sposito et al., 2007), have been observed that 48.7% of patients have mixed hyperlipidemia, 32.9% hypertriglyceridemia, low HDL-C 10.5% and 7.9% isolated hypercholesterolemia (Table 1 and 2). In the assessment of cardiovascular risk by Framingham Risk Score was found that more than 30% of the sample had medium and high cardiovascular risk.

Variables	Total Sample	n	%
Male		52	67.5
Female		25	32.5
Smoking	77	14	18.2
Alcoholism	77	31	40.3
Sedentary	77	55	71.4
Diabetes mellitus	77	17	21.1
SH *	77	19	24.7
Family history			
Diabetes	77	37	48.1
Hypertension	77	55	71.4
Dyslipidemia	72	28	38.9
Hepatic steatosis	66	30	45.5
Nutritional status**	76		
Thinness**		05	6.6
Eutrophic		44	57.9
Overweight/Obesity		27	35.5
Lipodystrophy	77		
Lipoatrophy		27	35.1
Hypertrophy		8	10.4
Mixed		42	54.5
Classification of dyslipidemia***	76		
Mixed Hyperlipidemia		37	48.7
Hypertriglyceridemia		25	32.9
Low HDL		8	10.5
Isolated hypercholesterolemia		6	7.9

Legend: SH - systemic hypertension; ** WHO, 1995; *** Sposito et al., 2007

Table 1. Patients profile with lipodystrophy and dyslipidemia accompanied by the Assistance Service of Metabolic Diseases Secondary to Antiretroviral Therapy, João de Barros Barreto University Hospital, Pará, Brazil.

Variable	Total Sample	Mean ± SD	Median
Age (years)	77	44.5 ± 9.6	45.0
ART Time (years)	77	6.9 ± 4.1	7.0
Time of HIV (years)	77	8.3 ± 5.4	8.0
BMI (kg/m²)	76	24.5 ± 4.2	23.9
Fasting glucose (mg/dL)	72	103.4 ± 27.7	98.5
Total Cholesterol (mg/dL)	76	218.9 ± 59.7	220.0
Triglycerides (mg/dL)	76	373.3± 393.8	280.5
HDL-c (mg/dL)	60	40.8 ± 13.34	39
Male HDL-c	36	37.4 ± 11.7	37.0
Female HDL-c	24	46.0 ±14.2	46.5
LDL-c (mg/dL)	58	115.6 ± 45.4	117.9

Legend: ART – Antiretroviral Therapy, BMI – body mass index, SD standard deviation.

Table 2. Distribution of mean and median values of some variables in patients with lipodystrophy and dyslipidemia accompanied by the Assistance Service of Metabolic Diseases Secondary to Antiretroviral Therapy, João de Barros Barreto University Hospital, Pará, Brazil.

The ambulatory care authors conducted an intervention study with outpatient HIV-positive with lipodystrophy syndrome, in use of HAART in the period October 2006 to December 2007. Patients were evaluated every quarter for four visits. This study followed all the guidelines contained in Resolution 196/1996 of the National Committee for Ethics in Research (CONEP), being approved by the Ethics in Human Research of the Center for Tropical Medicine, Federal University of Para, according to opinion of approval No. 058/2006, to date of October 19, 2006. The sample consisted of patients with positive serology for HIV, use of HAART for at least 12 months, with clinical diagnosis of lipodystrophy. We selected only adult patients, aged 20 to 60 years, of both sexes. All were invited and agreed to participate by reading and signing the Free and Informed Consent Term - FICT.

We excluded all patients with mental illness, malignant tumors, and chronic users of glucocorticoids, Diabetes Mellitus and dyslipidemia diagnosed before starting HAART and those who did not achieve at least three follow-up visits clinical and nutritional care at the Ambulatory care of Lipodystrophy HUJBB.

To collect data we used a treatment protocol for metabolic evaluation, nutritional counseling and patient outcomes, among several details registered there were: patient identification, socio-economic, personal and family morbidity history, time of HIV diagnosis, time of HAART treatment, clinical history and biochemical tests. Among the lipodystrophy syndrome metabolic changes were required tests to total serum cholesterol, LDL-C, HDL-C and triglycerides for dyslipidemia analysis (Sposito et al., 2007).

We studied 29 patients, 17 (59%) and 12 (41%), male and females, respectively, with an average age of 46.07 (± 9.04) years. In males, the average age was 47.59 (+ 7.66) years, median 46 years, whereas in females the mean age was 43.92 (± 10.67) years, median 44. The most prevalent age group for both sexes was 41 to 50 years.

In regarding to lipodystrophy syndrome classification, was observed that 11 (37.91%), 2 (6,9%) and 16 (55,17%) patients demonstrated lipoatrophy, lipohypertrophy and mixed syndrome, respectively. There is no sex association with lipoatrophy and mixed syndrome (p= 0.4138, OR= 0.3750, IC 95%= 0.0744 - 1.8891), whilst lipohypertrophy syndrome had predominance in females. It is assumed when calculating Odds Ratio to lipohypertrophy presence, was noted that female chance present lipohypertrophy is 2.66 times more, However, the results have not been significant (p=0.4130, IC 95% 0.5294 a 13.4334), data shown in Figure 2.

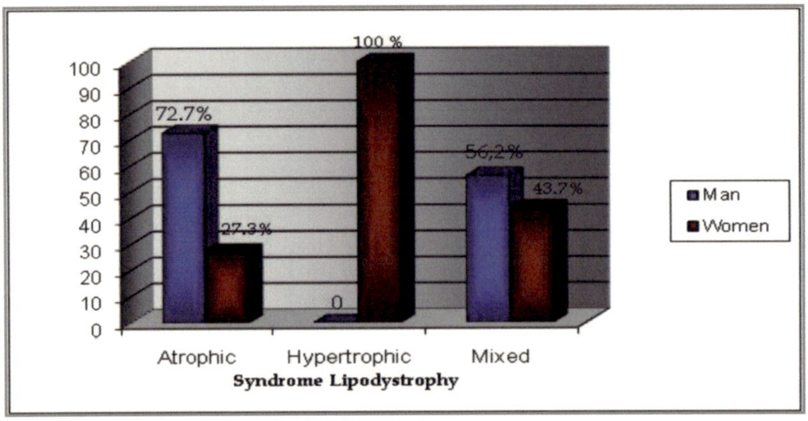

Fig. 2. Distribution of the lipodystrophy syndrome in relation to sex, Pará, Brazil 2006-2008.

The HAART temporal analysis showed that there was a growing evolution of lipoatrophy and lipohypertrophy presence in association with prolonged use of HAART ($p = 0.0485$, $p = 0.0393$, respectively).

Among the 29 patients, 6 were taking hypolipidemic. The lipid profile found in patient's evaluation, including those who had made use hypolipidemic therapy, was no statistically significant changes on the total cholesterol and LDL-C, however, for the HDL-C and triglycerides had significant differences between the first and last clinical follow-up nutritional (Figure 3).

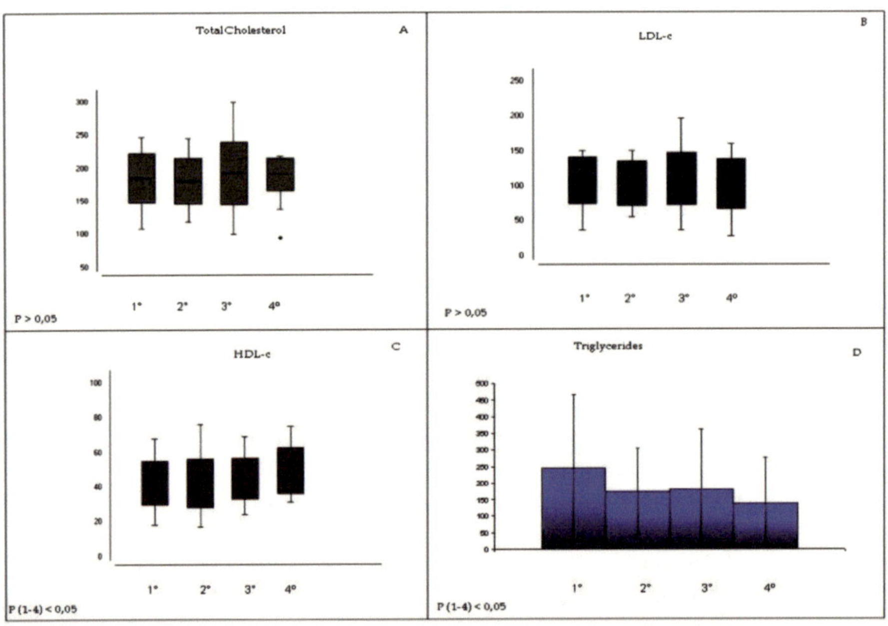

Legend: (A) Total cholesterol, (B) LDL-C, (C) and HDL-C (D) triglycerides, distributed by quarters. Dependent t-test for paired samples.

Fig. 3. HIV patients Serum lipids who did not use hypolipidemic, distributed by quarters, 2006-2008 Para-Brazil.

When analyzing only the sample of patients who were taking hypolipidemic (n = 7), there was no statistically significant changes in the levels of serum total cholesterol, LDL-C and triglycerides (Table 3).

Biochemical Tests	1°	2°	3°	4°	p value*
Cholesterol Total	207.7 (±40.2)	264.0 (±128.2)	216.7 (± 69.2)	219.3 (±60.9)	0.6626
LDL cholesterol	91.7 (±45.6)	136.6 (±56.3)	108.8 (±29.6)	89.7 (±46.04)	0.2539
Triglycerides	597.0 (±300.1)	996.0 (±1300.0)	488.3 (±637.6)	415.0 (±209.3)	0.0503

* Legend: *Friedman* test.

Table 3. Comparison of mean only of lipid profile of patients who were taking hypolipidemic therapy for the clinical follow-up of four nutritional consultations, Pará, Brazil 2006-2008.

In assessing relation between lipids and lipodystrophy syndrome, there was no significant association, as sample data in Table 4.

Lipodystrophy Syndrome				
	Lipoatrophy N (%)	Lipohypertrophy N (%)	Mixed N (%)	p value
Total Cholesterol				
Normal levels	3 (27.27)	0 (0.00)	7 (43.75)	0.3840
Abnormal levels	8 (72.73)	2 (100.00)	9 (56.25)	
LDL cholesterol				
Normal levels	9 (81.82)	1 (50.00)	14 (87.50)	0.4141
Abnormal levels	2 (18.18)	1 (50.00)	2 (12.50)	
HDL cholesterol				
Normal levels	1 (9.09)	0 (0.00)	5 (31.25)	0.2849
Abnormal levels	10 (90.91)	2 (100.00)	11 (68.75)	
Triglycerides				
Normal levels	3 (27.27)	1 (50.00)	5 (31.25)	0.3023
Abnormal levels	8 (72.73)	1 (50.00)	11 (68.75)	

Legend: N - number of patients. Test: Partitioning Chi-square.

Table 4. Association between lipid profile and lipodystrophy syndrome, Pará, Brazil 2006-2008.

In assessing comparison of mean of lipid profile of all patients before and after the clinical and nutritional intervention (first and fourth visit), there was a significant difference between the levels of total cholesterol, LDL-C, HDL-C and triglycerides between the lipoatrophy and mixed syndrome ($p > 0.05$) (Table 5). No analysis was performed on the lipohypertrophy syndrome due to be there of only two patients.

	Before			After		
	Lipoatrophy	Mixed	p-value	Lipoatrophy	Mixed	p-value
Total cholesterol	196.91 (±35.05)	183.00 (±41.84)	0.3744	198.14 (± 39.26)	185.58 (±45.97)	0.5538
LDL cholesterol	112.42 (±40.61)	94.54 (±34.67)	0.2308	110.37 (±50.44)	86.33 (±32.10)	0.2313
HDL cholesterol	37.91 (±11.65)	40.28 (±15.92)	0.6809	42.14 (±9.25)	44.92 (±14.64)	0.4504
Triglycerides	299.36 (±27.77)	310.75 (±259.21)	0.9133	220.86 (±193.46)	218.90 (±179.92)	0.9829

Table 5. Comparison of mean of lipid profile of all patients, including who were taking hypolipidemic therapy before and after the intervention in lipodystrophy syndrome, Pará, Brazil 2006-2008.

The manifestation of lipodystrophy syndrome with regard to gender did not present significant differences for lipoatrophy or mixed syndrome. However, the syndrome was related to female lipohypertrophy corroborating other studies (Galli et al., 2002; Heath et al., 2002) and disagreeing with most published data has been shown increased risk of lipoatrophy syndrome among women. Tien et al. (2003) in prospective study of lipodystrophy syndrome risk among HIV-infected women and non-infected observed a risk 2,1 times more of develop lipoatrophy in infected women with virus than non-infected, whereas it did not differ lipohypertrophy syndrome between the two groups and the most prevalent de form lipodystrophy was mixed syndrome (81%). Van Griensven et al. (2007) evaluated the lipodystrophy syndrome prevalence among patients using stavudine in antiretroviral therapy and found lipoatrophy syndrome prevalence in 9.8% of patients on stavudine and 4.9% with lipohypertrophy syndrome. The HAART temporal analysis showed that there was a growing evolution of the appearance of lipoatrophy and lipohypertrophy associated with HAART prolonged use, as demonstrated by studies of Lichtenstein et al. (2005) and Goujard et al. (2003).

As regards the evaluation of metabolic changes associated with use of HAART coupled with the treatment of nutritional guidance, it must be pointed out that some factors may have affected the outcome of this work as the low adherence to medical treatment, nutrition, failure to follow the previous recommendations for achieving of biochemical tests and the small sample size of patients available for this study. This difficulty in adhering to medical treatment and/or diet therapy was also found by other authors (Quintaes & Garcia, 1999; Ceccato et al. 2004; Parenti et al., 2005; Barros et al. 2007; Chencinski & Garcia, 2006). The reluctance of patients to nutritional treatment may be related to low purchasing power (Barros et al., 2007), cultural and dietary habits proper to the Amazon region, who abuse food that are rich in lipids. In addition to psychosocial factors of patients, where the prejudice, social isolation and emotional disorders such as anxiety and depression

commonly observed in patients infected with HIV make it difficult to change lifestyle (personal and food) as suggested by Quintaes & Garcia (1999) Chencinski & Garcia (2006).
There was also that patients profile evaluated before intervention reflected increase in serum total cholesterol and triglycerides, and lowering HDL-C as described in the literature (Caar et al. 1998; Hadigan et al. 2006; Having Hofstede et al., 2003; Abreu et al., 2006), disagreeing with main studies analyzed only about LDL-C, where most patients remained within normal range. Lipid disorders and association with lipodystrophy syndrome were common in all patients, especially in mixed syndrome, according to studies by Thiebaut et al. (2000) and Haugaard et al. (2005).
The lipid abnormalities evolution in patients after clinical and nutritional intervention during study noted significant changes of lowering triglycerides and increase in HDL-C, regardless of hypolipidemic use. The increased levels of HDL-C have been associated with decreased cardiovascular risk, as has been discussed in the work of Manninen et al. (1988). Where was reported that for every 1% increase in HDL-C was 3% reduction in coronary events and Pedersen et al. (1998) who said that for each 1% increase in HDL-C there was 1% reduction in coronary events, both independently of changes in LDL-C levels.
The lipid profile of patients before and after nutritional intervention clinically observed that patients who had shown serum levels of triglycerides, total cholesterol and fractions (LDL-C and HDL-C) normal at first, had increasing them at the end of treatment. These patients had borderline values facilitating risk of increased total cholesterol, LDL-C and triglycerides and decreased HDL-C associated with nutrition acceptance less than 75%. Other patients in the first consultation showed values above the reference levels for total cholesterol, LDL-C and triglycerides as well as lowering HDL-C, reaching normal values due to good acceptance to nutritional care. The remaining patients showed levels of total cholesterol, LDL-C fractions, HDL-C and triglycerides changed during the research; probably was not able to perceive the importance of nutritional treatment. There were also cases of patients who had their lipid profile within the normal range, suggesting that not only the use of HAART interfered with these metabolic changes, but also other factors may be implicated as genetic predisposition.
In regarding to lipodystrophy syndrome, the cholesterol and LDL-C means demonstrated it more significant in lipoatrophy than mixed syndrome compared before and after intervention. Triglyceride levels showed independent growing in despite to lipodystrophy syndrome, while HDL-C showed changed levels in mixed syndrome.
The physiopathology by which HAART determines HIV lipodystrophy syndrome, dyslipidemia therefore remains unknown. Second Andrade & Hutz (2002), the lipid serum levels are multifactorial characteristics, determinate by genetic and environmental factors, highlighting the genetic variability found in those genes that can affect the response to drugs used in hyperlipidemia treatment.
The authors of the lipodystrophy ambulatory care are developing a research paper about a case-control study conducted from December 2009 to July 2012. For data collection is being performed a clinical, epidemiological and nutritional evaluation where are registered information about patient identification, socio-economic conditions, personal and family history of morbidity, time of HIV diagnosis, HAART treatment duration, medication used - HAART, viral load, CD4 counts, clinical history, biochemical tests for dyslipidemia classification, anthropometric analysis and, APOAI and APOAV apolipoprotein polymorphism evaluation. This study aims to investigate these polymorphisms in an attempt to discover the main causes responsible for this metabolic disorder, the dyslipidemia.

6. Conclusion

The HAART has as one of its major collateral effect the lipodystrophy syndrome. There is necessity of more studies to deep into physiopathology of this syndrome; and metabolic and cardiovascular complications secondary to HAART. Dyslipidemia stands out as one of the most prevalent metabolic changes in patients with HIV, what makes it essential to feasibility of research in therapeutic care to clarifying of the clinical management. It is noted that nutritional guideline and/or hypolipidemic use, when have there been acceptance to treatment, takes place improvements of the lipid profile, can also there be normalization of those levels, in particular of the triglyceride levels. However, the adherence neither always takes place, what difficult the management of those patients.

7. References

Abreu, L., Escosteguy, C., Sodré, C., Godomiczer, A., Passoni, L., & Menezes, J. (2006). Tratamento anti-retroviral e hipercolesterolemia em população HIV positiva. *Revista da Sociedade de Cardiologia do Estado do Rio de Janeiro*, Vol. 19, No. 3, (Mai-Jun 2006), pp. (219-24), ISSN 2177-6024.

Almeida, L., Giudici, K., & Jaime, P. (2009). Consumo alimentar e dislipidemia decorrente da terapia antirretroviral combinada para infecção pelo HIV: uma revisão sistemática. *Arquivos Brasileiros de Endocrinologia & Metabologia*, Vol. 53, No. 5, (Jul 2009), pp. (519-527), ISSN 0004-2730.

American Heart Association. (2002). Third Report of the National Cholesterol Education Program (NCEP) Expert Panel on Detection, Evaluation, and Treatment of High Blood Cholesterol in Adults (Adult Treatment Panel III) Final Report. *Circulation*, Vol. 106, No. 25, (Dec 2002), pp. (3143-3421), ISSN 0009-7322.

Andrade, F., & Hutz, M. (2002). O componente genético da determinação dos lipídeos séricos. *Ciência & Saúde Coletiva*, Vol. 7, No. 1, (2002), pp. (175-182), ISSN 1413-8123.

Aouizerat, B., Kulkarni, M., Heilbron, D., Drown, D., Raskin, S., Pullinger, C., Malloy, M., & Kane, J. (2003). Genetic analysis of a polymorphism in the human apoA-V gene: effect on plasma lipids. *Journal of Lipid Research*, Vol. 44, No. 6, (Jun 2003), pp. (1167-1173), ISSN 1539-7262.

Assmann, G., Schmitz, G., Funke, H., & von Eckardstein, A. (1990) Apolipoprotein A-I and HDL deficiency. *Current Opinion in Lipidology*, Vol. 1, No. 1, (1990), pp. (110-115), ISSN: 0957-9672.

Baldini F, Di Giambenedetto S, Cingolani A, Murri R, Ammassari A, De Luca A (2000). Efficacy and tolerability of pravastatin for the treatment of HIV-1 protease inhibitor-associated hyperlipidaemia: a pilot study. *AIDS*, Vol. 14, No 11, (Jul 2000), pp. (1660-1662), ISSN: 0269-937.

Barros, E., Araujo, A., Freitas, M., & Liberato, E. (2007). Influencia da alimentação na lipodistrofia em portadores de HIV-Aids praticantes de atividade física regular. *Revista Brasileira de Prescrição e Fisiologia do Exercício*, Vol. 1, No. 2, (Mar-Abr 2007), pp. (13-18), ISSN 1981-9900.

Boccara, F., Auclair, M., Cohen, A., Lefèvre, C., Prot, M., Bastard, J.P., Capeau, J., & Caron-Debarle, M. (2010). HIV protease inhibitors activate the adipocyte renin angiotensin system. *Antiviral Therapy*, Vol. 15, No. 3, (2010), pp. (363-375).

Blanco Vaca, F., Ordóñez Llanos, J., Pérez Pérez, a., Sánchez Quesada, j. L., & Wägner Fahlin A. (2000). Lípidos, lipoproteínas y apolipoproteínas. Nuevas indicaciones en el diagnóstico, evaluación y prevención del riesgo cardiovascular. Roche Diagnóstica. S. L. In: Diaz, J. I.S. (2007). Guia practica. Marcadores Bioquimicos Cardiacos. Prologo, indice y presentacion. Acesso em 20 jun 2011. Disponível em: http://www.portalesmedicos.com/publicaciones/articles/828/2/Marcadores-cardiacos.-Factores-de-riesgo-cardiaco-en-la-aterosclerosis.-Recopilacion-de-datos-de-revisiones-bibliograficas-y-conclusiones

Caar, A., Sâmaras, K., Burton, S., Law, M., Freund, J., Chisholm, D., & Cooper, D. (1998). A syndrome of peripheral lipodystrophy, hyperlipidaemia and insulin resistance in patients receiving HIV protease inhibitors. *AIDS*, Vol. 12, No. 7, (Mai 1998), pp.51-58, ISSN: 0269-937.

Cahn, P., Leite, O., Rosales, A., Cabello, R., Alvarez, C., Seas, C., Carcamo, C., Cure-Bolt, N., L'Italien, G., Masntilla, P., Deibis, L., Zala, C., & Suffert, T. (2010). Metabolic profile and cardiovascular risk factors among Latin American HIV-infected patients receiving HAART . *Brazilian Journal of Infectious Diseases*, Vol. 14, No. 2, (Mar-Abr 2010), pp. (158-166), ISSN 1413-8670.

Carr, A., & Cooper, D. (2000). Adverse effects of antiretroviral therapy. *The Lancet*, Vol.356, No. 9232, (Oct 2000), pp. (1423-1430), INSS 0140-6736.

Ceccato, M., Acurcio, F., Bonolo, P., Rocha, G., & Guimarães, M. (2004). Compreensão de informações relativas ao tratamento anti-retroviral entre indivíduos infectados pelo HIV. *Caderno de Saúde Pública*, Vol. 20, No. 5, (Set-Out 2004), pp. (1388-1397), ISSN 0102-311X.

Chen, D., Misra, A., & Garg, A. (2002). Lipodystrophy in Human Immunodeficiency Virus-Infected Patients. *The Journal of Clinical Endocrinology & Metabolism*, Vol. 87, No. 11, (Nov 2002), pp. (4845-4856).

Chencinski, J., & Garcia, V. (Abr-Jun 2006). Dislipidemia em pacientes HIV/AIDS. In: Conselho Regional de Nutrição-3 Notícias. n.82, Acesso em 10 Mar 2008. Disponível em: <http://www.crn3.org.br/atualidades/revistas/arquivos/edicao_082_atualidades.pdf>.

Coté, H. (2007). Mechanisms of antiretroviral therapy-induced mitochondrial dysfunction. *Current Opinion in HIV and AIDS*, Vol. 2, No. 4, (Jul 2007), pp. (253-260), ISSN 1746-630X.

Diehl, L., Dias, J., Paes, A., Thomazini, M., Garcia, L., Cinagawa, E., Wiechmann, S., & Carrilho, A. (2008). Prevalência da Lipodistrofia Associada ao HIV em Pacientes Ambulatoriais Brasileiros: Relação com Síndrome Metabólica e Fatores de Risco Cardiovascular. *Arquivos Brasileiros de Endocrinologia e Metabologia*, Vol. 52, No. 4, (Jun 2008), pp. (658-667), ISSN 0004-2730.

Dubé, M., Stein, J., Aberg, J., Fichtenbaum, C., Gerber, J., Tashima, K., Henry, W., Currier, J., Sprecher, D., & Glesby, M. (2003). Guidelines for the evaluation and management of dyslipidemia in human immunodeficiency virus (HIV)-infected adults receiving antiretroviral therapy: Recommendations of the HIV Medicine Association of the Infectious Disease Society of America and the Adult AIDS Clinical Trials Group. *Clinical Infectious Diseases*, Vol. 37, No. 5, (Sep 2003), pp. (613-627), ISSN 378131.

Dutra, C. & Libonati, R. (2008). Perfil metabólico e nutricional de pacientes HIV positivos com lipodistrofia submetidos à terapia anti-retroviral: Orientação Nutricional. Dissertação de mestrado. Universidade Federal do Pará. Belém-Brazil. (Abr 2008), 151pp.

Eichenbaum-Voline S., Olivier, M., Jones, E., Naoumova, R., Jones, B., Gau, B., Patel, H., Seed, M., Betteridge, D., Galton, D., Rubin, E., Scott, J., Shoulders, C., & Pennacchio, L. (2004). Linkage and association between distinct variants of the APOAI/C3/A4/A5 gene cluster and familial combined hyperlipidemia. *Arteriosclerosis, Thrombosis and Vascular Biology*, Vol. 24, No. 1, (Jan 2004), pp. (167-174), ISSN 10795642.

Friis-M øller, N., Reiss, P., Sabin, C. A., Weber, R., Monforte, A., El-Sadr, W.,Thiebaut, R.,

De Wit, S., Kirk, O., Fontas, E., Law, M. G., Phillips, A., & Lundgren, J. D. (Mai 2003). Cardiovascular disease risk factors in HIV patients - association with antiretroviral therapy. In: *Official Journal of International AIDS Society*, Acesso em 06 Jun 2011, Disponível em: <http://discovery.ucl.ac.uk/6830/1/6830.pdf>

Friis-Møller, N; Weber, R., Reiss, P; Thiébaut, R., Kirk, O., Monforte, A., Pradier, C., Morfeldt, L., Mateu, S., Law, M., El-Sadr, W., De Wit, S., Sabin, C., Phillips, A., Lundgren, J. (2003). Cardiovascular disease risk factors in HIV patients - association with antiretroviral therapy. Results from the DAD study. *AIDS*, Vol 17, No 8,(May 2003), pp. (1179-1193), ISSN: 0269-937.

Furtado, J., Zambrini, H., Neto, D., Scozzafave, G., & Brasileiro, R. (2007). Ambulatório de Lipodistrofia do Hospital Heliópolis - Uma experiência com as correções cirúrgicas em dois anos de atendimento. *Prática hospitalar*, Vol. 58, No. 28, (Set-Out IX), pp. (28-32), ISSN 1679-5512.

Galli, M., Cozzi-Lepri, A., Ridolfo, A., Gervasoni, C., Ravasio, L., Corsico, L., Gianelli, E., Vaccarezza, M., Vullo, V., Cargnel, A., Minoli, L., Coronado, O., Giacometti, A., Antinori, A., Antonucci, G., D'Arminio Monforte, A., & Moroni, M. (2002). Incidence of adipose tissue alterations in first-line antiretroviral therapy: the LipolCoNa Study. *Archives of Internal Medicine*, Vol. 22, No. 162, (Dez 2002), pp. (2621-2628), ISSN 00039926.

Garg, A. (2000). Lipodystrophies. *The American Journal of Medicine*, Vol. 108, No. 2, (Feb 2000), pp. (143-152), ISSN: 0002-9343.

Gidding, S. S. Preventive pediatric cardiology(1999). *The Pediatric Clinics North America*. Vol. 46, No 2 (abr. 1999), pp. (253-262), ISSN:0031-3955.

Gkrania-Klotsas, E., & Klotsas, A. (2007). HIV and HIV treatment: effects on fats, glucose and lipids. *British Medical Bulletin*, Vol. 84, No. 1, (Nov 2007), pp. (49-68), ISSN 0007-1420.

Goujard, C., Vincent, I., Meynard, J., Choudet, N., Bollens, D., Rousseau, C., Demarles, D., Gillotin, C., Bidault, R., & Taburet, A. (2003). Steady-state pharmacokinetics of amprenavir coadministered with ritonavir in human immunodeficiency virus type 1-infected patients. *Antimicrobial agents and chemotherapy*, Vol. 47, No. 1, (Jan 2003), pp. (118-123), ISSN 0066-4804.

Grinspoon, S., & Carr, A. (2005) Cardiovascular Risk and Body-Fat Abnormalities in HIV-Infected Adults. *New England Journal of Medicine*, Vol. 352, No. 1, (Jan 2005), pp. (48-62), ISSN 0028-4793.

Grunfeld, C., Pang, M., Doerrler, W., Shigenaga, J., Jensen, P., & Feingold, K. (1992). Lipids, lipoproteins, triglyceride clearance, and cytokines in human immunodeficiency virus infection and the acquired immunodeficiency syndrome. *Journal of Clinical Endocrinology & Metabolism*, Vol. 74, No. 5, (May 1992), pp. (1045-1052), ISSN 0021-972X.

Hadigan, C., Kamin, D., Liebau, J., Mazza, S., Barrow, S., Torriani, M., Rubin, R., Weise, S., Fischman, A., & Grinspoon, S. (2006). Depot-specific regulation of glucose uptake and insulin sensitivy in HIV-lipodystrophy. *American Journal of Physiology, Endocrinology & Metabolism*, Vol. 2, No. 290, (Feb 2006), pp. 289-298, ISSN 0193-1849.

Haugaard, S., Andersen, O., Dela, F., Holst, J., Storgaard, H., Fenger, M., Iversen, J., & Madsbad, S. (2005). Defective glucose and lipid metabolism in human immunodeficiency virus-infected patients with lipodystrophy involve liver, muscle tissue and pancreatic beta-cells. *European Journal of Endocrinology*, Vol. 152, No. 1, (Jan 2005), pp. (103-112), ISSN 0804-4643.

Heath, K., Chan, K., Singer, J., O'shaughnessy, M., Montaner, J., & Hoogg, R. (2002). Incidence of morphological and lipid abnormalities: gender and treatment differentials after initiation of first antiretroviral therapy. *International Journal of Epidemiology*, Vol. 31, No. 5, (Oct 2002), pp.1016-1020, ISSN *0300-5771*.

Henry K, Melroe H, Huebesch J, Hermundson J, Simpson J. Atorvastatin and gemfibrozil for protease-inhibitor–related lipid abnormalities (1998). *Lancet.* Vol. 352, No 9133(Sep. 1998), pp. (1031–1032), ISSN 0140-6736.

Jones SP, Doran DA, Leatt PB, Maher B, Pirmohamed M (2001). Short-term exercise training improves body composition and hyperlipidaemia in HIV-positive individuals with lipodystrophy . *AIDS* . Vol. 15, No 15, pp. (2049–2051), , ISSN: 0269-937.

Kotler D. (2008). HIV and Antiretroviral Therapy: Lipid Abnormalities and Associated Cardiovascular Risk in HIV-Infected Patients. *Journal of Acquires Immune Deficiency Syndromes*, Vol. 53, No. 3, (Sep 2008), pp. (79-85), ISSN *1525-4135*.

Kramer, A., Lazzarotto, A., Sprinz, E., & Manfroi, W. (2009). Alterações metabólicas, terapia antirretroviral e doença cardiovascular em idosos portadores de HIV. *Arquivos Brasileiros de Cardiologia*, Vol. 93, No. 5, (Nov 2009), pp. (561-568), ISSN 0066-782X.

Liang, J., Distler, O., Cooper, D., Jamil, H., Deckelbaum, R., Ginsberg, H., & Sturley, S. (2001). HIV protease inhibitors protect apolipoprotein B from degradation by the proteasome: a potential mechanism for protease inhibitor-induced hyperlipidemia. *Nature Medicine,* Vol.7, No. 12, (Dec 2001), pp. (1327-1331), ISSN 1078-8956.

Licht, C., Vreeburg, S., van Reedt Dortland, A., Giltay, E., Hoogendijk, W., DeRijk, R., Vogelzangs, N., Zitman, F., de Geus, E., & Penninx, B. (2010) Increased sympathetic and decreased parasympathetic activity rather than changes in hypothalamic-pituitary-adrenal axis activity is associated with metabolic abnormalities *Journal of Clinical Endocrinology & Metabolism*, Vol. 95, No. 5, (May 2010), pp. (2458-2466), ISSN 0021-972X.

Lichtenstein, K. (2005) Redefining Lipodistrophy Syndrome: Risks and Impact on Clinical Decision Making. *Journal of Acquired Immune Deficiency Syndromes*, Vol. 39, No. 4, (Aug 2005), pp. (395-400), ISSN *1525-4135*.

Lihn, A., Richelsen, B., Pedersen, S., Haugaard, S., Rathje, G., Madsbad, S., & Andersen, O. (2003) Increased expression of TNF-α, IL-6, and IL-8 in HALS: implications for reduced adiponectin expression and plasma levels. *American Journal of Physiology Endocrinology & Metabology*, Vol. 285, No. 5, (Nov 2003), pp. (1072-1080), ISSN 0193-1849.

Maagaard, A., & Kvale, D. (2009). Mitochondrial toxicity in HIV-infected patients both off and on antiretroviral treatment: a continuum or distinct underlying mechanisms? *Journal of Antimicrobial Chemistry*, Vol. 64, No. 5, (Sep 2009), pp. (901-909), ISSN 0929-8673.

Mallewa, J., Wilkins, E., Vilar, J., Mallewa, M., Doran, D., Back, D., & Pirmohamed, M. (2008) HIV-associated lipodystrophy: a review of underlying mechanisms and therapeutic options. *The Journal of Antimicrobial Chemotherapy,* Vol. 62, No. 4, (Oct 2008), pp. (648-660), ISSN *0305-7453.*

Mallon, P., Miller, J., Cooper, D., & Carr, A. (2003). Prospective evaluation of the effects of antiretroviral therapy on body composition in HIV-1-infected men starting therapy. *AIDS,* Vol. 17, No. 7, (May 2003), pp. (971–979), ISSN 0269-9370.

Manninen, V., Elo, M., Frick, M., Haapa, K., Heinonen, O., Heinsalmi, P., Helo, P., Huttunen, J., Kaitaniemi, P., & Koskinen, P. (1988). Lipid alterations and decline in the incidence of coronary heart disease in the Helsinki Heart Study, *The Journal of the American Medical Association,* Vol. 260, No. 1, (1988), pp. (641-651), ISSN 00987484.

Marshall, H., Morrison, L., Wu, L., Anderson, J., Corneli, P., Stauffer, D., Allen, A., Karagounis, L., & Ward, R. (1994). Apolipoprotein polymorphism fail to define risk of coronary artery disease. Results of a prospective, angiographically controlled study. *Circulation,* Vol. 89, No. 2, (Feb 1994), pp. (567-577), ISSN 0009-7322.

Mello, A., Reis, E., & Ribeiro, R. (2008). Lipodistrofia no uso da Terapia Antiretroviral com Inibidores da Protease no HIV. *Saúde & Ambiente em Revista,* Vol. 3, No. 1, (Jan-jun 2008), pp. (66-75), ISSN 1980-2676.

Miller J, Brown D, Amin J, et al (2002). A randomized, double-blind study of gemfibrozil for the treatment of protease inhibitor–associated hypertriglyceridaemia. *AIDS.* Vol 16, No 16 (Nov. 2002), pp. (2195–2200), ISSN: 0269-937.

Ministério da Saúde do Brasil. (2008). Recomendações para terapia anti-retroviral em adultos infectados pelo HIV: manual de bolso. In: *Série A. Normas e Manuais Técnicos,* Data de acesso: Jun 2011, Disponível em: http://www.crt.saude.sp.gov.br/resources/crt_aids/arquivos_transmissao_vertical/transmissao_vertical_hiv/portarias_manuais_recomendacoes_outros/consenso_adulto_2008.pdf>.

Moyle GJ, Lloyd M, Reynolds B, Baldwin C, Mandalia S, Gazzard BG (2001). Dietary advice with or without pravastatin for the management of hypercholesterolemia associated with protease inhibitor therapy. *AIDS.* Vol. 15, No 12 (Aug 2001), pp. (503–508), , ISSN: 0269-937.

Mooser, V. & Carr, A. (2001). Antiretroviral therapy-associated hyperlipidaemia in HIV disease. *Current Opinion in Lipidology.,* Vol. 12, No. 3, (Jun 2001), pp. 313-319, ISSN 0957-9672.

Mulligan, K. (2003). Metabolic Abnormalities in Patient with HIV Infection. *Journal of the International Association of Physicians in Aids Care (Chicago),* Vol. 2, No. 2, (Apr-Jun 2003), pp. (66-74), ISSN 1545-1097.

Noor, M. (2007). The role of protease inhibitors in the pathogenesis of HIV-associated insulin resistance: cellular mechanisms and clinical implications. *Current HIV/AIDS Reports,* Vol.4, No. 3, (Dec 2007), pp. 126-134, ISSN 1548-3568.

Palacios R, Santos J, Gonzalez M, et AL (2002). Efficacy and safety of atorvastatin in the treatment of hypercholesterolemia associated with antiretroviral therapy. *Journal of Acquired Immune Deficiency Syndromes.* Vol. 30, No 5 (Aug. 2002), pp. (536–537), ISSN 1525-4135.

Parenti, C., Pereira, L., Brandão, Z., & Silvério, A. (2005). Perfil dos pacientes com AIDS acompanhados pelo Serviço de Assistência Domiciliar Terapêutica do Município de Contagem, Estado de Minas Gerais, Brasil, 2000-2003. *Epidemiologia e Serviços de Saúde,* Vol. 14, No. 2, (Jun 2005), pp. (91-96), ISSN 1679- 4974.

Pedersen, T., Olsson, A., Faergeman, O., Kjekshus, J., Wedel, H., Berg, K., Wilhelmsen, L., Haghfelt, T., Thorgeirsson, G., Pyörälä, K., Miettinen, T., Christophersen, B., Tobert, J., Musliner, T., & Cook, T. (1998). Lipoprotein changes and reduction in the incidence of coronary heart disease events in the Scandinavian Simvastatin Survival Study (4S). *Circulation*, Vol. 97, No. (1), (1998), pp. (1453-1461), ISSN 0009-7322.

Quintaes, D., & Garcia, R. (1999). Adesão de pacientes HIV positivos à dietoterapia ambulatorial. *Revista de Nutrição*, Vol. 12, No. 2, (Mai-Ago 1999), pp. (175-181).

Rasmusson, A., Schnurr, P., Zukowska, Z., Scioli, E., & Forman, D. (2010). Adaptation to extreme stress: post-traumatic stress disorder, neuropeptide Y and metabolic syndrome. *Experimental Biology and Medicina (Maywood)*, Vol. 235, No. 10, (Oct 2010), pp. (1150-1162), ISSN 1535-3702.

Riddle, M., Kuhel, D., Woollett, L., Fichtenbaum, C., & Hui, D. (2001). HIV protease inhibitor induces fatty acid and sterol biosynthesis in liver and adipose tissues due to the accumulation of activated sterol regulatory element-binding proteins in the nucleus. *Journal of Biological Chemistry*, Vol. 276, No. 40, (Oct 2001), pp. 37514-37519, ISSN 0021-9258.

Samaras, K., Wand, H., Law, M., Emery, S., Cooper, D., & Carr, A. (2009). Dietary intake in HIV-infected men with lipodystrophy: relationships with body composition, visceral fat, lipid, glucose and adipokine metabolism. *Current HIV Research*, Vol. 7, No. 4, (Jul 2009), pp. (454-461), ISSN 1570-162X.

Santos, C., Felipe, Y., Braga, P., Ramos, D., Lima, R., & Segurado, A. (2005). Self-perception of body changes in persons living with HIV/AIDS: prevalence and associated factors. AIDS, Vol. 4, No. 1, (Oct 2005), pp. (14-21), , ISSN: 0269-937, ISSN: 0269-937.

Sattler, F. (2008). Pathogenesis and Treatment of Lipodystrophy: What Clinicians Need To Know. *Topics in HIV Medicine*, Vol. 16, No. 4, (Oct-Nov 2008), pp. (127-133), ISSN 1542-8826.

Segarra-Newnham, M. (2002). Hyperlipidemia in HIV-positive patients receiving antiretrovirals. *The Annals of Pharmacotherapy*, Vol. 36, No. 4, (Apr 2002), pp. (592-595), ISSN 1060-0280.

Seidl, E., & Machado, A. (2008). Bem-estar psicológico, enfrentamento e lipodistrofia em pessoas vivendo com HIV/aids. *Psicologia em estudo*, Vol. 13, No. 2, (Apr-Jun 2008), pp. (239-247), ISSN 1413-7372.

Shahmanesh, M., Jaleel, H., DeSilva, Y., Ross, J., Caslake, M. & Cramb, R. (Jun 2001) Protease inhibitor related type III hyperlipoproteinaemia is common and not associated with apolipoprotein-E E2/E2 phenotype. In: *Sexually Transmitted Infections*, Acesso em 04 Jun 2011, Disponível em: < http://sti.bmj.com/content/77/4/283.abstract>

Smith P, DiCenzo R, Morse G (2001). Clinical pharmacokinetics of nonnucleosidereverse transcriptase inhibitors. *Clinical Pharmacokinetics*, Vol. 40, No 12, (2001), pp. (893–905), ISSN 0312-5963.

Sposito, A., Caramelli, B., Fonseca, F., & Bertolami, M. (2007). IV Diretriz Brasileira sobre Dislipidemias e Prevenção da Aterosclerose: Departamento de Aterosclerose da Sociedade Brasileira de Cardiologia. *Arquivos Brasileiros de Cardiologia*, Vol. 88, No. 1, (Abr 2007), pp. (2-19), ISSN 1678-4170.

Sprinz, E., Lazzaretti, R., Kuhmmer, R., & Ribeiro, J. (2010). Dyslipidemia in HIV-infected individuals. *Brazilian Journal of Infectious Diseases*, Vol. 14, No. 6, (Nov 2010), pp. (575-588), ISSN 1413-8670.

Stankov, M., & Behrens, G. (2010) Contribution of Inflammation to Fat Redistribution and Metabolic Disturbances in HIV-1 Infected Patients. *Current Pharmaceutical Design*, Vol. 16, No. 30, (Out 2010), pp. (3361-3371), ISSN 1381-6128.

Tall, A. (1990) Plasma high density lipoproteins. Metabolism and relationship to atherogenesis. *The Journal of Clinical Investigation*, Vol. 86, No. 2, (Aug 1990), pp. (379-384), ISSN 00219738.

Ter Hofstede, H., Burger, D., & Koopmans, P. (2003). Antiretroviral therapy in HIV patients: aspects of metabolic complications and mitochondrial toxicity. *The Netherlands Journal of Medicine*, Vol. 61, No. 12, (Dec 2003), pp. (393-403), ISSN 0300-2977.

The HIV/Aids Treatment Information Service (ATIS). (Sep 2002). *Glossary of HIV/AIDS-Related Terms*, The HIV/Aids Treatment Information Service (ATIS), Retirado de <http://www.hiv.gov.gy/edocs/glossary.pdf>.

Thiébaut, R., Daucourt, V., Mercié, P., Ekouévi, D. K., Malvy, D., Morlat, P., Dupon, M., Neau, D., Farbos, S., Marimoutou, C., & Dabis, F. (2000). Lipodystrophy, metabolic disorders, and human immunodeficiency virus infection: Aquitaine cohort, France, 1999. Groupe d'Epidémiologie Clinique du Syndrome d'Immunodéficience Acquise en Aquitaine. *Clinical Infectious Diseases*. Vol. 31, No. 6 (Dec 2000), pp. (1482-7), ISSN 1058-4838.

Tien, P., Cole, S., Williams, C., Li, R., Justman, J., Cohen, M., Young, M., Rubin, N., Augenbraun, M., & Grunfeld, C. (2003). Incidence of lipoatrophy and lipohypertrophy in the women's interagency HIV study. *Journal of Acquired Immune Deficiency Syndromes*, Vol. 34, No. 5, (Dec 2003), pp. (461-466), ISSN 1077-9450.

Tovar, J., & Schering, D. (2006) Management of Dyslipidemia in Special Populations. *Journal of Pharmacy Practice*, Vol. 19, No. 2, (Apr 2006), pp. (63-78), ISSN 0897-1900.

Valente, A., & Valente, O. (2007). Síndrome Lipodistrófica do HIV: Um Novo Desafio para o Endocrinologista. *Arquivos Brasileiros de Endocrinologia e Metabologia*, Vol. 51, No. 1, (Fev 2007), pp. (3-4), ISSN 0004-2730.

Van Griensven, J., De Naeyer, L., Mushi, T., Ubarijoro, S., Gashumba, D., Gazielle, C., & Zachariah, R. (2007). High prevalence of lipoatrophy among patients on stavudine-containing first-line antiretroviral therapy regimens in Rwanda. *Transactions of the Royal Society of Tropical Medicine and Hygiene*, Vol. 101, No. 8, (Ago 2007), pp. (793-798), ISSN 0035-9203.

World Health Organization (CH), United Nations Programme on HIV/Aids - UNAIDS (CH). (2009). Aids epidemic update: November 2009, In: *WHO Library Cataloguing-in-Publication Data*, Date of access: Jun 2011, Available from: <http://data.unaids.org/pub/Report/2009/jc1700_epi_update_2009_en.pdf>.

World Health Organization. (1995). Physical Status: The Use and Interpretation of Antropometry. In: *WHO Technical Report Series 854*, Date of Access: May 2011, Available from: <http://whqlibdoc.who.int/trs/WHO_TRS_854.pdf>.

Yarasheski KE, Tebas P, Stanerson B, et al (2001). Resistance exercise training reduces hypertriglyceridemia in HIV-infected men treated with antiviral therapy. *Journal of Applied Physiology*; Vol. 90, No. 1 (april 2001),. pp. (133–138), ISSN 8750-7587.

Yu, P., Calderaro, D., Lima, E. & Caramelli, B. (2005). Terapia hipolipemiante em situações especiais - Síndrome de Imunodeficiência Adquirida. *Arquivos Brasileiros de Cardiologia*, Vol. 85, No. 5, (Oct 2005), pp. (58-61).

22

Fenofibrate: Panacea for Aging-Related Conditions?

Makoto Goto
Division of Anti-Ageing & Longevity Sciences, Faculty of Medical Technology, Department of BioMedical Engineering, Toin University of Yokohama, Japan

1. Introduction

Fenofibrate, a selective peroxisome proliferator-activated receptors alpha (PPAR-α) activator, has been primarily developed to treat human dyslipidemia. PPAR modulate the expression of genes involved in lipid metabolism through peroxisome proliferator response elements (Willson et al., 2000). Although fenofibrate became commercially available in 1974 (Fournier, Inc., France), its lipid-lowering action mechanism has not been clarified until the late 1990's, contributing to open new research doors. With respect to the mechanisms of action, the drug with pleiotropic activity may be regarded as a "21st-century agent" (Staels et al., 1995).

Fenofibrate as a ligand of PPAR-α exhibits lipid-lowering effects by activating PPAR-α.

PPAR-α activators stimulate the β-oxidation of fatty acids in the liver resulting in a decreased availability of fatty acids for triglyceride (TG) synthesis (Schoonjans et al., 1995, 1996a, 1996b). In addition, fenofibrate enhances the production of apo-AI and apo-AII: the major component of HDL by activating PPAR-α and increases plasma level of HDL-C directly (Vu-Dac, 1994, 1995). Thus, the lipid-lowering action mechanism of fenofibrate involves potent TG-reducing and HDL-C-increasing actions. Statins, another type of lipid-lowering agent do not show such actions, though statins can inhibit hydroxymethylglutaryl (HMG)-CoA reductase (Endo A, 1992).

Furthermore, fenofibrate decreased the level of low-density lipoprotein cholesterol (LDL-C), especially "small dense LDL", which may be a powerful metabolic contributor to arteriosclerosis (Superko, 2000).

PPAR-α regulates the transcription of lipid-associated genes and various genes involved in homeostasis, suggesting the PPAR-α-mediated pleiotropic activities of fenofibrate. The reports on the pleiotropic activities of fenofibrate has been accumulated in a variety of large-scale, randomized, controlled trials (RCTs).

The studies presumably associated with the anti-aging actions of fenofibrate are reviewed in this article.

2. Clinical efficacy

The pleiotropic activities other than the lipid-lowering actions reported in clinical practice: the anti-inflammatory, antioxidant, and serum uric acid-reducing actions of fenofibrate are reviewed in this section. These activities may be tightly associated with anti-aging actions of fenofibrate. Three large-scale, randomized, comparative clinical studies of fenofibrate ("DAIS", "FIELD" and "ACCORD"), in which intervention was performed in patients with type II diabetes mellitus (DM), were published since 2000.

2.1 Anti-aging activities

Previous studies reported the involvement of various clinical parameters in anti-aging actions of fenofibrate (Schlesinger et al., 2009). In particular, chronic, systemic, silent, low-grade inflammation, named inflammaging is the target for intensive research in aging study (Goto, 2008b). Ross et al. defined arteriosclerosis as "chronic vascular inflammation" resulting from an interaction between oxidized lipid and macrophages (Ross, 1999). Inflammation is involved in the onset of arteriosclerotic disorders and acute coronary syndrome. Furthermore, oxidative stress that can induce a vicious cycle of chronic inflammation has been believed to be the major driving force to promote aging (Yu & Chung, 2001; Romano et al., 2010).

Uric acid has recently been considered to be a prognostic factor for the onset of DM and dementia that may accelerate aging (Hikita et al., 2007; Abate et al., 2004; Martinon et al., 2006), although an excess level of uric acid is the primary incite for gouty attack (Schlesinger et al., 2009).

2.1.1 Anti-inflammatory actions

The anti-inflammatory actions of fenofibrate were reported in Nature in 1998 (Staels et al., 1998). PPAR-α ligand: fenofibrate inhibited cyclooxygenase-2 (COX-2) expression and prostaglandin production by suppressing the transcription of COX-2 genes through the inhibition of nuclear factor κB (NF-κB: transcription factor) signals. Fenofibrate administration decreased the inflammatory parameters including serum levels of IL-6, fibrinogen, and C-reactive protein (CRP) in coronary disease patients and the patients with hypertriglyceridemia (Tsimihodimos et al., 2004; Muhlestein et al., 2006).

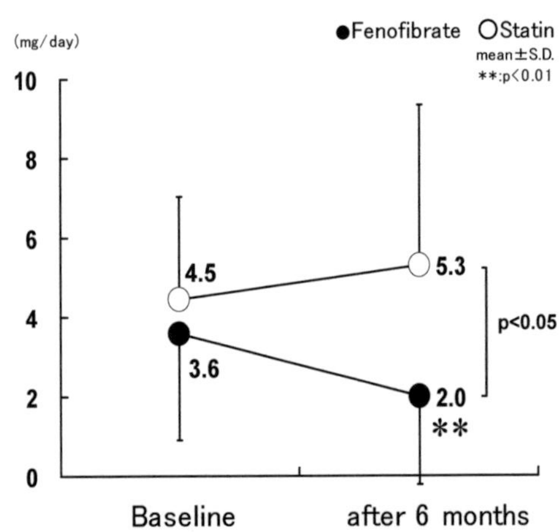

Closed circles represent fenofibrate; open circles represent statins. mean ± S.D.
Wilcoxon signed rank test versus baseline, ** P <0.01, Mann-Whitney U test versus group

Fig. 1. Changes in prednisolone (PSL) dosage.

We compared the anti-inflammatory effects of fenofibrate and statins in 44 patients with a chronic inflammatory disorder: rheumatoid arthritis (RA) (Goto, 2010). Japanese patients with RA and dyslipidemia were randomly divided into 2 groups: fenofibrate (Lipidil, Kaken Pharmaceutical Co., Ltd., micronized fenofibrate at 200 mg/day, n=23) and statins (n=21) groups. After 6-month administration, the laboratory data were compared, and pain was evaluated using the visual analogue scale (VAS) and dose change of prednisolone (PSL) was monitored. The VAS scores significantly decreased in the fenofibrate (from 49.1 to 14.7 mm, $p<0.0001$) and statin (from 47.4 to 20.2 mm, $p<0.001$) groups. The dose of PSL significantly reduced only in the fenofibrate group (from 3.58 to 2.00 mg/day, $p<0.01$). The reduction rate was also significantly better than in the statin group (Fig. 1).

In the fenofibrate group, a significant correlation was between the rate of change in the ΔVAS score and that in the ΔCRP level (Fig.2. $p<0.05$). The results suggest that, in patients with RA, fenofibrate exhibits more potent anti-inflammatory effects compared to statins.

Correlation with ΔVAS

	r	p
ΔHDL-C	-0.042	0.8495
ΔRF	-0.174	0.4274
ΔCRP	0.480	0.0207
ΔESR	0.278	0.1987
ΔPSL	-0.539	0.0705

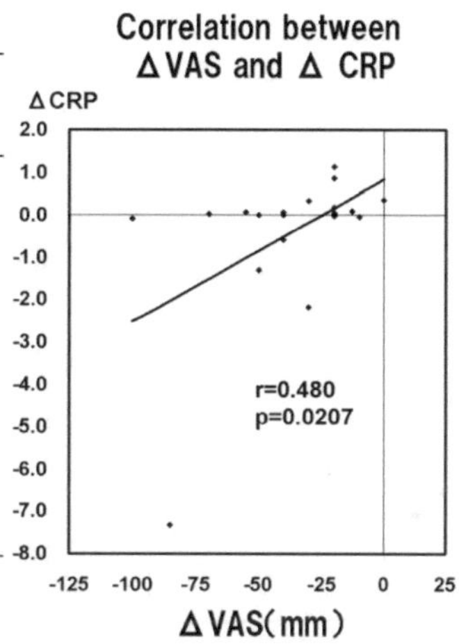

Spearman rank correlation coefficient
VAS visual analogue scale; HDL-C high-density lipoprotein-cholesterol; RF rheumatoid factor; CRP C-reactive protein; ESR erythrocyte sedimentation rate; PSL prednisolone

Fig. 2. Fenofibrate administration group: correlation between anti-inflammatory markers and ΔVAS.

2.1.2 Antioxidant actions

Oxidative stress has been considered to promote aging (Harman, 1978; Yu & Chung, 2001; Romano et al., 2010). As for oxidative stress markers that can be measured on clinical examination, serum lipids, MDA-LDL and Ox-LDL, and urinary lipids, 8-OHdG and 15-isoprostane F2t: 8-epi-PGF2α/8-isoPGF2α, are employed (Harman, 1978; Yu& Chung, 2001). Coenzyme Q10 (CoQ10), also known as ubiquinone shows antioxidant actions and has been monitored as an in vivo marker of oxidative stress.

CoQ10 is biosynthesized from mevalonic acid in the liver. As the pathway of CoQ10 biosynthesis is partially overlapped with that of cholesterol synthesis, the administration of an HMG-CoA reductase inhibitor, statins, reduces the production of CoQ10. Therefore, statins, represented by atorvastatin, also inhibit CoQ10 biosynthesis in vivo, leading to the increase in oxidative stress (Mabuchi et al., 2005).

The administration of standard fenofibrate at 150 mg/day to 18 Japanese type II DM with dyslipidemia for 12 weeks significantly decreased the triglyceride (TG) level (from 232±109 to 145±74 mg/dL, -37%, $p<0.01$), and significantly improved the HDL-C level (from 45±8.7 to 52±9.8 mg/dL, +14%, $p<0.01$) (Asano et al., 2006).

The plasma ubiquinol-10 level in fenofibrate group increased significantly after 8 weeks (from 768±265 to 886±310 nM, $p<0.05$) and after 12 weeks (from 768±265 to 894±336 nM, $p<0.05$). However, total plasma CoQ10 level (ubiquinol-10 plus ubiquinone-10) as an oxidative stress marker, decreased in statin group, elevated in fenofibrate group after 12 weeks administration (from 1010±296 to 1070±285 nM, +6%). In addition, plasma ubiquinone-10 in fenofibrate group decreased insignificantly. Fenofibrate treatment elevates plasma CoQ10, especially plasma ubiquinol-10 level.

In the wild-type mice administered by diethylhexylphthalate (DEHP: PPAR-α activator), elevation of plasma ubiquinone was significant, but the elevation was not observed in the PPAR-α-null mice (Turunen et al., 2000). In addition, the expression of PPAR-α gene was regulated in the liver of SAMP1 (senescence accelerated mouse prone 1) mice given ubiquinol for long term (Schmelzer et al., 2010a, 2010b). Although the antioxidant action mechanisms of fenofibrate remained unclear in human, mice studies suggested the direct interaction between CoQ10 and PPAR-α.

Fenofibrate not only restores the serum lipid profiles, but also suppresses oxidative stress. Fenofibrate with a variety of pleiotropic activities may protect the pathogenesis and progression of aging-associated atherosclerosis.

2.1.3 Serum uric acid-reducing actions

Hyperuricemia, a common co-morbidity in the patients with metabolic syndrome and dyslipidemia has recently been emphasized as an independent risk factor for cardiovascular disease (Lippi et al., 2008).

Kodama et al. performed a meta-analysis of 11 clinical studies, and reported that a 1-mg/dL increase in the serum uric acid level significantly elevated the relative risk of type II DM by 1.17-fold (Kodama et al., 2009). Schretlen et al. investigated 96 persons aged 60 to 92 years, and indicated that the information-processing capacity and memory were reduced in persons with high uric acid level, suggesting that the serum uric acid level may be a prognostic factor for dementia (Schretlen et al., 2007). Thus, hyperuricemia may play a role not only in the onset of cardiovascular disease but also in the promotion of dementia and aging.

Fenofibrate has been known to reduce the serum levels of lipids and also uric acid (Schlesinger et al., 2009). The serum uric acid-reducing action mechanism of fenofibrate, independent of lipid-profile changes, involves the promotion of uric-acid excretion (Liamis et al., 1999).

Urate Transporter 1 (URAT1), the target molecule of uric acid-reducing agents such as benzbromarone was identified which is responsible for the reabsorption of uric acid in the proximal uriniferous tubule (Enomoto et al., 2002). Furthermore, URAT1 inhibition was involved in the serum uric acid-reducing action mechanism of fenofibrate (Uetake et al., 2010). According to their study, the single-dose administration of standard fenofibrate at 300 mg to healthy adults decreased the serum uric acid level by approximately 1.5 mg/dL. In Japan, fenofibrate has been administered to metabolic syndrome patients with hyperuricemia, leading to the decrease in the serum uric acid level by approximately 2 mg/dL.

2.2 Randomized controlled trial (RCT)

Large-scale, randomized, controlled clinical trials of fenofibrate involving type II DM, that is, high-risk patients for arteriosclerosis, were conducted. The representative 3 studies were reviewed in this section: "DAIS" study, regarding coronary arteriosclerosis retraction, "FIELD" study, in which the inhibitory effects on cardiovascular events were examined, and "ACCORD" study, in which the inhibitory effects of lipid-intensified therapy with statins on cardiovascular events were investigated.

2.2.1 Diabetes Atherosclerosis Intervention Study (DAIS)

The DAIS is a placebo-controlled, double-blind, comparative study to verify whether the deterioration of coronary arteriosclerosis can be prevented by restoring abnormal lipid metabolism with fenofibrate in type II diabetics employing quantitative coronary angiography (DAIS investigators, 2001). This international, interventional study was conducted based on the World Health Organization (WHO)'s request and cooperation. This study is the first interventional study in which it was prospectively evaluated whether the correction of disturbance of lipid metabolism in type II DM prevents the deterioration of arteriosclerosis. It was carried out in Canada, Finland, Sweden, and France. Four-hundred and eighteen patients with type II diabetes in whom blood sugar control was favourable were randomly divided into fenofibrate (micronized fenofibrate, 200 mg/day, n=207) and placebo (n=211) groups to evaluate the deterioration of coronary arteriosclerosis using quantitative coronary angiography after 38-month (mean duration) administration.

In the fenofibrate group, a decrease in the minimum lumen diameter and an increase in the percent stenosiswere significantly suppressed in comparison with the placebo group (by 40%), confirming the inhibitory effects of fenofibrate on the deterioration of coronary arteriosclerosis in type II DM.

In the continuing study of DAIS, fenofibrate reduced the small dense LDL level, leading to the inhibition of the deterioration of diabetic nephropathy (DAIS investigators, 2003, 2005), confirming that fenofibrate inhibited the deterioration of macro- and micro-angiopathy in type II DM.

2.2.2 Fenofibrate Intervention and Event Lowering in Diabetes Study (FIELD)

The FIELD is a study to verify the inhibitory effects of fenofibrate on cardiovascular events involving approximately 10,000 patients with type II DM (FIELD investigators, 2005). It was conducted in Finland, Australia, and New Zealand. The subjects were 9,795 type II diabetics with mild dyslipidemia. They were randomly divided into fenofibrate (micronized fenofibrate, 200 mg/day, n=4,895) and placebo (n=4,900) groups. Each agent was administered for 5 years.

In the fenofibrate group, this agent inhibited the incidence of coronary events by 11% in comparison with the placebo group. Unfortunately, there was no significant difference between two groups. This was possibly because statins were combined with the placebo/fenofibrate in 32% of patients receiving the placebo and in 16% of patients receiving fenofibrate, reducing the effects of fenofibrate alone. Fenofibrate decreased the incidence of non-fatal myocardial infarction by 24% ($p<0.05$) and that of total cardiovascular events by 11% ($p<0.05$), confirming its efficacy.

In primary prevention patients without a history of cardiovascular disease, accounting for approximately 80%, fenofibrate significantly inhibited the incidences of coronary (by 25%) and total cardiovascular (by 19%) events in comparison with the placebo group. Furthermore, in the FIELD, fenofibrate inhibited the onset of diabetic nephropathy, deterioration of diabetic retinopathy, proportion of patients undergoing lower-limb amputation, and deterioration of diabetic neuropathy (FIELD investigators, 2005, 2007, 2009, 2010, 2011). As fenofibrate reduced DM-associated 3 major complications (retinopathy, nephropathy and neuropathy), this agent may be useful for treating diabetic complications.

Study name	Micro/macro-angiopathy	Rate of decrease in the relative risk	p value	Reference
DAIS	Diabetic nephropathy	progression in albumin excretion fenofibrate 8%, Placebo 18%	$p<0.05$	DAIS investigators, 2005
FIELD	Diabetic nephropathy	-14%	$p=0.002$	FIELD investigators, 2005, 2011
	Diabetic retinopathy	-31%	$p<0.001$	FIELD investigators, 2007
	Lower-limb amputation	-36%	$p=0.02$	FIELD investigators, 2009
	Diabetic neuropathy	-40%	$p=0.009$	FIELD investigators, 2010
ACCORD-Lipid	Diabetic nephropathy	incidence of microalbuminuria fenofibrate 38.2%, Placebo 41.6%	$p=0.01$	ACCORD Study Group, 2010
		incidence of macroalbuminuria fenofibrate 10.5%, Placebo 12.3%	$p=0.04$	
ACCORD-EYE	Diabetic retinopathy	-40%	$p=0.006$	ACCORD Study Group; ACCORD Eye Study Group, 2010

Table 1. Inhibitory effects of fenofibrate on diabetic angiopathy in a large-scale clinical study involving type II DM

2.2.3 ACCORD-Lipid & ACCORD-EYE study

In the ACCORD-Lipid study, the inhibitory effects of 3 intensified/standard medicinal therapies (blood sugar, blood pressure, lipids) on compound cardiovascular events were investigated in approximately 10,000 type II diabetics with mild dyslipidemia and the high risk of cardiovascular disease (CVD) under the auspices of the National Institutes of Health (NIH). Lipid intervention was performed in 5,518 patients: intensified (simvastatin 20mg + micronized fenofibrate 200mg) and standard (simvastatin 20mg + placebo) therapies. The mean follow-up was 4.7 years. In the fenofibrate-combined group, the incidence of cardiovascular events was inhibited by 8%, although there was no significant difference. In patients with a pre-treatment TG level of 204 mg/dL or more and HDL-C level of 34 mg/dL or less, significant inhibitory effects on events were confirmed (-31% ($p<0.05$), NNT=20) (ACCORD Study Group et al., 2010).

In the ACCORD–EYE study, the deterioration of diabetic retinopathy was evaluated in 2,856 patients from whom informed consent was obtained (lipid intervention: 1,593 patients) among type II DM who participated in the ACCORD-Lipid study (ACCORD Study Group; ACCORD Eye Study Group et al., 2010). In the fenofibrate-combined group, intensified therapy significantly inhibited the deterioration of diabetic retinopathy (by 40%) in comparison with the simvastatin group ($p=0.006$). The ACCORD–EYE study, the second large-scale clinical study following the FIELD, demonstrated the inhibitory effects of fenofibrate on the deterioration of diabetic retinopathy, supporting its efficacy for diabetic retinopathy.

The inhibitory effects of fenofibrate on diabetic microangiopathy are summarized below (Table 1). In a large-scale clinical study of lipid-lowering agents, no statin exhibited any inhibitory effects on diabetic microangiopathy. Only fenofibrate inhibited the complication. Thus, fenofibrate should be recognized as a "prophylactic drug for diabetic complications", and not solely as a lipid-lowering agent.

3. Conclusion

Fenofibrate is a generalized, PPAR-α-mediated, serum lipid-lowering agent. In this chapter, the pleiotropic effects of fenofibrate other than serum lipid-lowering actions were primarily reviewed. Concerning to the anti-inflammatory actions, we examined the effects of fenofibrate in patients with a representative inflammatory disorder, RA. Although there were no significant changes in inflammation parameters including CRP and ESR, improvement in the ΔVAS and PSL dose was achieved in patients receiving fenofibrate. In particular, improvement in the ΔVAS was significantly correlated with a reduction in the ΔCRP level, suggesting that the anti-inflammatory effects of fenofibrate may contribute the improvement in the patient's quality of life (QOL).

In Japan, infectious diseases have been the major causes of death in patients with RA (Souen, 2007; Shinomiya et al., 2008). However, the proportion of cardiovascular events represented by cerebral/myocardial infarction has been increasing, probably because of the changes in life-style (Goto et al., 2008a). So, fenofibrate with lipid-lowering, anti-inflammatory and anti-oxidant actions may be appropriate for reducing disturbances of lipid metabolism and also homeostasis in Japanese patients with RA.

With respect to antioxidant actions, fenofibrate, but not statin increased the plasma level of ubiquinol-10: a family of CoQ10. As fenofibrate exhibits antioxidant actions, combination therapy with fenofibrate and statins may be useful for achieving anti-aging effects and reducing oxidative stress. However, the evaluation methods for antioxidant activity in human should be strictly reviewed in the near future.

The serum uric acid-reducing actions of fenofibrate are regarded as one of its characteristic pleiotropic effects. The action mechanism may be mediated by a uric acid transporter, URAT1, but not by PPAR-α. This may suggest that among fibrate preparations fenofibrate may be favorably administered to the patients with high serum TG and high uric acid levels, as no other fibrate preparations can reduce the serum level of uric acid.

The large-scale clinical study of fenofibrate (FIELD) showed that early administration to "primary prevention" diabetics without a history of cardiovascular events inhibited the onset of cardiovascular events. Furthermore, the DAIS, FIELD, and ACCORD-EYE studies suggested that early fenofibrate administration to all diabetics with dyslipidemia should inhibit the deterioration of diabetic complications regardless of the duration of disease or risk of events.

Fenofibrate shows pleiotropic actions, especially a variety of clinical effects that may not be achieved by statins. This agent may be useful for inhibiting the deterioration of arteriosclerosis, and may play a role as an anti-aging panacea if properly used.

4. References

Abate, N., Chandalia, M., Cabo-Chan, A.V. Jr., Moe, O.W. & Sakhaee, K. (2004). The metabolic syndrome and uric acid nephrolithiasis: novel features of renal manifestation of insulin resistance. *Kidney Int,* Vo.65, No.2, (Feb 2004), pp.386-392, ISSN 0085-2538

ACCORD Study Group. (2010). Effects of combination lipid therapy in type 2 diabetes mellitus. *N Engl J Med,* Vol.362, No.17, (Apr 2010), pp.1563-1574, ISSN 0028-4793

ACCORD Study Group, ACCORD Eye Study Group. (2010). Effects of medical therapies on retinopathy progression in type 2 diabetes. *N Engl J Med,* Vol.363, No.3, (Jul 2010), pp.233-244, ISSN 0028-4793

Asano, A., Kobayashi, J., Murase, Y., Nohara, A., Kawashiri, M.A., Inazu, A., Shimizu, M. & Mabuchi, H. (2006). Effects of fenofibrate therapy on plasma ubiquinol-10 and ubiquinone-10 levels in Japanese patients with hyperlipidemia and type 2 diabetes mellitus. *Pharmacotherapy,* Vol.26, No.4, (Apr 2006), pp.447-451, ISSN 0277-0008

DAIS investigators. (2001). Effect of fenofibrate on progression of coronary-artery disease in type 2 diabetes: the Diabetes Atherosclerosis Intervention Study, a randomised study. *Lancet,* Vol.357, No.9260, (Mar 2001), pp.905-910, ISSN 0140-6736

DAIS investigators. (2003). Relationships between low-density lipoprotein particle size, plasma lipoproteins, and progression of coronary artery disease: the Diabetes Atherosclerosis Intervention Study (DAIS). *Circulation,* Vol.107, No.13, (Apr 2003), pp.1733-1737, ISSN 0009-7322

DAIS Investigators. (2005). Fenofibrate reduces progression to microalbuminuria over 3 years in a placebo-controlled study in type 2 diabetes: results from the Diabetes Atherosclerosis Intervention Study (DAIS). *Am J Kidney Dis,* Vol.45, No.3, (Mar 2005), pp.485-493, ISSN 0272-6386

Endo, A. (1992). The discovery and development of HMG-CoA reductase inhibitors. *J Lipid Res,* Vol.33, No.11, (Nov 1992), pp.1569-1582, ISSN 0022-2275

Enomoto, A., Kimura, H., Chairoungdua, A., Shigeta, Y., Jutabha, P., Cha, S.H., Hosoyamada, M., Takeda, M., Sekine, T., Igarashi, T., Matsuo, H., Kikuchi, Y., Oda, T., Ichida, K., Hosoya, T., Shimokata, K., Niwa, T., Kanai, Y., & Endou, H. (2002). Molecular identification of a renal urate anion exchanger that regulates blood urate levels. *Nature,* Vol.417, No.6887, (May 2002), pp.447-452, ISSN 0028-0836

FIELD study investigators. (2005). Effects of long-term fenofibrate therapy on cardiovascular events in 9795 people with type 2 diabetes mellitus (the FIELD study): randomised controlled trial. *Lancet,* Vol.366, No.9500, (Nov 2005), pp.1849-1861, ISSN 0140-6736

FIELD study investigators. (2007). Effect of fenofibrate on the need for laser treatment for diabetic retinopathy (FIELD study): a randomised controlled trial. *Lancet,* Vol.370, No.9600, (Nov 2007), pp.1687-1697, ISSN 0140-6736

FIELD study investigators. (2009). Effect of fenofibrate on amputation events in people with type 2 diabetes mellitus (FIELD study): a prespecified analysis of a randomised controlled trial. *Lancet,* Vol.373, No.9677, (May 2009), pp.1780-1788, ISSN 0140-6736

FIELD study investigators. (2010). Fenofibrate reduces peripheral neuropathy in type 2 diabetes: The frnofibrate intervention and event lowering in diabetes (FIELD) study. *Atherosclerosis Supplements,* Vol.11, No.2, (Jun 2010), pp.219-220, ISSN 1567-5688

FIELD study investigators. (2011). Effects of fenofibrate on renal function in patients with type 2 diabetes mellitus: the Fenofibrate Intervention and Event Lowering in Diabetes (FIELD) Study. *Diabetologia,* Vol.54, No.2, (Feb 2011), pp.280-290, ISSN 0012-186X

Goto, M. & Matsuura, M. (2008a). Secular trends towards delayed onsets of pathologies and prolonged longevities in Japanese patients with Werner syndrome. *Biosci Trends,* Vol.2, No.2, (Apr 2008), pp.81-87, ISSN 1881-7815

Goto, M. (2008b). Inflammaging (inflammation-aging): A driving force for human aging based on an evolutionarily antagonistic pleiotropy theory? *Biosci Trends,* Vol.2, No.6, (Dec 2008), pp.218-230, ISSN 1881-7815

Goto, M. (2010). A comparative study of anti-inflammatory and antidyslipidemic effects of fenofibrate and statins on rheumatoid arthritis. *Mod Rheumatol,* Vol.20, No.3, (Jun 2010), pp. 238-243, ISSN 1439-7595

Harman, D. (1978). Free radical theory of aging: nutritional implications. *Age,* Vol.1, No.4, (Oct 1978), pp.143-150, ISSN 0161-9152

Hikita, M., Ohno, I., Mori, Y., Ichida, K., Yokose, T. & Hosoya, T. (2007). Relationship between hyperuricemia and body fat distribution. *Intern Med,* Vol.46, No.17, (Sep 2007), pp.1353-1358, ISSN 0918-2918

Kodama, S., Saito, K., Yachi, Y., Asumi, M., Sugawara, A., Totsuka, K., Saito, A. & Sone, H. (2009). Association between serum uric acid and development of type 2 diabetes. *Diabetes Care,* Vol.32, No.9, (Sep 2009), pp.1737-1742, ISSN 0149-5992

Liamis, G., Bairaktari, E.T. & Elisaf, M.S. (1999). Effect of fenofibrate on serum uric acid levels. *Am J Kidney Dis,* Vol.34, No.3, (Sep 1999), pp.594, ISSN 0272-6386

Lippi, G., Montagnana, M., Franchini, M., Favaloro, E.J. & Targher, G. (2008). The paradoxical relationship between serum uric acid and cardiovascular disease. *Clin Chim Acta,* Vol.392, No.1-2, (Jun 2008), pp.1-7, ISSN 0009-8981

Mabuchi, H., Higashikata, T., Kawashiri, M.,Katsuda, S., Mizuno, M., Nohara, A., Inazu, A., Koizumi, J. & Kobayashi, J. (2005). Reduction of serum ubiquinol-10 and ubiquinone-10 levels by atorvastatin in hypercholesterolemic patients. *J Atheroscler Thromb,* Vol.12, No.2, (Jun 2005), pp.111-119, ISSN 1340-3478

Martinon, F., Pétrilli, V., Mayor, A., Tardivel, A. & Tschopp, J. (2006). Gout-associated uric acid crystals activate the NALP3 inflammasome. *Nature,* Vol.440, No.7081, (Mar 2006), pp.237-241, 0028-0836

Muhlestein, J.B., May, H.T., Jensen, J.R., Home, B.D., Lanman, R.B., Lavasani, F., Wolfert, R.L., Pearson, R.R., Yannicelli, H.D. & Anderson, J.L. (2006). The reduction of inflammatory biomarkers by statin, fibrate, the combination therapy among diabeteic patients with mixed dyslipidemia: the DIACOR (Diabetes and Combined Lipid Therapy Regimen) study. *J Am Coll Cardiol,* Vol.48, No.2, (Jul 2006), pp.396-401, ISSN 0735-1097

Romano, A.D., Serviddio, G., de Matthaeis, A., Bellanti, F. & Vendemiale, G. (2010). Oxidative stress and aging. *J Nephrol,* Vol.23, No.suppl 15, (Sep-Oct 2010), pp.S29-S36, ISSN 1121-8428

Ross, R. (1999). Atherosclerosis--an inflammatory disease. *N Engl J Med,* Vol.340, No.2, (Jan 1999), pp.115-126, ISSN 0028-4793

Schlesinger, N., Dalbeth, N. & Perez-Ruiz, F. (2009). Gout-what are the treatment options? *Expert Opin Pharmacother,* Vol.10, No.8, (Jun 2009), pp.1319-1328, ISSN 1465-6566

Schmelzer, C., Kubo, H., Mori, M., Sawashita, J., Kitano, M., Hosoe, K., Boomgaarden, I.,Döring, F. & Higuchi, K. (2010a). Supplementation with the reduced form of Coenzyme Q10 decelerates phenotypic characteristics of senescence and induces a peroxisome proliferator-activated receptor-alpha gene expression signature in SAMP1 mice. *Mol Nutr Food Res,* Vol.54, No.6, (Jun 2010), pp.805-815, ISSN 1613-4133

Schmelzer, C., Okun, JG., Haas, D., Higuchi, K., Sawashita, J., Mori, M. & Döring, F. (2010b). The reduced form of coenzyme Q10 mediates distinct effects on cholesterol metabolism at the transcriptional and metabolite level in SAMP1 mice. *IUBMB Life,* Vol.62, No.11, (Nov 2010), pp.812-818, ISSN 1521-6551

Schoonjans, K., Watanabe, M., Suzuki, H., Mahfoudi, A., Krey, G., Wahli, W., Grimaldi, P., Staels, B., Yamamoto, T. & Auwerx, J. (1995). Induction of the acyl-coenzyme A synthetase gene by fibrates and fatty acids is mediated by a peroxisome proliferator response element in the C promoter. *J Biol Chem,* Vol.270, No.33, (Aug 1995), pp.19269-19276, ISSN 0021-9258

Schoonjans, K., Peinado-Onsurbe, J., Lefebvre, A.M., Heyman, R.A.; Briggs, M., Deeb, S., Staels, B. & Auwerx, J. (1996a). PPARalpha and PPARgamma activators direct a distinct tissue-specific transcriptional response via a PPRE in the lipoprotein lipase gene. *EMBO J,* Vol.15, No.19, (Oct 1996), pp.5336-5348, ISSN 0261-4189

Schoonjans, K., Staels, B. & Auwerx, J. (1996b). Role of the peroxisome proliferator-activated receptor (PPAR) in mediating the effects of fibrates and fatty acids on gene expression. *J Lipid Res*, Vol.37, No.5, (May 1996), pp.907-925. ISSN 0022-2275

Schretlen, D.J., Inscore, A.B., Jinnah, H.A., Rao, V., Gordon, B. & Pearlson, G.D. (2007). Serum uric acid and cognitive function in community-dwelling older adults. *Neuropsychology*. Vol.21, No.1, (Jan 2007), pp.136-140, ISSN 0894-4105

Shinomiya, F., Mima, N., Nanba, K., Tani, K., Nakano, S., Egawa, H., Sakai, T., Miyoshi, H. & Hamada, D. (2008). Life expectancies of Japanese patients with rheumatoid arthritis: a review of deaths over a 20-year period. *Mod Rheumatol*, Vo.18, No.2, (Apr 2008), pp.165-169, ISSN 1439-7595

Souen, S. (2007). Mortality and causes of death in RA patients. *Rheumatology*, Vol.37, No.2, (Feb 2007), pp.164-168, ISSN 0915-227X

Staels, B., Vu-Dac, N., Kosykh, V.A., Saladin, R., Fruchart, J.C., Dallongeville, J. & Auwerx, J. (1995). Fibrates downregulate apolipoprotein C-III expression independent of induction of peroxisomal acyl coenzyme A oxidase. A potential mechanism for the hypolipidemic action of fibrates. *J Clin Invest*, Vol.95, No.2, (Feb 1995), pp.705-712, ISSN 0021-9738

Staels, B., Koenig, W., Habib, A., Merval, R., Lebret, M., Torra, I.P., Delerive, P., Fadel, A., Chinetti, G., Fruchart, J.C., Najib, J., Maclouf, J. & Tedgui, A. (1998). Activation of human aortic smooth-muscle cells is inhibited by PPARalpha but not by PPARgamma activators. *Nature*, Vol.393, No.6687, (Jun 1998), pp.790-793, ISSN 0028-0836

Superko, H.R. (2000). Small, dense, low-density lipoprotein and atherosclerosis. *Curr Atheroscler Rep*, Vol.2, No.3, (May 2000), pp.226-231, ISSN 1523-3804

Tsimihodimos, V., Kostoula, A., Kakafika, A., Bairaktari, E., Tselepis, A.D., Mikhaikidis, D.P. & Elisaf, M. (2004). Effect of fenofibrate on serum inflammatory markers in patients with high triglyceride values. *J Cardiovasc Pharmacol Ther*, Vol.9, No.1, (Mar 2004), pp.27-33, ISSN 1074-2484

Turunen, M., Peters, J.M., Gonzalez, F.J., Schedin, S. & Dallner, G. (2000). Influence of peroxisome proliferator-activated receptor alpha on ubiquinone biosynthesis. *J Mol Biol*, Vol.297, No.3, (Mar 2000), pp.607-614, ISSN 0022-2836

Uetake, D., Ohno, I., Ichida, K., Yamaguchi, Y., Saikawa, H., Endou, H. & Hosoya, T. (2010). Effect of fenofibrate on uric acid metabolism and urate transporter 1. *Intern Med*, Vol.49, No.2, (Jan 2010), pp.89-94, ISSN 0918-2918

Vu-Dac, N., Schoonjans, K., Laine, B., Fruchart, J.C., Auwerx, J. & Staels, B. (1994). Negative regulation of the human apolipoprotein A-I promoter by fibrates can be attenuated by the interaction of the peroxisome proliferator-activated receptor with its response element. *J Biol Chem*, Vol.269, No.49, (Dec 1994), pp.31012-31018, ISSN ISSN 0021-9258

Vu-Dac, N., Schoonjans, K., Kosykh, V., Dallongeville, J., Fruchart, J.C., Staels, B. & Auwerx, J. (1995). Fibrates increase human apolipoprotein A-II expression through activation of the peroxisome proliferator-activated receptor. *J Clin Invest*, Vol.96, No.2, (Aug 1995), pp.741-750, ISSN 0021-9738

Willson, T.M., Brown, P.J., Sternbach, D.D. & Henke, B.R. (2000). The PPARs: from orphan receptors to drug discovery. *J Med Chem,* Vol.43, No.4, (Feb 2000), pp.527-550, ISSN 0022-2623

Yu, B.P. & Chung, H.Y. (2001). Oxidative stress and vascular aging. *Diabetes Res Clin Pract,* Vol.54, No.2, (Dec 2001), pp.S73-S80, ISSN 0168-8227

23

Predictors of the Common Adverse Drug Reactions of Statins

Hadeer Akram AbdulRazzaq[1], Noorizan Abd Aziz[2], Yahaya Hassan[2], Yaman Walid Kassab[1] and Omar Ismail[3]
[1]*Department of Clinical Pharmacy, School of Pharmaceutical Sciences, Universiti Sains, Penang,*
[2]*Faculty of Pharmacy, UiTM, Puncak Alam Campus, Bandar Puncak Alam, Selangor DE,*
[3]*Department of Cardiology, Hospital Pulau Pinang, Penang, Malaysia*

1. Introduction

Statins are common lipid lowering agents to reduce elevation of cholesterol or as prophylaxis against other cardiac diseases. It estimated that 62.5% to 91.7% of dyslipidemic patients in United State of America are using statins[1] These agents widely used among cardiovascular patients in Malaysia[2]. In other countries, for example in UK, it has found that most patients who use statins are older than 35 years old and more of them are males (56%)[3]. In Canada, about 90% of cardiac patients are using statin, while in US, at least one third of all cardiac patients are using statins[4]. About 60% of American patients who older than 60 years old are using statin[5]. Thus, high number of users contributed to increase the risk of adverse drug reactions (ADRs).

The Food and Drug Administration (FDA) has determined that common statin-associated ADRs are fatigue, muscle pain, joints pain, back pain, visual disturbance and insomnia[6,7]. Previous studies have examined the incidence of these ADRs, and their results showed that more than half of the reported cases of muscle pain were related to statin use[8,9]. Clearfield et al found that fatigue, muscle pain, and bone pain were common and frequent ADRs in UK, and related to atorvastatin and rosuvastatin use[10]. Other studies exploring ADRs in patients using atorvastatin and lovastatin in the US found that muscle pain and fatigue were the most common statin-related ADRs[11]. The UK Committee on Safety of Medicines, as well as other studies, have reported that these symptoms should consider as early signs for more serious ADRs[8,12-15]. However, from our knowledge, no data available on the common ADRs statin-related and their predictors for Asian patients. Only a few studies (not related with Asian patients) have found out the predictors of the statin-related ADRs[8,9,10,16,17]. As health care professional, they should find methods to ensure patients not only receive effective medication but also feel comfortable with the therapy. Thus, the objectives of this study was to determine the common statin-related ADRs and their predictors in one of the referral hospital in Malaysia (one of country in South East Asia).

2. Method

Cross-sectional with convenient sampling study conducted for volunteer outpatients from the cardiac clinic of Penang Hospital in Pulau Pinang State of Malaysia. Study protocol was approved by Clinical Research Committee of Penang General Hospital, and signed consent forms were obtained from all participants. The patients included in this study were at least 18 years old and voluntarily to participate in this study. They have to used statins and could understand Malay Language (the National Language of Malaysia) or English Language, since Malaysia is a multiracial country. Patients who allergies to statin, pregnant or lactating women, or changing in types or dosage of statin used were excluded from this study. These types of patients excluded because their conditions may affected outcomes of the study. The study period was 5 months, and 1900 patients presented in the cardiac clinic within this study period. Depending on inclusion and exclusion criteria, 500 patients voluntarily agreed to participate in this study. A validated questionnaire form (Cronbach's alpha is 0.853) were used for reporting of ADRs. The patients were asked whether they have experience of common statin-related ADRs while they were on statin therapy and give their answers on the self-report questionnaire forms. This questionnaire form has some questions on demographic data and undesired symptoms that patients had during statin therapy. There were 27 ADRs of statin listed in the questionnaire form. They were required to tick yes or no on these listed ADRs. They can tick more than one ADR. In order to ensure these ADRs really related with statin therapy these patients had to indicate in the questionnaire form that these ADRs occurred while they were receiving statin therapy and these symptoms should continuously occurred at least for 3 months.

3. Statistics

Statistical Package for Social Science software (SPSS) version 18 used to analyze the data for this study. Odd ratio and Chi-square and logistic regression tests were used to ensure these ADRs were related with stain therapy and to determine their predictors. The results with p value less than 0.05 was considered statistically significant.

4. Results

Male patients (70%) were the more frequent users of statins, with mean age 60±10 years. The most frequent race that used statins was Chinese (37.6%), followed by Malays (34.4%), Indians (26.6%) and foreigners (1.4%). Small numbers of patients were cigarette smoker (12%) and alcohol consumers (9%).

Higher number of patients had dyslipidemia with primary type (51.5%) based on the Friedewald et al[18] and Stone et al[19] classifications. For primary subtypes of dyslipidemia, the most common subtype was IIa (50.6%), while common subtype of secondary dyslipidemia was diabetes (86.3%). The common type of statin used was lovastatin (81%), followed by simvastatin (9.4%) and atorvastatin (8%). The low dose (20 mg) of statin was the common prescribed to these patients. The mean duration of statin therapy was 3.5 years and the most frequent range of duration was 1-5 years (52.5%), as shown in Table 1.

Statistical regression analysis was used to exclude symptoms related to other medications and diseases. It found only few symptoms from 27 ADRs that correlated significantly with statins were; fatigue (59.4%), muscle pain (53.6%), joint pain (53.4%), back pain (47.8%), insomnia (44.8%) and visual disturbances (44.2%).

Demographics	Variables	No (%)
Gender	Male	351 (70%)
	Female	149 (30%)
Race	Malay	172 (34.4%)
	Chinese	188 (37.6%)
	Indian	133 (26.6%)
	Foreign	7 (1.4%)
Age (mean 60±10)year	28-50 year	94 (19%)
	51-65 year	258 (51%)
	66-92 year	148 (30%)
Smoke	Yes	59 (12%)
	No	441 (88%)
Alcohol consuming	Yes	47 (9%)
	No	453 (91%)
Dyslipidiemia type	Primary	247 (51.5%)
	Secondary	233 (48.5%)
Primary dyslipidemia subtype	I	13 (5.3%)
	IIa	125 (50.6%)
	IIb	59 (23.9%)
	III	7 (2.8%)
	IV	32 (13%)
	V	11 (4.5%)
Secondary dyslipidemia subtype	Renal	17 (7.3%)
	Diabetes	201 (86.3%)
	Nephrotic syndrome	1 (0.4%)
	Liver	1 (0.4%)
	Drugs	2 (0.9%)
	Hypothyroidism	11 (4.7%)
Type of statin	Atorvastatin	40 (8%)
	Simvastatin	47 (9.4%)
	Lovastatin	405 (81%)
	others	8 (1.6)
Combination therapy	Yes	35 (7%)
	No	465 (93%)
Duration of therapy Mean (3.5±3.0) year	3months or less	16 (3.2%)
	3months -1 year	133 (26.7%)
	1-5 years	262 (52.5%)
	5-20 years	89 (17.6%)

Table 1. Demographic data of 500 cardiac outpatients in Penang General Hospital

Predictors	**ADRs (percentage, P value, OR, CI)**					
	Fatigue	**Muscle pain**	**Joint pain**	**Back pain**	**Insomnia**	**Visual disturb-ances**
Gender (female)	NS	NS	61.74%, P=0.007, OR= 1.864, CI= 1.18-2.94	56.38%, P= 0.02, OR= 1.73, CI= 1.09-2.75	NS	NS
Race (Indian)	68.42%, P=0.027, OR= 1.81, CI= 2.14-2.75)	66.92%, P= 0.016, OR=1.94, CI= 1.13-3.32)	NS	62.4%, P=0.007, OR= 2.18, CI= 1.23-3.72	NS	49.62%, P=0.016, OR= 1.74, CI= 1.11-2.73)
Smokers	NS	NS	NS	NS	NS	NS
Alcoholic	76.60%, P= 0.011, OR= 3.0 CI= 1.29-7.01)	NS	NS	65.96%, P= 0.003, OR= 3.58, CI= 1.53-8.38	59.57%, P=0.006, OR= 2.89, CI= 1.36-6.15	NS
Age	NS	NS	NS	NS	NS	NS
Duration More than 5 years	53.41%, P=0.036, OR= 1.83, CI= 1.04-3.23)	60.23%, P=0.016, OR=1.96, CI= 1.133-3.39	NS	57.95%, P=0.001, OR=2.61, CI= 1.50-4.54)	NS	NS
Primary subtypes (type IIb)	NS	NS	NS	33.90%, P= 0.014, OR= 2.50, CI= 1.21-5.19)	NS	NS
Secondary subtypes (renal disease)	NS	NS	NS	NS	64.71%, P= 0.33, OR= 3.7, CI= 1.11-12.33	NS
Statin types	NS	NS	NS	NS	NS	NS
Atorvastatin doses (20mg)	NS	NS	NS	NS	NS	NS

Simvastatin dose (40mg)	NS	NS	NS	NS	NS	NS
Lovastatin doses (60mg)	72.73%, P=0.003, OR= 1.90, CI= 1.25-2.89)	NS	NS	NS	NS	NS
Combination therapy	NS	NS	NS	NS	NS	NS

NS= no significant

Table 2. Relationship between statin related ADRs and predictors

In term of predictor, females significantly had joint pain (61.74%, OR = 1.864) and back pain (56.38%, OR = 1.73). However, there was no significant relation between gender with fatigue, muscle pain, insomnia and visual disturbance. Indian patients had significantly higher incidence of fatigue (68.42%, OR= 1.81), muscle pain (66.92%, OR =1.94), back pain (62.4 %, OR = 2.18), and visual disturbances (49.62 %, OR = 1.738) when compared to other races. No significant relationship found between smoking and statin related-ADRs. Patients who consumed alcohol significantly had fatigue (76.6%, OR = 3.0), back pain (65.96%, OR = 3.584) and insomnia (59.57%, OR = 2.893). Age was without effect on incidence of statin related-ADRs. Patients used statins for more than 5 years significantly had fatigue (53.41%, OR = 1.83) and muscle pain (60.23%, OR =1.958), as shown in Table 2.

For secondary dyslipidemia types, renal induced dyslipidemia significantly caused higher incidence of insomnia when compared to the other secondary subtypes (64.71%, OR = 3.7). For subtypes of primary dyslipidemia, subtype IIb patients had significantly back pain (81.82%, OR = 2.5).

No significant relationship found between statin related-ADRs and statin types, the patients used simvastatin had a higher incidence of fatigue (65.96%), joint pain (57.45%), back pain (55.32%) and visual disturbance (53.19%). Patients used lovastatin had insomnia (45.68%), while patients used atorvastatin had higher incidence of muscle pain (52.17%). No significant relationship found between doses of statins and other ADRs except for lovastatin dose. Patients used 60 mg dose of lovastatin had significantly fatigue than patients used lower doses (72.73%, OR = 1.904). No significant relation found between the combination with other lipid lowering agents and incidence of ADRs (as shown in Table 2).

5. Discussion

After two decades of statin marketing, significant incidences of adverse drug reactions still presented during therapy. Number of studies of medications' ADRs always increased after first years of launching, but it found this matter is different with type of statin used[20]. Most of previous studies focused on serious ADRs of statin like muscle toxicity, elevation of liver enzymes, renal toxicity and polyneuropathy[21,22]. Although serious ADRs caused mortalities and death to patients, but their incidences are lower than other adverse reactions of statin symptomatic related ADRs. Kashani A. et al. [23] found that incidences of patients discontinued their therapy because of symptomatic ADRs of statin (5.6%) were higher than patients had rhabdomyolysis (0.2%), hepatotoxicity (1.4%), and creatine kinase (CK) elevations (0.9%). Therefore, self-reporting of ADRs are useful to determine and predict the toxicities induced by medication[24]. There are few studies done on the common statin-related ADRs that use patient self-report. There was a previous study that focused on the common ADRs during statin therapy and their predictors in cardiac outpatients. They reported the use of a self-report questionnaire form is suitable approach to assess the common undesired symptoms found during statin therapy[25]. In the real-life practice, doctors are more focusing on dyslipidemia and its complications than statin-related ADRs of their patients. Furthermore, self-report approach allows the patients to express directly their unwanted problems associated with statin therapy. In addition, patients sometimes feel uncomfortable or inappropriate telling their doctor about these undesired symptoms of statin[26,27]. The finding in this study showed a higher incidence of fatigue and muscle pain in this cardiac outpatients setting, which consistent with previous studies[8,10].

In this study, females reported having back and joint pain significantly more than males did. Female patients are more sensitive to ADRs than males possibly because of pharmacokinetic and pharmacodynamic differences between genders[28]. Not all ADRs of statin related to gender, this finding supported by FDA, Bayer reports and previous studies[29-32]. When compared to other races, Indian patients had significantly higher incidence of some common ADRs (fatigue, muscle pain, back pain and visual disturbance). This is because genetics also has contributed in adverse drug reactions[23]. This result was supported by FDA reports in which ADRs were different among races[7]. Cigarette smokers had increased incidence of these ADRs than nonsmokers, however this finding was not statistically significant. Alcohol consumers had significant problems with fatigue, back pain and insomnia, and increased incidence of ADRs in general[30]. This is because alcohol causes mitochondrial dysfunction, which would increase the risk of muscle disorders caused by statins[33]. There was no relationship between age and ADRs, as shown in Table 2, which supported by Kucukarslan et al study[34]. There was a relationship between duration of statin used and ADRs in previous studies[29,35,36]. Their finding were consistent with this present finding, where the duration of statin therapy has related to fatigue, muscle pain and back pain.

Based on our knowledge, no previous studies reported the relationship between dyslipidemia types and the common ADRs. Significant relationship was found in this study between dyslipidemia type (primary and secondary) and common ADRs. Patients who had secondary dyslipidemia type had increase frequency of insomnia than with primary type. Patients with subtype IIb and renal induced dyslipidemia were significantly more likely to have back pain and insomnia than other subtypes.

Although statins differ in their pharmacokinetic properties[37,38], there is no significant relationship found between statin types and common ADRs. However, simvastatin was more likely to cause fatigue, joint pain, back pain and visual disturbance than other statins. Although there is no significant relation found between atorvastatin and common ADRs. Atorvastatin found to cause muscle pain more often than other statin types, this finding also proved by Clearfield et al. and Golomb et al. [10,11]. Patients on lovastatin therapy had higher incidence of insomnia than other types of statin. Higher doses for all types of statins have resulted in a higher incidence of ADRs. The higher dose of lovastatin (60 mg) significantly associated with fatigue. The dose of statins used did not have significant relationship with other symptoms of common ADRs. This result is consistent with other studies[12,39]. Finally, there was no significant relationship between combination therapy and ADRs. This relationship could not be seen possibly due to small number of patients receiving more than one type of antilipidemic agent.

The finding of this study showed that significant number of patients feel undesired effects of statin therapy and their predictors. Adjustment or manipulating of these preventable predictors such as to change type of statin used, reduce dose and duration are recommended to the prescribers. For example, based on the odd ratio, fatigue was the highest for patients who are alcohol consumers, followed by lovastatin dosage, duration and race. Therefore, steps needed to reduce the incidence of fatigue by avoiding or reducing the preventable predictors that related to these common ADRs like cessation of alcohol and changing in type or dose of statin used.

6. Conclusion

This paper explained that significant number of cardiac outpatients were experienced common ADRs related-statin through self-report approach and their predictors. Common ADRs of statin were fatigue, muscle pain, joint pain, back pain, insomnia and visual disturbances. The main predictors or contributing factors of common statin-related ADRs were gender, race, alcohol consumption, duration of statin used, renal induced-secondary dyslipidemia, subtype IIb of primary dyslipidemia and lovastatin dose. These predictors are useful in clinical practice to determine the likelihood of ADRs and to manage the common ADRs of statin in cardiac outpatients. Finding from this study was suggested appropriate dose and type of statin use and also adjustment of the preventable predictors may minimize common ADRs of statin in cardiac outpatients. Appropriate prospective study design with multicenter sites recommended determining the actual effects of these preventable predictors on common ADRs of statin.

7. References

[1] Avorn J, Monette J, Lacour A, Bohn RL, Monane M, Mogun H, LeLorier J.(1998). Persistence of Use of Lipid-Lowering Medications: a cross-national study. Journal of the American Medical Association 279:1458-1462

[2] National Cardiovascular Disease Database (NCVD) (2006), Malaysia

[3] Dewilde S, Carey IM, Bremner SA, Richards N, Hilton SR, Cook DG (2003). Evolution of statin prescribing 1994–2001: a case of agism but not of sexism? Heart 89:417–421

[4] National Cholesterol Education Program (NCEP) (2002). Expert panel on detection, evaluation, and treatment of high blood cholesterol in adults (adult treatment panel III). Third report of the national cholesterol education program (NCEP) expert panel on detection, evaluation, and treatment of high blood cholesterol in adults (Adult Treatment Panel III) final report 106:3143–3421

[5] Farahani P, Gaebel K, Lelorier J, Perrault S, Gillis J, Soon J, Levine M (2005). Assessment of patient characteristics associated with statin use. The Canadian Journal of Clinical Pharmacology 12: e41-e149: 31

[6] AHFS (2007). HMG-CoA Reductase Inhibitors (Statins) - Safety Overview. Drug Information Service, University of Utah.
[7] U.S food and drug administration: Rosuvastatin Calcium (marketed as Crestor) Information Patient information sheet. (2005) [Online]. [10th March 2008] available from World Wide Web: http://www.fda.gov/cder/drug/ infopage/rosuvastatin/default.htm
[8] Thompson PD, Clarkson P, Karas RH. (2003). Statin associated Myopathy. Journal of the American Medical Association 289:1681–1690
[9] Ballantyne CM, Corsini A, Davidson MH, Holdaas H, Jacobson TA, Lieitersdorf E, Marz W., Reckless, J PD, Stein EA (2003). Risk for myopathy with statin therapy in high-risk patients. Archive of Internal Medicine 163: 553-564.
[10] Clearfield MB, Amerena J, Bassand JP, Hernández García HR, Miller SS, Sosef FF, Palmer MK and Bryzinski BS (2006). Comparison of the efficacy and safety of rosuvastatin 10 mg and atorvastatin 20 mg in high-risk patients with hypercholesterolemia - prospective study to evaluate the use of low doses of the statins atorvastatin and rosuvastatin (PULSAR). Licensee Biomed Central Ltd. Trial 7:35
[11] Golomb BA, Yang E, Denenberg J, Criqui M (2003). Statin-associated adverse events. Circulation 107; e7001-e7039, 95
[12] Pasternak RC, Smith SCJ, Bairey-Merz CN, Grundy SM, Cleeman JI, Lenfant C (2002). ACC/AHA/NHLBI Clinical advisory on the use and safety of statins. Journal of the American College of Cardiology 106: 567–572
[13] Hamilton CI (2003). Statins and muscle damage. Australian Prescriber 26:74-75
[14] Gaist D, Jeppesen U, Andersen M, García Rodríguez LA, Hallas J, Sindrup SH (2002). Statins and risk of polyneuropathy: a case-control study. Neurology 14; 58(9):1321-2.
[15] Committee on safety of medicines (2001). Cerivastatin (lipobay) withdrawn. Current Problem in Pharmacovigillance 27: 9
[16] Shepherd J, Cobbe SM, Ford I, Isles CG, Lorimer AR, MacFarlane PW, McKillop JH, Packard CJ (1995). Prevention of coronary heart disease with pravastatin in men with hypercholesterolemia. West of Scotland Coronary Prevention Study Group (WOSCOPS). The New England Journal of Medicine 333:1301-1307
[17] Cheryl A (2007). HMG-CoA Reductase Inhibitors/Statins, PHARMD, UCSF School of Pharmacy, University of California at San Francisco.
[18] Friedewald WT, Levy RI, Fredrickson DS (1972). Estimation of the concentration of low-density lipoprotein cholesterol in plasma without use of the preparative ultracentrifuge. Clinical Chemistry 18:499-502.
[19] Stone NJ and Blum CB (2008). Management of Lipids in Clinical Practice. Professional Communications p80
[20] Brown WV (2008). Safety of statins. Curr Opin Lipidol 19(6):558-62
[21] Zipes DP, Zvaifler NJ, Glassock RJ, Gilman S, Muñoz A, Gogolak V, Gordis L, Dedon PC, Guengerich FP, Wasserman SI, Witztum JL, Wogan GN (2006). Rosuvastatin: an independent analysis of risks and benefits. MedGenMed 8(2):73.

[22] Silva MA, Swanson AC, Gandhi PJ, Tataronis GR (2006). Statin-related adverse events: a meta-analysis. Clin Ther 28(1):26-35.

[23] Kashani A, Phillips CO, Foody JM, Wang Y, Mangalmurti S, Ko DT, Krumholz HM (2006). Risks associated with statin therapy: a systematic overview of randomized clinical trials. Circulation 114(25):2788-97.

[24] Grundy SM (2005). The issue of statin safety: where do we stand? Circulation 111:3016-3019

[25] Gholami K., Ziaie S., and Shalviri G (2008). Adverse drug reactions induced by cardiovascular drugs in outpatients. Pharmacy Practice 6(1):51-55.

[26] Golomb BA, Kane T and Dimsdale JE (2004). Severe irritability associated with statin cholesterol-lowering agents. The Quarterly Journal of Medicine 97:229-235.

[27] Golomb BA, Mcgraw JJ, Evans MA and Dimsdale JE (2007). Physician response to patient reports of adverse drug effects. Drug Safety 30(8): 669-675.

[28] Sigonda N (2003). guidelines for monitoring and reporting adverse drug reactions (ADRs) made under section 5 (c) of the Tanzania food, drugs and cosmetics Act 2003

[29] Alsheikh-Ali AA, Ambrose MS, Kuvin JT, Karas RH (2005). The safety of rosuvastatin as used in common clinical practice: a postmarketing analysis. Circulation 111:3051-3057.

[30] Hanston PD, and Horn JR (1998). Drug interactions with HMG CoA reductase inhibitors. Drug Interactions Newsletter 103-6

[31] EMEA (2002) Scientific conclusion and ground for withdrawal of the marketing authorization presented, CPMP/811/02

[32] Gray SL, Mahoney JE, Blough DK (1999). Adverse drug events in elderly patients receiving home health services following hospital discharge. The Annals of Pharmacotherapy 33:1147-1153

[33] Mabuchi H, Nohara A, Kobayashi J, Kawashiri MA, Inazu A (2007). Coenzyme Q10 Reduction with Statins: Another Pleiotropic Effect Current Drug Therapy 2: 39-51

[34] Kucukarslan SN, Peters M, Mlynarek M, Nafziger DA (2003). Pharmacists on rounding teams reduce preventable adverse drug events in hospital general medicine units. Arch Intern Med 22;163(17):2014-8.

[35] Corrao G, Zambon A, Bertù L, Botteri E, Leoni O, Contiero P (2004). Lipid lowering drugs prescription and the risk of peripheral neuropathy: an exploratory case-control study using automated databases. Journal of Epidemiology Community Health 58:1047–1051.

[36] Agostini JV, Tinetti ME, Ling H, Mcavay G, Foody JM and Concato J (2007). Effects of Statin use on muscle strength, Cognition, and Depressive Symptoms In older adults. The American Journal of Geriatric Cardiology in Society 55:420–425

[37] Jones P, Kafonek S, Laurora I, Hunninghake D (1998). Comparative dose efficacy study of atorvastatin versus simvastatin, pravastatin, lovastatin, and fluvastatin in patients with hypercholesterolemia (The Curves Study). The American Journal of Cardiology 81:582–587

[38] Corsini A, Bellosta S, Baetta R, Fumagalli R, Paoletti R, Bernini F (1999). New insights into the pharmacodynamic and pharmacokinetic properties of statins. Pharmacology and Therapeutic 84:413-428

[39] Ravnskov U, Rosch PJ, Sutter MC, Houston MC (2006). Should we lower cholesterol as much as possible? BMJ 332(7553):1330-1332.